MOSBY'S
COMPREHENSIVE
REVIEW OF
DENTAL
ASSISTING

MOSBY'S
COMPREHENSIVE
REVIEW OF
DENTAL
ASSISTING

BETTY LADLEY FINKBEINER
CDA, RDA, BS, MS

Chairperson, Dental Assisting Program
Washtenaw Community College
Ann Arbor, Michigan

CLAUDIA SULLENS JOHNSON
RDA, BS

Clinical Instructor, Dental Assisting Program
Washtenaw Community College
Ann Arbor, Michigan

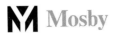 Mosby

St. Louis Baltimore Boston Carlsbad Chicago Naples New York Philadelphia Portland
London Madrid Mexico City Singapore Sydney Tokyo Toronto Wiesbaden

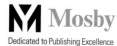
Mosby
Dedicated to Publishing Excellence

**A Times Mirror
Company**

Publisher: Don Ladig
Executive Editor: Linda L. Duncan
Managing Editor: Penny Rudolph
Project Manager: Linda McKinley
Production Manager: Rich Barber

Printed in the United States of America

Composition by Clarinda
Printing/binding by Maple Vail Book Mfg. Group

Mosby-Year Book, Inc.
11830 Westline Industrial Drive
St. Louis, Missouri 64146

Library of Congress Cataloging in Publication Data
Finkbeiner, Betty Ladley, 1939-
    Mosby's comprehensive review of dental assisting / Betty Ladley Finkbeiner, Claudia
Sullens Johnson.
        p.   cm.
    Includes index.
    ISBN (invalid) 0-8151-2695-7 (alk. paper)
    1. Dental assistants—Examinations, questions, etc.   2. Dentistry—Examinations, questions,
etc.   I. Johnson, Claudia, Sullens.   II. Title.
    [DNLM: 1. Dental Care—methods—examination questions.   2. Dental
Assistants.   3. Practice Management, Dental—examination questions.
WU 18.2 F499m 1997]
RK60.5.F54   1997
617.6′0076—dc21
DNLM/DLC   96-45090
for Library of Congress   CIP
International Standard Book Number: 0-8151-3303-0

97 98 99 00 01 / 9 8 7 6 5 4 3 2 1

This book is dedicated to our beloved spouses,
Charles Finkbeiner and David Johnson,
for their continued support and caring.

Preface

This textbook is written by dental assisting educators for dental assistants of varying career levels who are about to take a credentialing examination. The authors bring to this book the results of their broad backgrounds in test and measurement systems and clinical evaluation. Betty Finkbeiner has served as a test writer for the Dental Assisting National Board and consultant and staff member to the Commission on Dental Accreditation of the American Dental Association. In addition, she has had extensive course work in competency based education and test and measurement methodology. For nearly two decades, Claudia Johnson has performed clinical evaluation for dental assistants in an ADA accredited Dental Assisting Program. In addition, she has considerable experience in infection control and has been an examiner for the Michigan State Board Dental Assistant Registry examination.

This book is designed to enable an examination candidate to gain confidence to take a national or state credentialing examination by providing suggested approaches to studying. In addition, a broad overview of question styles is provided for the reader, with examples of these types of questions. While each chapter provides questions with rationales for the correct answers, the book concludes with a mock examination, allowing the reader to simulate an actual examination experience. A computer scantron style sheet is even provided to make this experience more realistic. Used in a school setting, this test could serve as an actual review for a major examination. The textbook is arranged in a logical sequence, beginning with the basic cognitive knowledge and progressing to the application of these concepts in clinical dentistry. The latter part of the textbook includes more complex laboratory and specialty areas.

For valid self-evaluation, the reader is encouraged to progress through the book in a logical sequence; answer the questions, review the rationales, and if difficulty is experienced, refer to standardized reference texts suggested in this textbook. The references are not all encompassing but should provide the reader with a comprehensive review of the literature.

The authors realize that each reader learns in a different manner. The reader is encouraged not to use this textbook to memorize questions, but to use it as a stimulus to evaluate his or her base of knowledge or as an incentive to continue to study for future credentialing examinations.

This book certainly has not been completed by our efforts alone. We would like to extend special thanks to our colleague Kathy Weber, RDA and to Phyllis Grzegorczyk, PhD, Dean of Allied Health and Public Service for surviving yet another manuscript while working with us. A special thanks to Linda Duncan, Executive Editor, and Penny Rudolph, Managing Editor, who continuously support us with their enthusiasm and wisdom and yet understand that deadlines are meant to be flexible.

Contents

CHAPTER 1

Preparing for an Examination— Guidelines for the Student

Preparing for a credentialing examination can be a satisfying yet stressful experience. The satisfaction comes from the confidence of accepting a challenge that will verify your professional credibility. On the other hand, stress may come from the fear of the unknown: what knowledge will be tested, what depth of knowledge will be tested, how will the questions be formatted, what is the length of the test, and how can I prepare?

Preparing for any test or board examination requires that you carefully plan, review and study, organize your schedule, and develop a positive attitude toward the experience. In fact, for most candidates preparation for a credentialing examination seldom differs from the routine you have conscientiously followed as a student or practicing dental assistant.

This text will provide an overview of common knowledge that is needed to successfully complete a credentialing examination. Suggestions will be offered for preparing, planning, and organizing yourself to take a national or state board examination.

CLASSIFICATION OF EXAMINATIONS

The dental assistant today may be eligible for two classifications of examinations; the Dental Assisting National Board examination or a state examination for a specific credential that is granted by an individual state board of dentistry.

National Board Examinations

The Dental Assisting National Board (DANB) assumes the responsibility for national dental assistant certification. Successful completion of the DANB examination enables an assistant to use the credential of Certified Dental Assistant (CDA), to wear the official certification pin, and to display the certificate. Three pathways lead to this national credential. Each of these pathways is outlined in the box.

Credentialing examinations provided by the DANB include the general chairside, radiographic hygiene, and infection control tests, as well as specialty examinations in dental office management, oral maxillofacial surgery, and orthodontics. More information on this credential is available by writing to the Dental Assisting National Board, 216 East Ontario St., Chicago, IL 60611.

State Credentialing

Credentials for dental assistants vary from state to state. The credentials may be granted in the form of a license, registration, or a certification for a single task or a series of tasks. Educational and examination requirements will also vary with each state. In some states, certification from the DANB is a prerequisite to eligibility for a state credential, while in other states specific

PATHWAYS TO DENTAL ASSISTANT CERTIFICATION THROUGH THE DANB
PATHWAY I
Graduate of an accredited dental assistant or dental hygiene program Current CPR card
PATHWAY II
High school graduation or equivalent Current CPR card Two years, or 3500 hours, of full-time employment Recommendation of dentist employer
PATHWAY III
Previous certification with a lapsed status of 18 months Current CPR card

course work or employment may be the criterion. For information about legal duties, educational requirements, and qualifications for credentialing, an assistant may write to the state board of dentistry in the state for which this information is desired.

Each credential verifies to patients and an employer a person's professional credibility in a specific area. A credential builds self-esteem and provides an assistant with bargaining power during salary negotiations. It is important that an assistant seek to obtain as many credentials as possible.

CREDENTIALING AGENCIES

The two agencies responsible for dental assistant credentials are the DANB and the board of dentistry in each state. Some dental assistants are unaware of the credentialing process, because not all candidates have had formal education or graduated from a dental assisting program accredited by the American Dental Association. It is important that a dental assistant have an understanding of the role of the various credentialing agencies, how the agency functions, the interrelationship between agencies, and the authority of the agency to administer examinations and to issue, verify, maintain, and revoke credentials.

The Dental Assisting National Board

The Dental Assisting National Board (DANB) is comprised of a board of directors, an executive director, and consultants. This agency is a national, independent, nonprofit credentialing agency that was established in 1948 for the sole purpose of determining competence of dental assistants. The board of directors includes representation from the American Association of Dental Examiners, the American Association of Dental Schools, the American Dental Assistants Association, the American Dental Association, DANB certificants, and the public. Consultants who serve the DANB are representative dentists, dental assistants, and scientific specialists.

State Board of Dentistry

The primary authority for recognizing a credential rests with the state board of dentistry. Each state has a dental practice act that regulates the practice of dentistry, dental assisting, and dental hygiene within that jurisdiction. Commonly the statutes within this act provide for a regulatory agency to enforce the law, conduct examinations, and regulate the practice of dentistry, dental assisting, and dental hygiene. The state board of dentistry is a government agency that is established by law and functions under the direction of the state legislature to regulate the practice of dentistry. The terms *state board* and *state board of dentistry,* when used in this text, refer to this regulatory agency.

It is common for each state to have a licensing agency that is responsible for creating, administering, and validating the examination. This office is responsible for maintaining records on the candidates and licensed professionals in the state.

A state dental or dental assistant organization is a voluntary organization, but frequently has input into membership on the board of dentistry. Membership on the state board varies from state to state but is commonly representative of practitioners within the state.

Unlike dentists and dental hygienists, the dental assistant at this time is not recognized in all dental practice acts. Therefore, it is vital that the dental assistant contact the state board of dentistry to obtain a copy of the dental practice act to ensure that the duties being performed in the office are legally delegable to him or her and that the educational and credentialing requirements have been met.

The Canadian Dental Assistants' Association

The Canadian Dental Assistants' Association (CDAA) provides a National Board examination in two forms. The level I examination emphasizes basic knowledge in professional conduct, dental health education, patient care procedures, clinical support procedures, practice management, and laboratory procedures. The level II category test focuses on knowledge in radiography and intraoral duties. Specific requirements are necessary for each of these examinations. Through national certfication, the CDAA is promoting the recognition of a standard of education across Canada in conjunction with recent government initiatives established to improve employment mobility for dental assistants between provinces.

National certification does not provide provincial registration. Each province in Canada defines its own legally delegable skills that a dental assistant may perform, as well as the education required for each task. Applicants must register with the provincial certification or licensure authority and inquire about provincial regulations for dental assistants.

Additional information about credentialing in Canada can be obtained by contacting the Canadian Dental Assistants' Association, 1785 Alta Vista Drive, Suite 105, Ottawa, Ontario KIG 3Y6.

TEST DEVELOPMENT

Credentialing examinations for dental assistants are developed by persons who know how different types of tests are developed for different purposes; but most of the tests are developed by those knowledgeable about dentistry. Most tests are developed from a test outline. The outline is a result of a detailed survey, commonly referred to as a task analysis, of dental professionals who identify common tasks and techniques in the field.

The members of the test construction committees represent various disciplines and often include educators with strong curriculum background, as well as persons with expertise in basic sciences, radiography, chairside assisting, dental materials, dental specialties, infection control, and practice management.

Because questions are developed by a committee, it is likely the tasks and knowledge will be categorized according to a set of questions:

Is this a task the dental assistant will perform frequently or infrequently?

Is the task simple or complex to perform?

Is the task easy or hard to learn?

Does this task require recall, application, or problem analysis?

What base of knowledge is needed to perform the task?

What references are available to validate the accepted method of performance?

What references are available to validate basic cognitive knowledge?

The test construction committee assumes the responsibility for creating new examinations, reviewing examination drafts, and reviewing inappropriate test items after an examination has been administered. The committee works with a test bank of questions that is maintained by the agency staff. Items are solicited for a test bank from the profession and all questions are reviewed, classified, and then sorted in the test bank with the assistance of the agency staff.

This information should serve as a guide for your examination preparation. For instance, there will be some tasks that the test construction committee feels every assistant should know because they are performed frequently. If a task is simple to perform and easy to learn, it is likely that fewer questions will be asked regarding this subject, yet if it is vital to every procedure some questions may be allocated to the task. That information should serve as a guide for your examination preparation. If 50 questions are going to be asked on one topic, such as chairside assisting, then that topic deserves more study time than a topic to be covered by only five questions. It is important for the candidate to be aware of the allocation of questions on the test and to review the references, because they will make up the criteria for acceptable performance on the examination.

PREPARATORY INFORMATION

Unlike the National Board examination, state board examinations vary greatly, and thus it is not possible to describe a standardized board examination. However, the following discussion will present a variety of factors that are common to various examinations.

The Application

The examination application is provided by the credentialing agency to explain the examination process to the candidate and to seek information about the candidate. It is a road map that describes the steps you must take to travel from point A to point B. The application will seek information about you, ask you to document certain data that might include information about your employment, type of education, graduation data (high school and dental assistant program), vital personal data, and CPR verification.

When completing the application it is important that you review it thoroughly before beginning. Most applications require you to complete the form in ink or type it. It may also require a notary's seal. A candidate for the DANB examination has an option to take a written or computerized version of the examination.

Examination Procedures

Information about the examination procedure may be included in the application or it may be a separate informational brochure or letter. It will likely include one or more of the following:

- Application deadlines that are strictly enforced
- The fee for the examination and the method of payment
- Method of notification of acceptance as a candidate
- The location of the examination site
- A listing of materials to be brought to the examination site, if applicable
- Prerequisite information for a clinical patient, if applicable
- The address to which all correspondence should be sent
- Transcript requirements
- Verification of malpractice insurance
- Verification of CPR

Examination Outline

Whether a state or national board examination, you will be provided with some form of test outline. The outline may be simple or extensive. An examination may be designed as two components, written and clinical. Each component will have identifiable sections.

The following is a descriptive outline of the written component of a typical statewide licensing examination. Some outlines may be even more detailed than this one.

I. WRITTEN SECTION
    The written examination consists of 200 multiple choice questions covering the following areas:

Category	Recall	Complexity level distribution Application	Analysis	Total questions
A. Data collection and recording	10	14	0	24
B. Chairside dental procedures	2	2	2	6
C. Patient management	2	2	0	4
D. Prevention of disease	4	6	4	14
E. Prevention and management of emergencies	0	2	2	4
F. Occupational safety	0	2	2	4
G. Legal aspects of dentistry	4	8	0	12
H. Dental radiography	18	28	0	46
I. Intraoral functions	34	52	0	86
Totals	74	116	10	200

Written/Computerized Examinations

The DANB examination is available in computerized or written format. Though the format in which the examination is taken may vary, it is likely you will encounter similar question formats. In the examination you will probably be given various styles of questions in a test booklet with a separate answer sheet for recording your choice of *a, b, c, d,* or *e* or whatever letters or numbers are used as an alternative response. The mechanics of recording your choice of the answer are simple; they just require *accurate* execution. Do not make responses hurriedly or carelessly. A test scoring machine reads responses exactly where you put them. In a written examination, if you put an answer on the wrong line or in the wrong column, there is no way that a machine can give you credit for a correct response.

When responding to a multiple-choice question it is important to keep in mind that you can arrive at the answer in two different ways, that is, by "knowing" the answer and finding it among the alternatives offered, or by eliminating incorrect responses by either knowing they are wrong or being able to figure it out. Both methods are perfectly legitimate. Both methods are based on knowing what is correct and/or what is incorrect. You must arrive at the one correct or one "best" answer by whatever method you use, or you must choose the one answer that seems *best to you.* Be certain to mark an answer for each question. Do not omit any. If you must, *guess* between two alternatives after eliminating two or three because you *know* they are wrong. Very few widely used tests apply a correction-for-guessing formula. Even if they do, the correction is only for completely random guessing across all alternatives offered. If you can eliminate any responses as incorrect based on your knowledge, you will *not* be guessing randomly but will be exercising *informed guessing.* If you are having difficulty understanding the question, skip it, and return to it later.

As mentioned previously there are a variety of types of questions, including one best answer, complex multiple choice, negative format, true or false, cause and effect, and matching.

One Best Answer

This is actually a multiple-choice type question, in which the item stem is followed by several responses, including one that is the only acceptable or most correct answer of the choices offered. An example of this type of question is illustrated in the following:

The abnormal opening of the anterior teeth caused by thumb sucking or tongue thrusting is referred to as

A. *Open bite*
B. *Closed bite*
C. *Cross bite*
D. *Retrognathism*

Complex Multiple Choice

In this style, the question stem is generally followed by four or five responses, at least one of which is correct. The candidate is directed to choose only one answer that is correct. Commonly a national or state test using this type of question will use a standardized format for the answers and provide directions as follows:

Fill in only one space on your answer sheet for each question. On the answer sheet fill in the space provided that corresponds to the choices listed below:

A if only 1, 2, and 3 are correct
B if only 1 and 3 are correct
C if only 2 and 4 are correct
D if only 4 is correct
E if all are correct

An example of this type of question is shown below:

What aids are used to diagnose caries?

1. A sharp explorer
2. A periodontal probe
3. Bitewing radiographs

4. A ball burnisher
5. Periapical radiographs

Negative Format

This type of question is used when several correct answers exist for a given question, but the exception is important to know (i.e., what is *not* true). The stem of the question is followed by several correct responses and one response that is *not* correct, or is the exception to the rule. The candidate must select this exception. Two examples of this type of question are illustrated below:

All of the following will result in the sterilization of an instrument EXCEPT

A. Dry heat
B. Steam under pressure
C. Unsaturated chemical vapor
D. Isopropyl alcohol

Which of the following is NOT found in a bitewing radiograph?

A. Restoration
B. Periapical abscess
C. Bone level
D. Teeth of two arches

Matching

In these questions, the candidate is asked to match an item in one column with its function or verbal or pictorial description in another column. An example of this type of question follows. The directions for this question will include:

Match each instrument in Column A with its primary use in Column B.

Column A	Column B
1. Periodontal probe	A. Planes roots of tooth
2. Periosteal elevator	B. Smooths alveolar process to promote healing
3. Rongeur forceps	C. Lifts and raises mucous membrane and underlying tissue covering bone
	D. Measures gingival sulcus depth
	E. Removes pathologic tissue and spicules of bone

True or False

Though this is not a common type of question used on credentialing examinations, it may be used in some situations. Typically a list of statements will be provided, and you are to determine if the statement is true or false. The difficulty in this type of question is that the candidate often anticipates the tester is trying to trick him or her. The candidate therefore reads more into the statement than is intended. The instructions will likely tell you to choose A for a true statement and B for a false statement.

A more complex type of true or false question is a paired true or false item, though this type of question does not appear frequently in credentialing examinations. In this type of question the stem is the only portion of the question that varies. The item consists of two statements about the same topic. The answer options always provide all possible true or false combinations. An example of this type of question follows:

Acquired immunodeficiency syndrome is transmitted through blood and other body secretions. A patient with this disease requires that you double glove.

a. Both statements are TRUE
b. Both statements are FALSE
c. The first statement is TRUE; the second is FALSE
d. The first statement is FALSE; the second is TRUE

Cause and Effect

Cause and effect questions are very similar to paired true or false questions in that the only part of the question that varies is the stem. In this type of question a stem will contain a statement and a reason that are written as a single sentence and connected by *because*. In some questions the statements may even be preceded by a case study about a clinical situation. The answers are always the same as shown below:

Placement of a sealant is more successful on a maxillary tooth because these teeth are more accessible than mandibular teeth.

A. Both statement and reason are correct and related
B. Both statement and reason are correct but NOT related
C. The statement and reason are correct but NOT related
D. The statement is NOT correct, but the reason is an accurate statement
E. NEITHER statement nor reason is correct

Hints for Answering Questions

Though many suggestions could be made to aid you in answering questions, the best suggestion is to be well prepared with a sound base of knowledge. There are, however, several sound pieces of advice that the authors feel should be considered by a candidate taking a credentialing examination; some are common sense and some result from research in test and measurements.

Some people say that it is best when answering a multiple-choice question to mark your first ''hunch'' and then stick with it. Others suggest that examinees should review questions carefully after finishing marking the answers to all questions. The rather limited research available suggests that ''abler'' students tend to increase their test scores a bit by carefully reviewing items, whereas lower scoring students do not. Perhaps the more appropriate procedure is to first mark responses to all questions that you ''know'' and then eliminate all wrong responses that you can for other questions and make your best estimate among the remaining choices. Go back over questions primarily to check that you have not made some obvious error in such things as reading or marking answers. Agonizing over choices does not seem to be a particularly successful approach.

Read questions and directions carefully. Do *not* add or delete information provided. Do not read into items information that is not there or construct situations that do not exist in the question as it is stated. Pay attention to words in the stem that are underlined, capitalized, or italicized. When the negative format is used be certain to look for the *exception,* not the correct answer.

Occasionally a candidate will try to second-guess the authors of a test by looking for response patterns such as a ''run'' of answers or answers in a particular response pattern (alternative C). Although it may be true that amateur test writers sometimes inadvertently give students such clues, professional authors of credentialing examinations will not fall into that trap. A credentialing examination is not a test of wits between you and the author; it is an attempt to allow you to demonstrate the knowledge and skill you have attained and to determine if it meets a minimal standard of practice.

Clinical Examinations

It is difficult to describe the content of clinical examinations for dental assistants since each test varies from state to state and the content is frequently revised. Some of the skills tested in a clinical examination include one or more of the following:

- Inspecting the oral cavity
- Performing preliminary oral examinations
- Applying topical anesthetics
- Topically applying anticariogenic agents
- Polishing coronal surfaces of the teeth
- Exposing radiographs
- Placing and removing wedges and matrices
- Placing, condensing, and carving amalgam restorations
- Placing and removing periodontal dressings
- Placing and finishing composite resin restorations
- Placing and removing sedative temporary restorations or crowns
- Applying cavity liners and bases
- Removing excess cement from the coronal surfaces of teeth
- Removing sutures

Evaluation Criteria

As in the written examination, there will be an outline to describe the clinical examination, and it will include the criteria for evaluation. The outline likely will include specific criteria for each of the clinical tasks. For instance, in one state examination, in which a model is used for the procedure, the evaluation criteria for placement of a temporary intracoronal restoration includes:

1. Margin adaptation. Cement must be flush or within 0.5 mm of margins of the MO preparation.
2. Proximal contact and contour. There must be visual contact with the adjacent tooth. Contact area must be at least 1 mm in width buccolingually. Contour should follow the anatomy of the tooth. Contour must extend from contact area to margins of the proximal box. (Please note: use of dental floss may cause an unacceptable open contact.)
3. Finish. Cement must not encroach into the gingival area or be excessive on the occlusal surface of the prepared tooth. Surface of intracoronal restoration should be smooth and free of voids.
4. Occlusion. Casts will be hand-articulated in centric occlusion with opposing arch. ML cusp of #2 or lingual cusp of #5 must contact #31 and #28 respectively.

Clinical Facilities

In most areas of the country where clinical examinations are given, provisions are made for access to modern clinical facilities. Often a dental school or a dental assistant program facility is used. A dental school is an ideal setting since more candidates can be tested at one time due to the large number of treatment areas. The state boards do not own these facilities, but rather reserve them for a specific period of time.

It is important to remember that, like you, the examiners assigned to the examination site may not be familiar with the facility. You generally can be assured, however, that the facility will have adequate lighting, water, evacuation systems, and functional equipment. You will, in most instances, be required to bring with you your own sterilized instruments and materials.

Patient Selection

Most testing agencies do not provide patients for candidates taking a clinical examination. This is your responsibility. The key to successful patient recruitment begins with advanced planning and a professional attitude. Within most test outlines the testing agency will identify specific patient requirements. One state includes the following patient criteria, which are common to most examinations:

1. 18 or more years of age
2. At least 18 fully erupted teeth
3. Good oral hygiene
4. The enclosed Patient Health/Consent Form must be completed and signed by the patient at the examination site.
5. The patient will *not* be acceptable if he or she presents with medical, health, or tissue conditions that would contraindicate providing the dental procedure or care to be evaluated.
6. The patient health questionnaire should be completed *by the patient* **before** the testing date and brought to the examination site.
7. Current written clearance must be obtained from the patient's physician if health conditions exist that indicate a need to consult the physician. This clearance must be presented to the examiner before beginning a clinical procedure.
8. The candidate must follow Centers for Disease Control and Prevention guidelines for aseptic techniques.
9. The candidate must bring all equipment and supplies to the examination site. All instruments used intraorally must be sterile.

Before beginning to recruit candidates for an examination follow these guidelines:

1. Review the criteria for patient selection.
2. Determine the availability of the patient for the date and time of the examination. Remember, clinical examinations will require long treatment sessions and periods of waiting for examiners and patients.
3. Practice basic treatment with the patient to ensure the patient's cooperation.
4. Inform the patient of the expected responsibilities.
5. Consider the attitude and degree of cooperation of the patient.
6. Maintain good rapport with the patient.
7. Advise the patient of the purpose of the examination and its importance to you.

Professional Liability

During clinical examinations you will be required to provide proof of liability coverage. If you are working in a dental office or if you have a student liability card, check immediately to ensure that the insurance carrier will cover you during the clinical examination. If you are not covered, you will be required to obtain the liability insurance before the clinical examination. You should obtain this coverage at the earliest possible date

to ensure that you will receive the necessary proof in time for the clinical examination.

Scoring System

It is common for most credentialing agencies to use a norm-referenced scoring system to ensure equivalent meaning of scores from edition to edition of the tests. The score that is reported is known as the standard score, and this score indicates how the candidate score relates to the average. This score results from two factors: a raw score, or the number of correct answers the candidate selects, and the distribution of raw scores from a norm-referenced group of candidates. A mean raw score of the norming group is assigned a standard score such as 85. Then the raw score 1.5 standard deviations below the mean raw score is assigned the standard score of 75. All other standard scores are computed by using the relationship between these two scores. The norm-referenced scoring system eliminates inconsistences in the results that may be caused by differences in difficulty between editions of the examination.

A testing agency will also perform an item analysis on each of the questions to determine potential errors in test question construction. Any questions that consistently are answered erroneously may be taken back to the test construction committee for evaluation, rewriting, or elimination. When such a question has been determined to be a problem on an examination, appropriate action is taken to ensure it does not jeopardize a candidate's score.

Time Schedule

Both types of examinations, written and clinical, are designed around a time constraint. You will be informed in the examination outline what this time limitation will be and how it is applied. Two factors are involved in time constraints: when the examination begins and how long it extends. It is important that you appear before the examination time and check in with the appropriate person to verify your attendance. Examinations start promptly. The penalty for tardiness can range from not hearing the directions, loss of time for completion, to nonadmission to the examination. *It is better to be 20 minutes early than 2 minutes late.*

It is wise to budget your time on any examination. Make a quick overview of the number of tasks required in a practical examination or the number of questions to be answered in a written examination and then think of the pace you will need to follow to allow appropriate amounts of time for each section. If one part has 30 questions and the other has 50 questions, you will likely need to spend more time on the latter.

Even though you do think about budgeting your time,

some tasks or questions may require more of your time than other tasks or questions because they are more difficult. Therefore, most test takers find it wise to work all the way through a written examination at a fairly rapid but cautious pace by answering first all the questions that they "know" or to which they can work out the answer fairly quickly. This method suggests skipping the difficult or unknown questions the first time through and coming back to them.

There are several good reasons for doing this. You will build on your own success. This success can help lessen any fears or concerns that you may have about the testing situation. This method also leaves time available for the tougher questions for which you need more time. Sometimes as you progress through the examination other questions or answers may trigger your mind to respond with the answer or may provide a cue for an earlier question. Mental "germination" works well for some people. They "know" the answer but cannot latch onto it immediately.

When you use this approach of moving through the test at a fairly rapid pace and skipping some questions, you must be particularly cautious in locating accurately the answer space for each question on your answer sheet. Inaccuracies in spacing on your answer sheet could create a problem that you might not locate until later, and having to make spacing corrections is a time-wasting and sometimes costly activity. It is wise to cross-check to ensure you have left a space for the missing answer on the answer sheet and circle the question in the test booklet.

For some candidates, it is helpful to take a break every now and then. You will not be allowed to leave an examination for a leisurely cup of coffee, but there is no reason why you cannot put your pencil down, close your eyes, take a deep breath, and relax for a few minutes. Your own personal style of working will dictate whether this technique will work for you.

Release of Examination Results

Typically, it takes 6 to 8 weeks to process and report examination results. The candidate receives an individual score report and in the case of the DANB examination the school of graduation receives a blind report. In some state board examinations, the results also are released to the schools.

In most instances you may retake an examination, but in some state board examinations you are limited to the number of retakes before you will be required to obtain some formal education. In some states there is a requirement to complete a written examination successfully before you are eligible to take a clinical examination. You should always understand the prerequisites to any credential before you begin the examination process.

Examination Availability

The DANB written examination is offered four times each year: February, June, August, and November. Each site that offers examinations generally provides two or more examination periods, but each site will set up its own schedule. Computerized testing is available continuously.

Rules for Examination Administration

A discipline policy exists within each agency that offers a credentialing examination for dental assistants. Such a policy is used to identify any irregularities or cheating on an examination. This commonly is done by a computer during the scoring process to compare answers to detect improbable similarities. In some testing agencies, alternate forms of the examination are used so that different test booklets have the same questions but in a scrambled order. It should be understood that a credentialing agency such as the DANB and a state board of dentistry is committed to maintaining the integrity of each candidate's results and will use a reasonable system to control any irregularities in the testing process.

In the DANB application form, a well-defined discipline policy is provided. Such a policy will define the grounds, the procedure, and the sanctions that will be placed on a candidate for national certification. Similar policies also exist with state licensing agencies. In all cases the candidate has an opportunity to a hearing and appeal.

Request for Examination Review

If you fail a portion or all of an examination and feel that there has been an error, it is likely there is a provision for an examination review. For instance, if you are informed that you failed the placement of an intracoronal temporary restoration on a model, you could request a review. This review is often set up with an examiner and another objective reviewer. During the review you can see the model, the temporary restoration, and the evaluation. You may challenge the results, but you should be prepared to rebut any questions asked during the interview.

Study Hints

A myriad of suggestions could be made to a candidate about to take a credentialing examination. The following 10 hints for studying should get you off to a good start.

1. Develop a thorough understanding of the body of knowledge and concepts to be covered by the examination.
2. Develop a reasonable study schedule for preparing for the examination at least 3 to 4 months before the testing date. This requires you to set aside specific times to review specific material. If

studying with a friend or group, be sure that the study group is serious and reliable.

3. Obtain copies of former credentialing examinations if available or a copy of a mock examination.

4. Grade yourself with a key that is included with the examination.

5. Identify areas where you have weaknesses. Use your past school experience or results of study examinations to help you determine your areas of greatest need. Dental assistants who have had no formal education should focus on basic science material and any developments in dental technology or assisting that they may not have had exposure to in their work experience.

6. Create a resource library for ready reference throughout the review process. This could be shared with a study group of other reliable candidates.

7. Once you have formulated a study plan, adhere to your schedule. If the plan meets obstacles, reassess the plan and modify it to avoid future deterrents. It may be necessary to work with your family and friends so they realize how important your study time is to your success.

8. Prepare yourself psychologically. Take some time the day before the examination to rest and relax. Eliminate potential distractions or immediate concerns on the day of the examination. Place all your energy into your concentration.

9. On the day of the examination arrive on time, thoroughly read the examination instructions, carefully read each question to understand exactly what is being asked, carefully enter your answers, pace yourself, relax as necessary, and maintain your self-confidence.

10. Take breaks as they become available, take time out to refresh yourself and restore your energy, and concentrate on the remaining parts of the examination.

HOW TO USE THIS BOOK FOR STUDYING

This book is designed to provide you an overview of the basic knowledge and procedures common to dental assisting throughout the United States. Take time to review one section of content at a time. First study the outlined material in the chapter. Then refer to recommended references and textbooks to research areas that are unclear. See the list of suggested readings at the end of this chapter.

After you have reviewed the contents of the chapter and completed your review of other literature, answer the review questions in the last part of the chapter. If you are unsure of an answer or guess at an answer, note this in the question section and review it later. Attempt to analyze each question, eliminate answers you are certain are incorrect, and then make a knowledgeable choice or an educated guess. It is wiser to make a guess than to leave an empty space on the answer sheet. Finally, compare your answers with those at the end of each chapter. If you answered an item incorrectly or you were uncertain about an answer, refer to recommended text materials for further review.

After several days have elapsed, review the chapter again and reanswer the review questions. If you continue to miss the same questions, you should continue further study or contact a resource person with knowledge in the area of concern.

Some candidates rely on a review book such as this as the sole reference. That is an unwise decision. As mentioned earlier, you need to create a good resource library. This book is not designed as a singular text for any credentialing examination but rather as an impetus to confirm your knowledge and stimulate you to seek more education in areas where you are weak. The authors of this text commend you for your decision to accept the challenge of a credentialing examination and wish you good luck!

SUGGESTED READINGS

Exposure and processing for dental radiography, pamphlet #N-413, Rochester, NY, 1994, Eastman Kodak Company, 1-800-933-8031.

Glossary of dentofacial orthopedic terms, St. Louis, 1988, American Association of Orthodontists.

Infection control in modern dental practice, (see pp. 14, 15, 23 for radiography-related information), pamphlet #N-419, Rochester, NY, 1992, Eastman Kodak Company, 1-800-933-8031.

Radiation safety in dental radiography, pamphlet #N-414, Rochester, NY, 1994, Eastman Kodak Company, 1-800-933-8031.

Successful intraoral radiographs, pamphlet #N-418, Rochester, NY, 1990, Eastman Kodak Company, 1-800-933-8031.

Successful panoramic radiography, pamphlet #N-406, Rochester, NY, 1994, Eastman Kodak Company, 1-800-933-8031.

X-Rays in dentistry, book #D1-5, Rochester, NY, 1985, Eastman Kodak Company, 1-800-933-8031.

AAOMS office anesthesia evaluation manual, ed 4, Chicago, 1991, AAOMS Publications.

AAOMS office anesthesia evaluation videotape, ed 2, Garden Grove, CA, 1991, Infomedix.

ADA Council on Dental Materials, Instruments and Equipment; ADA Council on Dental Practice; ADA Council on Cental Therapeutics: Infection control recommendations for the dental office and dental laboratory, JADA 123(8)(suppl S-246), August 1992.

An introduction to basic concepts in dental radiography, Chicago, January 1991, marketed by the American Dental Assistants Association, 312-541-1550.

Boucher CO: *Boucher's clinical dental terminology: glossary of accepted terms in all disciplines of dentistry,* ed 4, St. Louis, 1993, Mosby.

Centers for Disease Control and Prevention: Controlling exposures to nitrous oxide during anesthetic administration, NIOSH Alert, Publication 94-100, April 1994.

Centers for Disease Control and Prevention: Recommended infection control practices for dentistry, *MMWR* 41(RR-8): 1-12, May 28, 1993.

Cleveland JL, et al: TB infection control recommendations from the CDC, 1994: considerations for dentistry, *JADA* 126:593-600, May 1995.

Cottone JA, Terezhalmy GT, Molinari JA: *Practical infection control in dentistry,* Philadelphia, 1996, Williams & Wilkins.

Davis K: *Training manual for anesthesia assisting in the oral and maxillofacial surgery office,* ed 2, Burlington, 1988, Training Manual Publishing Company.

DeLyre WR: *Essentials of dental radiography for dental assistants and hygienists,* ed 5, Norwalk, CT, 1995, Appleton and Lange.

Dofka CM: *Competency skills for the dental assistant,* Albany, 1996, Delmar Publications.

Edwards C, et al: *Radiation protection for dental radiographers,* Denver, 1984, Multi-Media Publishing.

Ehrlich A, Torres H: *Essentials of dental assisting,* Philadelphia, 1995, WB Saunders.

Ehrlich A: *Nutrition and dental health,* Albany, 1987, Delmar Publications.

Evers H, Haegerstam G: *Introduction to dental local anesthesia,* St. Louis, 1991, Mosby.

Finkbeiner BL, Johnson CS: *Comprehensive dental assisting,* St. Louis, 1995, Mosby.

Finkbeiner BL, Finkbeiner CA: *Practice management for the dental team,* ed 4, St. Louis, 1996, Mosby.

Frommer HH: *Radiology for dental auxiliaries,* ed 6, St. Louis, 1996, Mosby.

Giaquinto C, Albano R: *Dental assisting test preparation,* Upper Saddle River, NJ, 1996, Brady/Prentice Hall.

Gragg PP, Young JM, Cottone JA: Handpiece sterilization: establishing an office protocol, *The Dental Assistant* 33-40, Second Quarter 1993.

Little JW, Falace DA: *Dental management of the medically compromised patient,* ed 4, St. Louis, 1993, Mosby.

Malamed SF: *Handbook of local anesthesia,* ed 4, St. Louis, 1996, Mosby.

Malamed SF: *Handbook of medical emergencies in the dental office,* ed 4, St. Louis, 1993, Mosby.

Malamed SF: *Sedation, a guide to patient management,* ed 3, St. Louis, 1991, Mosby.

Miles D, Van Dis M, Jensen C, Ferretti A: *Radiographic imaging for dental auxiliaries,* ed 2, Philadelphia, 1993, WB Saunders.

Miller CH, Palenik C: *Infection control and management of hazardous materials for the dental team,* St. Louis, 1994, Mosby.

Miyasaki-Ching C: *Chasteen's essentials of clinical dental assisting,* ed 5, St. Louis, 1997, Mosby.

Moreland N: Infection control in the age of AIDS: the dental assistant's role, *The Dental Assistant,* Third Quarter 1993.

Phillips RW, Moore BK: *Elements of dental materials for dental hygienists and dental assistants,* ed 5, Philadelphia, 1994, WB Saunders.

Reynolds JM: *Welcome to the world of orthodontics,* Lubbock, 1984, Zulauf, Inc.

Smith RG, et al: *Dental surgery assistants' handbook,* ed 2, St. Louis, 1993, Mosby.

Sonis ST: *Dental secrets,* Philadelphia, 1994, Hanley and Belfus.

Textbook of advanced cardiac life support (also known as the *ACLS provider text*), ed 2, Chicago, 1987-1990, American Heart Association.

The American Dental Assistants Association is marketing ICE PACK, a packet of the following and 16 other articles recommended by DANB's Infection Control Test Construction Committee. ICE PACK is available for purchase. Call ADAA at 312-541-1550.

Torres H, Ehrlich A: *Modern dental assisting,* ed 5, Philadelphia, 1995, WB Saunders.

US Department of Health and Human Services: *Practical infection control in the dental office: a workbook for the dental team,* October 1993.

US Department of Labor; Occupational Safety and Health Administration: *Controlling occupational exposure to bloodborne pathogens in dentistry,* OSHA Publication 3129, 1992.

US Department of Labor; Occupational Safety and Health Administration: *Hazard communication guidelines for compliance,* OSHA Publication 3111.

US Department of Labor; Office of Health Compliance Assistance: OSHA Hazard Communication Standard, Code of Federal Regulations, #29, Part 1910 et al, February 9, 1994.

US Federal Government: Occupational Exposure to Bloodborne Pathogens; Final Rule, Federal Register, 56(235), 64175-64182, December 6, 1991, 64175-64182.

CHAPTER 2

The Profession: Evolution and Ethics

OUTLINE

Dentistry as Health Care System
State Board of Dentistry
The Dentist
Dental Specialties

Dental Assistant
Dental Hygienist
Dental Laboratory Technician
Professional Organizations
The Dental Health Team

Societal Impact on Dentistry
Evolution of Dental Assisting
Ethical and Legal Aspects of
   Dentistry

KEY TERMS

Abandonment
Advanced functions
American Association of Dental
   Schools (AADS)
American Dental Assistants Associ-
   ation (ADAA)
American Dental Association
   (ADA)
Assault
Assignment
Battery
Certified Dental Assistant (CDA)
Certified Dental Practice Manage-
   ment Assistant (CDPMA)
Certified Dental Technician (CDT)
Certified Oral and Maxillofacial
   Surgery Assistant (COMSA)
Certified Orthodontic Assistant
   (COA)
Chairside assistant
Civil law
Commission on Dental Accredita-
   tion (CDA)

Consent
Council on Dental Education
   (CDE)
Credential
Defamation of character
Defendant
Dental assistant
Dental Assisting National Board
   (DANB)
Dental Auxiliary Teacher Education
   (DATE)
Dental Auxiliary Utilization (DAU)
Dental health team
Dental laboratory technician
Dental practice act
Dental public health
Dentist
Dentistry
Direct supervision
Doctor of Dental Surgery (DDS)
Doctor of Dental Medicine (DMD)
Endodontics

Ethics
Etiology
Expert witness
Fact witness
Felony
Four-handed dentistry
Fraud
General practitioner
Implied consent
Oral maxillofacial surgery
Oral pathology
Orthodontics
Pediatric dentistry
Periodontics
Prosthodontics
Registered Dental Assistant (RDA)
Registered Dental Assistant Ex-
   panded Functions (RDAEF)
Registered Dental Hygienist (RDH)
Specialty
State Board of Dentistry

The **dental health team** is the primary care unit within the profession of dentistry. The team consists of the **dentist,** the dental assistant, the dental hygienist, and the dental laboratory technician. **Dentistry** is a healing art and science that is concerned with the teeth, oral cavity, and associated structures. The objectives of dentistry include the following:

- Provide relief of pain from dental origin
- Help prevent pain by practicing preventive dentistry
- Help maintain personal appearance
- Help masticate food throughout a lifetime
- Maintain good oral health

The dentist, as a professional, has the privilege of self-government; however, he or she also has an obligation to the public to maintain a standard of quality care and ethical conduct. The mission of the profession is to encourage the improvement of the public's health, to promote the art and science of dentistry, and to represent the interests of the dental profession, as well as the public it serves.

The educated **dental assistant** has become a vital member of the dental health team in modern dental practice. Studies have proven that a highly skilled assistant at chairside can reduce stress on the patient, the dentist, and the assistant; can increase productivity; and can improve the quality of care. As dentists delegate more advanced functions to chairside dental assistants, such as specific intraoral clinical functions that go beyond basic chairside skills, and as they continue to place more management responsibilities on assistants in the business office, the dental assisting profession will become even more vital to dentistry. Keep in mind two important factors about the dental assistant's job: (1) the dental assistant should perform only duties that do not require the dentist's professional skill and judgment and (2) the dental assistant should perform only those duties that are delegable by the state dental practice act in the state in which the dentist practices.

The primary role of the dental hygienist is preventive care. Traditionally, this important role includes such duties as the oral prophylaxis (scaling and polishing the teeth), charting oral conditions, polishing restorations, applying anticariogenic agents, providing patient education in oral hygiene and nutrition, and exposing, processing, and evaluating dental radiographs. The individual state dental practice act determines if the dental hygienist may perform additional intraoral duties that are recognized as advanced functions.

A **dental laboratory technician** performs extraoral functions in a private dental office, a commercial laboratory, or a dental school. This dental team member's primary duty is the construction of prosthetic devices and restorations (i.e., crowns, bridges, or dentures). The dental laboratory technician works according to the written prescription of a licensed dentist.

Each day dental professionals are faced with issues involving the legal requirements and voluntary standards in the delivery of dental treatment. The **dental practice act** of each state defines the legal requirements necessary to practice dentistry and the scope of dental practice. The legal standards for dental care are derived from both common law (judicial decisions) and statutory law, such as the dental practice act, which was enacted by a legislative body.

The dental professional is governed in practice not only by the dental practice act of each state and by the legal standards derived from common law, but also by the voluntary standards, such as the principles of **ethics** that were developed and implemented by the dental profession itself. Both legal requirements and voluntary or professional standards are implemented for the protection of society and, ultimately, the patient.

Membership in a professional organization is voluntary and, thus, the standards of these organizations are considered voluntary but are used as guidelines in peer review. Professional organizations continually reassess the functions of their standards and the qualifications of their members.

DENTISTRY AS HEALTH CARE SYSTEM

I. The objectives of dentistry include the following:
   A. Maintaining dental health
   B. Diagnosing and treating oral diseases
   C. Preventing dental diseases
   D. Restoring defective teeth
   E. Replacing missing teeth and oral tissues
   F. Preventing, intercepting, and maintaining proper occlusion
   G. Providing function in mastication and speech
   H. Providing aesthetics

STATE BOARD OF DENTISTRY

I. Each state's practice act defines the **state board of dentistry**–the body that supervises the practice of dentistry.
   A. State government has a direct control over the practice of dentistry and the function and status of the dentist and the dental auxiliaries.
   B. States have written dental practice acts to protect the health of the public by providing standardized safe dental care.
   C. Dentists and dental hygienists are licensed in all states; however, dental assistants may receive some form of credential in some states and yet not be legally recognized in other states.

D. The composition of the state board of dentistry varies from state to state, but generally it includes several dentists who have varying dental and geographic backgrounds, hygienists, assistants (if they are included in the state practice act), and public members.

THE DENTIST

I. The dentist, as a professional, has the privilege of self-government; however, he or she also has an obligation to the public to maintain a standard of quality care and ethical conduct.

    A. A dentist must complete a specified program of study and successfully pass the appropriate examinations, thereby earning a license to practice within a specific state.

    B. A dentist may be in a partnership, a group practice, or a clinic or diversified unit. A dentist may receive a commission and practice in various branches of the armed forces.

    C. A dentist may provide a variety of treatments, limit the practice to a specialty, or become involved in hospital dentistry or dental public health.

    D. Except for Delaware, each state requires that a dentist pass a written national board examination administered by the Joint Commission on National Dental Examinations. The dentist must also pass a clinical examination.

        1. A licensed dentist must adhere to the state dental practice act or to other state or federal laws that govern a dental practice.

        2. Failure to abide by these laws can result in a fine or license revocation.

DENTAL SPECIALTIES

I. The **American Dental Association** recognizes eight dental **specialties.**

    A. ***Dental public health*** is a form of dental practice that considers the community as the patient rather than the individual, controlling dental disease and promoting dental health.

    B. ***Endodontics*** is concerned with the morphology, physiology, and pathology of the dental pulp and associated tissues.

    C. ***Oral pathology*** is the specialty that deals with the nature of the diseases that affect the oral cavity and the adjacent structures.

    D. The specialty of ***oral maxillofacial surgery*** is responsible for the diagnosis and surgical treatment of diseases, injuries, and defects of the oral and maxillofacial region.

    E. ***Orthodontics*** is concerned with the supervision, guidance, and correction of the growing or mature dentofacial structures, including those conditions that require moving the teeth to correct a malocclusion or a malformation of the jaw.

    F. The specialty of ***pediatric dentistry*** is defined as the practice and teaching of comprehensive preventive and therapeutic oral health care of children from birth through adolescence, including care for special patients beyond the age of adolescence who demonstrate mental, physical, and/or emotional problems and require specialized care.

    G. ***Periodontics*** includes the diagnosis and treatment of diseases of the supporting and surrounding tissues of the teeth.

    H. ***Prosthodontics*** pertains to the restoration and maintenance of oral functions, comfort, appearance, and health of the patient by the restoration of natural teeth or by the replacement of missing teeth or oral structures with artificial devices (dental prostheses).

DENTAL ASSISTANT

I. Studies have proven that a highly skilled dental assistant is a vital member of the dental health team in the modern dental practice. The dental assistant can reduce stress on the patient, the dentist, and the assistant; increase productivity; and improve the quality of care.

    A. Dental assistants should always consider two important factors about the job.

        1. They must perform only duties that do not require the dentist's professional skill and judgment.

        2. They must perform only those duties that are delegable by the state dental practice act in the state in which the dentist practices.

    B. **Credentials** that may identify a dental assistant's legal and/or educational achievement are illustrated in the box on page 14.

    C. A dental assistant may assume any of the following roles:

        1. Clinical **chairside assistant**

        2. Office manager

        3. Generalist

        4. Advanced functions practitioner

    D. Accredited educational programs vary in length from 1 to 2 years.

DENTAL HYGIENIST

I. The primary role of the dental hygienist is preventive care.

    A. The traditional role includes such duties as the oral prophylaxis (scaling and polishing the

ACRONYMS FOR IDENTIFICATION OF DENTAL ASSISTANTS
CDA
Certified Dental Assistant
National credential granted by the DANB to recognize successful completion of the national certification examination. This credential may be recognized as a licensure requirement for dental assistants in some state practice acts.
CDPMA
Certified Dental Practice Management Assistant
National credential granted by the DANB to recognize successful completion of the specialty examination in Dental Practice Management.
COA
Certified Orthodontic Assistant
National credential granted by the DANB to recognize successful completion of the specialty examination in Orthodontics.
COMSA
Certified Oral and Maxillofacial Surgery Assistant
National credential granted by the DANB to recognize successful completion of the Oral and Maxillofacial Surgery specialty examination.
RDA
Registered Dental Assistant
A credential given by some states to indicate that specific requirements have been met to practice expanded and advanced functions for that state.
RDAEF
Registered Dental Assistant in Expanded Functions
A credential given by some states to indicate specific requirements have been met to practice expanded and advanced functions in that state.
OJT
On-the-job trained assistant
This is *not* a credential but a status of level of knowledge, learned *on the job*.

teeth), charting oral conditions, polishing restorations, applying anticariogenic agents, providing patient education in oral hygiene and nutrition, and exposing, processing, and evaluating dental radiographs.

B. The individual state dental practice act determines if the dental hygienist may perform additional intraoral duties recognized as advanced functions.
C. Formal education of a dental hygienist requires at least 2 years of postsecondary education.
D. The dental hygienist is licensed in all states.

DENTAL LABORATORY TECHNICIAN

I. A dental laboratory technician performs extraoral functions in a private dental office, a commercial laboratory, or a dental school.
   A. Primary duties of this professional include the construction of prosthetic devices and restorations (i.e., crowns, bridges, or dentures).
   B. The dental laboratory technician works according to the written prescription of a licensed dentist.
   C. Education is attained through ADA-accredited programs, apprenticeships, postsecondary schools, the armed forces, or proprietary schools.
   D. An individual may receive a credential as a **Certified Dental Technician (CDT)**, but no state licensure is available for this dental auxiliary.

PROFESSIONAL ORGANIZATIONS

I. Voluntary educational organizations are available for each member of the dental health team at national, state, and local levels.
   A. The acronyms for each of the organizations are derived from the state and local districts of residence or practice as shown in the box on page 15.

THE DENTAL HEALTH TEAM

I. Members of the dental team must ensure that productivity is met with quality assurance by adhering to a set of professional guidelines.
   A. They must perform only those duties that are legally delegable to them.
   B. They must obtain skills and credentials for all legally delegable duties in the state.
   C. They must participate in professional activities.
   D. They must be willing to assist other staff members in performing their duties; the hygienist, the assistant, and the office manager help one another to get the job done.
   E. They must participate in staff meetings for the purpose of improving the overall dental practice.
   F. They must be team players who give others credit and respect for their various roles on the team.

PROFESSIONAL ORGANIZATIONS FOR THE DENTAL HEALTH TEAM

DENTIST

American Dental Association (ADA)
Michigan Dental Association (MDA)
Central District Dental Society (CDDS)*

DENTAL ASSISTANT

American Dental Assistants Association (ADAA)
Michigan Dental Assistants' Association (MDAA)
Central District Dental Assistants' Society (CDAAS)*

DENTAL HYGIENIST

American Dental Hygienists' Association (ADHA)
Michigan Dental Hygienists' Association (MDHA)
Central District Dental Hygienists' Society (CDDHS)

DENTAL LABORATORY TECHNICIAN

National Association of Dental Laboratories (NADL)†

*These acronyms are based on cities, counties, or districts.
†Membership is based on laboratory membership rather than individual membership.

G. They must promote the dental practice and be committed to its objectives.

SOCIETAL IMPACT ON DENTISTRY

I. Dental programs
   A. Dental labor shortages from 1950 through the 1960s were addressed with federal programs for **Dental Auxiliary Utilization (DAU),** Training in Expanded Auxiliary Management (TEAM), and Expanded Functions Dental Auxiliary (EFDA).
   B. These programs placed emphasis on increasing the production of the dental profession, maintaining quality of care, and providing cost containment for the consumer.
   C. In 1965 the Office of Economic Opportunity (OEO) enacted the Head Start Program to provide educational health and social services to preschool children in need.
   D. The 1970s was the decade of dental insurance, which today is considered one of the most desirable employee benefits.
   E. The 1970s brought consumerism to state dental boards as many states changed the composition of the dental boards to include laypersons.
   F. The 1980s and 1990s are known for the impact of renewed safety, including infection control and radiography regulations.

EVOLUTION OF DENTAL ASSISTING

I. The demographics of the profession include high employability and varied salaries, benefits, and responsibilities.
   A. The average national wage of a dental assistant in 1992-1993 was approximately $10 per hour.
   B. Dental assistants possessing formal education and certification or registration may receive significantly higher salaries.
   C. Dental assistants can receive varied benefit packages, including one or several of the following options: health (medical and dental) and disability insurance, membership in professional organizations, uniform or clothing stipends, hepatitis vaccine, paid vacations, wellness days, day care allotments, educational stipends, retirement plans, and profit sharing.
   D. Dental assisting provides an opportunity for full- or part-time employment; working on holidays is rare, and working on weekends is done only on an optional basis.
II. Early times
   A. Dr. C. Edmund Kells is credited with hiring the first dental assistant.
   B. In 1921 the **American Dental Assistants Association** was organized by Juliette Southard.
      1. This national organization represents the interests of dental assistants while promoting education.
      2. In 1933 *The Dental Assistant* was adopted as the official publication of the ADAA.
      3. An official pin representing membership in the ADAA displays the organization's motto, "Education, Efficiency, Loyalty, and Service."
III. Formal education for dental assistants
   A. In 1947 the certifying board of the ADAA was established to administer examinations and to certify dental assistants. In 1948 programs known as the 104-hour study courses were designed by the ADAA to be offered by local ADAA chapters throughout the country; their aim was to prepare an employed dental assistant for certification. These courses provided the dental assistant with basic skills and cognitive knowledge about dentistry and required a minimal employment time before taking the certification examination, which included written and clinical elements.
   B. The University of North Carolina (UNC) can be credited with some of the greatest contributions in promoting education for the dental assistant.
      1. In 1954 Dr. John Brauer, dean of the Uni-

versity of North Carolina, headed a program that designed a correspondence course for dental assistants.

2. In the same year UNC became one of five institutions that inaugurated an educational program for training dental assistants in the School of Dentistry.

C. In 1967 a model curriculum leading to a bachelor of science degree in **Dental Auxiliary Teacher Education (DATE)** was developed by the University of North Carolina School of Dentistry.

D. By 1979 a master of science degree was implemented in the DATE program, adding another step on the ladder of education for the dental assistant.

E. The ADA's **Commission on Dental Accreditation (CDA)** is responsible for accrediting dental schools and educational programs in dental assisting, dental hygiene, and dental laboratory technology.

F. The Dental Assisting National Board (DANB) assumes the responsibility for dental assistant certification and is independent of the ADAA.

1. Successful completion of the DANB examination enables an assistant to use the credential of Certified Dental Assistant (CDA).

2. The box shows the three pathways that lead to this national credential.

3. Credentialling examinations provided by DANB include the general chairside, radiographic hygiene, and infection control tests, as well as specialty examinations in dental office management, oral maxillofacial surgery, and orthodontics.

4. Examinations may be taken at accredited dental assistant program sites or at Sylvan Testing Centers throughout the country.

G. State credentialing varies from state to state.

1. Minnesota was the first state to license dental assistants.

2. Each state establishes educational prerequisites for eligibility for a state examination.

H. Dental Auxiliary Utilization movement

1. In 1956 the federal government provided funds for a few dental schools to expand the use of chairside assistants.

2. By 1960 the project was so successful and the desire to increase the productivity of dentists was so evident that the federal government provided Dental Auxiliary Utilization (DAU) grants to all dental schools in the United States.

3. Dental assistant educational programs began to develop at a greater rate within dental schools, as well as within postsecondary and technical institutions.

4. These programs, like those for dental hygienists and dental laboratory technicians, are eligible for accreditation by the ADA's CDA.

5. In the early 1970s DAU was phased out and the inception of Training in Expanded Auxiliary Management (TEAM) grants were made available on a limited basis, but these too were later phased out.

I. Varied employment opportunities exist for dental assistants in dental practice, and now the field offers employment in many settings, including:

1. Private dental offices
2. Dental schools
3. Public/state or federal clinics
4. Corporate/department store clinics
5. Hospitals
6. Armed forces
7. Teaching
8. Publishing/public relations
9. Insurance companies
10. Dental manufacturers and suppliers

PATHWAYS TO DENTAL ASSISTANT CERTIFICATION THROUGH THE DANB
PATHWAY I
Graduate of an accredited dental assistant or dental hygiene program Current CPR card
PATHWAY II
High school graduation or equivalent Current CPR card Two years, or 3500 hours, of full-time employment Recommendation of dentist employer
PATHWAY III
Previous certification with a lapsed status of 18 months Current CPR card

ETHICAL AND LEGAL ASPECTS OF DENTISTRY ■

I. Law consists of enforceable rules governing relationships among individuals and between individuals and their society.

A. Law can be divided into two classifications.
1. **Civil law** relates to duties between persons or between citizens and their government.
2. Criminal law deals with wrongs committed against the public as a whole.
3. A crime is a wrongdoing against society as a whole and is prosecuted by a public official.
   a. Criminal liability requires performing or committing a prohibited act with a specific state of mind showing intent on the part of the actor.
   b. In some cases the omission of performing an act can be a crime if the person has a legal duty to perform the act (e.g., failure to maintain patient records).
4. A tort is a civil wrongdoing that is a breach of a legal duty owed by one person to another.
   a. Torts generally are resolved through a civil trial with a monetary settlement for damages.
   b. Torts include areas of assault and battery, infliction of mental distress, defamation, and fraud.
   c. Torts may involve an intentional or unintentional act of wrongdoing.
   d. Intentional tort means the person intended to commit the act.
   e. Unintentional torts involve a particular mental state that results in a failure to exercise a standard of care, treatment that the reasonable person would exercise in similar circumstances when someone suffers injury; the professional failed to live up to a particular standard of care.
   f. There are four elements that determine the unintentional tort of negligence.
      (1) Was there a duty to follow a standard of care?
      (2) Was this duty breached?
      (3) Did the plaintiff suffer injury?
      (4) Was that injury a direct result of that breach of duty?
   g. Common negligent acts in a dental office are listed in the box.
   h. Malpractice is considered negligence by professionals, but it can mean any wrongdoing by a professional.
      (1) Malpractice can refer to any professional misconduct, evil practice, or illegal or immoral conduct and is not just limited to acts of negligence.

COMMON NEGLIGENT ACTS IN A DENTAL OFFICE

Abandonment
Burns
Mistaken identity
Foreign objects left in patients after surgical procedures
Defects in equipment
Failure to observe patient reactions and to respond appropriately
Medication errors
Drug administration errors
Failure to exercise good judgment
Failure to communicate
Loss of or damage to patient's personal property
Disease transmission

---

      (2) Malpractice can be either unintentional or intentional.
5. Statutes are laws enacted by a legislative body that conform to state and federal constitutions.
   a. A dental practice act is a statutory law.
B. Litigation involves the entire legal process encompassing a lawsuit, whereas the lawsuit itself is the legal action in a court.
1. The person or party who initiates the lawsuit is the plaintiff, the injured party.
2. The person being accused of the wrongdoing is the **defendant.**
3. A **fact witness,** when placed under oath, can and must provide only firsthand knowledge testimony, not hearsay (rumor or speculation).
4. An **expert witness** is called to testify and explain to the judge and jury what happened based on the patient's record and to offer an opinion as to whether or not the dental care, as administered, met acceptable standards.
C. The state board of dentistry in each state is responsible for regulating the practice of dentistry in the individual state.
1. Members of this board are commonly appointed by the governor of the state and generally include dentists, dental hygienists, and assistants in those states in which assistants are licensed or credentialed by the board.
2. Consumer members who have no relationship to dentistry may also be included.
3. Board membership represents a cross-section of the profession to obtain geographic, spe-

cialty, academic, and private sector representation.

D. Professional standards ensure the competence of its practitioners.
   1. Credentialing refers to the ways in which a professional can ensure and maintain competence.
   2. Accreditation is the process by which an educational program is evaluated and recognized by an outside agency such as the Commission on Dental Accreditation (CDA) of the American Dental Association (ADA) for having attained a predetermined set of standards.
   3. National certification in dental assisting is a voluntary procedure and may be achieved through the **Dental Assisting National Board (DANB).**
   4. Licensure is the credential granted to a candidate by the state after the candidate has met the necessary requirements to practice in the profession.
   5. Ethics in daily professional practice challenge a practitioner to differentiate between right and wrong.
   6. Voluntary standards are shaped by personal morals and reflect the challenges and needs of society.

E. Dental assistant liability
   1. Assignments for intraoral duties that involve direct patient care increase the dental assistant's need for liability insurance.
   2. The doctrine of respondeat superior holds an employer liable for the negligent acts of an employee when carrying out the employer's orders or when serving the employer's interest.
      a. This doctrine applies to an employee/employer relationship and is applicable only when a negligent act is committed within the scope of employment.
      b. This doctrine does not relieve the negligent employee of liability but opens the door for the injured person, commonly the patient, to sue another party.
   3. A dental assistant's best legal safeguard is competent practice, but with the increasing numbers of malpractice claims, it is wise for the practicing dental assistant to carry some form of liability insurance.

F. Risk management programs
   1. Educational programs for the dental professional illustrate cases in which dental professionals have been found liable in the past and try to teach them ways to avoid exposing themselves to such liability.
   2. They aid dental professionals in identifying, analyzing, and dealing with risks in their dental offices.
   3. They generally include information on operating safety, product safety, quality assurance, and waste disposal.

G. Assignment of duties
   1. According to the dental practice act, it is the responsibility of the licensed dentist.
   2. If a duty that is not legal within the state is assigned to the dental assistant, the dentist is liable for this illegal action.
   3. If a dental assistant performs a procedure that cannot be legally delegated to be performed by the assistant, the assistant is liable for such action.

H. **Consent** is the voluntary acceptance or agreement of what is planned or done by another person.
   1. To examine or treat a patient without consent constitutes unauthorized touching and makes the person committing the act guilty of battery as discussed below.
   2. Two forms of consent exist in the delivery of dental care: informed and implied.
   3. Informed consent requires the presence of specific elements.
      a. Consent *must be* given freely.
      b. Treatment and diagnosis *must be* communicated in understandable language.
      c. Risks and benefits of the proposed treatment, estimate of success of treatment, prognosis if no treatment is elected, and alternative treatment plans *must be* given.
      d. Rights of the patient to ask questions and have them answered *must be* part of informed consent.
      e. If these elements of informed consent are not met, the courts may conclude that the patient did *not* consent to the operation and therefore the doctor may be guilty of battery or negligence (depending on the individual state).
      f. Patients under the influence of alcohol, drugs, or severe stress may not have sufficient capacity to give consent for treatment.
      g. When treating a minor, only the parent or guardian may grant consent.
   4. **Implied consent** refers to the duties or ac-

IMPLIED DUTIES OWED BY THE DENTIST TO THE PATIENT

1. Use reasonable care in the provision of services as measured against acceptable standards set by other practitioners with similar training in a similar community.
2. Be properly licensed, registered, and meet all other legal requirements to engage in the practice of dentistry.
3. Obtain an accurate health (medical and dental) history of the patient before a diagnosis is made and treatment is begun.
4. Employ competent personnel and provide for their proper supervision.
5. Maintain a level of knowledge in keeping with current advances in the profession.
6. Use methods that are acceptable to at least a respectable minority of similar practitioners in the community.
7. Do not use experimental procedures.
8. Obtain informed consent from the patient before instituting an examination or treatment.
9. Do not abandon the patient.
10. Ensure that care is available in emergency situations.
11. Charge a reasonable fee for services based on community standards.
12. Do not exceed the scope of practice authorized by the license nor permit any person acting under his or her direction to engage in unlawful acts.
13. Keep the patient informed of his or her progress.
14. Do not undertake any procedure for which the practitioner is not qualified.
15. Complete the care in a timely manner.
16. Keep accurate records of the treatment rendered to the patient.
17. Maintain confidentiality of information.
18. Inform the patient of any untoward occurrences in the course of treatment.
19. Make appropriate referrals and request necessary consultations.
20. Comply with all laws regulating the practice of dentistry.
21. Practice in a manner consistent with the codes of ethics of the profession.
22. Use universal precautions in the treatment of all patients.

IMPLIED DUTIES OWED BY THE PATIENT TO THE DENTIST

1. Cooperate in the care by following home care instructions, prescriptions, recalls, and any other reasonable instructions related to care.
2. Keep appointments and notify the office should an appointment not be kept or if the appointment will be delayed.
3. Provide honest answers to questions asked on the history form and by the doctor and the office personnel.
4. Notify the office staff or doctor of a change in health status.
5. Pay a reasonable fee for the service if no fee is agreed on either in writing or verbally.
6. Remit the fee for services within a reasonable period of time.

tions that flow automatically from the relationship between the patient and the dental professional.

   a. There are implied duties that the dentist owes to the patient and duties that the patient owes to the dentist.

   b. When a dentist accepts a patient for treatment, this implies that he or she agrees to accept certain responsibilities for that patient's dental care.

   c. If a patient agrees to accept treatment by the dentist, that patient is assuming certain implied responsibilities to the dentist. The boxes list the implied responsibilities for each of these parties.

I. Acts that can result in potential liabilities

  1. Assault and battery is any unexcused, harmful, or offensive physical contact intentionally performed.

   a. **Assault** is the threat of touching another person without his or her consent.

   b. **Battery** is the actual carrying out of such a threat, such as the unlawful touching of a person's body.

  2. **Abandonment** is the severance of a professional relationship with a patient who is still in need of dental care and attention without adequate notice to the patient.

  3. False imprisonment involves the interference with that individual's freedom to move without restraint.

  4. **Fraud** is a form of deception that is deliberately practiced to secure unfair or unlawful gain.

5. Defamation of character is the communication of false information to a third party about a person that results in injury to a person's reputation.
6. Negligence is an act of omission or commission (neglecting to do something that a reasonably prudent person would do or doing something that a reasonably prudent person would not do).
   a. To prove negligence requires proof that a deviation from the standard of care has occurred, and it is often necessary to provide expert testimony.
   b. The plaintiff must show the following:
      (1) There was an obligation to provide care according to a specified standard.
      (2) There was failure to meet that standard.
      (3) This failure to meet the standard led to injury.
      (4) There was in fact an actual injury to the patient.
7. Invasion of privacy refers to the publishing, otherwise making known, or using information related to the private life and affairs of a person without that person's approval or permission.

J. Records management
   1. Thorough, accurate, and objective documentation are the most valuable documents in potential litigation situations.
   2. Record the exact treatment date, the type of treatment performed, any materials used, whether or not complications arose, and any special notations about that treatment.
   3. Note any unusual or unruly incidences created by the patient's comments or reactions.
   4. Include the initials of the treating operator(s) and recorder.
   5. Update records routinely.
   6. Maintain records relating to incidences that occur between patients, employee, and employer.
   7. Employee reports must be retained in employee records and may include episodes of accidental needle punctures that require a report, including the name of the employee, the patient being treated, and the date and time of the injury.
   8. Other employee reports may include performance, unusual behavior on the part of a patient, or a verbal confrontation between staff members.

K. Good Samaritan law
   1. Every state has passed some form of legislation that grants immunity for acts performed by a person who renders care in an emergency situation.
   2. The Good Samaritan law was considered necessary to create an incentive for health care providers to provide medical assistance to the injured in cases of automobile accidents or other disasters without the fear of potential litigation.
      a. There is no intent for the provider to seek compensation for the act.
      b. The provider is solely interested in providing care to the injured in a caring, safe manner, with no intent to do bodily harm.
      c. The law does not provide protection for a negligent health care provider who is being compensated for services.
L. Factors to consider in making ethical decisions are outlined in the box.

TWELVE STEPS TO MAKING ETHICAL DECISIONS

1. Is the task I am performing legally delegable to me?
2. Do I have the necessary credential to perform this task?
3. Am I competent to perform this task, both physically and emotionally?
4. Am I performing this procedure in a safe working environment that meets the standards of OSHA?
5. Has the patient been informed about his or her treatment?
6. Am I respecting the patient's right to privacy and confidentiality?
7. Do I maintain complete and accurate records, and have I documented any special problems arising with patients, employees, and the employer?
8. Do I maintain professional liability insurance?
9. Do I participate in risk management programs?
10. Am I willing to compromise my standards for the lack of ethics or legal responsibility on the part of an employer or fellow employees?
11. Do I maintain current knowledge of changes in dental practice acts, occupational safety, and reporting methods?
12. Do I actively participate in my professional organization and contribute to community dental health?

Questions

The Profession: Evolution and Ethics

1 What is the prime function of a state dental practice act?
   a. Describing illegal practice of dentistry
   b. Encouraging licensing of dentists and hygienists
   c. Differentiating dentistry from other health professions
   d. Defining and regulating the practice of dentistry

2 Which of the following is not a recognized dental speciality?
   a. Forensics
   b. Prosthodontics
   c. Periodontics
   d. Endodontics

3 The definition of the acronym ADA is
   a. American Dentist Association
   b. American Dental Association
   c. American Dietetic Association

4 The definition of the acronym CDA is
   a. Commissioned Dental Assistant
   b. Certificate of Dental Assisting
   c. Certified Dental Assistant

5 The definition of the acronym COA is
   a. Certified Office Assistant
   b. Certified Orthodontic Assistant
   c. Credential of Office Assistant

6 The national professional organization for a dental assistant is the
   a. ADA
   b. ADAA
   c. ADHA
   d. NADA

7 The group responsible for establishing regulations that govern the practice of dentistry within a state is the
   a. American Dental Association
   b. Dental Assistant National Board
   c. Commission on Dental Accreditation
   d. Board of dentistry

8 The definition of the acronym DANB is
   a. Division of the American National Board
   b. Dental Assisting National Board
   c. Dental Assistant National Board

9 The definition of the acronym RDA is
   a. Recognized Dental Assistant
   b. Registered Dental Assistant
   c. Licensed Dental Assistant

In each of the following situations match the name of the specialist to whom a general dentist might refer a patient for treatment.
   a. Periodontist
   b. Public health dentist
   c. Pediatric dentist
   d. Endodontist
   e. Orthodontist

_____ **10** A person is interested in starting a clinic for children with special needs in a local school district

_____ **11** The patient has severe malocclusion

_____ **12** The patient has an identified disease within the pulp of a tooth

_____ **13** The supporting tissues around a patient's tooth are severely inflamed, and the bone support is in jeopardy

_____ **14** A child displays severe emotional problems and needs extensive dental treatment

15 The most important person/people in the dental office is/are
   a. The dentist
   b. The team
   c. The patient

16 What is the suffix used to identify the science or study of a specialized area in dentistry?
   a. ics
   b. ist
   c. ant

17 What is the suffix used to identify the person who practices a specialized area of dentistry?
   a. ics
   b. ist
   c. ant

From the list below choose the one best term that defines each of the following statements.
   a. CDT
   b. CDA
   c. DDS
   d. RDH
   e. RDAEF

_____ **18** A person with a credential granted from the DANB

_____ **19** Licensed person whose primary role is preventive treatment

_____ **20** Performs extraoral functions, primarily the construction of prosthetic devices

_____ **21** Meets the requirements in some states to perform intraoral duties

From the list below choose the one best term that defines each of the following statements.
   a. OJT
   b. RDH
   c. DDS
   d. RDA
   e. EFDA

_____ **22** Licensed to diagnose and cut hard and soft tissues

_____ **23** An auxiliary licensed in each state in the United States

_____ **24** An acronym that defines a status of intraoral techniques but not licensure

_____ **25** An acronym that indicates that a person has no formal education or dental credential

Rationales

The Profession: Evolution and Ethics

1 D The dental practice act of each state is intended to define the responsibility of a dentist and dental auxiliaries. The dental practice act protects the health of the public by providing the elements required to practice standardized safe dental care.

2 A Currently there are eight recognized dental specialties, forensics is not one of them. The specialties include dental public health, endodontics, oral pathology, oral maxillofacial surgery, orthodontics, pediatric dentistry, periodontics, and prosthodontics.

3 B The American Dental Association (ADA) is the national professional organization for dentists.

4 C The acronym, *Certified Dental Assistant (CDA)*, is a national credential granted by the Dental Assistant National Board (DANB) to recognize successful completion of the national certification examination.

5 B Certified Orthodontic Assistant (COA), is a national credential granted by the DANB to recognize successful completion of the specialty examination in orthodontics.

6 B The American Dental Assistants Association (ADAA) is the national professional organization for dental assistants.

7 D The state board of dentistry is the body in each state that supervises the practice of dentistry. The composition of the board will vary from state to state.

8 B The Dental Assisting National Board (DANB) assumes responsibility for dental assistant certification and is independent of the ADAA.

9 B Registered Dental Assistant (RDA) is a credential given by some states to indicate that specific requirements have been met to practice expanded or advanced functions in that state.

10 B Public health dentistry is concerned with public education, applied dental research, and the administration of group dental care programs, as well as the prevention and control of dental diseases on a community-wide basis.

11 E The specialty of orthodontics is concerned with the supervision, guidance, and correction of the growing or mature dentofacial structures, including those conditions that require moving the teeth to correct a malocclusion or to correct a malformation of the jaw.

12 D The specialty of endodontics is concerned with the morphology, physiology, and pathology of the dental pulp and associated tissues.

13 A The diagnosis and treatment of diseases of the supporting and surrounding tissues of the teeth are the focus of the specialty of periodontics.

14 C Pediatric dentistry is defined as the practice and teaching of comprehensive preventive and therapeutic oral health care of children from birth through adolescence, including care for special patients beyond the age of adolescence who demonstrate mental, physical, and/or emotional problems.

15 C The patient is the most important person in the dental office. Without the patient there is simply no need for the dental team.

16 A The suffix *ics* describes the specialty of dentistry.

17 B The suffix *ist* is used to describe the person who practices the specialty.

18 B See #4.

19 D A primary duty of a dental hygienist is to perform an oral prophylaxis and legally delegable periodontal treatment in the prevention of oral disease.

20 A A dental laboratory technician is responsible to construct extraoral devices such as dental protheses.

21 E See #9.

22 C Only a dentist is licensed to cut hard or soft tissue in a state dental practice act.

23 B A dental hygienist is licensed in all states in the United States.

24 E EFDA is a status and is not treated as a license in most states. It refers to an Expanded Functions Dental Assistant.

25 A The acronym OJT is used to indicate that a person has been trained on the job. It does not indicate formal education or dental credential.

To enhance your understanding of the material in this chapter, refer to the illustrations in Chapter 12 of Finkbeiner/Johnson: *Mosby's Comprehensive Dental Assisting: A Clinical Approach.*

Basic Anatomy and Physiology

OUTLINE

Prefixes and Suffixes
Anatomy
Descriptive Anatomic Terms

Physiology
Cells
Tissues

Organs and Body Systems
Oral Facial Structures and the Oral
  Cavity

KEY TERMS

Alveolar process
Anatomic position
Anatomy
Anomalies
Anterior
Artery
Atria
Blood
Body plane
Bone
Canal
Cells
Condyle
Cranial bones
Deglutition
Distal
Dorsal
Extrinsic
Facial bones
Foramen
Fossa
Frenum
Frontal

Gingiva
Inferior
Insertion
Intrinsic
Lateral
Longitudinal
Mandible
Maxilla
Meatus
Medial
Meniscus
Mesial
Muscles of facial expression
Muscles of mastication
Neuron
Orbit
Organ
Origin
Osteoblast
Osteoclast
Papilla
Periosteum
Physiology

Posterior
Process
Protuberance
Proximal
Ramus
Sagittal
Salivary glands
Septum
Sinus
Superior
Suture
Symphysis
Synovial
System
Temporomandibular joint
Tissue
Transverse
Tubercle
Vein
Ventral
Ventricle
Vestibule

To develop a thorough understanding of oral and dental anatomy, it is first necessary to develop an understanding of basic human anatomy. This chapter provides an overview of basic anatomic terms and the systems of the body as they relate to dentistry. In addition, a thorough review of head and neck anatomy will be presented as it relates to the role of the dental assistant.

To communicate effectively in the dental profession the dental assistant must have a general understanding of terminology that relates to the anatomy and physiology of the human body and specifically of the head and neck regions. An understanding of anatomic terminology enables a dental assistant to communicate with other professionals and to identify specific locations of anatomic structures in a universal professional language. This section will present various body systems, the body planes, anatomic structures, and key terminology.

PREFIXES AND SUFFIXES

I. A prefix is a single letter or group of letters placed at the beginning of a word, and a suffix is a single letter or group of letters placed at the end of a word.
A. It is common in dentistry to add both a prefix and a suffix to a root word.
B. A suffix can modify a prefix or the root word.
C. Review the list of common prefixes, suffixes, and root words in the box on page 25.

ANATOMY

I. **Anatomy** is the science of the shape and structure of the body.
A. Gross anatomy is the study of structures that can be identified with the naked eye; it commonly involves the use of cadavers (corpses).
B. Microscopic anatomy (histology) is the study of cells that compose tissues and organs; it involves the use of a microscope to study the specimen details.
C. Comparative anatomy is the comparative study of animal structure in regard to similar organs or regions.
D. Developmental anatomy (embryology) is the study of an individual as a single cell through birth.

DESCRIPTIVE ANATOMIC TERMS

I. Anatomic position
A. **Anatomic position** refers to the body when it is in a vertical position, with the face and the palms of the hands facing forward.
B. When the body is in the anatomic position, specific descriptive terms can be used to locate ar-

---

COMMON ANATOMIC TERMS USED IN DESCRIBING BODY LOCATIONS

Anterior—situated in front, toward the front of the body

Distal—away from the midline of the body, structure, or organ, or the median sagittal plane

Dorsal—toward the back surface or posterior of an organ

Inferior—below or lower part, farthest from the head on the body

Lateral—toward the outside of the body or to the left or right of the midsagittal plane

Medial—toward the midline or middle line of the body

Mesial—toward the midline or middle line of the body

Posterior—toward the back of the body, structure, or organ

Proximal—part closest to the source, part of limb closest to the trunk

Superior—area or part closest or nearest to the head

Ventral—front or abdominal area of the body

---

eas on the body. The box above contains a list of common terms.

II. Body plane or section
A. A **body plane** or section is formed by an imaginary line that extends through an axis, dividing the body into segments.
B. The planes are referenced relative to the body in the anatomic position. The box on page 26 defines these planes.

III. Body cavities
A. **Dorsal** cavity (contains the brain and spinal cord)
1. Cranial cavity (formed by bones of the skull)
2. Vertebral cavity (formed by the vertebrae)
B. **Ventral** cavity
1. Thoracic cavity
a. The pericardial cavity contains the heart.
b. The pleural cavity contains the lungs.
c. The trachea, bronchi, esophagus, and thymus lie between these subdivisions.
2. Abdominopelvic cavity
a. The upper cavity contains the liver, small and large intestines, stomach, spleen, pancreas, and gallbladder.
b. The lower cavity contains the bladder, rectum, sigmoid colon, and reproductive organs.

COMMON PREFIXES AND SUFFIXES

PREFIXES

a, ab—away from
a, an—without
adeno—gland
album—white
ante—before, preceding
ant, anti—against
bi, bin, bis—two, twice
bio—relating to living organism
blast—formative cell
cardio—heart
cephal—head
cheil—lip
chemo—relating to chemistry
contra—against
crani—skull
cyano—blue
cyst—sac, bladder, bag
cyt—cell
de—away
deci, deca—ten
dento, denti—tooth, dental
dermato, dermo—skin
di—two
dis—free of, separation, reversal
dys—difficult, painful, faulty
e, ex—out, away from, without
ecto, exo, extra—without, on the
    outside
encephal—brain
erythro—red
galact—milk
gastro—stomach
glosso—tongue
hemato, hemo, hema—blood
hepato, hepatico—liver

histo—tissue, weblike
homo—alike, same
hydro—water
hypo—below
infra—under
inter—between
intro—into
kerato—horn, corn
kin—movement
labia—lip
latero—to the side of
lith—stone
macro—great
mast—breast
media, medial—middle
meta—change
micro—small
milli—thousand
mono—one
morpho—form
myo—muscle
narco—numbness
naso—nose
necro—dead
neo—new
neuro—nerve
nona—ten
octo—eight
odonto—tooth, teeth
ortho—straight, correct
osteo—bone
oti—ear
para—beside, alongside of
path—disease
penta—five
pedo—child

per—between, through, across
peri—around
pharm—drugs
phlebo—vein
pneum—air
poly—many
post—behind, after
pre—before
pro—in front
pros—toward
pseudo—false
psycho—soul, mind
pyo—pus
re, retro—behind, backward, again
rhino—nose
rube—red
semi—half
septa—seven
septic—poison
sial—saliva
sphygmo—pulse
sub—less, deficient
super, supra—above, over, excess
tachy—fast, swift
ter, tri—three
tetra—four
thermo—heat
thrombo—clot
toxi, toxo—poison
tracheo—windpipe, air passageway
trans—across, through
uni—mono, one
utlra—beyond, excess
vaso—vessel
xero—dry

SUFFIXES

-al—act, process
-algia, -algesia—pain
-agra—seizure, acute pain
-ago, -igo—disease
-cide—destroyer, killer
-eal, -eous—of the nature of
-ectomy—to excise, to remove
-emesis—vomiting
-emia—condition of the blood
-gnosis—knowledge
-ia, -iasis, -id, -ism—abnormal,
    diseased
-iasis—a condition

-ics—science or art of
-ist—person who does
-itis—inflammation
-ize—action, treatment
-less—without
-lith—stone
-logy—study of
-oid, -oides—like, resembling
-oma—tumor
-osis—condition, state
-oscopy—inspection of
-ostomy—an opening
-otomy—incision, cut

-pathy—disease
-phagy, -phage—swallowing
-phonia—voice, sound
-phylaxis—protection
-plasty—repair, reconstruction by
    surgery
-pnea—breathing
-rrhage—excessive flow
-rrhaphy—suture
-stasis—stopping the flow
-staxis—dripping, oozing
-therapy—treatment, healing
-uria—condition of the urine

BODY PLANES

The **transverse** or *horizontal* plane divides the body into two portions, superior and inferior, by cutting across the long axis of the body, thereby creating a *cross-section*. The superior portion of the body is above the horizontal plane and the inferior beneath it.

The **sagittal** plane is a vertical plane from the top of the body down that creates right and left segments.

The **midsagittal** plane is a sagittal plane that divides the body into equal segments, running from the front to the back through the sagittal suture of the skull down through the body.

The **longitudinal** plane runs the length of the long axis of the body with the body in the anatomic position.

The **frontal** or *coronal* plane is a vertical plane at a right angle to the sagittal plane that divides the body into anterior and posterior segments.

PHYSIOLOGY

I. **Physiology** is the study of mechanisms by which the body performs various functions; it attempts to explain vital processes by using principles outlined in biologic, chemical, or physical sciences.
    A. Comparative physiology is the study of comparing and contrasting the vital processes in different organisms.
    B. Developmental physiology is the study of the vital processes related to embryonic development.
    C. General physiology studies the functions of the vital processes.
    D. Human physiology studies the functions within the human body.
    E. Pathologic physiology studies the diseases that relate to an imbalance in function.

CELLS

I. **Cells** are the smallest structures and functionally self-contained units in the body. They vary in size, shape, and surface, depending on their individual function.
    A. Cells exhibit similar common physiologic properties that permit:
        1. Growth and reproduction
        2. Reaction to external stimuli
        3. Assimilation and synthesis of materials
    B. Cells are the basic units of tissue formation.

C. Each human cell is surrounded by a membrane consisting of organelles, which are specialized structures with specific functions. The cell membrane allows passage of molecules and provides direction for the organelles' functions.
D. Components of cells include:
    1. Cytoplasm (ground substances of colloidal solution)
    2. Nucleus (the control center for cell activity)
    3. Inclusions
    4. Organelles

Cell Membrane

I. The cell membrane, also known as the plasma membrane, provides a barrier between the inside and the outside of the cell.
    A. The membrane allows passage of certain molecules to and from the cytoplasm; thus, the membrane is considered selectively permeable.
    B. Passage through the membrane of lipid-soluble molecules, including gases and water, occurs by diffusion, which is the movement from an area of greater concentration to one of lesser concentration to attain equilibrium.
    C. Osmosis is another form of molecular movement. When a greater concentration of water exists on one side of a permeable membrane, water crosses to the side of lesser water concentration until equilibrium is reached.
    D. To achieve homeostasis, or an internal stability within a living structure, an organism of any form must undergo change. The change of conditions may be from within or from an external environment to maintain balance and ensure survival of the organism.

TISSUES

I. Individual cells multiply and differentiate to perform specialized functions; groups of cells with similar morphologic characteristics and functions come together and form tissues.
    A. A **tissue** is a combination of cells, crystals, fibers, and fluids that have similar shape and function.
    B. Tissues in the human body can be classified into four types:
        1. Epithelial tissue
        2. Connective tissue
        3. Nerve tissue
        4. Muscle tissue
    C. Each of the four basic tissues may be further subdivided into several variations.

Epithelial Tissue

I. Epithelial tissue consists of cells held together by specialized cell junctions with very little intercellular material between the cells; cells rest on an underlying connective tissue.
   A. Epithelial cells form continuous sheets (tissues) and serve the following functions:
      1. Protection—cover all outer surfaces of the body (e.g., skin)
      2. Absorption—line all inner surfaces of the body (e.g., digestive tract)
      3. Secretion—form glands (glandular tissue)
   B. Epithelium can be classified according to shape or number of cell layers.
      1. Squamous (flat)
      2. Cuboidal
      3. Columnar
      4. Simple (one cell layer)
      5. Stratified (several cell layers)
      6. Combination of each of the above (e.g., simple squamous or stratified squamous)
   C. Epithelium lining the oral cavity (oral mucosa) and the skin (dermis) are examples of stratified squamous epithelium.

Connective Tissue

I. All connective tissue proper develops from embryonic menenchume.
   A. Two primary functions of connective tissue:
      1. Provides mechanical and biologic support
      2. Provides pathways for metabolic substances
   B. Types of connective tissue:
      1. Loose connective tissue
      2. Bone
      3. Cartilage
      4. Bone marrow
      5. Lymphoid tissue (tonsils and lymph nodes)
      6. Fat
      7. Dental tissues
         a. Pulp
         b. Dentin
         c. Cementum

ORGANS AND BODY SYSTEMS

I. An **organ** is made of a group of tissues that work together to carry out a specific function; the tooth is an organ made of connective, blood, and nerve tissues. A body **system** is a similar group of tissues or organs that perform like functions. Eleven systems of the human body are listed in Table 3-1. Many of the systems are directly related to dentistry, while others are more abstract in their relationship.
   A. Skeletal system
      1. The skeleton provides the underlying structure or frame for the body.
      2. The skeleton shapes and supports the body and provides protection for internal organs.
      3. The skeleton is the framework to which muscles are attached, and it also stores certain chemicals for use by the body.
      4. With regard to the relationship of the skeletal system to dentistry, the skeleton provides the **maxilla** (upper jaw) and the **mandible** (lower jaw), which support the teeth. The cranium and facial structure are formed by the skeletal system.
   B. Muscular system
      1. The muscular system provides the tissue that allows movement of all the parts of the body.
      2. The human body contains three kinds of muscle fibers: smooth, striated, and heart, or cardiac.
      3. With regard to the relationship of the muscular system to dentistry, muscles aid in talking, chewing, swallowing, eating, and smiling. They provide a person the ability to change facial expressions.
      4. Muscles that are not exercised regularly can become weak, soft, and flabby. This is evidenced in dentistry when individuals lose their teeth and become edentulous. The muscles of the face begin to sag from loss of support and normal use, often causing these people to look older than their chronologic age.
   C. Nervous system
      1. The nervous system is a combination of the brain, spinal cord, and nerve cells, or neurons, that run through the body.
      2. A **neuron** is the structural and functional unit of nervous tissue.
      3. Nerves carry messages back and forth between the brain and the rest of the body.
      4. The muscles of the body are controlled by the nervous system.
      5. With regard to the relationship of the nervous system to dentistry, nerves innervate and control the senses emanating from the area of the head and neck. Each tooth is supplied with one or more nerves, depending on its anatomic structure. When a patient complains of certain types of pain, the dentist will seek to determine if there has been trauma, disease, or degeneration of the nerve.
   D. Circulatory system
      1. The major parts of the human circulatory,

Table 3-1 Organ systems

Organ system	Function/responsibility	Relationship to dentistry
Muscular	Responsible for body movement and heat.	Assists in deglutination, phonetics.
Nervous	Regulates all body activity, learning, and memory.	Major nerve affecting the area of head and neck; includes the trigeminal nerve.
Respiratory	Exchanges gaseous substances between the environment and the blood.	The head is the first source of breathing for both internal and external respiration; mouth breathing as a source of respiration causes complications in the oral cavity.
Circulatory	Transports life-necessary substance to cells and removes metabolic waste from cells.	Use of a vasoconstrictor to obtain anesthesia in the oral cavity may have an effect when the patient has contraindications to this therapy. Hematologic studies would verify systemic disease.
Skeletal	Provides framework and supports structures and flexibility for movement of the body; produces blood cells.	The skull as part of the skeletal system includes the only movable part, which is the mandible working on a hinge. Anomalies in skeletal development relate to malocclusion and facial development.
Lymphatic	Provides body immunity, drains body fluids, and absorbs fats.	It is important to protect the lymphatic system, particularly the area of head and neck, from radiation exposure. This system produces fluids at the site of infection.
Urinary	Filters blood and maintains the volume as well as chemical composition of blood.	Secretions from this system are used to test for systemic diseases.
Endocrine	Secretes hormones for regulation with chemicals in the body.	Radiation to the thyroid during diagnostic radiography can cause abnormal behavior in the gland.
Digestive	Continues the function of breaking down and absorbing food.	Digestion begins in the oral cavity through mastication. A patient with dental pain may not be able to masticate easily.
Male reproductive	Produces sperm and transfers the sperm to the female reproductive system.	Radiation used in the diagnosis of oral anomalies can cause damage to male reproductive ability.
Female reproductive	Produces ova and receives sperm from the male; area where fertilization of ovum, implantation, and development of embryo to fetus and delivery of the fetus take place.	Radiation used in the diagnosis of oral anomalies can cause damage to female reproductive ability. Diet during pregnancy may affect the development of the fetus.

or cardiovascular, system are the blood, blood vessels, heart, and lymph system.

2. This system is responsible for moving food, water, and oxygen through the body to sustain life and growth.

3. The heart is a pump that forces blood out to the tissues of the body through blood vessels.

4. Blood vessels include arteries, veins, and capillaries.

5. An **artery** carries blood away from the heart; a **vein** carries blood to the heart; and capillaries are small vessels that connect arteries to veins.

6. Arteries have thick, elastic walls; veins have thin walls with valves to prevent the backflow of blood; and capillaries have walls that are only one cell thick.

7. **Blood** is the fluid that transports all of the body substances; it is a special type of connective tissue that consists of a solid part, called blood cells, and a nonliving substance called plasma.

8. Three types of blood cells exist.
   a. Red cells, or erythrocytes, are shaped like discs and do not have a nucleus. They contain a red pigment called hemoglobin, a protein substance that is essential to life.
   b. White cells, or leukocytes, are larger than red cells, have a nucleus, contain no hemoglobin, are colorless, and are

capable of ameboid movement. The body contains fewer white cells than red cells, with approximately one white cell for every 600 red cells. White blood cells are an important defense against infection.

   c. Platelets, or thrombocytes, are much smaller than red blood cells, are shaped irregularly, and are colorless. They are formed in the red marrow and are incapable of moving on their own and simply float along in the bloodstream. Platelets are important in forming blood clots.

  9. Plasma is composed of water, proteins, digested food, mineral salts, organic nutrients, and cell wastes.

  10. Circulation is vital to dentistry. The fluctuation of blood pressure, which is the measure of the pressure of blood in arteries, from normal can be a contraindication or negative factor in the treatment of a patient.

   a. Other factors such as poor circulation, coronary disease, clotting anomalies, or other blood diseases can be reasons to carefully examine the patient before beginning treatment.

   b. A patient's blood count can be important when a surgical procedure is undertaken; a person who is taking blood-thinning medication may have inadequate amount of platelets to promote clotting.

   c. Blood is supplied to each tooth and provides nourishment. When trauma occurs to a tooth, the blood supply may be reduced or lost, possibly causing the loss of tooth vitality.

E. Respiratory system

  1. The respiratory system includes the nose, pharynx, larynx, trachea, bronchi, sinuses, and lungs. Body cells need a continuous supply of oxygen that is carried to the cells by the circulatory system from the air a person breathes.

  2. Functions of the respiratory system include:
   a. Breathing
   b. Supplying the blood with oxygen
   c. Removing carbon dioxide from the blood

  3. The respiratory system is closely linked to dentistry. Blockage of the nose and sinuses can force a person to become a mouth breather, possibly damaging the oral tissues over a long period of time. Sinus pain can also be confused with dental pain because of the location of the sinuses. The use of nitrous oxide analgesia must be followed up with an appropriate inhalation of oxygen to prevent damage to the lungs.

F. Digestive system

  1. The mouth, teeth, salivary glands, pharynx, esophagus, stomach, intestines, liver, gallbladder, and pancreas are organs of the digestive system that work together to process food for use by the body.

  2. Digestion begins in the mouth. The teeth break off and grind the food as the salivary glands secrete enzymes that begin the digestive process.

  3. As foods move through the digestive tract, they undergo a series of chemical changes. During each step, a specific enzyme is secreted.

  4. The digestive system is vital to dentistry. Without teeth and salivary glands to aid in mastication, the digestive process is inhibited.

G. Excretory/urinary system

  1. The kidneys, ureters, urinary bladder, urethra, and skin are the organs of the excretory system, which is also referred to as the urinary system. This system is responsible for eliminating waste products from the body. Waste fluid flows to the bloodstream and is carried to the excretory organs for elimination.

  2. The kidneys are the primary excretory organs. Wastes are brought to the kidneys through the bloodstream, and, after an elaborate filtering process, the waste, or urine, passes to the ureters.

  3. The ureters carry the urine to the urinary bladder, and the urine is then excreted through the urethra.

  4. The skin is also an excretory organ made of the epidermis (outer layer) and the dermis (the layer beneath the epidermis). Excretion through the skin is in the form of perspiration, which helps to regulate body temperature.

  5. The excretory system does not have a primary relationship to dentistry. However, the oral cavity aids in the beginning of the digestive processes that ultimately produce the wastes excreted from the body. A patient with systemic diseases of the organs of this

system may be taking medication that could potentially contraindicate dental treatment.

H. Reproductive system
1. The reproductive system provides new life through the combination of ovaries, fallopian tubes, uterus, vagina, mammary glands, testes, and penis. The primitive germ layers—the ectoderm, mesoderm, and endoderm—actively form structures of skin, cartilage, nervous system, lining of the mouth to the pharynx, connective tissue, bone, muscles, blood and vessels, lymphatics, trachea, and other structures.
2. With regard to the relationship of the reproductive system to dentistry, genetic anomalies (abnormalities) that develop from this system may be identified in the dental arches of the child. Toxins from dental infections of the mother can endanger a fetus.
3. Care should be taken to protect pregnant patients from exposure to dental radiography during the second week through the sixth week of gestation to safeguard the development of the fetus.

I. Endocrine system
1. The endocrine system contains the glands that secrete hormones to promote growth and metabolism. This system integrates and coordinates the activities of various body organs.
2. Glands such as salivary glands have ducts that emit secretions into an organ; these duct glands are referred to as exocrine glands.
3. Endocrine glands are ductless, and secretions from these glands go directly into the bloodstream.
4. Endocrine gland secretions are known as hormones.
5. Glands that are in this system include the thyroid, parathyroid, pituitary, adrenal, pancreas, thymus, ovaries, testes, and hypothalamus.
6. The relationship of this endocrine system to dentistry is both direct and indirect. Directly, this system is responsible for the metabolism of sugars and starches that takes place during the digestive process, which of course begins in the oral cavity; indirectly, this system affects the practice of dentistry when a patient presents for treatment and has a disease in any of the organs of this system such as diabetes mellitus.

J. Sensory system

1. Organs that provide the sense of vision, hearing, touch, smell, and taste are included in the sensory system.
2. Special sense organs called receptors are located in the skin.
3. There are five different kinds of receptors:
   a. Touch
   b. Pressure
   c. Pain
   d. Heat
   e. Cold
4. The sense of taste is in a person's mouth, specifically involving the taste buds on the tongue.
5. The four flavors that can be recognized—sweet, sour, salty, and bitter—originate from papillae on the tongue.
6. The sense of smell, like the sense of taste, results from a chemical stimulation of certain nerve endings; these are located in the nose.
7. The sense of hearing is derived from the ear—a complex organ.
8. Vision comes from the eye.
9. This system is closely related to dentistry because many of the organs responsible for these senses are located within close proximity to the oral cavity. When a patient has lost complete use of any of these senses, special attention must be given to the patient (e.g., communication with vision or hearing impairment).

K. Lymphatic system
1. Lymph fluid, a tissue fluid, carries nutrients and oxygen to the cells and also removes wastes and other products from the cells. Tiny lymph vessels group together, forming larger vessels that enlarge to create lymph nodes or glands.
2. The function of lymph nodes is to cleanse lymph fluid before it returns to the blood. The area of the head and neck contains many lymph nodes such as the tonsils and adenoids.
3. This system has both a direct and an indirect relationship to dentistry. The tonsils, which are found in the oral cavity, may become inflamed and swollen with infection, making dental treatment uncomfortable, if not difficult, for the patient. Lymph nodes that are found to be enlarged during an extraoral examination may prompt the dentist to refer the patient to a physician for further examination.

L. Skeletal system
1. The skeletal system consists primarily of a hard connective tissue called bone that forms the framework of the body. **Periosteum** is a form of connective tissue that covers bones throughout the body.
2. There are two types of **bone.**
   a. Compact, or cortical, bone is strong, hard, and dense.
   b. Cancellous, or spongy, bone is not as strong and weighs less than compact bone.
3. Both of these types are formed by cells called **osteoblast.** *Osteo* means bone and *blast* refers to former.
4. Bone may be destroyed by cells called **osteoclasts.** *Clast* means something that destroys.
   a. Under certain conditions, particularly orthodontic treatment, the two cells may work together in response to stress.
   b. Bone may be disturbed during the movement of teeth through osteoclast activity, while osteoblasts assist in forming new bone growth around the new position of the teeth.
5. Bones of the skull
   a. The bones of the skull consist of **cranial** and **facial bones** (a total of 22). They are found in pairs or as single bones. Table 3-2 lists the name of the bones found in both categories.
6. Anatomic terms that pertain to the location of the bones of the skull:
   a. **Canal**—a long tube opening through bone
   b. **Condyle**—a rounded surface at the articular end of a bone
   c. **Foramen**—a short opening in a bone or other structure
   d. **Fossa**—a pit, hollow, or depression in bone
   e. **Meatus**—an opening or tunnel through the body
   f. **Process**—a distinct projection of bone
   g. **Septum**—a thin bony layer separating two areas such as the nasal cavities
   h. **Sinus**—a hollow space or opening, a cavity
   i. **Suture**—a rigid joint formed between two bones by cartilage, connective tissue, or bone
   j. **Tubercle**—a rounded elevation on the surface of tissue

Table 3-2 Cranial and facial bones

Name of bone	Number of bones
CRANIAL BONES	
Ethmoid	1
Frontal	1
Occipital	1
Parietal	2
Sphenoid	1
Temporal	2
Total	8
FACIAL BONES	
Inferior nasal conchae	2
Lacrimal	2
Mandible	1
Maxilla	2
Nasal	2
Palatine	2
Vomer	1
Zygomatic	2
Total	14

7. Cranial bones
   a. Ethmoid—single bone
   b. Frontal—single bone
   c. Occipital—single bone
   d. Parietal—paired bones
   e. Sphenoid—single bone divided into two segments: the greater wing and the lesser wing
   f. Temporal—paired bones
8. Facial bones
   a. Inferior nasal conchae—paired bones
   b. Lacrimal—paired bones
   c. Mandible—single bone
   d. Maxilla—paired bones
   e. Nasal—paired bones
   f. Vomer—single bone
   g. Palatine—paired bones
   h. Zygomatic—paired bones
9. Hyoid bone
   a. The hyoid bone is an integral aspect of the skull. Suspended between the mandible and the larynx, it provides support for the tongue and other muscles.
   b. It is not always considered a portion of the skull but is a necessary bone to several functions.
10. Sutures of the skull
    a. Coronal—union of the parietal, frontal, and sphenoid bones

b. Squamosal—union of the temporal and parietal bones

c. Lambdoidal—union of the parietal and occipital bones

M. Muscular system

1. The **muscles of mastication** and those muscles that are responsible for facial expression allow movement in the skull.

2. The muscle origin is the end of the muscle that is attached to a nonmovable structure.

3. The insertion is the end of the muscle that is attached to a movable structure.

4. The body of the muscle is the area between the origin and the insertion.

5. The origin and insertion of the muscles normally attach to bone, but in some circumstances the attachments may be to soft tissue.

6. Muscles of mastication

   a. Four pairs of muscles are grouped as the muscles of mastication:

   (1) Masseter muscle

   (2) Temporal muscle

   (3) Medial pterygoid muscle

   (4) Lateral pterygoid muscle

   b. Accessory muscles of mastication include the hyoid muscles.

   (1) The suprahyoid muscles are the digastric, mylohyoid, geniohyoid, and stylohyoid muscles.

   (2) The infrahyoid muscles are the omohyoid, sternohyoid, sternothyroid, and thyrohyoid muscles.

   c. Muscles are responsible for chewing, tearing, and grinding food.

   d. Muscles are attached to the mandible (insertion) and the upper two thirds of the skull (origin).

   e. They provide protrusion, retrusion, elevation, and lateral movement of the mandible.

   f. The four sets of muscles are paired and work in conjunction to contract, allowing the mandible to open and close. The box defines the functions of the muscles of mastication.

7. **Muscles of facial expression**

   a. They are responsible for movement of the cheeks and lips to reveal emotions, as well as motion during mastication and speech.

   b. These muscles include:

   (1) Orbicularis oris

   (2) Depressors of the lip (a combination of muscles: the mentalis, depressor labii inferiorus, depressor anguli oris, and platysma muscles)

   (3) Elevators of the lip (levator labii superioris, levator labii superioris alaeque nasi, levator anguli oris, zygomaticus minor, and zygomaticus major muscles)

   (4) Risorius muscle

   (5) Buccinator muscle

8. **Temporomandibular joint** (TMJ)

   a. This joint is responsible for movement of the mandible.

   b. It is the only movable joint that exists in the skull, with the hinging of the mandible to both temporal bones.

   c. The hinged joint allows a gliding motion, as well as the hinge action.

   d. It is attached to the cranium by ligaments.

   e. Muscles of mastication assist in maintaining position of the joint.

   f. The temporomandibular joint is composed of a combination of structures.

   (1) Mandible, particularly the condyle

   (2) Glenoid or mandibular fossa in the temporal bone

   (3) The articular disc, or meniscus, between the mandibular condyle and the temporal bone (the articular eminence) and in the glenoid or mandibular fossa

   (4) **Synovial** cavities

   (5) Articular capsule

N. Paranasal sinuses, nasal cavity, and the orbits of the eyes

1. The paranasal sinuses are located in the areas surrounding the nasal cavity.

2. The nasal cavity is divided in half by the nasal septum.

3. Each half is the opening of the nasal cavity

FUNCTIONS OF MUSCLES OF MASTICATION

Elevation	Moves the mandible up or in closing
Protrusion	Moves the mandible forward
Retrusion	Moves the mandible back
Depression	Lowers or opens the mouth
Lateral excursion	Moves the mandible sideways

into the skull and is referred to as the nasal aperture.

4. **Superior** to the nasal cavity toward the lateral area are the orbits, the bony openings of the eyes.

5. Some of the same bones that make up segments of the nasal cavity are also included in the orbit.

6. Paranasal sinuses are paired and are found within many of the previously mentioned structures.

7. The main functions of the sinuses are to:
   a. Lighten the skull
   b. Provide resonance chambers for the voice
   c. Warm inspired air for the respiratory system

8. The sinuses are covered with an epithelial lining called the respiratory epithelium.

9. The sinuses
   a. Maxillary sinuses are the largest and are found in the body of the maxilla.
   b. Frontal sinuses are located superior to the orbit of the eye within the frontal bones.
   c. Sphenoid sinuses are found in the area of the pituitary fossa in the sphenoid bone.
   d. Ethmoid sinuses are not paired but are divided into the anterior, middle, and posterior ethmoids and are referred to as ethmoid air cells.

O. **Salivary glands**

1. Saliva, the fluid of the oral cavity, is secreted from salivary glands.

2. The purpose of saliva is to cleanse the oral cavity and to moisten food during mastication, protect the mucosal lining from dryness, and moisten tissues for ease in speech.

3. The consistency of saliva may vary from serous, or watery, to mucous, which is thick and may be ropelike.

4. Three major glands secrete the majority of fluid into the oral cavity, but smaller additional glands also exist.

5. Major salivary glands
   a. The parotid gland is the largest of the glands. Saliva exits into the oral cavity through the parotid duct, or Stensen's duct, and is of serous consistency.
   b. The submandibular or submaxillary gland is the second largest of the salivary glands. Secretions enter the oral cavity by way of the submandibular duct, or Wharton's duct.

c. The sublingual gland is the smallest of the major salivary glands. The sublingual gland exits into the oral cavity by way of Bartholin's duct into the submandibular duct and other openings along the lingual surface of the tongue.

6. Minor salivary glands
   a. Minor salivary glands are located throughout the rest of the oral cavity, labially, buccally, palatally, lingually, and glossopalatally.
   b. They are primarily responsible for secreting small amounts of saliva to maintain moisture on the mucosal surfaces.
   c. They are found in clusters rather than in a duct pattern as are the major salivary glands.
   d. The glands are the labial, buccal, palatine, glossopalatine, and lingual glands.
   e. The lingual glands are divided into groups: the anterior lingual glands, the lingual glands of von Ebner, and the posterior lingual glands.

P. Circulatory system

1. This system is a network of channels through which blood flows within the body.

2. The three parts of the circulatory system:
   a. Heart
   b. Blood
   c. Blood vessels

3. The heart is divided into chambers: two **atria,** or upper chambers; and two ventricles, or lower chambers. The atria and ventricles are further divided into the right and left, with the right receiving blood and the left carrying blood.

4. Blood is moved from the atria and ventricles via blood vessels called arteries, veins, and capillaries.
   a. A vein carries blood to the heart from all areas of the body.
   b. An artery carries blood away from the heart.
   c. A capillary connects the venous and arterial systems and slows the movement of blood by dispersing it into smaller vessels over a greater area.

5. Major arteries in the head and neck area:
   a. The aorta extends from the left ventricle of the heart and provides blood for the common carotid artery, which is divided into the internal and external carotid vessels.

BRANCHES OF THE ARTERY

Ascending pharyngeal—pharynx and surrounding muscles

Superior thyroid—thyroid gland and surrounding muscles

Lingual—floor of mouth, sublingual gland, mylohyoid muscles, tonsils, soft palate, and epiglottis

Facial—soft palate, pharynx, pharyngeal muscles, tonsils, sublingual and submandibular glands, mylohyoid muscles, mandibular lip, chin, maxillary lip, facial skin, muscles and skin of nose, and eyelids

Occipital—scalp, surrounding muscles, and muscles of the neck

Posterior auricular—outer ear and surrounding scalp

Superficial temporal—temporalis muscle

Maxillary—facial structures

---

    b. The internal carotid artery does not supply blood to the mouth, rather it branches off to supply the brain and the eyes.

    c. The external carotid artery extends throughout the head and neck, supplying blood to eight branches serving various anatomic structures.

    d. The external carotid artery rises from the heart to the mandible, crossing the face and scalp.

    e. The eight branches of the artery and the areas supplied are shown in the box.

    f. One of the most important arteries arising from the external carotid artery is the maxillary artery; it provides the blood supply to the mandibular and maxillary teeth, the palate, the masticatory muscles, and the nasal and oral cavities.

    g. Veins of the head and neck basically correspond with the arteries and have similar names (e.g., the maxillary vein, which drains blood into the internal jugular vein).

Q. Nervous system

  1. The nervous system communicates with the body by carrying messages to and from the brain.

  2. Messages from the brain to a body structure to perform an action or function are referred to as motor, or efferent, messages.

  3. Messages that originate in a body structure and are then transferred to the brain are referred to as sensory, or afferent, messages.

  4. The central nervous system is a combination of the brain and the spinal cord.

  5. The peripheral nervous system includes the cranial and spinal nerves.

  6. Neurons are the cells working in each of these systems to transmit messages via a small electrical current into information, depending on the type of neuron that delivers the message, whether motor or sensory.

  7. The cranial nerves are 12 pairs of nerves that act as sensory or motor nerves; they are named according to the area or type of function they assist and are referred to by name and/or Roman numeral. Table 3-3 identifies the 12 pairs of cranial nerves and the function of each.

  8. The trigeminal and facial nerves are the most vital to the dental profession.

  9. The terminal branches of the trigeminal and facial nerves interrelate, explaining why, when the division of the trigeminal nerve is anesthetized, motor capabilities may be reduced on the patient's face.

  10. The trigeminal nerve divides into three branches: the mandibular, the maxillary, and the ophthalmic.

    a. The mandibular division is separated into the buccal nerve, which supplies the buccal mucous membrane, the mucoperiosteum of the molars, and the lingual nerve, which supplies the anterior two thirds of the tongue, the lingual mucosa, and the mucoperiosteum.

    b. The third branch of the mandibular division of the trigeminal nerve is the inferior alveolar nerve, which branches into four subdivisions.

      (1) The mylohyoid nerve supplies the mylohyoid and digastric muscles.

      (2) The incisive nerve breaks into small branches that supply the central and **lateral** incisors and the cuspids.

      (3) The mental nerve supplies the mucosa of the mandibular lip and the chin.

      (4) The small dental nerves supply the periosteum, alveolar process, molars, and premolars.

    c. The maxillary division of the trigeminal nerve branches into the anterior palatine nerve, which supplies the mucoperios-

Table 3-3 Cranial nerves

Nerve	Type	Function
OLFACTORY NERVE	Sensory	Provides sense of smell
OPTIC NERVE	Sensory	Provides sense of sight
OCULOMOTOR NERVE	Motor	Provides movement of the muscles of the eye
TROCHLEAR NERVE	Motor	Provides movement for a single muscle of the eye
TRIGEMINAL NERVE	Motor and sensory	Divided into three parts; largest and most important nerve to dentistry
OPHTHALMIC DIVISION	Sensory	Supplies the eyes and forehead
MAXILLARY DIVISION	Sensory	Supplies the maxillary arch and related structures and innervates the maxillary teeth
MANDIBULAR DIVISION	Motor and sensory	Supplies the mandibular arch and sensory-related structures and innervates the mandibular teeth
ABDUCENS NERVE	Motor	Provides movement for one muscle of the eye
FACIAL NERVE	Motor and sensory	Provides movement to facial muscles and salivary glands; supplies sense of taste
ACOUSTIC NERVE	Sensory	Provides hearing and sense of balance
GLOSSOPHARYNGEAL NERVE	Motor and sensory	Provides movement for muscles of soft palate, throat, and salivary glands; provides sense of taste, pain, temperature, and pressure
VAGUS NERVE	Motor and sensory	Provides movement for larynx and pharynx, muscles of the soft palate, and smooth and cardiac muscles; provides sense of taste from the root of the tongue and sensory information from the skin around the ear
ACCESSORY (SPINAL) NERVE	Motor	Provides movement for muscles of the shoulder
HYPOGLOSSAL NERVE	Motor	Provides movement for muscles of the tongue

teum, while combining with the naso-palatine nerve, which supplies the mucoperiosteum of the palate to the **anterior** teeth.

    d. The maxillary division also branches to include the anterior, middle, and posterosuperior alveolar nerves, which supply the following:

      (1) Anterior alveolar

        (a) Central and lateral cuspids

        (b) Periodontal membranes

        (c) Gingiva

      (2) Middle alveolar

        (a) First and second premolars

        (b) Mesiobuccal root of the first molar

        (c) Maxillary sinus

      (3) Posterosuperior alveolar

        (a) Rest of the first molar roots

        (b) Second and third molars

        (c) Lateral wall of the maxillary sinus

ORAL FACIAL STRUCTURES AND THE ORAL CAVITY

I. Oral cavity

  A. The oral cavity is where the first step in the digestive process takes place.

  B. The oral cavity participates in the respiratory system and contains the taste organs.

  C. The area of the oral cavity is bordered by the lips anteriorly, the anterior pillars posteriorly, the palate superiorly, and the muscles of the floor of the mouth inferiorly.

  D. The oral cavity commonly is divided into two segments.

    1. Vestibule

    2. Oral cavity proper

II. Vestibule

  A. The **vestibule** is the space or cavity that serves as the entrance to the oral cavity.

    1. The outer borders of the vestibule are the lips and cheeks.

    2. The inner borders are the facial surfaces of the teeth and the **alveolar processes,** which create a troughlike space.

    3. The skin that covers the face and stops at the edge of the lips is called keratinized stratified squamous epithelium.

    4. Mucosa is the tissue that covers the oral cavity and is termed parakeratinized stratified squamous epithelium.

    5. The area of the lips that appears redder, where the two kinds of epithelium join, is highly vascular and is called the vermilion border.

6. The contact point for the upper and lower lip in the corner of the mouth is referred to as the labial commissure.
7. Various landmarks of the lips and cheeks are shown in Fig. 3-1.

B. Muscle and fiber attachments found within the vestibule and oral cavity are named according to location.
1. The attachments are composed of connective tissue and are known as frena (singular *frenum)* and are responsible for connecting the lips, cheeks, and tongue to the alveolar processes.
2. These attachments include:
   a. Lingual frenum (Fig. 3-2)
   b. Maxillary labial frenum (Fig. 3-3)
   c. Maxillary buccal frena (Fig. 3-3)
   d. Mandibular labial frenum (Fig. 3-3)
   e. Mandibular buccal frena (Fig. 3-3)
3. The mucobuccal fold, or fornix, is where the alveolar buccal mucosa joins with the cheek mucosa.
   a. The mucolabial fold, or fornix, is found in the anterior segment of the maxillary and mandibular arches where the labial mucosa joins with the alveolar mucosa.
4. The oral mucosa that surrounds all the teeth is designated as **gingiva** (Fig. 3-3).
   a. The gingiva appears to differ in color from the lining mucosa of the lips and cheeks and from the alveolar mucosa that lies between the lining mucosa and the gingiva.
   b. Difference in color is attributed to the increased vascular supply, with the alveolar mucosa appearing redder than the gingiva, which is pink to brown, depending on genetic background.
5. The gingiva is divided into two parts.
   a. Free gingiva or marginal gingiva that covers the neck of the teeth and extends to a depth of 1 to 3 mm before it reaches the attached gingiva.
   b. Attached gingiva covers the alveolar bone and a portion of the cementum of the teeth. A detailed drawing of this area appears in Chapter 6.

III. Oral cavity proper
A. The oral cavity proper (Fig. 3-3) is bounded by the internal surface of the alveolar process and the teeth; it lies between the dental arches and includes the tongue.
B. The bony roof of the mouth, the maxilla, includes the palate, which is divided into the hard and the soft palates.
1. Both are covered by palatal mucosa, with the mucosa attached to the hard palate.
2. The hard palate is so named because the bone of the maxilla is superior to it, while the soft palate has no bone-based support.
3. Located on the hard palate, **posterior** to the maxillary central incisors, is a V-shaped tis-

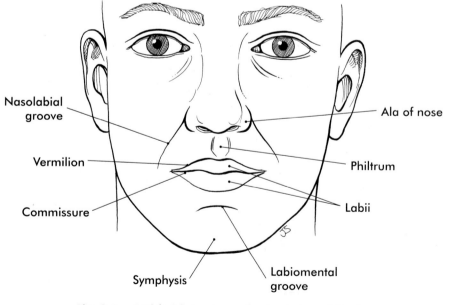

Fig. 3-1 Oral facial structures of a front view of the face.

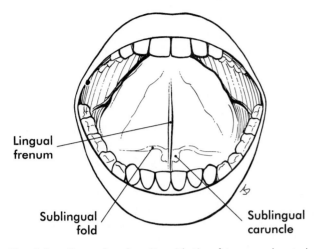

Lingual
frenum

Sublingual
fold

Sublingual
caruncle

Fig. 3-2   Opened oral cavity with tip of tongue elevated.

sue elevation, the incisive **papilla** or palatine papilla, which covers the maxillary incisive foramen.

4. Extending from the anterior portion of the maxilla down the palate's midline is a ridge called the palatine raphe.

5. The irregular folds or ridges of connective tissue extending from the anterior of the maxilla to the area of the maxillary first molars from the palatal raphe are the palatine rugae that aid in speech and mastication.

C. The soft palate is posterior to the hard palate and is referred to as soft because there is no bony support.

1. An extension of the soft palate is the uvula, a vertical segment of muscle, connective tissue, and glands that hang in the back of the throat and closes the nasopharynx and

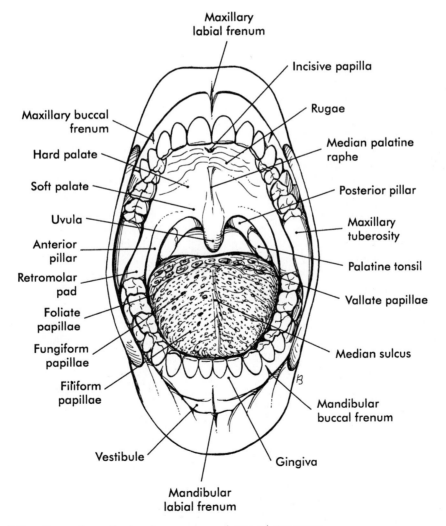

Maxillary
labial frenum

Incisive papilla

Maxillary buccal
frenum

Rugae

Hard palate

Median palatine
raphe

Soft palate

Posterior pillar

Uvula

Maxillary
tuberosity

Anterior
pillar

Palatine tonsil

Retromolar
pad

Vallate papillae

Foliate
papillae

Fungiform
papillae

Median sulcus

Filiform
papillae

Mandibular
buccal frenum

Vestibule

Gingiva

Mandibular
labial frenum

Fig. 3-3   Opened mouth showing numerous intraoral structures.

prevents the entry of objects into the nasal cavity.

D. Small pits in the mucosa may be visible, known as the palatine foveae, where the soft and hard palates meet and where some of the palatine salivary glands empty.

E. The posterolateral areas of the mouth house the posterior folds, which are two folds of muscle and tissue.

   1. The larger fold is referred to as the posterior pillar, or palatopharyngeal pillar or fold, which is located behind the palatine tonsil.

   2. Anterior to the palatine tonsil is the anterior pillar, or palatoglossal pillar or fold.

   3. The open area between the sets of pillars on either side of the mouth is referred to as the fauces. Here the oral cavity opens into the pharynx.

   4. Three sets of tonsils are located in the posterior segment of the oral cavity.

     a. Pharyngeal adenoid tonsils are superior and near the soft palate.

     b. Palatine tonsils are directly inferior to this area.

     c. Lingual tonsils are on the inferior lateral surface at the base of the tongue.

   5. Anterior to the tonsils on the maxilla and posterior to the third molars is a mass of bone called the maxillary tuberosity.

   6. **Inferior** to the maxillary tuberosity and posterior to the mandibular third molars is the retromolar pad that forms the inferior portion of the anterior border of the ramus and is a raised area of tissue.

IV. Tongue and floor of the mouth

A. The tongue is a highly muscular and vascular structure covered by epithelium.

   1. It is extremely well-coordinated and has acute tactile sense.

   2. Its functions include:

     a. Forming words for speech

     b. Assisting in mastication and swallowing

     c. Providing taste sensation from the taste buds located on its surface

   3. The tongue is divided into two portions: the posterior, or base, and the anterior, or body.

   4. The line on the dorsal surface of the body, called the median sulcus or fissure, divides the tongue into right and left segments.

   5. The median sulcus extends to the posterior of the tongue and then to the circumvallate papillae.

   6. Posterior to the circumvallate papillae is a developmental line called the terminalis sulcus, which divides the anterior from the posterior portion of the tongue (Fig. 3-3).

   7. Four types of papillae are found on the tongue (Fig. 3-3).

     a. Circumvallate are on the posterior segment of the tongue and form a V anterior to the terminalis sulcus. They receive bitter tastes.

     b. Fungiform cover the anterior two thirds of the tongue and appear as small raised areas of tissue. Buds on the dorsal surface of the tongue are responsible for detecting sweet sensations; those toward the lateral surface sense salty tastes.

     c. Filiform are somewhat hairlike in appearance and are located completely over the dorsal surface of the tongue in large quantities. They detect no taste sensations, but are sensitive to tactile sensations on the surface.

       (1) Pathologic conditions may develop in the area of the filiform papillae, such as hairy tongue and glossitis.

     d. Foliate are found on the posterior third and on the lateral surfaces of the tongue in the folds. They detect sour taste sensations.

     e. Papillae are elevated structures on epithelial tissues of the tongue responsible for the sensation of taste.

   8. Muscles of the tongue are divided into two groups: the **extrinsic** (outside the muscle) and the **intrinsic** (inside the muscle).

   9. The intrinsic muscles consist of four groups. These muscles function during mastication, speech, and deglutition.

     a. Superior longitudinal

     b. Transverse

     c. Vertical

     d. Inferior longitudinal

   10. The extrinsic muscles consist of four groups. These muscles suspend and anchor the tongue and also allow the tongue to move in a protruding or depressing movement.

     a. Genioglossus

     b. Hyoglossus

     c. Palatoglossus

     d. Styloglossus

Questions

Basic Anatomy and Physiology

1 Genetics is the study of
   a. The nervous system
   b. Heredity
   c. Tissue composition
   d. Intercellular fluids

2 Which tissue has the poorest regeneration capability?
   a. Epithelial
   b. Connective
   c. Nerve
   d. Muscle

3 The function of bone marrow is to
   a. Add resiliency to bones
   b. Produce blood cells
   c. Decrease the weight of bones
   d. Aid in muscular attachments

4 Muscle tissue is present in which system?
   a. Circulatory
   b. Digestive
   c. Respiratory
   d. All of the above

5 A nerve impulse is transmitted from nerve to nerve via the
   a. Myoneural junction
   b. Ligaments
   c. Synaptic junction
   d. Foramina

6 The central nervous system is covered by a membrane called the
   a. Hyaline membrane
   b. Meninges
   c. Nasmyth membrane
   d. Primary cuticle

7 The function of the epiglottis is to
   a. Regulate the carbon dioxide and oxygen ratio of inspired air
   b. Control the volume of air
   c. Support the thyroid gland
   d. Prevent liquids and solids from entering the respiratory system

8 Inspiration is caused by
   a. A decrease in size of alveoli
   b. Expansion of the pleural cavity
   c. Relaxation of the diaphragm
   d. Contraction of the chest

9 The function of hemoglobin is to
   a. Transport nutrients
   b. Fight infection
   c. Transport oxygen
   d. Stimulate endocrine glands

10 Leukocytes are
   a. A defense mechanism of the body
   b. Part of the oxygen transport system
   c. Formed by bone marrow
   d. Part of the excretory system

11 The rhythmic movement of the esophagus that moves the food bolus onward is known as
   a. Digestion
   b. Churning
   c. Swallowing
   d. Peristalsis

12 Absorption of most nutrients occurs in the
   a. Stomach
   b. Esophagus
   c. Small intestine
   d. Large intestine

13 The presence of bacteria in the urine indicates
   a. A possible infection of the urinary tract
   b. Normal functioning
   c. Bacteremia
   d. Hypotension

14 The most important function of saliva is its
   a. Action on fats
   b. Action on proteins
   c. Ability to break down sugars
   d. Lubrication that facilitates swallowing

15 The main group of deep cervical lymph nodes forms a chain along the
   a. Anterior jugular vein
   b. External jugular vein
   c. Internal jugular vein
   d. Internal carotid artery
   e. External carotid artery

16 Which main artery supplies the teeth?
   a. Brachial
   b. Occipital
   c. External carotid
   d. Superior vena cava

17 The immunity that a newborn infant acquires from its mother is
   a. Natural active immunity
   b. Natural passive immunity
   c. Artificial active immunity
   d. Artificial passive immunity

18 Which of the following is not a function of the buccinator muscle?
   a. Open the jaw
   b. Aid in mastication
   c. Aid in facial expression
   d. Close the mandible
   e. Protrude the mandible

19 The enzyme secreted by a salivary gland is
   a. Protease
   b. Ptyalin
   c. Protaglase

20 The paranasal sinuses that have the greatest significance in dentistry are
   a. Maxillary
   b. Ethmoid
   c. Frontal
   d. Lacrimal

21 Which of the following is not a function of the paranasal sinus?

a. Lighten the skull
b. Provide voice tone
c. Increase ability to breathe
d. Warm inhaled air

22 The branch of the external carotid artery that supplies the teeth is the
a. Facial branch of the external carotid artery
b. Lingual branch of the external carotid artery
c. Lingual branch of the internal carotid artery
d. Facial branch of the internal carotid artery

23 The _____ nerve innervates the muscles of mastication.
a. Ocular
b. Trachlear
c. Trigeminal
d. Temporal

24 The size of salivary glands based on secretion amount in ascending order is
a. Parotid, submandibular, and sublingual
b. Submandibular, parotid, and Bartholin's
c. Sublingual, parotid, and submandibular

25 The tissue of the mouth categorized as parakeratinized stratified squamous epithelium is
a. Vermilion
b. Frenum tissue only
c. Mucosa
d. Gingival tissue only

Rationales

Basic Anatomy and Physiology

1 B Genetics pertains to reproduction, birth, or origin that evolves from parents to offspring.

2 C Nerve regeneration may occur when the damaged nerve fibers are aligned. If not aligned, regeneration is reduced and nerve muscle function is not likely.

3 B Bone marrow is the connective tissue in the spaces of spongy bone where blood cell production occurs.

4 D Each of these systems contains muscle tissue. The circulatory contains cardiac and smooth muscle tissue; the digestive is comprised of smooth and skeletal muscles; and the respiratory contains smooth muscle.

5 C The synaptic junction is the region around two nerve ends or the nerve end and an organ that allows nerve impulse transmission through the work of a neurotransmitter.

6 B The meninges is a combination of three layers that encloses the brain and the spinal cord.

7 D The epiglottis lies over the larynx, preventing food and fluids from entering the larynx and the trachea.

8 B Air drawn into the lungs for the exchange of oxygen and carbon dioxide occurs during inspiration. The diaphragm contracts allowing the pleural cavity to expand and inward air flow.

9 C Hemoglobin carries oxygen to cells from the lungs and carbon dioxide away from the cells to the lungs.

10 A Leukocytes are white blood cells that squeeze through intercellular spaces to work as phagocytes of bacteria, fungi, and viruses to protect the body.

11 D The wavelike contraction of smooth muscle that occurs in hollow tubes in the body is referred to as peristalsis. Such action can force food through the esophagus at the beginning of the digestive tract.

12 C Small glands exist in the area of the small intestine and allow the greatest amount of absorption in the digestive process.

13 A The excretory system, from which urine is derived, is the filtering system of the body. When an infection is present, this system would throw off the bacteria in the waste.

14 D Saliva softens and moistens food allowing it to be swallowed with greater ease and comfort.

15 C The right lymphatic duct aligns by the internal jugular vein and drains into it. Since these are deep cervical nodes it indicates they are within or near the internal jugular vein.

16 C The external carotid artery supplies blood to the head and neck as well as eight branches of various anatomic structures, which supply the head and neck.

17 B The transfer of antibodies from a mother to a child is known as natural passive immunity. The mother is exposed to antigens throughout life and has antibodies against many antigens. These antibodies are passed through the placenta and enter the fetal circulation, thus giving the newborn infant natural passive immunity.

18 E The buccinator muscle maintains the cheek position over the mandible and the maxilla. It controls a tautness as the mouth is opened and closed thus aiding in mastication and facial expression.

19 B Ptyalin is a starch-digesting enzyme that is secreted by salivary glands to aid in digestion.

20 A The maxillary sinuses are the largest and are in close proximity to maxillary root structures. A patient may indicate discomfort in this area that may relate to a sinus condition rather than a dental problem.

21 C The sinuses decrease the weight of the skull and provide for the resonance of voice quality. During respiration, the sinuses warm the air that is inhaled through the nose, but do not increase the ability to breathe.

22 B The lingual branch of the external carotid artery supplies the mouth, tongue, and submandibular and sublingual glands. The maxillary artery also supplies the arches and the teeth.

23 C The trigeminal nerve is responsible for innervation of the muscles of the face, eyes, nose, mouth, and jaws.

24 A The parotid gland is the largest of the salivary glands followed by the submandibular and the sublingual glands.

25 C The oral mucosa is the smooth tissue that lines the mouth and consists of the gingival and frenum tissues as well. This tissue is parakeratinized stratified squamous epithelium.

To enhance your understanding of the material in this chapter, refer to the illustrations in Chapter 3 of Finkbeiner/Johnson: *Mosby's Comprehensive Dental Assisting: A Clinical Approach.*

Intraoral Structures

OUTLINE

The Dental Arches
Dentition
Permanent Dentition
Mixed Dentition
Tooth Morphology

Tooth Numbering Systems
Tooth Surfaces
Dental Anatomy
Oral Embryology and Histology
Parts of the Tooth

Tissues of the Tooth
Supporting Tissues of the Oral Cavity
Tooth Development and Eruption
Eruption Sequence for Primary and
  Permanent Dentition

KEY TERMS

Ameloblast
Angle
Apical foramen
Attrition
Axial
Bell stage
Buccal
Bud canine
Cap stage
Cementoblast
Cementum
Cingulum
Concave
Contact area
Convex
Crown
Curve of Spee
Cusp
Cuspid
Deciduous
Dentin
Dentinal tubule
Dentition
Diastema

Ectoderm
Embrasure
Embryology
Enamel
Enamel cuticle
Endoderm
Facial
Fibroblast
Fossa
Furcation
Gingiva
Groove
Incisal
Incisor
Histology
Labial
Lamina dura
Lingual
Lobe
Mamelon
Mandible
Maxilla
Mesoderm

Molar
Mucosa
Oblique ridge
Occlusal
Occlusion
Odontoblasts
Overbite
Overjet
Papilla
Periodontium
Permanent
Premolar
Primary
Primordium
Proximal
Pulp
Quadrant
Ridge
Secondary
Segment
Succedaneous
Sulcus
Supernumerary
Tubercle

A thorough knowledge of intraoral structures is required to perform basic clinical skills and complete the many records common to most dental patients.

THE DENTAL ARCHES

I. In a human mouth there are two dental arches: the **maxilla,** or maxillary arch, and the **mandible,** or mandibular arch.
  A. Lay terms refer to the maxillary arch as the upper jaw and the mandibular arch as the lower jaw.
  B. The arches support a combination of teeth that are referred to as **dentition.**
  C. Each half of the arch is referred to as a **quadrant** or one quarter of the mouth.
    1. Each arch has two quadrants, totaling four quadrants in a full dentition.
    2. Each quadrant extends from the midline of the arch to the most posterior area of the arch.
  D. Ideally each quadrant in a person's arch will be symmetric: the same number, type, and alignment of teeth in each quadrant.
  E. Each arch also can be divided into segments rather than quadrants.
    1. A **segment** is a section of the arch.
    2. Three segments are in each arch, totaling six segments in the dentition.
    3. A dental arch can be divided into an anterior segment and two posterior segments, right and left.

DENTITION

I. In a lifetime it is normal to have two sets of dentition.
  A. The **primary,** or **deciduous,** dentition (sometimes referred to as the baby teeth by the layperson) is the first to develop in an infant's mouth; it begins to erupt at approximately 6 months and consists of 20 teeth.
  B. The primary dentition is replaced by the secondary, or **permanent,** dentition, which includes a maximum of 32 teeth.
  C. The **secondary** teeth begin to erupt at approximately 6 years of age.
  D. The number of permanent teeth varies, depending on whether the third molars, or wisdom teeth, erupt.
  E. Each arch accommodates the same number of teeth.
    1. The primary dentition contains 10 teeth per arch (total of 20 teeth).
    2. The permanent dentition contains 16 teeth per arch (total of 32 teeth).
    3. A quadrant in the primary dentition will consist of five teeth, with eight teeth in each quadrant of the permanent dentition.
    4. The anterior segment consists of the anterior teeth, the four incisors, and the cuspids, or canines. The posterior segments consist of the remaining teeth of the arch: the premolars and molars.

PERMANENT DENTITION

I. Functions of the teeth:
  A. Provide aesthetics or good appearance
  B. Support other structures
  C. Aid in swallowing, mastication, and digestion
  D. Aid in producing speech and phonetics
  E. Provide a guide for the permanent teeth during development and eruption (function of the primary teeth)
  F. Allow the permanent dentition to assume its place in the arches (as the dental arches grow, the position of the primary teeth changes slightly)
  G. Prepare food for swallowing and digestion (during mastication, eating, and chewing, each tooth type has a specific purpose)
    1. **Incisors** have sharp biting edges that aid in cutting and incising food.
    2. **Cuspids,** or canines, have pointed cusps that aid in holding and tearing food.
    3. **Premolars** crush and tear food.
    4. **Molars** have broad biting surfaces that aid in chewing and grinding food. The box provides a diagram of each of these teeth, including the identifying characteristics of each type of tooth.

MIXED DENTITION

I. Mixed dentition usually exists in a person's oral cavity from approximately 6 to 12 years of age.
  A. Mixed dentition is a combination of primary and permanent dentition; it occurs as the permanent teeth begin to erupt within the oral cavity, while some of the primary teeth are still present.
  B. When primary dentition is naturally lost, it is replaced by the permanent teeth, which are called **succedaneous** teeth, a group of teeth that follows the first set.
  C. Any teeth of the permanent dentition that do not replace primary teeth are referred to as nonsuccedaneous teeth.

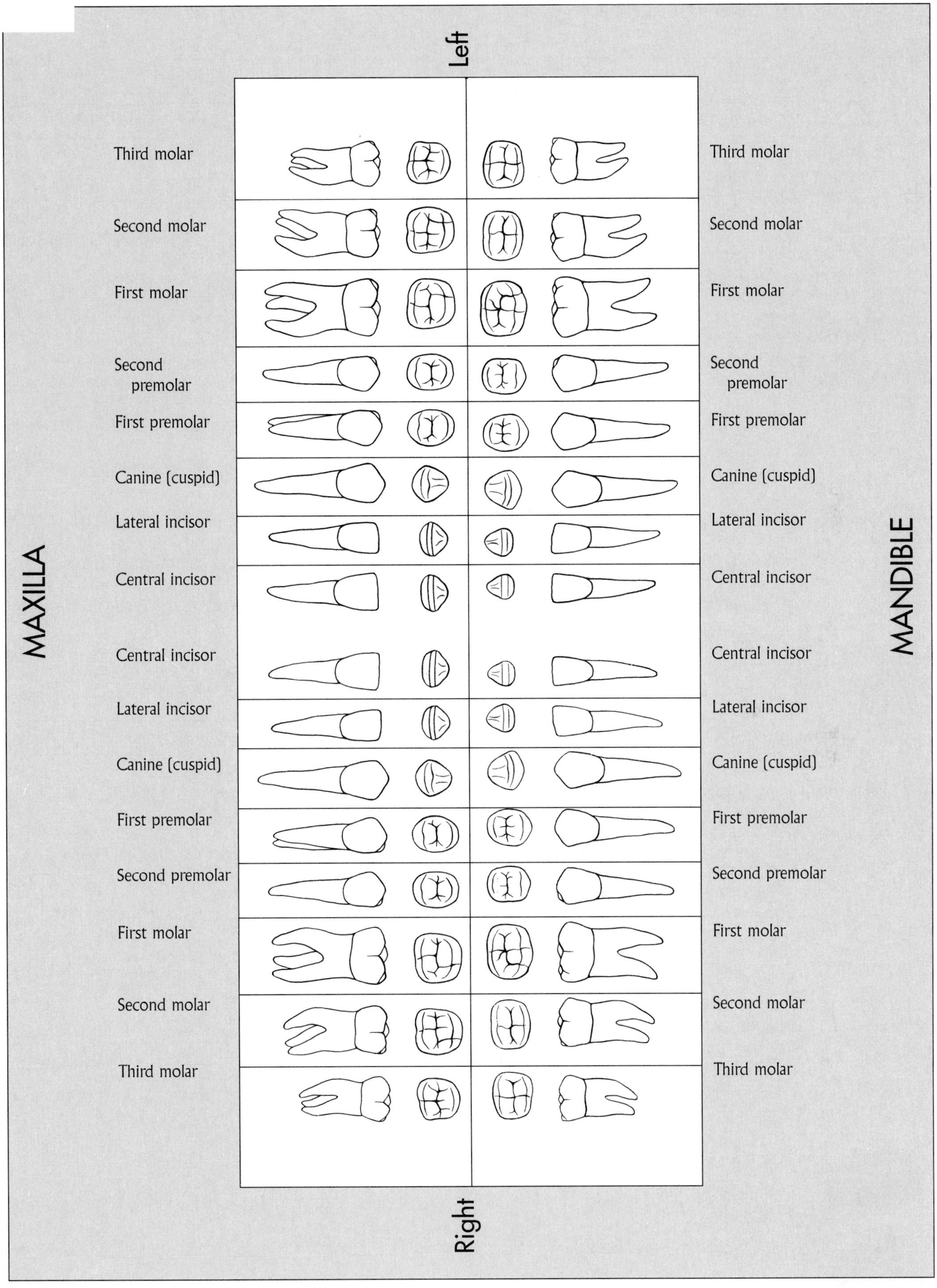

Left

MAXILLA

Third molar

Second molar

First molar

Second premolar

First premolar

Canine (cuspid)

Lateral incisor

Central incisor

Central incisor

Lateral incisor

Canine (cuspid)

First premolar

Second premolar

First molar

Second molar

Third molar

Right

Third molar

Second molar

First molar

Second premolar

First premolar

Canine (cuspid)

Lateral incisor

Central incisor

Central incisor

Lateral incisor

Canine (cuspid)

First premolar

Second premolar

First molar

Second molar

Third molar

MANDIBLE

CHARACTERISTICS AND DIAGRAM OF EACH TYPE OF TOOTH

MAXILLARY RIGHT AND LEFT CENTRAL INCISORS

Universal numbering system - #8 and #9
Palmer numbering system - 1| and |1
FDI numbering system - #11 and #21
Identifying characteristics:
  Largest and widest of the incisor teeth in the mouth
  Well-developed cingulum on lingual surface
  The mesioincisal point is more acute, while the distoincisal is more blunted in shape
  Has triangular-shaped root tipped toward the distal
  The mesial contact with the abutment tooth is near the mesioincisal angle
  Single root

MAXILLARY RIGHT AND LEFT LATERAL INCISORS

Universal numbering system - #7 and #10
Palmer numbering system - 2| and |2
FDI numbering system - #12 and #22
Identifying characteristics:
  Crown is smaller in size than the maxillary central incisor, but root length is similar
  Smaller cingulum than maxillary central incisor and has distinct lingual pit and fossa
  Mesioincisal point is more rounded than the maxillary central incisor
  Mesial contact with abutment tooth is near the incisal and middle third of tooth
  Distal contact with abutment tooth is near middle third of tooth
  Single root

MANDIBULAR CENTRAL INCISORS

Universal numbering system - #24 and #25
Palmer numbering system - 1| and |1
FDI numbering system - #31 and #41
Identifying characteristics:
  Usually is the smallest incisor in the mouth
  Usually smaller than the mandibular lateral incisors
  The mesial-distal crown width is small
  Has a flat cingulum
  The root is oval in shape in a cross-section
  Single root that may curve slightly towards the distal

MANDIBULAR LATERAL INCISORS

Universal numbering system - #23 and #26
Palmer numbering system - 2| and |2
FDI numbering system - #32 and #42
Identifying characteristics:
  The mesial contact is near the incisal third, and the distal contact is near the middle third
  The distal incisal edge slopes apically
  The mesial-facial line angle is longer than the distal-facial line angle
  The cingulum is positioned slightly towards the distal
  The incisal edge wears more towards the distal surface
  Single root

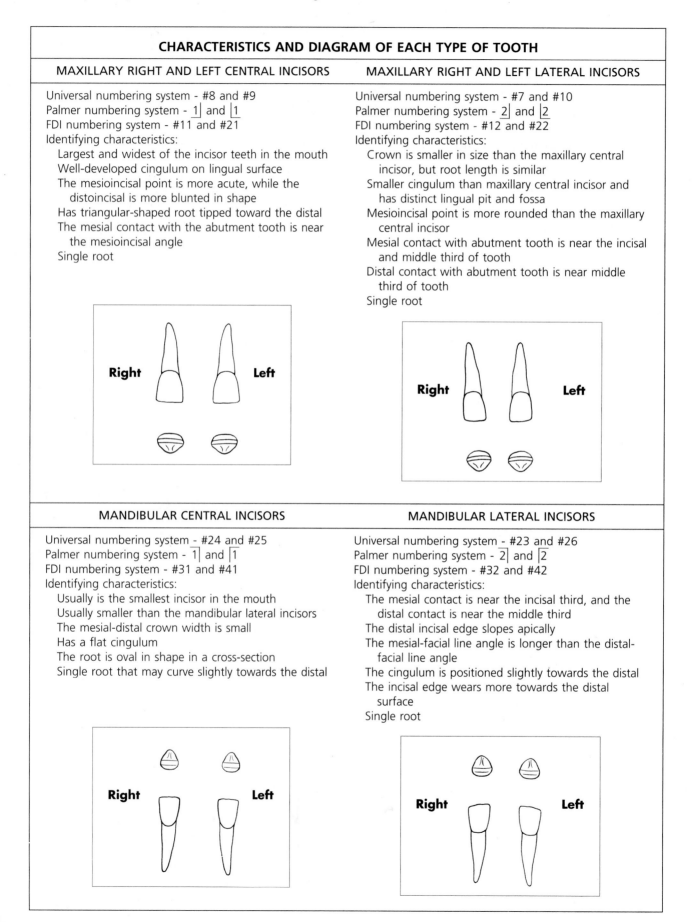

CHARACTERISTICS AND DIAGRAM OF EACH TYPE OF TOOTH

MAXILLARY RIGHT AND LEFT CUSPIDS (CANINES, SINGLE CUSP)

Universal numbering system - #6 and #11
Palmer numbering system - 3| and |3
FDI numbering system - #13 and #23
Identifying characteristics:
  Has no incisal edge, has a cusp instead
  Length of distal cusp ridge is longer than mesial cusp ridge
  Mesial contact with abutment tooth is near cusp apex
  Distal contact with abutment tooth is near cervical area
  Prominent cingulum in cervical half of clinical crown
  Longest single-rooted tooth in mouth

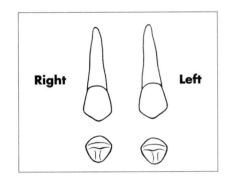

MAXILLARY RIGHT AND LEFT FIRST PREMOLARS (BICUSPIDS, TWO CUSPS)

Universal numbering system - #5 and #12
Palmer numbering system - 4| and |4
FDI numbering system - #14 and #24
Identifying characteristics:
  Crown of tooth has a hexagonal shape
  Has both a buccal and lingual cusp, with buccal cusp usually being longer
  Buccal cusp is wider from the mesial to distal than the lingual cusp
  Central occlusal groove crosses the mesial marginal ridge
  Buccal cusp ridge slopes towards the mesial of the tooth
  Usually double rooted with one buccal and lingual root, but may be single rooted

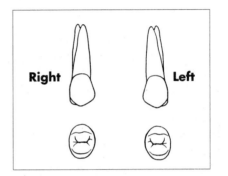

MANDIBULAR CUSPIDS (CANINES, ONE CUSP)

Universal numbering system - #22 and #27
Palmer numbering system - 3| and |3
FDI numbering system - #33 and #43
Identifying characteristics:
  Has smooth lingual anatomy with a cingulum in the cervical third
  Has cusp, no incisal edge
  The distal cusp ridge is longer than the mesial cusp ridge
  Has smaller mesiodistal width than the maxillary cuspids
  Receives much wear on facial surface
  Single root that curves toward the distal

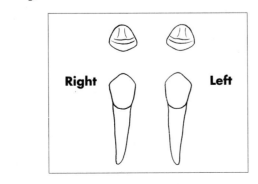

MANDIBULAR RIGHT AND LEFT FIRST PREMOLARS (BICUSPIDS, TWO CUSPS)

Universal numbering system - #21 and #28
Palmer numbering system - 4| and |4
FDI numbering system - #34 and #44
Identifying characteristics:
  Smaller in size compared to the mandibular second premolar
  Lingual cusp(s) are nonfunctional
  Has large cusp with one or two smaller and shorter lingual cusps
  Has transverse ridge across the occlusal surface
  Single root is smaller than the mandibular second premolar

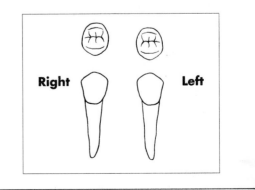

Continued.

CHARACTERISTICS AND DIAGRAM OF EACH TYPE OF TOOTH

MAXILLARY RIGHT AND SECOND LEFT PREMOLARS (BICUSPIDS, TWO CUSPS)

Universal numbering system - #4 and #13
Palmer numbering system - 5| and |5
FDI numbering system - #15 and #25
Identifying characteristics:
  Has buccal and lingual cusps that are similar in length
  No depression on the mesial or distal crown surfaces
  Size of crown wider from buccal to lingual than from mesial to distal
  Tooth has central groove that doesn't cross the marginal ridge
  Buccal cusp ridge is parallel to the central groove
  Single root

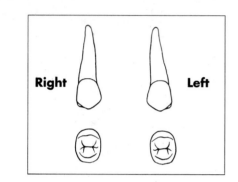

MAXILLARY RIGHT AND LEFT FIRST MOLARS

Universal numbering system - #3 and #14
Palmer numbering system - 6| and |6
FDI numbering system - #16 and #26
Identifying characteristics:
  Usually the largest maxillary tooth
  Has four defined cusps: mesiolingual, mesiobuccal, distobuccal, and distolingual, with the mesiolingual being the largest and the distolingual the smallest
  Has a supplemental cusp called cusp of Carabelli that is lingual to the mesiolingual cusp
  The crown shape is rhomboidal
  Has a strong and defined oblique ridge
  Has three roots being trifurcated—mesiobuccal, distobuccal, and lingual

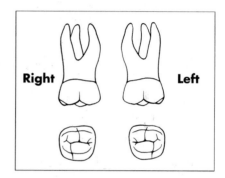

MANDIBULAR RIGHT AND LEFT SECOND PREMOLARS (BICUSPIDS, THREE CUSPS)

Universal numbering system - #20 and #29
Palmer numbering system - 5| and |5
FDI numbering system - #35 and #45
Identifying characteristics:
  Has single buccal cusp with one or two lingual cusps
  Lingual cusps are more functional than mandibular first premolar
  If the tooth has single lingual cusp, occlusal pattern is usually U or H shaped
  If the tooth has two lingual cusps, occlusal pattern is usually Y shaped
  Larger and longer root than the mandibular first premolar
  Has single root

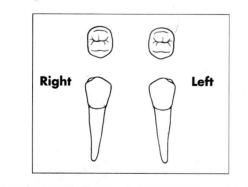

MANDIBULAR RIGHT AND LEFT FIRST MOLARS

Universal numbering system - #19 and #30
Palmer numbering system - 6| and |6
FDI numbering system - #36 and #46
Identifying characteristics:
  Usually the largest mandibular tooth
  Has five well-developed cusps: mesiobuccal, mesiolingual, distolingual, distobuccal, and distal
  Has two buccal grooves with three cusps
  Has one lingual groove and two cusps
  Crown shape is somewhat rectangular
  Has two roots, one mesial and one distal; they are spaced wide apart

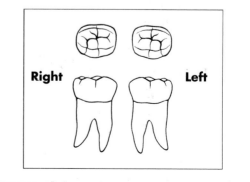

CHARACTERISTICS AND DIAGRAM OF EACH TYPE OF TOOTH

MAXILLARY RIGHT AND LEFT SECOND MOLARS

Universal numbering system - #2 and #15
Palmer numbering system - 7| and |7
FDI numbering system - #17 and #27
Identifying characteristics:

Has four defined cusps: mesiolingual, mesiobuccal, distobuccal, and distolingual

Also has oblique ridge, but it is crossed by the central groove

Crown of tooth is usually shorter in length than the maxillary first molar

The distolingual cusp usually is smaller than that of the maxillary first molar

The roots tend to be closer together than the maxillary first molar

Has three roots being trifurcated: mesiobuccal, distobuccal, and lingual; the roots are usually longer than the maxillary first molar roots

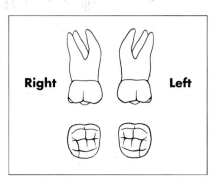

MAXILLARY RIGHT AND LEFT THIRD MOLARS

Universal numbering system - #1 and #16
Palmer numbering system - 8| and |8
FDI numbering system - #18 and #28
Identifying characteristics:

Usually no oblique ridge

Size, shape, and contour may differ greatly because the teeth are developmental anomalies

Roots curve toward the distal

Roots are often fused together

The number of roots may vary: one, two, or three

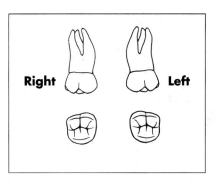

MANDIBULAR SECOND MOLARS

Universal numbering system - #18 and #31
Palmer numbering system - 7| and |7
FDI numbering system - #37 and #47
Identifying characteristics:

Has four cusps: mesiobuccal, mesiolingual, distobuccal, and distolingual

Has two buccal cusps and one groove

Lingual cusps are more pointed and longer than the buccal cusps

Has three occlusal pits

Buccal cusps tip toward the lingual

Has two roots, mesial and distal, that are not spread as far apart as the mandibular first molars

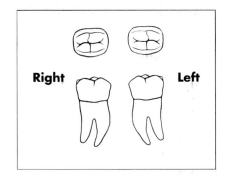

MANDIBULAR THIRD MOLARS

Universal numbering system - #17 and #32
Palmer numbering system - 8| and |8
FDI numbering system - #38 and #48
Identifying characteristics:

Size, shape, and contour may differ greatly because these are developmental anomalies

Roots are usually fused together

Roots are usually curved distally

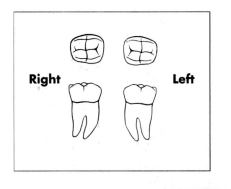

1. Teeth considered nonsuccedaneous are the permanent molars; they erupt distal to the primary teeth and do not replace any primary teeth.
   D. Teeth can also be congenitally missing, or the tooth bud may not be present at birth; this could occur with a primary or permanent tooth.
   E. A dental anomaly known as **supernumerary** teeth is the existence of additional tooth bud(s) that erupt as a third tooth or teeth on the dental arch(es).

TOOTH MORPHOLOGY

I. Morphology is the study of form and shape.
II. The sequence of tooth identification should be the dentition, then the arch, then the quadrant, and finally the specific tooth of reference (box).
   A. The permanent dentition has the same teeth in each quadrant from the most posterior area of the mouth to the midline of the mouth.
   B. The teeth in a quadrant of the permanent dentition include:
      1. Third molar
      2. Second molar
      3. First molar
      4. Second premolar (second bicuspid)
      5. First premolar (first bicuspid)
      6. Cuspid (canine)
      7. Lateral incisor
      8. Central incisor
   C. The primary dentition has the same teeth in each

quadrant from the most posterior area of the mouth to the midline of the mouth.
   D. The teeth in each quadrant of a primary dentition include:
      1. Second molar
      2. First molar
      3. Cuspid (canine)
      4. Lateral incisor
      5. Central incisor

TOOTH NUMBERING SYSTEMS

I. The objective of a numbering system is to name and code each tooth in the oral cavity, either numerically or alphabetically.
   A. This number or letter provides an abbreviated form of tooth reference and aids in consistency in records management.
   B. The most common types of numbering systems include:
      1. Universal numbering system
      2. Palmer notation system
      3. Federal Dentaire Internationale system

Universal Numbering System

I. The most popular of these systems is the Universal numbering system.
   A. It uses the Arabic numbering system 1 through 32 for the permanent dentition.
   B. It uses letters A through T for the primary dentition.
   C. Mixed dentition may include permanent and primary teeth, so this system may use numbers and letters in a charting sequence for a particular patient.
   D. Numbering begins with the most posterior tooth on the patient's maxillary right quadrant, the third molar, tooth #1, or the permanent maxillary right third molar; if the numbering is for the primary dentition, the tooth would be #A for the primary maxillary right second molar.
   E. The numbering continues toward the anterior midline to the right central incisor, tooth #8, of the permanent dentition or tooth #E for the primary dentition.
   F. The numbering continues to the maxillary left quadrant from the midline to the most posterior tooth, either #16 of the permanent or #J of the primary dentition.
   G. The numbering then drops to the mandibular left quadrant to permanent tooth #17, primary tooth #K, across the arch to the mandibular right most posterior tooth, #32 or #T.

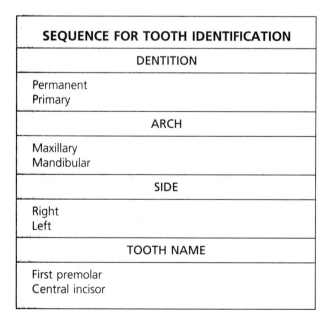

SEQUENCE FOR TOOTH IDENTIFICATION
DENTITION
Permanent Primary
ARCH
Maxillary Mandibular
SIDE
Right Left
TOOTH NAME
First premolar Central incisor

Palmer Notation System

I. The Palmer notation system assigns each of the four quadrants a bracket to designate the area of the mouth in which the tooth exists.

    A. Each permanent tooth in any quadrant is assigned the same number with #1 beginning at the midline and increasing to #8 distally.

    B. The direction of the bracket determines the arch, and the number within the bracket determines the tooth.

        Maxillary right central incisor = $1\rfloor$
        Maxillary left central incisor = $\lfloor 1$
        Mandibular left central incisor = $\lceil 1$
        Mandibular right central incisor = $1\rceil$
        Maxillary right third molar = $8\rfloor$
        Maxillary left second molar = $\lfloor 7$
        Mandibular right first premolar = $4\rceil$
        Mandibular left lateral incisor = $\lceil 2$

    C. The primary dentition uses the bracket system to assign a quadrant, but the teeth are designated by letters, A through E, instead of numbers; A specifies the central incisors and E the second molars.

The Federal Dentaire Internationale

I. The Federal Dentaire Internationale (FDI) system assigns a two-digit number to each tooth in any quadrant; the first number indicates the quadrant in which the tooth is positioned, and the second number identifies the specific tooth.

    A. The numbers 1 through 4 are assigned to the permanent dentition and 5 through 8 are assigned to the quadrants of the primary dentition.

    B. Number identification of quadrant:
        Permanent maxillary right = 1
        Permanent maxillary left = 2
        Permanent mandibular left = 3
        Permanent mandibular right = 4
        Primary maxillary right = 5
        Primary maxillary left = 6
        Primary mandibular left = 7
        Primary mandibular right = 8

    C. The second number identifies the specific tooth in the arch.

    D. Numbers 1 through 8 are the second digit assigned to the permanent dentition.

    E. Numbers 1 through 5 are for the primary dentition.

    F. #1 in both dentitions begins with the central incisors.

    G. Numbering of the teeth proceeds posteriorly so that the last tooth in the quadrant is the highest number in the sequence.

    H. This two-digit system indicates the following for the permanent dentition:

        1. Permanent maxillary right central incisor is #11, or #one one

        2. Permanent maxillary left central incisor is #21, or #two one

        3. Permanent mandibular left central incisor is #31, or #three one

        4. Permanent mandibular right central incisor is #41, or #four one

    I. The primary dentition is handled in the same manner, but because there are only five teeth per quadrant, the numbers would range from 1 through 5 for each tooth and from 5 through 8 for the quadrants.

    J. The two-digit system indicates the following for the primary dentition:

        1. Primary maxillary right first molar is #54, or #five four

        2. Primary mandibular left lateral incisor is #72, or #seven two

TOOTH SURFACES

I. All crowns of the teeth are divided into surfaces.

    A. These surfaces are identified by the anatomic position they take in relation to the oral cavity.

    B. The posterior teeth, premolars, and molars have five surfaces.

    C. The anterior teeth, incisors, and canines have four surfaces with a **ridge.**

    D. Of these surfaces, both anterior and posterior teeth have four axial surfaces.

        1. **Axial** surfaces are those surfaces that run vertically from the biting surface to the apex of a tooth.

        2. The posterior teeth have one additional surface, the occlusal surface, which is a horizontal surface running perpendicular to the other axial surfaces.

    E. The surfaces of the teeth are not only named but are also identified by letters or numbers.

        1. Surface annotation is used to chart notations and is used in all insurance claim reporting.

        2. The letter or number is commonly placed as a superscript (above the print line) next to the tooth number (e.g., the permanent maxillary left first molar involving the mesial surface using the universal numbering system is $\#14^m$ or $\#14^1$).

II. Surfaces of the teeth are identified with the following names and annotations:

A. **Mesial surface** (M or 1) is the axial surface of teeth that is closest to the midline of the mouth; it is directly opposite on the tooth from the distal surface.

B. **Distal surface** (D or 2) lies directly opposite the mesial surface on all teeth and is the axial surface furthest from the midline.

C. **Facial surface** (F or 3) is the surface of a tooth that faces the cheek and lips, or the exterior of the mouth.

D. **Labial** surface (LA or 3) is the same as the facial surface but is found facing only the lips on the anterior teeth.

E. **Buccal** surface (B or 3) is the same as the facial surface but is found on posterior teeth only facing the cheeks.

F. **Lingual** surface (L or 4) is the surface closest to the tongue on all teeth, anterior and posterior.

G. **Occlusal surface** (O or 5) is found only on posterior teeth on a vertical plane on the biting surface of the teeth.

H. **Occlusal surface** (O or 6) is found only on posterior teeth where a ridge divides the surface into two parts; the portion designated as surface 6 is the distal segment.

I. **Incisal ridge/edge/surface** (I or 5) is found only on anterior teeth where there is a biting edge.

J. The proximal area, or surface, is the surface where two teeth abut or face each other. On any given tooth, there are two proximal surfaces, the mesial and the distal; in third molars, only the mesial surface may be considered a proximal surface.

K. When more than one surface is involved, such as the mesial, occlusal, and distal surfaces, the surface annotations are placed in order from mesial to distal (e.g., #19^{MOD}).

L. The area where two surfaces on a tooth meet is a line **angle.** The angles on teeth are named by the two surfaces that meet. Examples of line angles for anterior and posterior teeth are seen in the box.

M. A point angle is the area where three surfaces meet at a point. Examples of point angles for anterior and posterior teeth are found in the box.

N. The names formed to describe either line or point angles are developed from the surfaces that are joined together; when the multiple surfaces are joined together to form one term, the *al* suffix is dropped and replaced with the letter *o*.

LINE ANGLES OF ANTERIOR AND POSTERIOR TEETH
ANTERIOR TEETH
Distolabial Mesiolabial Labioincisal Distolingual Mesiolingual Linguoincisal
POSTERIOR TEETH
Distobuccal Mesiobuccal Distolingual Mesiolingual Buccoocclusal Linguoocclusal Distoocclusal Mesioocclusal

DENTAL ANATOMY

I. Anatomic terminology related to dental anatomy is described in the boxes on pages 51-55. Each tooth has specific physical characteristics.

ORAL EMBRYOLOGY AND HISTOLOGY

I. **Embryology** is the science that deals with the origin and development of an individual organism. Oral embryology specifically examines the development of the tissues in the oral cavity.

II. **Histology** is the study of living tissues, their composition, and their function. The study of the tissues

POINT ANGLES OF ANTERIOR AND POSTERIOR TEETH
ANTERIOR TEETH
Mesiolabioincisal Distolabioincisal Mesiolinguoincisal Distolinguoincisal
POSTERIOR TEETH
Mesiobuccoocclusal Distobuccoocclusal Mesiolinguoocclusal Distolinguoocclusal

ANATOMIC TERMS

Cingulum - a prominence of enamel on the lingual surface of anterior teeth and referred to as a lobe

Concave - a curvature that leans inward, opposite of convex

Contact area - the area of a tooth that physically touches the abutment tooth; the contact areas occur on the proximal surfaces of the teeth

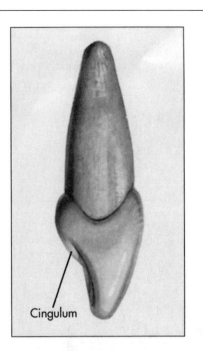

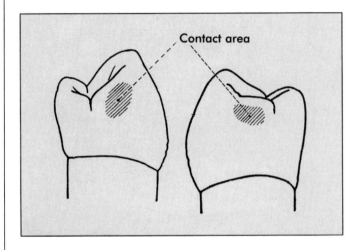

Convex - a curvature that extends outward, opposite of concave

Curve of Spee - the curve upward that the maxillary and mandibular arches form when the two are in occlusion

Cusp - a prominence of large tooth structure found on canines, premolars, and molars

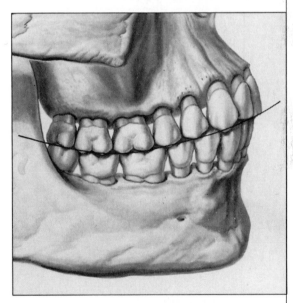

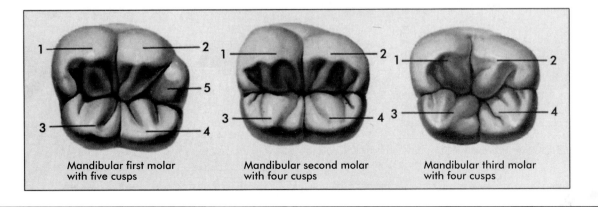

Mandibular first molar with five cusps

Mandibular second molar with four cusps

Mandibular third molar with four cusps

Continued.

ANATOMIC TERMS—cont'd

Developmental groove - a line on the surface of the tooth that separate distinct portions of the tooth from each other

Diastema - a spacing between two adjacent teeth

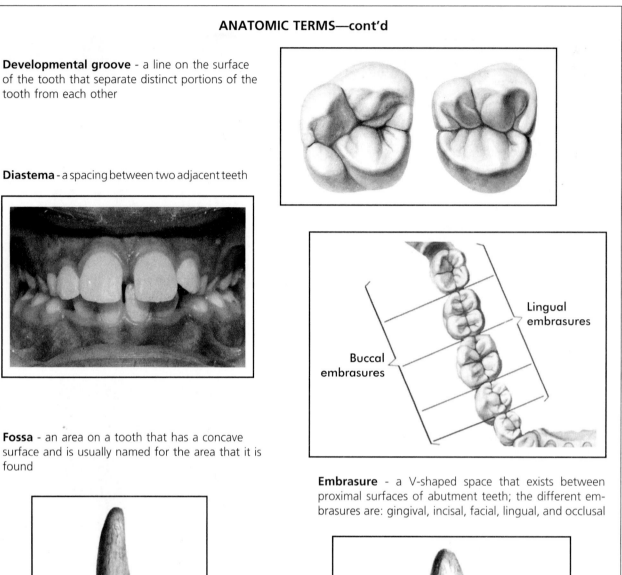

Fossa - an area on a tooth that has a concave surface and is usually named for the area that it is found

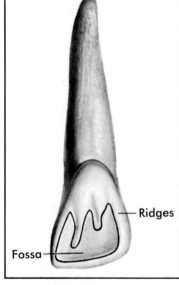

Lingual groove - a line that separates the cingulum from the other lobes that exist on the tooth

Embrasure - a V-shaped space that exists between proximal surfaces of abutment teeth; the different embrasures are: gingival, incisal, facial, lingual, and occlusal

ANATOMIC TERMS—cont'd

Lobes - a growth center that forms together with other developmental structures to combine as the crowns of teeth

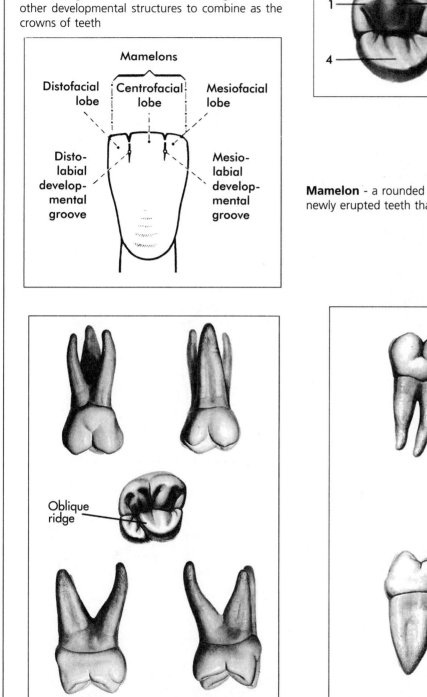

Oblique ridge - an elevated line on the occlusal surface crossing from mesiolingual cusp to the distobuccal cusp of maxillary molars

(Courtesy of Zeisz and Nuckolls.)

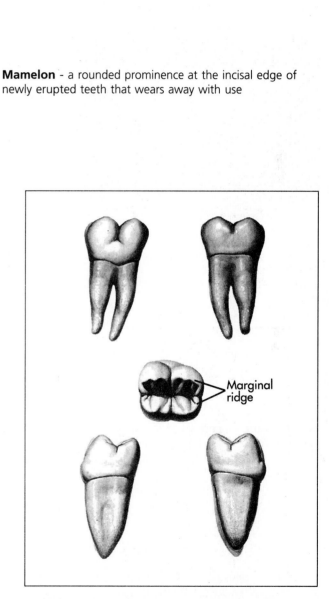

Mamelon - a rounded prominence at the incisal edge of newly erupted teeth that wears away with use

Marginal ridge - rounded areas on the proximal surfaces of teeth where contact may exist with the abutment teeth, creating embrasures

(Courtesy of Zeisz and Nuckolls.)

Continued.

ANATOMIC TERMS—cont'd

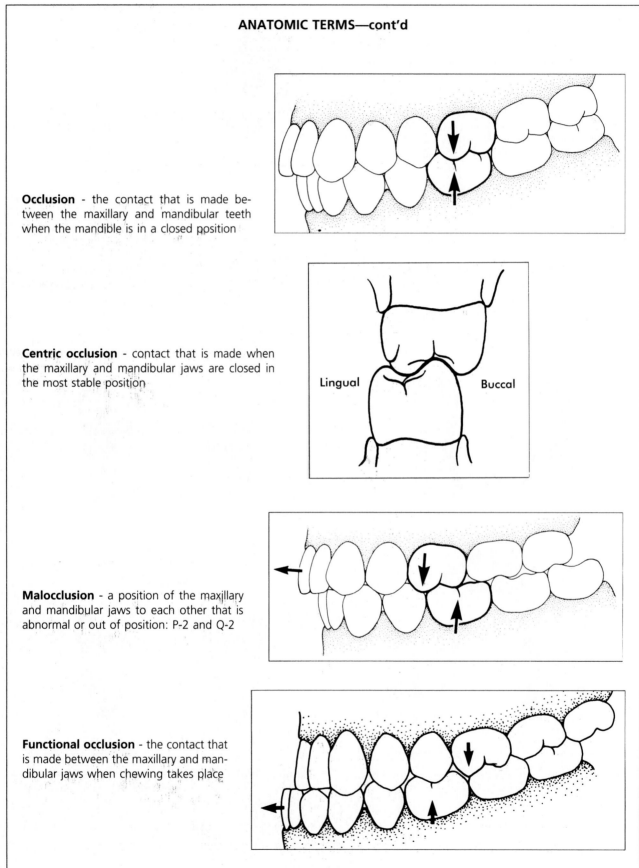

Occlusion - the contact that is made between the maxillary and mandibular teeth when the mandible is in a closed position

Centric occlusion - contact that is made when the maxillary and mandibular jaws are closed in the most stable position

Lingual   Buccal

Malocclusion - a position of the maxillary and mandibular jaws to each other that is abnormal or out of position: P-2 and Q-2

Functional occlusion - the contact that is made between the maxillary and mandibular jaws when chewing takes place

Overbite - the overlap of the maxillary teeth over the mandibular teeth when the mouth is closed

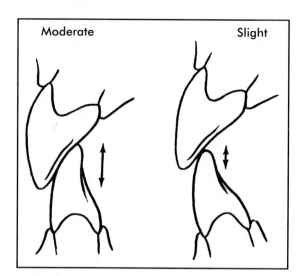

Moderate   Slight

Overjet - the horizontal projection of the maxillary teeth when they are occluded with the mandibular teeth

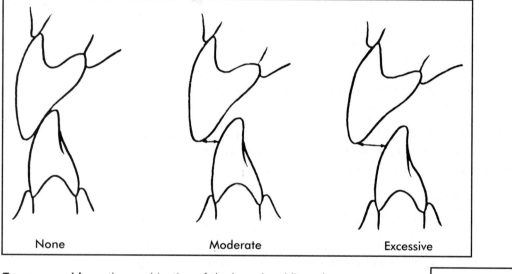

None   Moderate   Excessive

Transverse ridge - the combination of the buccal and lingual triangular ridge; this crosses the occlusal surface of posterior teeth, dividing it into two segments

Triangular ridge - a line that runs from the tip of a cusp to the occlusal surface

Tubercle - a small layer of enamel on the crown of the tooth

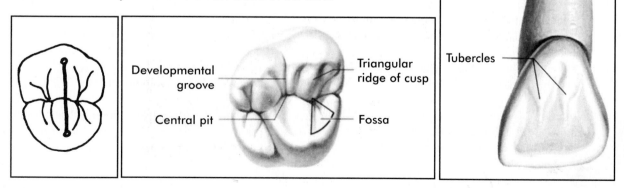

Developmental groove

Triangular ridge of cusp

Central pit

Fossa

Tubercles

of the teeth and the surrounding structures is called oral histology.

III. Long before the primary teeth of an infant have erupted into the oral cavity, development and growth have occurred in the body that allow tooth eruption to evolve.

A. Fetal cells are proliferating, differentiating, and integrating to form the primary embryonic cell layers that eventually become the human body.

B. The embryonic layers of the fetus are as follows:
1. Ectoderm
2. Endoderm
3. Mesoderm

C. **Ectoderm** forms the epithelium, nervous system, organs of special sense, mucosal tissues, tooth enamel, and hair and nails.

D. **Endoderm** produces lining for the cavities and passages of the body and internal organs.

E. **Mesoderm** forms the dentin, cementum, and pulp of the teeth, as well as circulatory and reproductive systems, kidneys, bones, connective tissue, muscles, blood, and abdominal lining.

F. The branchial arches, apparent during the fourth week of fetal development, are five defined areas that develop into structures of the head and neck.
1. The branchial arches produce the human face at approximately 5 to 8 weeks, with increased development of the dental arches and face.
2. During the fourth month the hard and soft palates of the fetus and the primary dentition have begun to form.
3. The increased growth activity and development of the fetus produce a head and face.
4. The oral cavity of the infant continues to change during the modeling or alteration that occurs during growth.

PARTS OF THE TOOTH

I. Each tooth has a **crown** and a root.
A. The crown is covered with enamel.
B. The root is covered with cementum.
C. The area where the enamel and cementum meet is the cementoenamel junction (CEJ), or cervical line.
D. The portion of the crown that is visibly seen above the gingival or tissue line is the clinical crown.
E. A portion of the crown that extends below the gingival line and includes the clinical crown is referred to as the anatomical crown.

1. Throughout the life cycle of the tooth, the anatomical crown remains the same, extending from the occlusal/incisal edge of the tooth to the CEJ.
2. The clinical crown may vary with age as soft tissue recedes.

F. The tooth must erupt through bone and gingival tissue for the crown to be visible.

G. The root remains within the alveolar process, specifically in the alveolus.
1. The root may be single or multiple.
2. The anatomic junction of the roots and crown is referred to as the **furcation.** If the tooth has multiple roots, this area is either a bifurcation (a division into two roots) or a trifurcation (a division into three roots).
3. Each root has an apex, or end, that is set in the dental arch.

TISSUES OF THE TOOTH

I. Tissues of the tooth (hard or soft)
A. Hard tissues include the enamel, dentin, and cementum.
B. Soft tissue is the pulp.

II. Enamel
A. The outer layer of the anatomic crown ends at the cervical line and is formed from **ameloblasts**—enamel-producing cells.
B. **Enamel** is a hard calcified tissue composed of 96% inorganic and 4% organic material and water.
C. The color of enamel varies from tooth to tooth, depending on the thickness and mineralization of the tissue.
1. The enamel appears whiter at a thick point, such as the middle of the crown.
2. As the enamel becomes thinner, the color and translucency vary, possibly showing the yellow of the underlying dentin.

III. Dentin
A. **Dentin** lies under the surrounding enamel and cementum that cover the crown and the root.
B. Dentin is the largest portion of tooth tissue.
C. Dentin is also a calcified tissue but is not as hard as enamel.
D. Dentin is yellow and contributes to the difference in tooth coloring because of the varying degrees of enamel translucency.
E. Dentin consists of approximately 70% inorganic and 30% organic material and water.
F. Dentin is formed from **odontoblasts**—dentin-producing cells—just as enamel is formed from ameloblasts.

G. Unlike enamel, dentin is able to repair itself after trauma; this occurs as the odontoblasts form secondary dentin, or reparative dentin, to protect the pulpal tissues in the area disturbed by the trauma.

H. Formation of this reparative tissue is unique in that dentin is the only tooth tissue that can be formed after the eruption process has been completed.

I. Dentin is also a porous tissue that forms as microscopic tubes (known as **dentinal tubules**).
   1. Dentinal tubules begin at the pulpal tissues and extend to the enamel or cementum junctions.
   2. As decay penetrates the enamel tissues to the dentin, the carious bacteria may travel quickly through the dentinal tubules to the **pulp.**

IV. Cementum
   A. **Cementum** covers the root of the tooth and the dentin of this area.
   B. Cementum consists of approximately 50% organic and 50% inorganic material, resulting in a tissue softer than enamel and dentin.
   C. The function of cementum is to provide an attachment for the periodontal fibers to the alveolar bone where the tooth rests in the alveolar socket.
   D. Cementum is similar to bone in its consistency; however, it does not have the same resorption ability as bone.
   E. Cementum is thinner at the cervical line, the point where the dentin and cementum meet, the dentinocemental junction, than it is at the apex of the root.
   F. Cementum is formed by **cementoblasts**—cementum-producing cells—that are acellular and cellular cementum.
      1. The acellular cementum forms and covers the complete root as it develops.
      2. The cellular cementum is found only in the apical third of the root and is able to regenerate, as does dentin.
      3. During a patient's life, attrition, or wearing of the crown surface, occurs; cellular cementum can lay down additional cell layers in the apical area, aiding in additional occlusal eruption and maintaining occlusal balance.

V. Pulp
   A. Blood and lymphatic vessels, nerve and connective tissues, and odontoblasts all combine to form the pulpal tissues.
   B. In a young person the pulp chamber (found in the coronal portion of the tooth) is larger than it is in that of an older individual.
   C. The odontoblasts (found immediately surrounding the pulpal tissues) continue to form layers of secondary dentin as trauma occurs, decreasing the size of the pulp.
   D. Parts of the pulp include:
      1. The coronal pulp, or pulp chamber (found in the crown of the tooth), has peaks that extend toward the cusps and are referred to as pulp horns.
      2. The pulp canal or root canal extends the length of the root, carrying the blood and nerve vessels to the apical foramen.
      3. The **apical foramen** is a channel connecting the blood, nerve, lymph, and connective tissues to the interior of the tooth to provide necessary nourishment.
   E. When the pulpal tissues are invaded by bacteria or when damage occurs by other means, the reparative dentin is formed for protection; if trauma is too severe, the vascular supply may diminish or disappear, causing subsequent death of the tooth.

SUPPORTING TISSUES OF THE ORAL CAVITY ■

I. A variety of tissues contribute to the function of the tooth within the oral cavity.
   A. The **periodontium** is the connective tissue found between the cementum of the root and the bony alveolar process.
      1. It is formed by cells called fibroblasts.
      2. The periodontium supports and suspends the tooth in the alveolus.
      3. It also protects the tooth and provides nourishment and sensory reception.
      4. The periodontium is also vascular with the supply arriving from the bone, proceeding through the alveolus and into the periodontal ligament.
      5. The parts of the periodontium are listed in the box on page 58.
   B. The bone of the alveolar process to which the periodontal ligament attaches is referred to as the **lamina dura.**
      1. The lamina dura can be seen as a radiopaque or dark line on a radiograph because of the dense nature of the bone.
      2. The blood and lymph vessels and the nerve supply of the tooth travel through openings in the lamina dura at the apex of the tooth.
      3. The periodontal ligament attaches to the lamina dura of the alveolar process; the fibers

---

THE PERIODONTIUM

The periodontal ligament supports and suspends the tooth in position with fibers that attach to the alveolar process or the cementum.

The cementum has fibers that attach to it from the periodontal ligament.

The alveolar process supports and stabilizes the tooth.

The attached **gingiva** is the keratinized (leathery) tissue that is firmly attached to bone and cementum. It connects to the free gingiva at the free gingival junction and extends apically until it meets the alveolar mucosa. It is the visible portion of the periodontium.

The free gingiva fills the interdental spaces by covering structures. It is the interdental papilla and creates the gingival sulcus. It is the visible portion of the periodontium.

---

that attach to the cementum are called Sharpey's fibers.

C. The oral **mucosa** consists of the lining mucosa and the masticatory mucosa.

1. The lining mucosa is found on the cheeks, lips, vestibule, and floor of the mouth, as well as on the soft palate and underside of the tongue.

   a. These tissues are highly vascular and flexible, allowing ease in movement during speech and mastication.

   b. Some tissues in the cheeks, lips, vestibule, and palate are smooth in appearance and are less susceptible to injury compared to the floor of the mouth and the underside of the tongue.

2. The masticatory mucosa is stronger than the lining mucosa to withstand trauma during the act of mastication.

   a. This tissue is not as flexible; it covers the free and attached gingiva, hard palate, and dorsal surface of the tongue.

TOOTH DEVELOPMENT AND ERUPTION ▬▬

I. The development of a tooth is seen in stages that begin during the fifth or sixth week in utero, with the formation of small tooth buds.

A. The thickening of the oral epithelium is the dental lamina.

1. The dental lamina is a U-shaped band of tissue on the future developing alveolar arches.

2. The thickening develops throughout the arches in different areas—10 in the maxillary and 10 in the mandibular.

3. This thickening eventually evolves into the enamel of the primary dentition.

4. The enamel forms from the ectoderm, which is the outer embryonic germ layer.

B. The stages of tooth development:

1. The bud stage pertains to the enamel organ, condensed areas of ectomesenchyme cells that are continuous with oral epithelium. The connection between the two is referred to as the dental lamina.

2. The **cap stage** determines the future shape of the tooth. Cells specialize to form the enamel organ.

3. The **bell stage** is when the primitive cells of the cap stage histodifferentiate, or change, and their functions become specialized. During the eighth week in utero, three main parts of the bud are formed: the dental organ, dental papilla, and dental sac.

4. Near the fourteenth week in utero, a fourth layer develops in the bell stage called the *stratum intermedium,* which is located between the inner enamel epithelium and the stellate reticulum.

5. During the bell stage, the inner enamel epithelium is producing cells—ameloblasts, or enamel-producing cells. The dental papilla converts some cells to odontoblasts, or dentin-producing cells. The dental lamina produces the **primordium,** superior to the primary tooth bud, which is the area responsible for the formation of the permanent tooth bud. This area is also referred to as the successional lamina. The dental sac cells differentiate into cementoblasts, cementum-producing cells, or **fibroblasts,** periodontal–ligament-producing cells. The alveolar bone is also developing around the tooth bud.

6. The advanced bell stage begins during the eighteenth week in utero. The ameloblasts and odontoblasts begin to produce enamel and dentin, which means that amelogenesis and odontogenesis are occurring, forming the crown of the tooth. The dental papilla develops into the pulp, which consists of blood vessels and lymphatic, nerve, and fibrous tissues, as well as odontoblasts. The dental lamina disappears at this time, and the primordium migrates to the lingual side of the continually developing bud.

C. The formation of the root of the tooth is the first stage of the eruption cycle and begins after the enamel and dentin have completely formed an outline of the crown.
   1. The dental organ has collapsed and the ameloblasts have reduced function to only the enamel cuticle, or Nasmyth's membrane —a thin coating on the surface of the tooth that abrades as the tooth enters the oral cavity.
   2. The outer enamel epithelium and the inner enamel epithelium form layers referred to as Hertwig's epithelial root sheath. The cells grow downward into the connective tissue, forming the root development.
   3. The dental papilla lies within the forming root structure and the dental sac outside, aiding in the formation and shaping of the root and allowing odontoblasts and cementoblasts to continue their functions.
   4. The root sheath grows inward, forming the epithelial diaphragm that develops the shape and the number of roots for each tooth.
   5. With the continued formation of dentin and cementum, the growth of the tooth, or apposition, occurs.
D. As the development of the tooth occurs, so does the development of the alveolar process.
   1. This combination action forces the tooth into the proper position in the oral cavity.
   2. As the tooth begins to erupt through the oral mucosa into the oral cavity, only a fragment of the root has actually formed.
   3. It takes 1 to 3 years for a deciduous tooth and nearly 3 years for a permanent tooth to completely erupt, with the deposition of the hard tissues of the root.

ERUPTION SEQUENCE FOR PRIMARY AND PERMANENT DENTITION ▬▬▬▬

I. The primary and permanent dentition erupt at different times in the life of a human, even though the teeth are forming in utero.
   A. The first eruption of the primary teeth usually occurs around 6 to 8 months of age.
   B. The succeeding teeth erupt at different times, depending upon the individual. The permanent teeth normally begin to erupt near age 6. Table 4-1 lists the common eruption sequence for both primary and permanent dentition.
   C. Active eruption process occurs as the teeth/ crowns become properly positioned in the dental arch.

Table 4-1 Tooth eruption sequence

Primary teeth	Normal eruption time in months
Mandibular central incisors	6
Mandibular lateral incisors	7
Maxillary central incisors	7½
Maxillary lateral incisors	8
Mandibular first molars	12 to 16
Maxillary first molars	14
Mandibular canines	16
Maxillary canines	18
Mandibular second molars	20
Maxillary second molars	24

Permanent teeth	Normal eruption time in years
Mandibular first molars	6 to 7
Maxillary first molars	6 to 7
Mandibular central incisors	6 to 7
Mandibular lateral incisors	7 to 8
Maxillary central incisors	7 to 8
Maxillary lateral incisors	8 to 9
Mandibular canines	9 to 10
Maxillary first premolars	10 to 11
Mandibular first premolars	10 to 12
Maxillary second premolars	11 to 12
Mandibular second premolars	11 to 12
Maxillary canines	11 to 12
Mandibular second molars	11 to 13
Maxillary second molars	12 to 13
Third molars	17 to 21

D. A second phase of eruption may occur, passive eruption, which arises when additional tooth structure is exposed supragingivally.
E. **Attrition,** the wearing away of the tooth structure caused by contact with other surfaces, may also occur, thereby causing passive eruption.

Questions

Intraoral Structures

1 The fold of tissue that attaches the lip to the oral mucosa above the maxillary central incisors is the
a. Labial frenum
b. Lingual frenum
c. Mucobuccal fold
d. Incisive papilla

2 The tissue of a tooth that most closely resembles bone is the
a. Pulp
b. Dentin

c. Enamel
d. Cementum

3 Each of the following is a muscle of mastication *except*
a. Temporal m.
b. Masseter m.
c. Anterior palatine m.
d. Median pterygoid m.

4 In the human embryo, during the third week of development, the first branchial arch divides to form the mandibular arch and the
a. Hyoid arch
b. Maxillary process
c. Branchial pouch
d. Thyrohyoid arch

5 The parotid duct opens on the inner surface of the cheek opposite the
a. Maxillary first molar
b. Mandibular first molar
c. Maxillary second premolars
d. Mandibular second premolars

6 In formation of a tooth the dental organ arises from the
a. Dental sac
b. Dental lamina
c. Dental papilla
d. Dental cuticle

7 A mixed dentition consists of the following:
a. Deciduous and permanent teeth existing simultaneously in a child's mouth
b. Deciduous teeth that are ankylosed
c. Permanent teeth that are rotated
d. Supernumerary permanent teeth

8 The relationship of the maxillary and mandibular teeth when they contact is called
a. Contact point
b. Vertical dimension at rest
c. Occlusion
d. Lateral excursion

Using the information provided below complete the following chart by indicating in the blank spaces the tooth number for each of the teeth within each system.

	Universal (ADA)	Palmer	FDI
9	#32	___	___

a. 8| and 48
b. |8 and 48
c. 8| and 48
d. |8 and 48

10	___	6|	___

a. 30 and 46
b. 19 and 42
c. 30 and 26
d. 46 and 30

11	#24	___	___

a. 1| and 11
b. 8 and 31
c. |1 and 31
d. 31 and 8

12	___	___	44

a. 22 and 4
b. |4 and 22
c. 28 and 4|
d. 20 and 6

13	#T	___	___

a. 10 and 85
b. E and 85
c. T and 85
d. 85 and 10

14	#8	___	___

a. 1| and 11
b. 21 and 8
c. 1 and 21
d. 21 and 1

15	___	___	#82

a. Q and B
b. Q and D
c. D and Q
d. B and Q

16 If a tooth is numbered 30 in the universal numbering system, what is the same tooth numbered in the opposite quadrant of the same arch?
a. 3
b. 14
c. 18

17 What is this same tooth (#30) numbered if it is on the same quadrant in the opposite arch?
a. 3
b. 14
c. 18

18 The cells responsible for the formation of enamel are
a. Ameloblasts
b. Odonotoclasts
c. Ameloclasts
d. Odontoblasts

19 The cells responsible for the formation of cementum are
a. Ameloblasts
b. Cementoblasts
c. Cementoclasts
d. Odontoblasts

20 The cells responsible for the formation of dentin are
a. Ameloblasts
b. Cementoblasts
c. Odontoblasts
d. Fibroblasts

21 Which of the following is not part of the enamel organ?
a. Outer enamel epithelium
b. Inner enamel epithelium
c. Stellate reticulum
d. Dental lamina

22 At what age do the permanent second molars normally erupt?
a. 8 years
b. 10 years
c. 12 years

23 At what age does all the primary dentition normally erupt?
   a. 2 to 24 months
   b. 6 to 12 months
   c. 6 to 24 months

24 At what age does the permanent maxillary incisors normally erupt?
   a. 4 years
   b. 5 years
   c. 7 years

25 At what age does the maxillary central incisor typically erupt.
   a. 4 years of age
   b. 7 years of age
   c. 10 years of age

Rationales

Intraoral Structures

1 A The labial frenum is positioned between the maxillary central incisors, while the lingual frenum is beneath the tongue. The mucobuccal fold is the area in which the lip connects to the mucosa and the incisive papilla is directly behind the maxillary central incisors.

2 D The cementum covers the root of the tooth and areas of the dentin. Cementum, a connective tissue, most closely resembles bone tissue in its composition.

3 C The anterior palatine muscle does not exist.

4 B The maxillary and mandibular processes form at the same time in utero during the third week of pregnancy.

5 A The parotid duct exits near the maxillary first molars; the mandibular premolars and molars are near the submandibular and sublingual glands. The maxillary second premolars are not positioned near a gland.

6 B The dental organ develops in the bud stage as the dental lamina extends downward into the tissue.

7 A A mixed dentition occurs when a child has not exfoliated all the primary dentition before the eruption of the permanent dentition. This may begin to occur at approximately 6 years of age as the permanent incisors erupt, causing both permanent and deciduous teeth to exist simultaneously in the oral cavity.

8 C The contact between the masticatory tooth surfaces of the maxillary and mandibular teeth during closure is known as occlusion.

9 A The permanent mandibular right third molar is known as #32 in the Universal, 8⌐ in the Palmer, and 48 in the FDI systems.

10 A The permanent mandibular right first molar is known as #30 in the Universal, 6⌐ in the Palmer, and 46 in the FDI systems.

11 C The permanent mandibular left central incisor is known as #24 in the Universal, ⌐1 in the Palmer, and 31 in the FDI systems.

12 C The permanent mandibular right first premolar is known as #28 in the Universal, 4⌐ in the Palmer, and 44 in the FDI systems.

13 B The primary mandibular right molar is known as #T in the Universal, E⌐ in the Palmer, and 85 in the FDI systems.

14 A The permanent maxillary right central incisor is known as #8 in the Universal, 1⌐ in the Palmer, and 11 in the FDI systems.

15 A The primary mandibular right cuspid is known as #Q in the Universal, B⌐ in the Palmer, and 82 in the FDI systems.

16 C Tooth #30 in the Universal Numbering system is the permanent mandibular right first molar, that same tooth in the opposite quadrant is #18. Also refer to definitions in Nos. 9–15.

17 A Since numbering begins with the maxillary right quadrant in the Universal system the maxillary right first molar is #3. Refer to definitions in Nos. 9–15.

18 A Ameloblasts form enamel, odontoclasts destroy dentin, ameloclasts destroy enamel and odontoblasts create dentin.

19 B Cells with the suffix -*blast* create and those with the suffix -*clast* destroy cells. Cementoblasts create cementum.

20 C Refer to No. 19. These cells form the surface layer of the dental papilla that is responsible for the formation of the dentin of a tooth.

21 D The dental lamina is the oral epithelium that is present at birth. The enamel organ continues a downward growth and consists of the stellate reticulum and inner and outer enamel epithelium.

22 C The maxillary and mandibular second molars erupt at approximately 12 years of age.

23 C The primary dentition normally beings eruption at approximately 6 months and is usually completed near 24 months.

24 C The permanent maxillary incisors usually erupt at approximately the same time as the mandibular lateral incisors at 6–7 years of age.

25 B Generally, the permanent maxillary central incisors erupt between the ages of 7 to 8 years. At about the same time the permanent maxillary and mandibular first molars will be present.

To enhance your understanding of the material in this chapter, refer to the illustrations in Chapter 4 of Finkbeiner/Johnson: *Mosby's Comprehensive Dental Assisting: A Clinical Approach.*

CHAPTER 5

Nutrition and Dental Health

OUTLINE

Digestion
Nutrition and Nutrients
Diet and Nutrition
Recommended Dietary Allowance

Food Pyramid
Energy-releasing Nutrients
Non–energy-releasing Nutrients
Nutritional Information

Carbohydrates and Dental Caries
Health Risks Related to Diet
Medicine, Drugs, and Nutrition

KEY TERMS

Calorie/kilocalorie

Carbohydrate

Disaccharide

Fat

Fat soluble

Fructose

Galactose

Glucose

Metabolize

Mineral

Monosaccharide

Nutrient

Polysaccharide

Protein

Saccharin

Sucrose

Vitamin

Water soluble

As a health care provider the dental assistant has a dual responsibility in the study of nutrition. First, understanding the way proper nutrition nourishes the body and maintains it in optimal condition is necessary. Second, the dental assistant is a resource person for the patient who seeks answers to nutritional questions. The study of nutrition changes rapidly as research continues to unfold new discoveries. Consequently, frequent reviews of nutritional literature and updates are necessary to remain current with trends. This chapter provides a basic knowledge of nutrition as it pertains to you, the patient, and good oral health.

DIGESTION

I. To use the food the body receives, it passes through several stages.

A. Breakdown
B. Digestion
C. Absorption
D. Metabolism
E. Two types of digestion:
   1. Mechanical
   2. Chemical

Mechanical Digestion

I. Mechanical digestion occurs in the oral cavity and stomach.
   A. The teeth and tongue break down the larger mass of food into smaller, easier-to-digest pieces.
   B. When the food reaches the stomach, it is further broken down mechanically for easier absorption into the system.

Chemical Digestion

I. Chemical digestion involves enzymes and other body chemicals.
   A. The enzyme ptyalin, or salivary amylase, combines with the food in the mouth. The function is to chemically digest carbohydrates.
   B. The partially digested food passes to the stomach through the pharynx and esophagus.
   C. In the stomach, mechanical mixing takes place with the gastric juice; it contains hydrochloric acid and enzymes such as protease (pepsin), which acts on proteins; rennin, which breaks down dairy products; and lipase, which helps digest emulsified fats.
   D. The small intestine continues the digestion process; bile, which is produced by the liver and stored in the gallbladder, is used to further chemically reduce the fat molecules.
      1. The pancreas also produces enzymes called *pancreatic juices* that are released into the small intestine during the digestion process; these include protease, lipase, and amylase and are used to break down proteins, fats, and carbohydrates, respectively.
      2. Additional enzymes are created by the small intestine itself, forming intestinal juices that are a blend of lactase, maltase, and sucrase, all of which act on carbohydrates, and peptidases, which aid in the digestion of proteins.
   E. The food products then progress to the large intestine where bacterial enzymes break down dietary fiber.
      1. The large intestine also absorbs water and minerals and synthesizes some of the B-complex vitamins and vitamin K.
      2. Digestion is completed in the large intestine.
      3. Any undigested products and waste materials are excreted from the body.
   F. When a food product has been sufficiently digested into usable molecules, it can be absorbed into the body, primarily through blood and lymph fluids.
      1. The small intestine is the primary site for this absorption.
      2. The intestinal walls are specifically designed to absorb nutrients into the blood and lymph fluids.
      3. Once absorbed, the nutrients are available to be metabolized or used by the body tissues to perform specific body functions.

NUTRITION AND NUTRIENTS

I. Nutrition is a science that relates diet to health.
   A. Nutrition is concerned with the way the body uses food for the growth, development, and maintenance of tissues and structures.
   B. **Nutrients** are the chemical parts of a food that are needed by the body to carry on its activities.
      1. A nutrient can be as simple as a molecule of water, which, although it furnishes no energy, is essential to life itself.
      2. A nutrient can be as complex as a protein molecule in hemoglobin; the nutrient protein, as with carbohydrate and fat nutrients, releases energy.
      3. As the body **metabolizes** food, heat is produced and energy is released, allowing the body to carry on its many functions.
      4. The heat produced is measured in units called **calories,** also known as **kilocalories** (kcal), which are units of 1000 calories.
      5. Some nutrients do not release energy or heat and therefore do not contain kcalories; these include vitamins, minerals, and water.
      6. Fat, the most concentrated form of energy, contains 9 kcal/g (1 oz equaling approximately 30 g).
      7. Carbohydrates and protein each contain 4 kcal/g.
      8. Although the other nutrients do not release any energy, they are essential to complete body health and aid in the overall metabolism of food and many other body functions.

DIET AND NUTRITION

I. *Diet* refers to the total food (or nutrient) intake and the consumption pattern of these foods
   A. Several factors relate to a person's diet
      1. Favorite foods
      2. Family tradition
      3. Religious beliefs
      4. Aging
      5. Socioeconomic status
      6. Food sensitivities
      7. Preference for vegetarian diet
      8. Availability and convenience of certain foods
      9. Interest in food

RECOMMENDED DIETARY ALLOWANCE

I. The recommended dietary allowance (RDA) was developed in 1941 as a guide for nutritional workers in national defense and the nutritional needs of the general population.
   A. A new edition of the RDA is published approximately every 5 years.
   B. The current 1989 revision of the RDA is contained in Table 5-1.

Table 5-1 Food and Nutrition Board,
National Academy of Sciences National Research Council Recommended Dietary Allowances[a]; Revised 1989

Category	Age (years) or condition	Weight[b] (kg)	Weight[b] (lb)	Height[b] (cm)	Height[b] (in)	Protein (g)	Fat-soluble vitamins Vitamin A (μg RE)[c]	Vitamin D (μg)[d]	Vitamin E (mg α-TE)[e]	Vitamin K (μg)
Infants	0.0-0.5	6	13	60	24	13	375	7.5	3	5
	0.5-1.0	9	20	71	28	14	375	10	4	10
Children	1-3	13	29	90	35	16	400	10	6	15
	4-6	20	44	112	44	24	500	10	7	20
	7-10	28	62	132	52	28	700	10	7	30
Males	11-14	45	99	157	62	45	1000	10	10	45
	15-18	66	145	176	69	59	1000	10	10	65
	19-24	72	160	177	70	58	1000	10	10	70
	25-50	79	174	176	70	63	1000	5	10	80
	51+	77	170	173	68	63	1000	5	10	80
Females	11-14	46	101	157	62	46	800	10	8	45
	15-18	55	120	163	64	44	800	10	8	55
	19-24	58	128	164	65	46	800	10	8	60
	25-50	63	138	163	64	50	800	5	8	65
	51+	65	143	160	63	50	800	5	8	65
Pregnant						60	800	10	10	65
Lactating	1st 6 months					65	1300	10	12	65
	2nd 6 months					62	1200	10	11	65

[a]The allowances, expressed as average daily intakes over time, are intended to provide for individual variations among most normal persons as they live in the United States under usual environmental stresses. Diets should be based on a variety of common foods in order to provide other nutrients for which human requirements have been less well-defined. See text for detailed discussion of allowances and nutrients not tabulated.
[b]Weights and heights of Reference Adults are actual medians for the US populations of the designated age, as reported by NHANES II. The use of these figures does not imply that the height-to-weight ratios are ideal.

C. The RDA offers guidelines for daily nutrient consumption for healthy individuals in the US population.
   1. It is not a requirement for each specific person.
   2. The amounts stated in the RDA include a margin of safety to cover most healthy people.
   3. The needs of medically compromised persons are not contained in this listing.
   4. The acronym USRDA represents the United States Recommended Daily Allowances, which are based on the RDA. The USRDA are used on food labels to help the consumer understand the content of the package and nutritional value obtained when the food is ingested.
   5. There are currently four different USRDA listings:
      a. Infants up to age 1 year
      b. Children from age 1 to 4 years
      c. Pregnant and lactating women
      d. Healthy individuals age 4 years and older

FOOD PYRAMID

I. In 1992 the **United States Department of Agriculture (USDA)** introduced the food guide pyramid.
   A. The pyramid contains five food groups:
      1. Bread, cereal, rice, and pasta
      2. Fruits and vegetables
      3. Dairy products and meat, poultry, fish, beans, eggs, and nuts
      4. Fats, oils, and sweets
   B. The concept in the pyramid suggests that the base of the pyramid is the foundation of the diet from which the greatest daily consumption should be derived.
      1. With the increase in the number of servings in the grain, fruit, and vegetable groups (which are naturally lower in fat and kilocalories) and inclusion of a notation at the peak of the pyramid to use fats, oils, and sweets sparingly, the public is encouraged to develop healthier eating habits.
      2. As the pyramid narrows at the top, so should the amounts from each of these groups decrease to provide a healthier diet.
      3. The latest development in nutritional guid-

Designed for the Maintenance of Good Nutrition of Practically All Healthy People in the United States

Water-soluble vitamins							Minerals						
Vitamin C (mg)	Thiamin (mg)	Riboflavin (mg)	Niacin (mg NE)[f]	Vitamin B_6 (mg)	Folate (µg)	Vitamin B_{12} (µg)	Calcium (mg)	Phosphorus (mg)	Magnesium (mg)	Iron (mg)	Zinc (mg)	Iodine (µg)	Selenium (µg)
30	0.3	0.4	5	0.3	25	0.3	400	300	40	6	5	40	10
35	0.4	0.5	6	0.6	35	0.5	600	500	60	10	5	50	15
40	0.7	0.8	9	1.0	50	0.7	800	800	80	10	10	70	20
45	0.9	1.1	12	1.1	75	1.0	800	800	120	10	10	90	20
45	1.0	1.2	13	1.4	100	1.4	800	800	170	10	10	120	30
50	1.3	1.5	17	1.7	150	2.0	1200	1200	270	12	15	150	40
60	1.5	1.8	20	2.0	200	2.0	1200	1200	400	12	15	150	50
60	1.5	1.7	19	2.0	200	2.0	1200	1200	350	10	15	150	70
60	1.5	1.7	19	2.0	200	2.0	800	800	350	10	15	150	70
60	1.2	1.4	15	2.0	200	2.0	800	800	350	10	15	150	70
50	1.1	1.3	15	1.4	150	2.0	1200	1200	280	15	12	150	45
60	1.1	1.3	15	1.5	180	2.0	1200	1200	300	15	12	150	50
60	1.1	1.3	15	1.6	180	2.0	1200	1200	280	15	12	150	55
60	1.1	1.3	15	1.6	180	2.0	800	800	280	15	12	150	55
60	1.0	1.2	13	1.6	180	2.0	800	800	280	10	12	150	55
70	1.5	1.6	17	2.2	400	2.2	1200	1200	300	30	15	175	65
95	1.6	1.8	20	2.1	280	2.6	1200	1200	355	15	19	200	75
90	1.6	1.7	20	2.1	260	2.6	1200	1200	340	15	16	200	75

[c]Retinol equivalents. 1 retinol equivalent = 1 µg retinol or 6 µg β-carotene.
[d]As cholecalciferol. 10 µg cholecalciferol = 400 IU of vitamin D.
[e]α-Tocopherol equivalents. 1 mg d-α tocopherol = 1 α-TE.
[f]1 NE (niacin equivalent) is equal to 1 mg of niacin or 60 mg of dietary trytophan.

ance by the USDA illustrates a positive addition to the health of the general public.

ENERGY-RELEASING NUTRIENTS

I. Energy-releasing nutrients contain fuel or kilocalories that the body can use for energy.
   A. These nutrients provide the energy to carry on daily activities and build and repair body cells and energy to simply digest the food eaten. Table 5-2 summarizes each of these energy-releasing nutrients as they apply to dentistry.
   B. Energy-releasing nutrients include carbohydrates, fats, and proteins.

Carbohydrates

I. **Carbohydrates** are the body's main source of energy.
   A. The brain and central nervous system depend on a constant supply of carbohydrates in the form of glucose to function.
   B. Without sufficient carbohydrates the body may use protein as an alternative energy source; the use of protein in this way interferes with protein's function to build and repair cells.

C. This nutrient group includes sugars, starches, and fiber.
D. Carbohydrates provide 4 kcal/g and usually make up approximately 50% of daily kilocalorie intake.
E. Carbohydrates themselves are not fattening, but when eaten in excess or when added to other high-fat ingredients, they tend to cause weight increase.
F. Carbohydrates consist of saccharide or sugar units. Saccharides can be categorized as:
   1. **Monosaccharides** (single sugars)
   2. **Disaccharides** (double sugars)
   3. **Polysaccharides** (multiple units of sugar)
G. Processed foods contain surprisingly large amounts of sugar and should be discussed with the patient when discussing the amount of sugar in common foods. Table 5-3 may be of assistance.

Monosaccharides

I. The single sugars, monosaccharides, are glucose, fructose, and galactose.
   A. These are the simplest units, which need no further digestion.

Table 5-2 Dental Nutrient Function/Effect Chart

Nutrient	Source	Function	Effect on dental health
Carbohydrates	Grains, fruits, vegetables, legumes, tubers	Primary energy source for the body, 4 kcal g	Main component in production of dental caries
Protein	Meats, poultry, fish, eggs, legumes, nuts	Building and maintenance of body tissues Components of hormones, enzymes, and antibodies, 4 kcal g	No cariogenicity Growth and proper development of teeth and oral structures Component of collagen, the protein glue that holds cells together and aids in healing Slow healing, for example, gingival treatment or periodontal and oral surgery (if deficient)
Fat	Red meat, butter, margarine, eggs, salad oils and dressings, nuts	Cushion for vital body organs Insulation to prevent body heat loss Transport of fat-soluble vitamins, 9 kcal g	No cariogenicity Acidic saliva buffer
Water	Drinking water, beverages	Transport of water-soluble vitamins Solvent and lubricant in numerous body functions No kilocalories of energy	Acidic saliva buffer Decreased flow of saliva, less tissue lubrication, and greater caries potential (if deficient)
Sodium	Table salt, processed foods	Electrolyte that helps maintain body fluid balance	Decreased saliva flow, greater caries potential, less tissue lubrication, and increased tissue irritation (in excessive amounts)
Potassium	Widely distributed in foods: legumes, grains, potatoes, green leafy vegetables, oranges, bananas	Electrolyte that helps maintain body fluid balance	Proper amount and quality of saliva
Chloride	Table salt, processed foods	Electrolyte that helps maintain body fluid balance	Proper amount and quality of saliva
Calcium	Milk, cheese, yogurt, dark green leafy vegetables	Blood coagulation and muscle contraction Strength and stability for bones and teeth	Major component of teeth and bones
Phosphorus	Widely distributed in foods: lean meat, milk	Mineralization and maintenance of bones Proper energy metabolism	Mineralization of teeth Second most abundant mineral in tooth structure
Magnesium	Dark green leafy vegetables, nuts, legumes, whole grains	Cell respiration Stabilization of bones	Stabilization of tooth components Third most abundant mineral in tooth structure Hypoplasia during tooth development and compromised formation of periodontium (if deficient)
Fluoride	Drinking water, tea, seafood	Source of strength to bone structure, reducing susceptibility to osteoporosis	Strength and caries resistance to developing teeth Endemic fluorosis (mottled enamel) (in excessive amounts)
Iron	Meat, eggs, enriched/ fortified grains	Manufacture of protein hemoglobin Cell respiration and oxygen transport	Glossitis, angular cheilosis, atrophy of oral tissues (if deficient)
Zinc	Meat, eggs, fish, legumes, whole grains	Component of numerous body enzymes, including insulin Tissue growth and wound healing	Healing of oral tissues, for example, in gingivitis, periodontal surgery, or oral surgery Slow/difficult healing of tissues (if deficient)

Table 5-2 Dental nutrient function/effect chart—cont'd

Nutrient	Source	Function	Effect on dental health
Iodine	Iodized table salt, seafood	Manufacture of thyroid hormone thyroxine	Late tooth eruption, small jaw size (if deficient)
Copper	Organ meats, shellfish, legumes	Component in manufacture of proteins hemoglobin and collagen	Collagen needed for growth and healing of epithelial cells in the oral tissues
Selenium	Seafood, meat, organ meats, legumes, milk products	Antioxidant	Part of protein component of the teeth
Vitamin A	Dark green leafy vegetables, bright orange/yellow fruits and vegetables, liver, egg yolks	Antioxidant Bone remodeling, proper vision, health of the mucous membranes	Maintenance of health and secretions of mucous membranes Development of ameloblasts during tooth formation
Vitamin D	Sunshine, liver oils, fortified milk	Absorption of calcium and phosphorus in bone mineralization	Proper tooth calcification and on-time eruption Hypoplasia (if deficient)
Vitamin E	Eggs, liver, vegetable oils, dark green leafy vegetables	Antioxidant Stabilization of red blood cell walls	Unknown
Vitamin K	Dark green leafy vegetables, liver, egg yolks, bacteria in gastrointestinal tract can synthesize vitamin K	Blood clotting Component in manufacture of protein prothrombin	Increased gingival bleeding (if deficient)
Vitamin B_1	Pork, legumes, whole/enriched grains	Coenzyme in nutrient metabolism, especially carbohydrates	A burning tongue, sensitive oral tissues (if deficient)
Vitamin B_2—riboflavin	Meat, fish, poultry, whole grains	coenzyme in nutrient metabolism	Glossitis, angular cheilosis, swollen lips (if deficient)
Niacin	Dairy products, whole grains, meat	Coenzyme in nutrient metabolism	Angular cheilosis, glossitis (if deficient)
Vitamin B_6—pyridoxine	Chicken, pork, fish, organ meats, whole grains	Coenzyme in nutrient metabolism, especially proteins	Glossitis, angular cheilosis (if deficient)
Folacin	Dark green leafy vegetables, legumes, liver	Manufacture of red blood cells	Burning of tongue and oral tissues, angular cheilosis, gingivitis (if deficient)
Pantothenic acid	Legumes, liver, eggs, whole grains	Coenzyme in nutrient metabolism	Unknown
Biotin	Organ meats, milk, egg yolks, intestinal bacteria able to synthesize biotin	Coenzyme in nutrient metabolism	Glossitis
Vitamin B_{12}—cobalamin	Liver, milk, eggs, cheese, fish	Coenzyme in nutrient metabolism Blood cell formation	Glossitis (atrophic)
Vitamin C—ascorbic acid	Citrus fruits, green and red peppers, broccoli, cabbage, spinach	Synthesis of protein collagen	Proper tooth and bone formation/maintenance Enlarged gingiva that bleeds easily, slow/difficult healing of oral tissues (if deficient)

B. **Glucose,** also called *dextrose*, is the blood sugar required by the brain and nervous system.

C. **Fructose** is the sweetest of all monosaccharides and is found in fruits and honey and is also converted to glucose by the body.

D. **Galactose** is not found as a single sugar unit in foods but is a component of the disaccharide lactose; similar to fructose, galactose can be converted by the body to glucose.

Disaccharides

I. Disaccharides, or double sugars, are combinations of two monosaccharides.

A. These must be metabolized by the body to single sugar units to provide energy.

B. White table sugar is actually disaccharide **sucrose;** one unit of glucose and one of fructose join to form one molecule of sucrose.

C. Other sources of sucrose are powdered and

Table 5-3 Sugar in processed foods

Food	Sugar content (tsp)
1.6 oz bran muffin	1.2
5 oz canned corn	3
½ c canned fruit	4
1 T ketchup	1
12 oz soft drink	8
¾ c beans and franks	3.3
8 oz yogurt (fruit on the bottom)	7
1 T creamer	2
2 oz chocolate	8

brown sugar, molasses, and some fruits and vegetables.
   D. Lactose, or milk sugar, is another type of disaccharide.
      1. It is the main carbohydrate in milk and can be the primary source for milk bottle caries.
      2. A single unit each of glucose and galactose combine to form this sugar.
   E. Maltose is composed of two glucose units.
      1. Also called *malt sugar,* it is found in germinating seeds, although it is not commonly found in the daily diet.
      2. Maltose is obtained by the body through starch metabolism.

Polysaccharides

I. Polysaccharides, sometimes called *complex carbohydrates,* include starch, glycogen, and cellulose.
   A. Many single units of sugar join to form these large molecules.
      1. One molecule of starch may contain 3000 single glucose units.
      2. Starches are an important part of the diet and are found in plant sources—especially grain products, such as rice, wheat, corn, barley, and oats.
      3. Peas and beans, known as *legumes,* and tubers, such as potatoes and yams, are also significant sources of this nutrient.

Glycogen

I. Glycogen is not found by itself in plant sources but is actually a storage product, made by the body from glucose and reserved in the liver and muscle tissue. The body can draw on glycogen reserves whenever additional or emergency energy is required.

Fiber

I. Dietary fiber, or cellulose, has been identified as an important component of diets today.
   A. Increasing the cellulose in the diet from a daily average of 10 to 15 g to 20 to 30 g is recommended for a healthier diet and better digestion and elimination.
   B. Cellulose is found in plant sources, particularly grains, legumes, fruits, and vegetables.
      1. These contain little or no fat but provide plenty of energy.
      2. The large cellulose molecules take more time to be metabolized, creating the feeling of fullness that lasts for a long time after eating cellulose.

Fats

I. **Fats** or lipids are the most concentrated form of the energy-releasing nutrients, providing 9 kcal/g.
   A. Fats are an alternative source of energy when carbohydrates are not available.
   B. Fat provides a cushion for vital organs.
   C. Fat acts as insulation under the skin to prevent body heat loss and aids the transport and absorption of vitamins A, D, E, and K (the **fat-soluble** vitamins).
   D. Fats can be further divided into smaller components called *essential fatty acids.*
      1. The essential fatty acids linolenic and arachidonic acid cannot be produced by the body in sufficient amounts for proper body function; these must be acquired from dietary sources.
      2. Technically, linolenic acid is the only true essential dietary fatty acid; when sufficient amounts are present, the body can synthesize the other two.
      3. Metabolism of other fats and cholesterol and cell membrane strength are associated with an adequate intake of these nutrients.
      4. Deficiency symptoms include dermatitis and compromised wound healing. Important sources of these nutrients include the oils: corn, cottonseed, peanut, soybean, and safflower.
   E. Foods that provide fat include meats, nuts, salad oils and dressings, olives, avocados, eggs, milk, butter, and margarine.
      1. The American diet contains an average of 40% to 45% fat.
      2. The American Heart Association has suggested lowering that amount to a healthier

30% to reduce the risks of some forms of cancer and heart disease.

Protein

I. The major functions of **protein** are building and maintaining body tissue and aiding in nutrient metabolism.
   A. Proteins are necessary components of the body hormones, enzymes, and antibodies.
   B. Protein provides 4 kcal/g.
   C. Protein can be used by the body as an optional energy source but only when carbohydrates and fats are not in ample supply.
   D. Amino acids are the building blocks of the protein molecule.
      1. There are 20 to 22 amino acids, 8 to 10 of which are classified as essential.
      2. Essential amino acids cannot be made or synthesized by the body and must be obtained from food.
   E. Proteins are classified as complete or incomplete. An egg is an example of a complete protein because it possesses all the essential amino acids.
   F. Complete and high-quality proteins are usually derived from animal sources, such as meat, fish, poultry, eggs, milk, and cheese. Plant sources such as legumes, grains, seeds, and nuts also provide essential amino acids but often not in the amounts needed; thus they are referred to as *incomplete proteins.*

NON–ENERGY-RELEASING NUTRIENTS ▄▄▄

I. Non–energy-releasing nutrients contain no kilocalories for use by the body.
   A. They are essential to many important body functions, including nutrient metabolism and formation of blood cells, enzymes, and healthy bones and teeth.
   B. If these nutrients are not obtained through the diet, numerous body functions will be impaired and deficiency symptoms will become evident. Table 5-2 summarizes the way each of these non–energy-releasing nutrients applies to dentistry.

Vitamins

I. **Vitamins** are essential nutrients that provide no energy, contain no kilocalories, and are needed in only small amounts (Table 5-2).
   A. The major function of vitamins is to assist in the metabolism of other nutrients to release energy for the body's use. Vitamins also aid in the prevention of certain dental anomalies such as glossitis, help prevent periodontal disease, and promote healing of oral tissues.
   B. **Water-soluble** vitamins include vitamins B_1 (thiamin), B_2 (riboflavin and niacin), B_6 (pyridoxine), B_{12} (cobalamin), B complex (folacin, pantothenic acid, and biotin), and C.
   C. All nine water-soluble vitamins share the following characteristics:
      1. Needed every day
      2. Not stored in the body
      3. Readily show deficiencies
      4. Are organic, contain nitrogen
      5. Easily destroyed in cooking and processing
      6. Not usually toxic unless taken in large doses
      7. Excreted in the urine (excess amounts)
   D. Fat-soluble vitamins include vitamins A, D, E, and K, and all possess the following characteristics:
      1. Not excreted
      2. Not needed every day
      3. Can be toxic (excess amounts)
      4. Are organic
      5. Stored in the body in liver and fatty tissue until used

Major Minerals

I. **Minerals** are categorized based on two factors: the amount of the mineral present in the body and the amount needed in the daily diet.
   A. A major mineral must be present in the body in amounts larger than 5 g, and the daily dietary requirement must be at least 100 mg per day. These include the following:
      1. Calcium
      2. Phosphorus
      3. Magnesium
      4. Sulfur
      5. Potassium
      6. Chloride
      7. Sodium
      8. Water
   B. Trace minerals, or microminerals, are so named because of the small amounts (less than 100 mg) needed daily by the body for proper function. Trace minerals include iron, zinc, iodine, selenium, copper, and fluorine.

NUTRITIONAL INFORMATION ▄▄▄

I. The American Diabetes Association, American Heart Association, and American Dietetic Association have provided specialized diet exchange menus

A. Cookbook publishers, the press, and the USDA have expended much expertise in providing nutritional information to the public concerning food labels and recipes, such as the one shown in the box below.

B. Food exchange diets are common in diet management.

    1. This concept is used by patients who are on specialized diets, such as individuals with di-

---

RECIPE
THREE-BEAN BAKED BEANS

½ lb bacon, diced   ½ tsp chili powder
½ lb ground beef   1 tsp black pepper
1 large onion, peeled   ½ tsp salt
  ends removed,   1 16 oz can butter
  chopped   beans, drained
½ c brown sugar   1 16 oz can kidney
½ c granulated sugar   beans, drained
¼ c ketchup   1 31 oz can pork
¼ c barbecue sauce   and beans, drained
2 tsp prepared mustard
2 tsp molasses

Preheat oven to 350° B. In a large skillet, brown bacon, beef, and onion over medium heat; drain. Transfer to a 3- to 4-quart baking dish, and mix in brown sugar, granulated sugar, ketchup, barbecue sauce, mustard, molasses, chili powder, pepper, salt, butter beans, kidney beans, and pork and beans.

Bake 1 hour. Remove from oven and serve. Serves 8 to 10 people. COOK'S NOTE: To reduce the calories, fat, and sodium, make these changes. Use ¼ lb bacon, ¼ lb ground beef, ¼ c granulated sugar, and ¼ low-sodium ketchup; omit the salt; drain and rinse the beans. Note the difference in the following nutritional information.

Nutritional details per serving

Original Recipe	Healthier Version
Calories.................449	Calories.................340
% of calories from fat 36%	% of calories from fat 27%
Fat Protein Carbohydrates	Fat Protein Carbohydrates
18 gm 16 gm 56 gm	10 gm 13 gm 51 gm
Cholesterol Sodium	Cholesterol Sodium
40 mg 1,070 mg	23 mg 590 mg
Diabetic Exchanges	Diabetic Exchanges
2½ starch, 1 lean meat	2¼ starch, ½ lean meat
½ vegetable, 1½ fruit, 3 fat	¼ vegetable, 1 fruit, 1½ fat

---

abetes and cardiovascular disease, or by individuals on a weight reduction diet.

    2. The concept refers to the exchange of various foods within one of the basic groups: milk or dairy, meat, bread or starch, vegetables, fruit, or fat. Table 5-4 illustrates the exchange concept.

II. The Nutritional Labeling and Education Act requires manufacturers to list all ingredients in the product.

A. Prepackaged products are required to use metric and standard units of measurement.

B. Various nutrients are listed on the labels, including total calories, calories from fat, total fat, saturated fat, cholesterol, sodium, total carbohydrates, dietary fiber, sugars, protein, vitamin A, vitamin C, calcium, and iron.

C. Nutritional labeling helps control manufacturers' specific health and food claims.

D. This labeling should also aid individuals with special dietary needs and make it easier to plan meals and snacks.

III. Most packaged food items purchased today contain a list of ingredients and USRDA labeling.

A. The ingredients are listed by their weight or predominance in the food product, with the most prevalent ingredient listed first and the other ingredients following according to their decreasing weight.

    1. This label lists additives that may include modified food starch, assorted seasonings, salt, flavorings, spices, soybean oil, and betacarotene.

    2. Salt has other names that may not be recognizable at first but include terms that are

Table 5-4 Food exchange lists

Exchange list	Carbohydrate (g)	Protein (g)	Fat (g)	Calories
Starch/bread	15	3	Trace	80
Meat				
Lean	—	7	3	55
Medium-fat	—	7	5	75
High-fat	—	7	8	100
Vegetable	5	2	—	25
Fruit	15	—	—	60
Milk				
Skim	12	8	Trace	90
Low-fat	12	8	5	120
Whole	12	8	8	150
Fat	—	—	5	45

related to sodium such as monosodium glutamate (MSG).

B. Sugar is another ingredient that has many names: sucrose, dextrose, fructose, corn syrup, and honey.

C. Use nutrition information to determine the percentage of calories, saturated fat, maximum daily cholesterol, and sodium as well as diet exchange information.

IV. Patients who eat fast foods must do the following:

A. Choose healthy options when eating in fast food restaurants.

B. Seek information about the nutritional value of foods served in the restaurant.

C. Use sugar-free syrups in place of honey or regular syrup when eating pancakes or similar types of foods.

D. Substitute snacks with low sugar and fat content.

E. Follow meals with tooth-cleansing vegetables or fresh fruits.

V. *Energy balance* refers to the number of kilocalories a person consumes in relation to the number of kilocalories the body uses.

A. Three factors influence the amount of energy needed for this balance:

1. Basal metabolic rate (BMR)—Controlled largely by the hormones produced in the thyroid gland, it is the amount of energy (kilocalories) required by the body to maintain life-supporting functions while the body is at rest; BMR is also called *resting energy expenditure (REE)*.

2. Specific dynamic action (SDA)—The energy needed for the digestion and absorption of food.

3. Activity level—The energy that the body expends during various levels of activity, such as typing, walking, or running.

CARBOHYDRATES AND DENTAL CARIES ▬▬

I. Various carbohydrates can be a factor in the onset of dental caries. Each carbohydrate has its own rate of caries production or level of cariogenicity.

A. This level is based on its texture, how sticky the food is, and what type of carbohydrate it is (polysaccharide, disaccharide, or monosaccharide).

B. A simplified formula for the formation of dental decay is as follows:

Sugar + Plaque = Acid

Acid + Tooth = Decay

C. Plaque, or more specifically *Streptococcus mu-*

tans (a bacterial component of plaque), is a necessary ingredient in caries formation.

D. This type of bacteria requires a carbohydrate energy source to produce the acid that leads to decay.

E. Fats and proteins do not provide a suitable alternative and are not considered cariogenic substances.

F. Acid formation takes place within 20 seconds after a carbohydrate has been broken down to sucrose in the mouth.

G. The normal pH of saliva ranges from 6.2 to 7.0; during an acid attack, the saliva pH decreases.

1. Enamel decalcification and dental decay occur in the critical pH level of 5.0 to 5.5.

2. Each repeated introduction of a suitable carbohydrate into the mouth causes the pH level to remain at this detrimental number for 20 to 30 minutes.

H. Frequent eating or snacking is damaging to the teeth because continuous exposures to sucrose add up to more acid production, longer subjection to acidic saliva, and increased tooth decay.

II. Evaluating carbohydrate intake for a patient is useful in the detection of cariogenic carbohydrates and hidden sugars in the patient's diet.

A. Ask the patient who is experiencing a high rate of decay to record food intake, including the amounts of food, the time of day that food is eaten, and the condiments that are used, for a specific number of days.

B. Review the diary with the patient and note carbohydrates that can easily promote acid production; include the following in the evaluation:

1. What carbohydrate is eaten? What is the texture of this food? Is it sticky and does it remain on the teeth for a long period like a caramel or raisins? Or does it have a high water content, such as fruit, and leave the mouth quickly?

2. When is the carbohydrate eaten? Is the carbohydrate eaten during a meal when the saliva is flowing freely? Or at bedtime when the saliva flow tends to slow down and less acid-buffering action is available?

3. What is eaten with the carbohydrate? Is the carbohydrate eaten alone or with other fats and proteins that offer some degree of acid neutralization? Certain cheeses are currently being studied and show some acid-buffering ability when eaten after a cariogenic food item.

4. How often are carbohydrates eaten? Does the patient eat three distinct meals, or is there a

pattern of frequent snacking during the day? With each additional incidence of carbohydrate intake comes the probability of subsequent acid production and tooth demineralization.

C. Suggest sugar alternatives for those who wish to decrease or totally avoid the use of sugar.

1. *Sugar free* or *no sugar added* labeling may indicate that sucrose or table sugar was not used as an ingredient in this product, but it also may mean that the food contains other forms of sugar such as fructose or honey.

2. Sorbitol, mannitol, and xylitol are sugar alcohols. These alternative sweeteners do not possess a high rate of cariogenicity.

3. Aspartame (NutraSweet) is derived from the essential amino acid phenylalanine and does not promote dental decay because of its amino acid composition.

4. **Saccharin** is used today as a table sweetener or an additive in some sodas; oral bacteria are unable to use it as an energy source to produce acid, so it is considered noncariogenic.

HEALTH RISKS RELATED TO DIET ■■■■■

I. Health risks related to diet can be attributed to environmental, behavioral, social, and genetic factors.

A. Improper diet can increase the probability of obesity and contraction of several diseases, including cancer, hypertension, diabetes, and atherosclerosis (Table 5-5).

B. Assessment and counseling for dental patients are a vital part of nutrition related to the prevention of oral disease.

C. Special diets may be needed for the following patients:

1. Pregnant patients
2. Older adult patients
3. Patients with food allergies
4. Vegetarian patients
5. Patients with heart disease
6. Diabetic patients
7. Surgery patients
8. Orthodontic patients

MEDICINE, DRUGS, AND NUTRITION ■■■■■

I. Drugs interact with each other and affect nutrition. Table 5-6 lists examples of food's effect on the absorption of certain drugs.

Table 5-5 Classic symptoms of poor nutritional status

Area examined	Symptom	Possible nutrient imbalance
Skin	Follicular hyperkeratosis (calloused dry, thickened)	↓ Vitamin A
	Petechiae (tiny, purple—red spots)	↓ Vitamin C
	Dark dermatitis in areas exposed to sunlight	↓ Niacin
	Flaky dermatitis	↓ Protein—energy
	Pallor	↓ Iron, folate, vitamin B_{12}, copper
Eyes	Xerosis (dry tissue)	↓ Vitamin A
	Keratomalacia (ulcerated cornea)	
	Bitot's spot (thick white deposits)	
	Inflamed conjunctiva	
Mouth and tongue	Cheilosis (scales and fissure on lips)	↓ Riboflavin
	Glossitis (magenta tongue)	↓ Niacin, folacin, iron
	Gingivitis (bleeding, spongy gingiva)	↓ Vitamin C
	Carious teeth	↓ Fluoride
		↑ Sugar
	Mottled enamel	↑ Fluoride
Glands	Thyroid, parotid enlargement	↓ Iodine
		↓ Protein
Hair	Depigmentation	↓ Protein—energy
	Thin, sparse, poor texture	↓ Protein—energy
Nails	Koilonychia (spoon nails)	↓ Iron
Subcutaneous fat	Little fat	↓ Protein—energy
	Excessive fat	↑ Energy nutrients
	Edema	↓ Protein—energy
Musculature	Wasted muscles	↓ Protein—energy, thiamin
	Paralysis at extremities	↓ Thiamin, vitamin B_{12}
Skeletal structure	Bowed legs, knock-knees	↓ Vitamin D
	Rosary beading of ribs	↓ Vitamin C

Table 5-6 Food effect on drug absorption

Absorption reduced by food	Absorption delayed by food
Amoxicillin	Acetaminophen
Ampicillin	Amoxicillin
Aspirin	Aspirin
Demethylchlortetracycline	Cephalexin
Doxycycline	Cephradine
Isoniazid	Digoxin
Levodopa	Furosemide
Methacycline	Sulfadiazine
Oxytetracycline	Sulfamethoxazole
Penicillin G, V(K)	Sulfamethoxypyridazine
Phenethicillin	Sulfanilamide
Phenobarbital	Sulfanilamide
Propantheline	Sulfisoxazole
Rifampin	
Tetracycline	

Adapted from Roe DA: Interactions between drugs and nutrients, *Med Clin North Am* 63:985, 1979; and Roe DA: *Diet and drug interactions*, ed 2, New York, 1989, AVI Books.

A. Foods can slow the absorption of drugs in the digestive system.
B. Drugs can make nutrients unavailable for absorption.
C. Drugs can modify taste or alter appetite.
D. Nutrients can interfere with the action or excretion of drugs.
E. Drugs can also interfere with the action or excretion of nutrients.

Questions

Nutrition and Dental Health

1 Which of the following nutrients are the most cariogenic?
a. Fats
b. Carbohydrates
c. Proteins
d. Amino acids

2 When considering the relationship of sugar consumption to dental caries, which of the following factors is most important?
a. Type of sugar consumed
b. Quantity of sugar consumed
c. Form in which the sugar is consumed
d. Frequency of sugar consumption

3 Which of the following are not defined categories in the food pyramid?
a. Sugar
b. Fruit
c. Grains
d. Fats, oils, and sweets
e. Bread and cereal

4 Which of the following are included in the peak of the food pyramid?
a. Citrus fruits and fruit juices
b. Green beans and corn
c. Cornmeal and rice
d. Butter and margarine

5 Which of the following are excellent food sources for calcium?
a. Fish, meat, and poultry
b. Yellow vegetables and citrus fruits
c. Egg yolk, liver, and bread
d. Milk, cheese, and green vegetables

In questions 6–9 match the fat-soluble vitamin in Column A with the function in Column B.

Column A	Column B
_____ **6** Vitamin A	a. Absorption of calcium in bone mineralization
_____ **7** Vitamin D	b. Coenzyme in nutrient metabolism
_____ **8** Vitamin E	c. Antioxidant
_____ **9** Vitamin K	d. Stabilization of red blood cell walls
	e. Essential to blood clotting

In questions 10–13 match the fat-soluble vitamin in Column A with the deficiency in Column B.

Column A	Column B
_____ **10** Vitamin A	a. Gingival bleeding
_____ **11** Vitamin D	b. Glossitis
_____ **12** Vitamin E	c. Needed to develop amelo-blasts
_____ **13** Vitamin K	d. Unknown
	e. Hypoplasa

A sample diet obtained from a patient receiving nutritional counseling includes the following:

Breakfast
8 oz grapefruit juice
2 cups of coffee
2 slices of rye toast with margarine
1 egg

Lunch
12 oz cola
Hot dog with sweet relish
Potato salad
3 tomato slices

Dinner
8 oz pork steak
1 cup of asparagus tips
1 small baked potato (dry)
Small tossed salad with vinagarette dressing
1 cup of fresh strawberries

The patient appears to have a relatively healthy diet, but has had several carious lesions lately. Some suggestions may be made for dietary improvement. Answer the following questions A for TRUE and B for FALSE.

_____ **14** The patient should substitute diet drink for the lunch beverage

_____ **15** The patient has sufficient vegetable servings for the day

_____ **16** An increase in the grains group would be helpful

_____ **17** An excess of the meat group was consumed

18 A riboflavin deficiency results
a. Malformation of dentinal tubules
b. Caries prone teenage years
c. Cheilitis
d. Herpetic lesion

19 Metabolism is
a. A steady heart beat
b. The changes in nutrients by the body
c. A combination of vascular changes
d. A respiratory difficulty

20 Which of the following is known as table sugar?
a. Sucrose
b. Maltose
c. Fructose
d. Lactose

For each level of the food pyramid listed below select the number of servings recommended each day.

_____ **21** Fats   a. 6-11
_____ **22** Vegetables   b. 2–3
_____ **23** Meat   c. 3–5
_____ **24** Milk   d. 2–4
_____ **25** Grains   e. Use sparingly

Rationales

Nutrition and Dental Health

1 B   Carbohydrates combined with plaque, acid and tooth surfaces will result in decay.

2 D   The constant bathing of the oral cavity with sugar is more detrimental than the amount, type and form of sugar that a person consumes.

3 A   There is no specific group for sugar or grains. The food groups on the pyramid include fruit; fats, oils and sweets; bread, cereal, rice, and pasta; meat, poultry, fish; vegetable; and milk, yogurt, and cheese.

4 D   Butter and margarine are included in the fats, oils, and sweets group, which is recommended to be used sparingly.

5 D   Besides milk, cheese, and yogurt, commonly thought to be high in calcium, green leafy vegetables are high in calcium.

6 C   Vitamin A does act as an antioxidant and aids in maintenance of health and secretions of mucous membranes.

7 A   Vitamin D is found in sunshine, liver oils, and fortified milk and does assist in the absorption of calcium in bone.

8 D   Vitamin E, found in eggs, liver, vegetable oil, and dark green leafy vegetables, assists in the stabilization of red blood cells.

9 E   Vitamin K, found in dark green leafy vegetables, liver, and egg yolks, can be synthesized in bacteria of the gastrointestinal tract. When deficient gingival bleeding can result.

10 C   Vitamin A is necessary in the development of ameloblasts, enamel producing cells, and a deficiency results in impaired tooth formation.

11 E   Vitamin D deficiency will cause hypoplasia, which may result in undeveloped bone and teeth.

12 D   Vitamin E deficiency is not really known since sources of the vitamin are obtained from so many foods.

13 A   Vitamin K is essential to proper blood clotting, and a deficiency will result in excess bleeding.

14 A   A diet beverage or water should be suggested as an alternative to reduce sugar consumption.

15 A   Three to five vegetable group servings are recommended each day and the food consumed met these recommendations.

16 A   Two or three servings of grains are recommended daily.

17 B   Two or three meat group servings are recommended per day.

18 C   Cheilitis is an inflammation and cracking of the lips. It may be caused by a riboflavin deficiency or excessive exposure to sunlight and allergic sensitivity to cosmetics.

19 B   Metabolism is the breaking down of nutrients into smaller units, reorganizing the units as tissue building blocks or as energy sources, and the elimination of waste products.

20 A   Glucose, fructose and galactose are single sugars and easier to digest, while sucrose, maltose and lactose are double sugars and must be metabolized to single sugars to provide energy.

21 E   Fats are recommended to be used sparingly on a daily basis.

22 C   Vegetables are recommended to be consumed in three to five servings per day.

23 B   Meat is recommended for consumption of two or three servings per day.

24 B   Two or three servings of the milk group are recommended per day.

25 A   Grains should be consumed in 6-11 servings per day.

To enhance your understanding of the material in this chapter, refer to the illustrations in Chapter 5 of Finkbeiner/Johnson: _Mosby's Comprehensive Dental Assisting: A Clinical Approach._

CHAPTER 6

Diseases of the Oral Cavity

OUTLINE

Systemic Diseases
Developmental Conditions
Diseases of the Teeth and
Supporting Tissues

Normal Periodontium
Etiology of Periodontal Disease
Inflammation
Periodontal Diseases

Diseases Affecting the Teeth
Forms and Classification of Cavities
Cavity Preparation
Questions

KEY TERMS

Abrasion
Acquired pellicle
Acute periodontal abscess
Acute herpetic gingivostomatitis
Acute necrotizing ulcerative gingivitis
Adenopathy
Atrophy
Attrition
Benign
Bilateral
Biopsy
Calculus
Carcinoma in situ
Caries
Cavity floor
Cavity preparation
Cavity wall
Clinical description
Congenital

Convenience form
Dysplasic
Erosion
Erythematous
Etiology
Extrinsic stain
Genetic
Gingivitis
Hyperkeratinization
Hyperplasia
Hypertrophy
Idiopathic
Inflammation
Innocuous
Intrinsic stain
Lesion
Leukoplakia
Line angle
Localized
Malignant

Materia alba
Metastasis
Neoplasm
Nodule
Nursing-bottle mouth
Obturator
Opportunistic
Oral pathology
Outline form
Palpation
Periodontitis
Point angle
Recurrent decay
Reparative dentin
Resistance form
Resorption
Retention form
Tumor
Unilateral

Oral pathology is defined as the study of disease that occurs in the mouth. A basic knowledge of oral pathology is necessary to differentiate between normal oral structures and abnormal findings in the oral cavity. The study of oral pathology includes discussion of diseases including common canker sores or aphthous ulcers, herpes virus, candidiasis, and oral cancer. Oral pathology includes descriptions of disturbances in the soft and hard tissues of the mouth as well as diseases of the oral cavity.

Diseases, including oral disease, may be caused by **genetic** changes or by external sources, such as microorganisms, drugs, chemicals, trauma, temperature change, radiation, inadequate nutrition, and immunologic causes.

SYSTEMIC DISEASES

I. Systemic diseases may involve the oral cavity, and the symptoms may become troublesome.
   A. *Mumps* and *measles* are often considered childhood diseases, but they can occur in adults.
      1. Mumps is an acute, contagious disease characterized by **inflammation** of the parotid glands and other salivary glands.
         a. Swelling of the glands is usually inferior and anterior to the ear.
         b. Movement of the jaw may be painful and restricted.
      2. Measles, a highly communicable disease, is characterized by various symptoms, such as fever, general malaise, and skin rash. Orally, bluish white spots on the buccal mucosa *(Koplik's spots)* may appear.
   B. *Tetanus* is an acute infectious disease resulting from the toxin of tetanus bacillus.
      1. Tetanus may occur at a wound site or in muscle or joints (e.g., the temporomandibular joint).
      2. The first symptom of tetanus in the head and neck is stiffness of the jaw, esophageal muscles, and some neck muscles.
   C. *Tic douloureux* is degeneration of or pressure on the trigeminal nerve.
      1. This disorder results in neuralgia.
      2. Acute and severe pain radiates from the angle of the jaw along one of the involved nerve branches.
II. Most pathologic conditions in the oral cavity result from inflammation, a normal immune response of the body.
   A. The four signs of inflammation are the following:
      1. Heat
      2. Redness
      3. Pain
      4. Swelling
   B. When a site becomes inflamed, the connective tissue cells encapsulate the inflamed site, forming a barrier of fibrin and fibrous tissue and localizing the inflammation.
      1. Healing begins with the development of granulation tissue—soft, fleshy projections of cells that form around the wound.
      2. If the immune system is not functioning properly, the body may be unable to protect itself and is then susceptible to invasion by other pathogens and disease.
III. Irregularities of the skin and oral mucosa are called **lesions.**
   A. Lesions are usually found below or above the surface and may be flat or raised.
   B. Categories and characteristics of lesions are listed (box on page 77).
   C. The specific cause of the lesion can be identified only after tissue is surgically removed and examined under the microscope; this procedure is called **biopsy.**
      1. The **clinical description** (features of the lesion that can be seen by the clinician) must always be recorded and submitted to the pathologist with the biopsy specimen.
      2. Clinical features of the lesion include its color, surface texture, location, and tissue consistency.
   D. Lesions should be examined according to the following general rules:
      1. Compare the affected side with the opposite side for similarities or differences.
      2. Remember that conditions that appear abnormal but look the same on both sides of the oral cavity are considered normal for that particular patient and are usually not pathologic.
      3. Obtain a history of the lesion from the patient that includes the following:
         a. Patient's perception of the cause of the lesion
         b. Duration of the lesion's presence
         c. Level of pain (if any) associated with the lesion
         d. Treatment used on the lesion

DEVELOPMENTAL CONDITIONS

I. Abnormal conditions include those that form during fetal development or develop after birth.

A. Genetic (inherited) disorders are transmitted through the genes.
B. Acquired malformations result from an occurrence during pregnancy that disrupts the development of the fetus.
   1. Acquired malformations can occur in the fetus if the mother ingests any of a variety of drugs or contracts a disease (such as German measles); they also can occur for **idiopathic** (unknown) reasons.
C. **Congenital** conditions are present at birth; they can be either inherited or acquired.

CATEGORIES OF ORAL LESIONS

BELOW THE MUCOSAL SURFACE

Cyst—Closed sac lined with epithelium containing fluid or semisolid material.
Ulcer—Craterlike lesion that may also involve inflammation and infectious or malignant activity.
Abscess—Cavity or area containing pus with inflammation or injury.

ABOVE THE MUCOSAL SURFACE

Vesicle—Small, thin-walled blister that contains clear serous fluid.
Plaque—Flat or raised patch.
Bulla—Thin-walled blister greater than 1 cm in diameter, containing clear serous fluid.
Pustule—Small, circumscribed elevation of the skin that usually contains fluid.
Hematoma—Collection of blood trapped in tissues; usually results from trauma.
Papule—Small, solid, raised lesion less than 1 cm in diameter.

FLAT SURFACE

Patch—Small spot of surface tissue that differs from surrounding tissue in color or texture (or both).
Petechia—Tiny purple or red spot that appears as a result of minute hemorrhage.
Purpura—Bleeding disorder that results in hemorrhage in tissues.
Macula—Small blemish or discoloration.

FLAT OR WITH RAISED SURFACE

Granuloma—Chronic inflammation lesion with a tumorlike mass or nodule of granulation tissue.
Nodules—Small node or rounded mass.
Tumors—Swelling or enlargement that occurs in inflammatory conditions; may be categorized as benign or malignant.

II. Lesions may be characterized as white, ulcerative, or pigmented.
   A. White lesions (box below) usually occur intraorally and may be a thickened surface layer of keratin, a thickened layer of epithelium, or edematous epithelial cells.
   B. Lesions of an abnormal color are divided into two primary groups:
      1. Pigmented lesions (box on page 78) usually are dark (brown to black) because of the production of melanin.
      2. Vascular lesions blanch under pressure.
         a. Mucocele
         b. Hemangioma composed of blood vessels
      3. Yellow lesions (box on page 78) contain lymphoid material, lipid, pus, or exudate.
III. Descriptions, **etiology,** and treatment are outlined for a variety of developmental conditions that occur in the oral cavity.
   A. *Foliate papillae:* These are part of the collection of normally occurring papillae on the tongue.
      1. Clinical appearance: Vertical folds of **erythematous,** or reddish, tissue are seen on both sides of the posterolateral aspect of the tongue. Their position is perpendicular to the dorsal surface and at a right angle. They are best seen when the tongue is extended and turned and the extreme posterior area of the side of the tongue is in view. They are mostly small and inconspicuous but may be enlarged and prominently red and may appear inflamed and swollen.

WHITE LESIONS

Genokeratoses
   Leukoedema
   White sponge nevus
   Hereditary benign intraepithelial dyskeratosis
Leukoplakia
   Focal hyperkaratosis
   Snuff dipper pouch
   Nicotine stomatitis
   Idiopathic leukoplakia
Candidiasis
Mucosal burns
Lichen planus
Geographic tongue

PIGMENTED LESIONS

PIGMENTATIONS—BROWN, BLUE, BLACK

Melanin
  Physiologic pigmentation
  Ephelis (freckle)
    Peutz-Jeghers syndrome
    Addison's disease
  Cafe au lait spots
    Neurofibromatosis
    Fibrous dysplasia
  Lentigo (age spot, liver spot)
  Nevus (mole)
    Intradermal
    Junctional
    Compound
    Blue
  Melanotic macule
  Melanoma
    Superficial
    Nodular
  Neuroectodermal tumor of infancy
Silver—Amalgam tattoo

YELLOW LESIONS

Fordyce granules
Ectopic lymphoid tissue (oral tonsil, lymphoepithelial
  cyst)
Lipoma
Xanthoma
Gingival cyst
Parulis

---

2. Etiology: Lymphoid tissue is found in the soft palate, pharynx, and posterior area of the tongue and is often reddish. When found in the area of the foliate papillae, it appears as an enlarged, red lesion. It is sometimes called *lingual tonsil* to denote the lymphoid tissue that is combined with the foliate papillae structure.

3. Treatment: Foliate papillae require no treatment but can be mistaken for **malignant** tissue. Compare the two sides of the tongue to determine whether the red enlargement is normal for the patient or is potentially pathologic.

B. *Varix:* A varix is a dilated blood vessel associated with the aging process.
  1. Clinical appearance: Varices appear as dark blue, purple, or black elevated lesions. They can occur in any mucosal location but are more likely to be found under the tongue or on the buccal mucosa.
  2. Etiology: A varix probably represents a distended vein weakened by the aging process—the oral counterpart of a varicose vein.
  3. Treatment: No treatment is required.

C. *Torus:* Torus is a **benign tumor** of bone when it occurs in the palate *(torus palatinus).* A torus located in the lingual aspect of the mandible apical to the canine-premolar region is called *torus mandibularis.* Tori also occur on the labial aspect of both the maxilla and the mandible *(exostoses).*
  1. Clinical appearance: Tori may be single or multiple **nodules,** or lumps, extending from the surface and covered by normal epithelium. **Palpation** reveals a hard consistency; mandibular tori are usually **bilateral.**
  2. Etiology: The cause is unknown, but tori are probably hereditary.
  3. Treatment: No treatment is indicated unless the patient needs a removable prosthetic appliance; then tori must be surgically removed to accommodate the appliance.

D. *Fissured tongue: This* is a common condition occurring on the dorsal surface of the tongue.
  1. Clinical appearance: Furrows or cracks can be seen on the dorsal surface of the tongue. The condition may be painful if it is secondarily infected by bacteria. Retained food can be caught in the fissures and promote the growth of microorganisms.
  2. Etiology: The cause is probably hereditary; some cases may be associated with irritation. The condition is more common in older individuals.
  3. Treatment: When pain is associated with a fissured tongue, instruct patient to clean retained food debris from the furrows.

E. *Fordyce granules:* This condition represents a common deviation from normal found in some individuals. It usually occurs at puberty.
  1. Clinical appearance: Multiple yellow, round structures are found in the oral mucosa; these appear just below the surface, most often on the buccal mucosa, but they can be found on any mucosal area.
  2. Etiology: These structures are sebaceous glands on the surface of the epithelium; they usually surround hair follicles but are not associated with hair follicles when they

occur in the mouth. It is not known why Fordyce's granules appear on oral mucosa—a location where hair is never found.

    3. Treatment: No treatment is required.

F. *Cleft lip and cleft palate:* These are the most common clefting disorders of the head and neck region. They can occur separately (cleft lip only, cleft palate only) or can occur combined. Combined cleft lip and cleft palate occur more frequently (1 in every 800 births) than does either condition separately.

    1. Clinical appearance: Cleft lip appears as an absence of tissue between the center of the lip and the adjacent lip area. It usually is **unilateral,** but the defect can affect both sides of the lip. The nose is often misshapen on the affected side. Cleft palate displays an open space anywhere from the uvula up through the median palatine raphe, depending on the severity of the cleft. *Bifid uvula* has been called the mildest form of cleft palate.

    2. Etiology: Heredity is considered the single most likely cause of clefting disorders, although not all cases are inherited. Cleft lip results from a failure of embryonic mesodermal cells to penetrate the epithelial groove between the medial and lateral nasal processes. Cleft palate occurs when the palatal processes fail to fuse at the median line.

    3. Treatment: Cleft lip is surgically repaired by 1 month of age; cleft palate, by 18 months of age. If the palatal cleft is large, an **obturator** is prepared to fill the defect. Complete treatment may take several years.

IV. Descriptions, etiology, and treatment are outlined for diseases of mucous membranes that occur in the oral cavity.

A. *Geographic tongue:* In this condition, filiform papillae **atrophy** in patches. It is also referred to as *benign migratory glossitis,* which describes the course of the disease in that lesions appear, heal, then seem to migrate to another area of the tongue.

    1. Clinical appearance: Geographic tongue is characterized by circular pink-to-red areas on the dorsal surface of the tongue that are surrounded by yellow borders of necrotic filiform papillae. It occurs most commonly on the tongue but can occur on other mucosal areas of the mouth. Persons of all ages are affected, and multiple or single lesions can occur at the same time. Symptoms range from a mild stinging sensation with tenderness to none at all.

    2. Etiology: The cause is unclear; some evidence supports hereditary transmission.

    3. Treatment: No treatment is required. Inform the patient of the **innocuous** nature of the condition to relieve any anxiety.

B. *Hairy tongue:* This condition consists of elongated filiform papillae, making the tongue appear coated and discolored. Tobacco products can stain the tongue a dark color; then the condition is called *black hairy tongue.*

    1. Clinical Appearance: Filiform papillae become elongated and are light colored unless they have been stained by substances taken into the mouth. The condition is not painful, but the papillae can become so long that they reportedly cause a gagging reflex.

    2. Etiology: The condition is related to irritation from several factors, such as inadequate tongue cleaning, frequent use of a hydrogen peroxide mouth rinse, tobacco, *Candida albicans* yeast infection, and antibiotics; other cases are idiopathic.

    3. Treatment: Advise the patient to improve tongue-brushing technique, which eventually causes the condition to resolve. If the cause is apparent, tongue brushing should be discontinued. Extremely long papillae can be clipped to reduce gagging.

C. *Traumatic (decubitus) ulcer:* This is the most common ulceration that occurs on oral mucosa. It results from an injury that cuts or abrades the epithelium.

    1. Clinical appearance: Decubitus ulcer resembles most oral ulcerations—it is a shallow, depressed, circular lesion that is usually covered by a yellow or white necrotic membrane and may have a red border. The ulcer is usually painful and lasts from a few days to several weeks; tongue-related ulcers often persist longer.

    2. Etiology: The ulcer can result from an injury caused by a variety of sources, such as cheek biting, sharp teeth or restorations, denture irritation, removal of dry cotton rolls from the vestibule after dental treatment, or burns from hot food.

    3. Treatment: It is important to remove the cause to prevent further injury and allow healing of the ulcer. Topical anesthetic

agents and corticosteroids to relieve pain is recommended. Ulcers that do not heal in 3 weeks should be biopsied to rule out malignancy.

D. *Recurrent aphthous ulcers:* These ulcers, commonly called *canker sores,* are common ulcerations that tend to recur throughout the patient's lifetime. They affect persons of both sexes and all ages but are more common in women.

1. Clinical appearance: Recurrent aphthous ulcers appear as shallow, circular ulcers with a yellow necrotic center where the epithelium has died. An erythematous halo often surrounds these ulcers, which range in size from 1 to 2 cm; smaller lesions (2 to 5 mm) appear more commonly. These ulcers appear on a moveable mucosa, such as the lip, cheek, **floor** of the mouth, vestibule, or soft palate. They are thought not to be preceded by blisters, they can be painful, and they last from 10 to 14 days.

2. Etiology: The cause is unknown, but these ulcers are thought to involve a disorder of the immune response. Recurrences are associated with hormonal changes, emotional stress, food or drug allergies, and hereditary predisposition.

3. Treatment: Treatment is primarily aimed at reducing pain; topical anesthetics are used for this purpose, and topical steroid preparations are used to reduce inflammation. Tetracycline rinses are reported to resolve the lesions in a few days. The condition is not contagious, but trauma should be avoided during dental treatment.

E. *Herpetic ulcers:* These ulcerations, caused by the herpes simplex I virus, resemble small aphthous ulcerations but are usually differentiated from aphthous ulcers in that they are found on mucosa bound to bone, such as gingiva or palatal attached mucosa. The viral infection is contagious and occurs in four forms: The *fever blister (herpes labialis)* on the lip; *intraoral recurrent herpetic ulceration,* the intraoral counterpart, which most often occurs on the palate; *primary herpetic gingivostomatitis,* the initial infection that usually occurs in children and is characterized by oral ulceration of all mucosa; and *herpetic whitlow,* infection of the finger. This condition has decreased since dental personnel wear gloves routinely.

1. Clinical appearance: On the lips, a herpetic ulcer appears as a solitary blister or collection of blisters. The intraoral recurrent lesion appears as a cluster of small pinpoint ulcers. The ulcer may or may not be covered with a necrotic membrane; it may be surrounded by an area of redness and inflammation. The ulcer in the primary infection is severe, covering intraoral mucosa, gingiva, and lips. Pain can be significant, preventing the patient from eating. Herpetic whitlow appears as a swelling close to the nailbed, with vesicles that break and form crusted, painful sores, which can recur throughout life.

2. Etiology: The *herpes simplex 1* virus causes herpetic ulcers. The virus is prevalent, and children can contract it from kissing family members who have fever blisters. Lesions are infectious in both the vesicular and the crusted stage. Precipitating factors that provoke recurrence include sun exposure, stress, trauma, fever, and menstruation.

3. Treatment: Topical application of acyclovir during the early stage of the lesion may reduce the severity of the episode and shorten the duration of the lesion. Patients with multiple lesions and fever should drink plenty of liquid to prevent dehydration. Pulling or stretching the lips while a lesion is present can cause the virus to spread and may be painful.

F. *Lichen planus:* This is a skin disease with oral manifestations. Lesions appear brown and crusted on legs, wrists, and ankles. Oral lesions appear in two main forms: Reticular, which is the mildest form and is often asymptomatic, with the patient unaware that it exists, and erosive, which results in loss of oral epithelium in affected areas that are painful.

1. Clinical appearance: The reticular form is characterized by white lines that intersect in a lacy fashion and a circular pattern; the buccal mucosa is a common location for these oral lesions. In the erosive form the reticular pattern is found along with ulcerated areas. Lesions can occur on the gingiva or mucous membranes; those that affect the gingiva are called desquamative **gingivitis.**

2. Etiology: The cause is related to an immunologic disorder; erosive lesions tend to

worsen when the patient is under emotional stress.

3. Treatment: No treatment is needed for asymptomatic lesions; painful erosive lesions are treated with topical application of antiinflammatory drugs. Patients should be reexamined twice a year because a small percentage of lesions become malignant.

G. *Angular cheilosis:* Cracking at the corners of the mouth has been called *angular cheilosis, angular cheilitis,* and *perleche.* The condition is associated with a fungal infection or the loss of vertical dimension in a denture patient when the occlusal plane is worn and the nose and chin become closer together.

1. Clinical appearance: Crusted and fissured areas occur at the corners of the mouth, usually bilaterally. Retained saliva in the corners of the mouth promotes colonization by microorganisms because of the warm, moist environment; pain is minimal.

2. Etiology: Loss of vertical dimension is a major predisposing factor in patients who wear worn dentures or no dentures at all. Vitamin-B deficiency is a cause in malnourished individuals. The fungal organism *Candida albicans* has been found in many lesions.

3. Treatment: Elimination of the causative factor will allow the area to heal. Candidal infections are treated with antifungal drugs.

H. *Thrush:* This form of fungal infection is found within the oral cavity of newborns or older adults. In adults the infection is called *candidosis.*

1. Clinical appearance: Mucous membranes develop a white, curdlike covering that represents colonies of yeast overgrowth mixed with necrotic epithelium. The white membrane can be removed by wiping with a gauze pad; it can occur on any mucous membrane.

2. Etiology: *C. albicans* can be introduced into a newborn's mouth during birth as the baby moves through the birth canal.

3. Treatment: Topical antifungal drugs are applied after wiping white colonies from the mouth.

I. *Amalgam tattoo:* Occasionally, during restoration placement or oral surgery, amalgam is embedded in adjacent soft tissue and the wound heals, entrapping the metals.

1. Clinical appearance: The condition is **localized** to the soft tissue and appears blue to gray. It is found adjacent to an area where amalgam was placed or removed. The condition is asymptomatic and innocuous.

2. Etiology: When amalgam particles are accidentally embedded in a wound, an amalgam tattoo can form.

3. Treatment: No treatment is required.

J. *Nicotine stomatitis:* This tobacco-related injury is not considered premalignant.

1. Clinical appearance: Palatal mucosa may be fissured with a light-colored hyperkeratinized appearance. Minor salivary glands are affected, and the orifice of the ducts is red and inflamed. Sometimes the gland is enlarged, giving a rolled appearance around the opening.

2. Etiology: Pipe smoking is a frequent cause, but the condition can occur with heavy use of all forms of smoking tobacco.

3. Treatment: No treatment is recommended, but dental personnel should inform the patient of the cellular damage that has occurred and suggest that the patient stop smoking. The condition usually disappears after cessation of smoking.

K. *Snuff lesion:* This fairly common tobacco-related injury is caused by smokeless tobacco. Snuff is frequently held in the oral vestibule, causing the lesion to form.

1. Clinical appearance: Mucosa under the smokeless tobacco product is wrinkled. Its opaque to white appearance is caused by **hyperkeratinization** from frequent irritation.

2. Etiology: Irritation from tobacco components that are applied on a frequent basis causes soft-tissue changes.

3. Treatment: No treatment is recommended, but dental personnel should show the patient the soft-tissue changes and advise the patient to stop the behavior. The lesion can become malignant but will disappear if the habit is discontinued.

V. Descriptions, etiology, and treatment are outlined for malignant and premalignant lesions in the oral cavity.

A. *Neoplasm:* The excessive growth of tissue in some of these lesions is called a **neoplasm.**

1. Neoplasms do not return to normal size after the stimulus for overgrowth has been removed.

2. Neoplasms can be benign or malignant.

B. *Leukoplakia:* **Leukoplakia** is a white patch. Other white lesions already discussed could technically be called *areas of leukoplakia.* White lesions of the mucosa are not associated with lichen planus or candidiasis. Biopsy is required to identify the cause of most areas of leukoplakia. This condition is considered premalignant because a small percentage of these lesions will become malignant.
  1. Clinical appearance: The white patch of leukoplakia can occur on any mucous membrane, will not wipe away with gauze, and often has a leathery surface. It can occur in a small, localized area or can cover a large surface.
  2. Etiology: Smoking is considered a major causative factor; other factors include excessive alcohol intake, trauma, and vitamin-A deficiency. Biopsy of most white patches reveals hyperkeratinization. A small percentage of biopsies reveal either **dysplasic** or malignant cells.
  3. Treatment: Treatment is dependent on biopsy results. No treatment is required for hyperkeratinized tissue, but dental personnel should advise the patient to discontinue the causative behavior. Dysplasic or malignant cells are surgically removed and followed by chemotherapy or radiation in some instances.
C. *Erythroplakia:* A velvety red lesion of oral mucosa, this lesion is likely to be malignant at the time of biopsy. It is considered dangerous.
  1. Clinical appearance: The velvety red surface may be rough or smooth. The lesion may cover a small or large area. Sometimes it is speckled or contains white areas. Usually the patient is unaware of its existence and reports no symptoms. Erythroplakia often occurs on the floor of the mouth or on the lateral borders of the tongue, areas considered at high risk for malignancy. It also occurs on other mucosal areas.
  2. Etiology: Erythroplakia has numerous causes, but alcohol and tobacco are highly rated as causative factors.
  3. Treatment: Treatment may include elimination of the cause or surgical excision, or, when **metastasis** or spreading of malignant cells into the body has occurred, appropriate chemotherapy and radiation.

D. *Squamous cell carcinoma:* The oral cavity is lined with stratified squamous epithelium; malignancy in this tissue is called *squamous cell carcinoma.* A lesion with malignant cells that have remained within the epithelial layer and have not metastasized past the basement membrane of epithelium is called **carcinoma** in situ. Cancer at this stage is easily removed with no chance of recurrence; the length of time a malignancy can exist before cells metastasize and infiltrate deeper tissues is not known.
  1. Clinical appearance: Squamous cell carcinoma is a white, red, or speckled ulcerated area that fails to heal. It most commonly occurs on the lateral borders of the tongue and floor of the mouth and is painless unless secondarily infected. It is more common in men older than 40 years and ranks as the ninth most common cancer in the United States.
  2. Etiology: Several factors are involved, but alcohol and tobacco are considered the prime factors. Viruses, such as the herpes and papillomavirus, may be the cause in some cases.
  3. Treatment: Treatment involves the surgical removal of malignant tissue and regional lymph nodes if metastasis is suspected, combined with radiation and chemotherapy.
E. *Basal cell carcinoma:* The most common malignant carcinoma, basal cell carcinoma is found most often in skin that has been exposed to sunlight. In the head and neck region these lesions are usually found on the face, nose, and lips. Unlike squamous cell carcinoma, malignant cells are not likely to metastasize; however, untreated basal cell carcinoma on the scalp could ultimately grow through the skull and invade the brain, causing death. It is most common in men older than age 40.
  1. Clinical appearance: Basal cell carcinoma most often appears as a painless crusted lesion with rolled borders, which represent tumor cells that are growing laterally.
  2. Etiology: Fair-complexioned people who have been frequently exposed to sunlight are most likely to develop basal cell carcinoma.
  3. Treatment: The tumor is surgically removed, and care is taken to excise all malignant cells. The area is checked at recall appointments to avoid recurrence. It is not

uncommon for persons who have had one basal cell lesion to develop others.

VI. Descriptions, etiology, and treatment are outlined for hyperplastic lesions in the oral cavity.

A. *Hyperplasia:* **Hyperplasia** is an increase in the number of cells; most hyperplastic overgrowths of tissue are benign and commonly occur in the mouth.

1. Hyperplastic overgrowths form as a result of chronic irritation.

2. Sometimes these overgrowths are referred to as *reactive lesions* because the cells react to irritation by forming more cells.

3. Hyperplasia is sometimes confused with **hypertrophy,** which is an increase in the size of a cell that occurs as part of the inflammatory response.

   a. Hypertrophy causes a temporary increase in size, which returns to normal after the inflammation resolves.

   b. Hyperplastic tissue usually does not resolve by itself but must be surgically removed.

B. *Irritation fibroma (fibroma):* Fibroma is the most common benign oral soft-tissue growth. It frequently occurs on the buccal mucosa where the teeth occlude—a location that is commonly exposed to irritation.

1. Clinical appearance: The fibroma is hyperplasia of connective tissue covered by normal epithelium. It most often occurs on the buccal mucosa; however, it can occur in other oral locations. Fibroma is dome shaped, pink, usually smaller than 1 cm, and painless.

2. Etiology: Connective tissue growth is stimulated in the presence of repeated trauma. Fibroma often occurs in patients with a habit of cheek biting.

3. Treatment: Surgical removal is recommended, but because the growth is benign, it is often left untreated.

C. *Epulis fissurata (redundant tissue):* This hyperplastic lesion occurs in the oral vestibule of a person with an ill-fitting denture.

1. Clinical appearance: The excess mass of hyperplastic tissue is covered by normal epithelium and is the same reddish color as vestibular mucosa. It grows over the flange of the ill-fitting denture.

2. Etiology: Chronic irritation from the flange of a denture that extends too far into the vestibule causes the lesion.

3. Treatment: Excess tissue is surgically removed, the denture is recast, and the tissue overgrowth does not recur.

D. *Papillary hyperplasia:* Irritation to palatal mucosa under a maxillary denture can result in a unique hyperplastic lesion of numerous polyps of tissue. This tissue does not become malignant.

1. Clinical appearance: In the early stage of disease the palate is red and inflamed; a pebbly texture appears in the central area of the palate as the condition progresses. In the late stage, numerous round red-to-pink papillary nodules fill the vault of the hard palate.

2. Etiology: A combination of factors is responsible for this lesion: *C. albicans* is usually cultured from the overgrowth of tissue and from the maxillary denture. Chronic irritation from the untreated infection causes the lesion to form under an appliance that fits poorly.

3. Treatment: Lesions are treated with topical antifungal drugs, such as nystatin or clotrimazole. The patient is instructed about proper denture hygiene and warned against wearing dentures during the night. Ill-fitting appliances are relined, or a new denture is constructed. If hyperplastic tissue is excessive, surgical removal may be necessary before the denture is remade.

E. *Pyogenic granuloma:* Pyogenic granuloma is a hyperplastic reactive lesion; it is more common in women and frequently develops during pregnancy. *Pyogenic* is a misnomer because pus is not associated with this hyperplasia.

1. Clinical appearance: The lesion is a red, rounded, painless growth of tissue that extends from the surface of the mucosa. The gingival papilla is a common site, followed by the lips, tongue, and lining mucosa of the mouth. The tumor is filled with capillaries and bleeds easily. Tumors range from 1 to 4 cm, making this growth fairly large. If not surgically removed, the inflammatory component can resolve or become scarred and form a lesion that looks like a fibroma.

2. Etiology: Chronic inflammation from bacterial plaque and local irritation from subgingival **calculus** may play a primary role in forming gingival lesions. Hormonal changes may cause an exaggerated inflammatory response. Lesions on the tongue,

lips, and other mucosal areas may form as a result of chronic mild trauma to the area.

3. Treatment: Lesions are surgically removed; a biopsy can provide a definite diagnosis because the pyogenic granuloma can resemble other soft-tissue tumors.

F. *Gingival hyperplasia:* This condition is overgrowth of the connective tissue component in gingivae. It is a reactive overgrowth of various causes. The area is examined for evidence of chronic irritation, and a history of the condition is obtained from the patient.

1. Clinical appearance: Overgrown gingivae cover a considerable portion of the adjacent teeth. The area is pale pink, and unless the marginal area is secondarily infected from retained bacterial plaque, the tissue does not bleed. In most cases the condition is painless.

2. Etiology: There are various causes for this condition. Chronic irritation can occur from retained plaque because of orthodontic appliances, malaligned teeth, etc. Another cause is side effects of some drugs, such as phenytoin (Dilantin), which is taken for epilepsy; nifedipine or diltiazem, which is taken for cardiovascular disease; and cyclosporine, which is taken by organ transplant patients to keep the body from rejecting the organ. Heredity is another cause.

3. Treatment: Treatment consists of removal of bacterial plaque on a regular basis. Hyperplastic tissue must be removed surgically. Drug-induced hyperplasia will resolve if the drug is discontinued. Removal of teeth has resulted in reduction of tissue size, called *atrophy,* although this is a drastic measure.

G. *Papilloma:* Another name for papilloma is *squamous papilloma,* which identifies the type of epithelium from which the tissue grows. This lesion is not hyperplastic because it does not occur from chronic irritation; it is classified as a reactive lesion that occurs after infection by a virus.

1. Clinical appearance: Papilloma extends from the surface as a cluster of papillary projections that resemble a mulberry. It occurs on any mucosal area but more frequently on the palate and uvula. It generally is white because the blood supply is minimal; pink lesions have a greater blood supply.

2. Etiology: The human papilloma virus may be responsible for this condition. Over 60 subtypes of this virus exist; several different subtypes have been discovered in growths that resemble the papilloma.

3. Treatment: Surgical removal usually results in no recurrence of the lesion.

VII. Descriptions, etiology, and treatment are outlined for lesions in the oral cavity that are associated with acquired immunodeficiency syndrome (AIDS).

A. AIDS results in destruction of T lymphocytes, which are immune cells that protect us from many infections. Individuals with AIDS contract numerous **opportunistic** infections, which are caused by microorganisms that cannot cause disease in individuals with healthy immune systems.

B. *Pseudomembranous candidosis:* Sometimes called *candidiasis,* this is the most common and the earliest oral manifestation of human immunodeficiency virus (HIV) infection. It occurs in patients who are immunocompromised for various other reasons, such as after cancer chemotherapy and head and neck radiation, and uncontrolled diabetes mellitus. It also can occur after long-term antibiotic therapy.

1. Clinical appearance: The lesion usually appears as a white membrane in a round or linear pattern on oral mucosa. Wiping with gauze removes the membrane, leaving a red, irritated surface; patients may complain of a burning sensation. Infection can occur on any oral mucous membrane and extend into the pharynx and esophagus.

2. Etiology: Candidosis is caused by *C. albicans,* the same fungal organism that causes lesions described as thrush.

3. Treatment: Antifungal drug therapy, both topical and systemic, is used.

C. *Hairy leukoplakia:* This unique lesion is associated with opportunistic infection in AIDS patients, but it can occur in immunocompromised patients who are not infected with HIV.

1. Clinical appearance: A corrugated pattern of white lines on the lateral borders of the tongue is the usual appearance of the lesion. It looks similar to candidosis but cannot be removed by wiping with gauze.

2. Etiology: The Epstein-Barr virus is considered the causative organism in hairy leukoplakia.

3. Treatment: No treatment is available; the clinician usually refers the patient for a blood test to evaluate for possible HIV infection.

D. *Kaposi's sarcoma:* This unique cancer is a malignancy of blood vessels; it affects about one third of AIDS patients.
   1. Clinical appearance: This malignancy occurs on the skin and in the oral cavity, usually on the palate. The lesion is purple, blue, or red; it may be flat or nodular. As the tumor grows, it forms a hemorrhagic mass; the cancer invades the tissue and causes bleeding and pain.
   2. Etiology: It is not known what occurs in the AIDS patient to cause malignant transformation of the endothelial cells that form the blood vessels.
   3. Treatment: Chemotherapeutic drugs and low-dose radiation have been used; no single treatment has been successful for all patients.

E. Gingival lesions in HIV-infected patients can be severe and progress to a stage of rapid bone loss within a short time.
   1. Clinical appearance: Gingivae may be red, inflamed, and bulbous. Necrotic areas (dead tissue) may occur on the marginal and papillary areas. The lesions are painful and bleed easily.
   2. Etiology: Gram-negative bacteria and spirochetes are found in large numbers in subgingival plaque, along with large numbers of yeast organisms.
   3. Treatment: Scaling and root planing, rinsing with chlorhexidine mouthwash to facilitate oral hygiene measures, and the antibiotic metronidazole have been used with varying degrees of success.

VIII. Descriptions, etiology, and treatment are outlined for miscellaneous conditions in the oral cavity (several common oral pathologic conditions fall outside the categories already identified).

A. *Mucocele:* Mucocele occurs as a result of trauma to a minor salivary gland. The patient may report a history of the lesion filling with fluid and enlarging and then shrinking when the fluid is expressed from the swelling.
   1. Clinical appearance: The mucocele is a blue elevation of the mucosa caused by fluid collection within the soft tissue when the duct has been severed from the minor salivary gland. It can occur anywhere that minor salivary glands are located, but the lower lip is often affected.
   2. Etiology: Usually trauma to the area causes the duct to be severed from the minor salivary gland, resulting in the mucocele. Less frequently a stone may form in a duct, resulting in fluid backup in the gland and causing elevation of tissue.
   3. Treatment: Removal of the affected gland and duct resolves the condition.

B. *Pleomorphic Adenoma:* This is the most common benign tumor of the salivary glands. It can occur in both minor and major salivary glands. The tumor most commonly occurs in the parotid salivary gland; however, when it occurs in minor salivary glands, the most common location is the palate.
   1. Clinical appearance: A slowly growing tumor produces an enlargement within the affected gland. When it occurs in the parotid, the enlargement is inferior and anterior to the ear; the skin overlying the gland is normal. When the tumor affects the intraoral minor salivary gland, it produces a painless, firm, dome-shaped enlargement that is covered by normal epithelium.
   2. Etiology: The cause is unknown.
   3. Treatment: The mass should be surgically removed and submitted for biopsy because a small percentage of these lesions become malignant. It is impossible to differentiate between benign and malignant salivary gland tumors in their early stages.

C. *Nasopalatine canal cyst:* This disorder has also been called *incisive canal cyst* and *nasopalatine duct cyst.* It occurs in the anterior or posterior section of the canal.
   1. Clinical appearance: The cyst usually is not seen clinically but is identified on a radiograph as a round radiolucency apical to the maxillary central incisor roots. It is frequently found in edentulous patients. Occasionally the cyst becomes large enough to cause swelling of tissue in the palate under the cyst. Cysts in the posterior portion of the canal occur in the midline of the palatal area.
   2. Etiology: The cyst forms from remnants of epithelium left by embryonic fusion of the premaxilla and lateral palatine processes. The stimulus for cyst formation from this tissue is not known.
   3. Treatment: The cyst is removed surgically; recurrence is rare.

D. *Periapical cemental dysplasia:* This condition (formerly called a *cementoma*) is not a tumor but an unusual reaction of normal bone.
1. Clinical appearance: The condition occurs within apical bone; the only way to identify it is with dental radiographs. No symptoms are associated with the condition. Pulp tissue is vital. The condition is usually discovered on routine radiographic survey. The lesion progresses through three stages. Initially, bone **resorption** occurs below the apices of roots, causing multiple radiolucencies that resemble periapical disease. In the next stage, new resorptive areas occur and older areas begin to calcify, leaving areas of radiolucency and radiopacity within the apical bone. In the last stage, bone calcifies, leaving radiopaque areas. The process usually takes years to complete. The condition is most common in the lower anterior area but can occur in other locations and is seen predominantly in African-American females.
2. Etiology: The cause is unknown.
3. Treatment: There is no treatment. The teeth are vital, and the condition is innocuous.

DISEASES OF THE TEETH AND SUPPORTING TISSUES

I. Diseases of the teeth and supporting tissues can be classified as follows:
A. Periodontium
B. Calcified portions of the teeth
C. Pulp (described in Chapter 22)

NORMAL PERIODONTIUM

I. The periodontium develops during the eruption of the teeth; its integrity is maintained through the forces of normal mastication.
A. The function of the periodontium is to attach the tooth to the alveolar bone of the mandible and maxilla.
B. Three factors contribute to changes in the periodontium:
1. Morphologic and functional changes
2. Changes in the oral environment
3. Age
C. The periodontium has four components (Fig. 6-1):
1. Gingiva
2. Periodontal ligament
3. Cementum
4. Alveolar bone
D. Physical characteristics of the periodontium are as follows (box).
1. Clinically, the gingiva is uniformly coral pink, but no single color can be considered normal.
2. The exact color of a healthy gingiva depends on the pigmentation of the individual.
3. A sharp distinction in color can be made between the gingiva from the alveolar mucosa at the mucogingival junction.
4. The gingival surface is fully keratinized, and the margin of the tissue is knife-edged and circumscribes the teeth in a collarlike fashion.
5. The depth of the healthy gingival sulcus is 0.5 to 1 mm.
6. When probed, the tissue does not bleed and exudate is absent.
7. In a radiograph, a healthy periodontium is indicated by the following:
a. An unerupted lamina dura *(darkened line)* surrounding the roots.
b. The alveolar crest bone is located slightly apical to the cementoenamel junction and appears pointed at the crest of the alveolar bone.

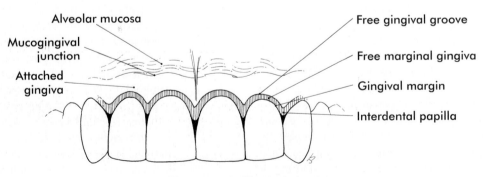

Alveolar mucosa

Mucogingival junction

Attached gingiva

Free gingival groove

Free marginal gingiva

Gingival margin

Interdental papilla

Fig. 6-1 Healthy periodontium.

CLINICAL APPEARANCE OF GINGIVAL TISSUES IN HEALTHY AND DISEASED STATES
COLOR
Normal
Uniform in color; variations in pigmentation may occur in different races and complexions; darker pigment evident in people with darker complexions
Diseased tissue
Subtle change occurs in interdental papilla from light pink to red Acute inflammation: bright red Chronic condition: bluish pink to bluish red; magenta or deep blue
SHAPE
Normal
Knife-edged marginal gingiva; follows contour of the tooth; papillae are pointed and fill the interproximal space
Diseased tissue
Swollen; edematous interdental papilla; marginal gingiva is rolled or rounded; papillae may be bulbous, blunted, or cratered
SIZE
Normal
Free gingiva flat, not enlarged; fits securely around the tooth
Diseased tissue
Enlarged; edematous
TEXTURE
Normal
Free gingiva is smooth; attached gingiva is stippled
Diseased tissue
Acute condition: smooth, shiny gingiva Chronic condition: firm stippling may be more pronounced
CONSISTENCY
Normal
Firm; attached gingiva securely adherent to underlying bone
Diseased tissue
Acute state: soft and spongy; bleeds easily on probing Chronic inflammation: firm gingiva; resists probing; bleeding in deeper part of a pocket, not near margin

ETIOLOGY OF PERIODONTAL DISEASE

I. The etiology or causative factors contributing to the development of periodontal disease can be classified into local and systemic factors.
    A. Local factors include inflammation and anomalies that contribute to the accumulation of plaque and trauma.
    B. Systemic factors are influenced by nutritional and hormonal deficiencies, metabolic disturbances, and the use of various medications or other substances.
    C. Terms used to describe these various factors include the following:
        1. Severity of the disease
            a. Slight
            b. Moderate
            c. Severe
        2. Distribution of the disease
            a. Localized: involves a small region, either a single tooth or a segment of teeth
            b. Generalized: exists throughout the mouth or is generalized to a specific arch or quadrant
            c. Marginal: confined to the free or marginal gingiva
            d. Papillary: involves a papilla but not the rest of the free gingiva around a tooth
            e. Diffuse: occurs when both the attached and free gingiva are involved; commonly, a diffuse change is localized rather than generalized

INFLAMMATION

I. *Inflammation* is the response of tissue to an irritant. Signs of inflammation include the following:
    A. Redness
    B. Heat
    C. Swelling
    D. Pain
II. Inflammation of the gingival tissues can be attributed to the following factors:
    A. Presence of plaque
    B. Calculus
    C. Stain
    D. Food impaction
    E. Mouth breathing
III. **Acquired pellicle** is composed primarily of non-bacterial acellular salivary glycoproteins.
    A. This deposit forms within minutes after a professional prophylaxis.
    B. It is a thin coating covering the teeth, restorations, calculus, and even the fixed and removable prostheses.

C. A disclosed pellicle takes on a light color and a filmlike appearance.

D. Acquired pellicle provides a primary attachment where the plaque bacteria form and colonize.

E. A professional prophylaxis is necessary for removal of this deposit.

IV. *Plaque* is a structured yellow-gray, transparent or near-transparent mass of colonizing bacteria that adheres to the acquired pellicle and supporting tissues.

A. Plaque is not visible to the patient.

B. Plaque that is coronally at or above the gingival margin is referred to as *supragingival plaque.*

   1. The main constituents of supragingival plaque are *Streptococcus mutans,* the acidogenic microorganism responsible for enamel **caries.**

   2. As the plaque remains for longer periods, changes take place in the bacterial structure that later can develop into dense pockets of spirochetes and vibrios, which can create a gingival inflammation.

C. Plaque that forms apically beneath the gingival margin within the sulcus is *subgingival plaque.*

   1. Subgingival plaque creates a different environment for microorganisms.

   2. The plaque may be either adherent or nonadherent, depending on the bacterial composition.

     a. Adherent plaque develops within the sulcus on the root surface of the tooth and can contribute to gingival irritation.

     b. Nonadherent plaque consists of anaerobic bacteria that are motile and move about freely on soft tissues, causing inflammatory lesions.

D. Plaque can contribute to the following conditions:

   1. Unsightly appearance

   2. Halitosis

   3. Development of caries

   4. Formation of calculus

   5. Inflammation of gingivae

   6. Periodontal disease

E. Plaque commonly occurs in the following areas:

   1. Cervical third of the tooth

   2. Proximal areas

   3. Lingual aspect of mandibular molars

   4. Pit and fissure areas

   5. Areas where it is difficult to maintain hygiene

V. **Materia alba** is a soft deposit with a composition different from that of plaque.

A. It is a loosely adherent mass of bacteria and cellular debris that covers plaque deposits.

B. It is white or gray, with no uniform structure, and can be removed by vigorous water irrigation and brushing.

C. Components include salivary proteins and food particles.

D. It appears thick and can feel fuzzy to the patient.

E. It is commonly found at the cervical third of the tooth and in the interproximal areas.

F. When a disclosing agent is used on materia alba, it acquires a dark hue.

G. This soft deposit may contribute to gingival irritation.

VI. *Calculus* is a chalky yellow or white crustaceous deposit.

A. It is found on the lingual aspect of mandibular anterior teeth and on the buccal surface of the maxillary molars.

B. It may also be found in the interproximal areas of the individual with inadequate flossing habits.

C. Calculus formation begins with the attachment of bacterial plaque to the acquired pellicle.

   1. Minerals from the saliva, most commonly calcium and phosphate, are deposited into the plaque matrix.

   2. The once-soft deposit then becomes mineralized.

   3. Calcification can take 10 to 20 days to form the mature calculus.

D. Calculus deposits can form both above the gingiva (supragingival calculus) and below the gingiva (subgingival calculus).

   1. Calculus is irritating to the soft tissue and supporting periodontium because of its bacterial content and rough surface texture.

   2. Subgingival calculus differs from the chalky yellow-white supragingival calculus in that it is usually darker because of blood pigments in the sulcus.

   3. Calculus formation can be reduced by brushing and flossing.

VII. *Food impaction* can contribute to periodontal disease.

A. When food is forced into the interdental space by normal mastication, it acts as an irritant and can cause inflammation of the tissues.

B. Factors that lead to food impaction include the following:
1. Open contacts
2. Fractured teeth
3. Defective restorations
4. Partially erupted teeth

VIII. *Mouth breathing* can contribute to potential gingival inflammation when a patient is unable to breathe effectively through the nasal opening. Mouth breathing can contribute to several conditions:
A. Dehydration
B. Chafing
C. Enlargement of the lips

IX. *Defective restorations* can contribute to the accumulation of plaque. An overhanging restoration creates an environment for the accumulation of plaque and food and ultimately for the formation of calculus.

X. Additional contributing factors that result in localized gingival inflammation may include the following:
A. Abnormally attached frenum or gingiva
B. Malalignment of teeth
C. Trauma to the gingival tissues from finger or nail biting, tongue thrusting, finger sucking, bruxism, or traumatic occlusion

XI. *Systemic deficiency,* including the lack of proper nutrition and metabolic and hormonal changes, can contribute significantly to periodontal health.
A. Two examples of hormonal changes that have an effect on oral tissues are puberty and pregnancy.
1. In pubertal enlargement the tissues are soft and bleed readily, but after the removal of local irritants and a reestablishment of hormonal balance, the tissues usually return to a healthy state.
2. Gingival irritation may occur during pregnancy, but once the irritants are removed and parturition occurs, the enlargement usually subsides.
B. The pubescent child and the pregnant woman are susceptible to changes in eating habits that may lead to nutritional deficiencies. The same nutritional deficiencies are evident in other patients, including older adult patients and anorexic, handicapped, and depressed patients.
C. The results of metabolic and chemical disturbances often occur concurrently in the oral cavity.
1. Metabolic disturbances, such as epilepsy,

may require drug therapy to control the disease.
2. Therapy may result in gingival enlargement that could eventually cover the teeth completely.
3. Factors contributing to the progression of the enlargement can be local irritations.
4. Plaque control and regular prophylaxis can minimize this disturbance of the gingival tissues.

PERIODONTAL DISEASES

I. *Periodontal disease* refers to diseases of the periodontium, which include the gingiva, the connective tissues, and the alveolar process.
A. Periodontal diseases are classified in two categories:
1. One category includes diseases that involve the gingiva alone.
2. The second category includes diseases that involve the gingival tissue and the periodontium. Table 6-1 describes changes in the tissue from a normal to an abnormal state.

II. *Gingivitis* is the term used when the gingiva alone is inflamed.
A. *Trench mouth, Vincent's gingivitis* or *inflammation, Vincent's gingivostomatitis,* and *necrotizing gingivitis* are also known as **acute necrotizing ulcerative gingivitis (ANUG).**
1. Most common in patients between the ages of 18 and 30 years
2. Associated with poor oral hygiene, smoking, and emotional stress
3. Clinical signs indicating ANUG: ulceration of the marginal gingiva and interdental papilla
a. Begins with a necrotic ulcer on the papilla
b. Rapidly progresses to destroy the papilla
c. Spreads to adjacent marginal gingiva
d. Continues to destroy other papillae
4. As ANUG spreads, the tissues become red, raw, and exposed, and cause the following problems:
a. Severe discomfort
b. Spontaneous bleeding
c. Foul odor
5. Initial treatment of ANUG includes the removal of local irritants.
a. When the pain and discomfort subside, the patient can be treated with further scaling and curettage.

Table 6-1 Gingival assessment: clinical characteristics

Clinical characteristic	Ideal/Normal	Abnormal
Color	Uniformly coral pink Variations may occur depending on patient's complexion and race	Acute—bright red Chronic—red, bluish red, dark pink Color changes may be restricted to papilla or extend to marginal and attached gingiva
Contour	Margins are knifelike Contour of free margin forms regular parabolic curve as it goes around teeth Papillae are pointed and fill embrasure space	Margins become rolled, bulbous, enlarged; irregular contour may be noted; clefting or festooning Papillae may be flattened, bulbous, blunted, or cratered
Size	Free margin is near cementoenamel junction (CEJ) Margin adheres closely to tooth	Enlarged because of excess fluid in tissues (edematous) or buildup of collagen fibers (fibrotic) Margin may be retracted away from tooth with air or instrument
Consistency	Firm	Edematous, soft, spongy; pressure on tissues with an instrument will leave a dent Fibrotic, firm, hard tissue
Surface texture	Smooth free gingiva Stippled attached gingiva	Acute——loss of stippling; smooth and shiny Chronic—stippling present; may increase in occurrence
Position of gingival margin	1 to 2 mm above CEJ in fully erupted teeth	May be enlarged so that margin is more coronal than CEJ May show apical recession so that root surface is exposed
Position of junctional epithelium	At CEJ in fully erupted teeth	Apical migration onto root surface
Mucogingival junction	Clear distinction between appearance of attached gingiva (pink, stippled, immobile, firm) and alveolar mucosa (red, shiny, smooth, mobile)	Lack of attached gingiva determined by 1. Loss of junctional line 2. Mobility of all existing tissues 3. Probing extends beyond mucogingival junction
Bleeding	No bleeding detectable with palpation or probing	Spontaneous bleeding Bleeding resulting from probing
Exudate	No exudate with palpation or probing	Increase in amount of clear crevicular fluid Presence of white fluid (pus) with palpation

From Woodall IR *Comprehensive dental hygiene care,* ed 4, St Louis, 1993, Mosby. Compiled from Goldman HM, Chohen DW *Periodontal therapy,* ed 6, St Louis, 1980, Mosby; and Wilkens E: *Clinical practice of the dental hygienist,* ed 5, Philadelphia, 1989, Lea & Febiger.

b. Interim treatment requires improving home care, including the following:
1. Thorough plaque control through gentle brushing
2. Flossing
3. Rinsing the mouth often with warm water and hydrogen peroxide or other recommended oral rinses

B. **Acute herpetic gingivostomatitis** is an infection caused by the herpes simplex virus.
1. Clinically identified by the following:
   a. Edema
   b. Pain
   c. Redness of the mucosa
2. Lasts 2 to 3 days in its acute stage
3. Resolves in approximately 7 to 10 days
4. More common in young children but may occur in adolescents and adults

C. *Pericoronitis* is a localized gingivitis that occurs around a partially erupted tooth.
1. Food and plaque become impacted under the gingival tissue that lies over the partially erupted crown.
2. Severity of the inflammation may range from acute to chronic.
3. The condition is characterized by the following:
   a. Edema
   b. Redness
   c. Exudate
   d. Foul odor
   e. Pain radiating from the point of origin to the ear, throat, or floor of the mouth
   f. Tenderness of the lymph nodes
   g. Facial edema

h. Difficulty in closing the mouth

i. Possible increase in body temperature

4. Treatment typically involves the removal of the bacteria and local irritants.

5. Surgical removal of the gingival tissue or the involved tooth may be necessary, especially in the case of third molars.

D. **Acute periodontal abscess** is an acute purulent infection of the soft tissues of the periodontium and is typically treated in a dental office as an emergency procedure.

1. Symptoms of this condition include the following:

a. Swelling and pain

b. Exudate (may distend the gingival tissues)

c. **Adenopathy,** extrusion of the tooth involved

d. Loosening

e. Tenderness to slight percussion

2. A periodontal abscess may be an extension of chronic periodontal disease.

3. The primary objective of treatment is to relieve pain by establishing a route of drainage for the site. To accomplish this, locate the opening of the periodontal pocket and gently force the release of the exudate or make an incision to provide drainage.

E. If neglected, gingivitis can progress to periodontal disease.

III. **Periodontitis** results when the gingival disease has progressed to the deeper structures of the periodontium.

A. Periodontitis is a chronic disease that can result from gingival inflammation and evolves into a variety of conditions, such as the following:

1. Periodontal pocket formation

2. Bleeding and exudate from the pocket

3. Tooth mobility

4. Resorption of the alveolar process

5. Tooth loss if the disease is not treated

B. The progression of periodontitis includes the following:

1. Resorption of the alveolar bone

2. Loss of gingival attachment

3. Eventual formation of periodontal pockets

C. A normal periodontal depth measured in the gingival sulcus is expected to be 1 to 3 mm.

D. The space between the detached gingiva and the tooth is called a *pocket*. As periodontal disease advances, the pocket depth increases and the alveolar bone resorbs.

E. Mild periodontitis is indicated by the following:

1. Red and swollen gingival tissues

2. Evident bleeding

3. Periodontal pockets 3 to 5 mm

F. The progression to chronic moderate periodontitis is indicated by the following:

1. More definitive loss of the attached gingiva

2. Pocket depths 6 to 7 mm

G. Advanced periodontitis is indicated by the following:

1. Severe bleeding

2. Exudate

3. Tooth mobility

4. Radiographic evidence of loss of the alveolar process

H. Treatment of periodontal disease may require several different approaches.

1. Initial treatment is the thorough removal of all local irritants from the gingival sulcus and around the teeth.

2. Home care instructions are given to the patient.

3. Periodic follow-up of the patient is necessary.

4. If the patient does not improve, additional treatment is necessary, including the following:

a. Root planing to smooth rough root surfaces

b. Gingival surgery to remove and eliminate periodontal pockets

c. Occlusal adjustment to eliminate excessive trauma

d. Orthodontic treatment to improve occlusal alignment

e. Restorative procedures to remove faulty restorations and establish proper contacts and contours of the teeth

IV. *Juvenile periodontitis* is a disease of the periodontium that occurs in relatively healthy young persons.

A. The disorder often is associated with a genetic etiologic pattern.

B. The condition is best identified by the rapid loss of alveolar bone around one or more teeth.

C. Although the condition appears to be generalized, the most common areas of the mouth in which bone loss occurs are the incisors and the first molar regions.

DISEASES AFFECTING THE TEETH ▰▰▰▰

I. The calcified portions of the teeth are affected by several conditions and external factors, including the following:

A. **Attrition,** the physiologic loss of the surfaces of the teeth through mastication, can have an effect.
   1. Factors that facilitate attrition include the following:
      a. Bruxism
      b. Premature centric or eccentric contacts
      c. Teeth that are abnormal in shape, size, and position
B. **Abrasion** can be caused by external sources in addition to the normal loss of tooth structure attributed to attrition.
   1. It is clinically difficult to distinguish abrasion from attrition.
   2. If wear can be attributed to an external source, the condition can be considered abrasion.
   3. Abrasion may be caused by the vigorous use of a toothbrush and dentifrice on tooth surfaces. Tobacco chewing or holding objects between the teeth regularly, such as toothpicks, bobby pins, or a pipe, may cause the same condition.
C. **Erosion,** which is the loss of calcified tooth surface caused by an abnormal substance in the mouth, is usually caused by the wearing away of a tooth or surface by acid. It may occur in the mouths of individuals who regularly eat lemons or are bulimic.
D. **Stains,** which refers to the discoloration of the teeth, can have an effect.
   1. Stains of the teeth emanate from two sources:
      a. **Intrinsic** (from within the tooth), in which case the stain is usually the result of a medical condition or medication given to treat a medical condition or disease.
      b. **Extrinsic** (from outside the tooth), which most often occurs when oral hygiene is not maintained properly.
E. Root fractures, which usually occur as a result of trauma, can have an effect.
   1. Root fractures are difficult to diagnose.
   2. A periapical radiograph is used to identify root fractures.
   3. A root fracture below the dentogingival attachment may heal without additional treatment, although immobilization of the crown may be necessary.
F. Resorption (internal or external), which results from a pathologic process that causes loss of some structure, can have an effect.
   1. Internal resorption involves a change in tooth structure within the tooth, enamel, dentin, or pulp.
   3. External resorption other than that seen in primary teeth causes changes in the root structure.
G. Dental caries, an abnormal condition of the tooth characterized by decay, are caused by various microorganisms (such as *S. mutans* or *S. sobrinus* and *S. lactobacilli*) that cause a breakdown in the integrity of enamel, dentin, or cementum surfaces.
   1. Areas of the teeth that are normally susceptible to dental caries are usually deep occlusal pits and fissures, interproximal surfaces, areas surrounding gingival margins that are exposed because of recession, and defective surfaces.
   2. If decay reaches the dentin layer of the tooth, it will progress into the internal tissues at a much quicker pace, sometimes leading to pulpal involvement.
   3. Involvement of the pulpal tissues during the decay process may require extensive dental treatment.
   4. As decay invades the tooth beyond the enamel, dentinal calcification, sclerosis, or **reparative dentin** begins to provide protection from the invasion of decay.
   5. During the aging process, odontoblastic activity continues in the pulp chamber through the protective layering of dentin on the pulpal surfaces; this is referred to as *secondary dentin.*
   6. **Recurrent decay** under existing dental restorations is often caused by incorrectly designed **cavity preparations,** improperly placed restorations, and/or poor oral hygiene, with subsequent bacterial invasion.
   7. **Nursing-bottle mouth** is decay caused by the constant bathing of the mouth with sweetened liquid throughout the day, but particularly during sleep. The liquid containing sugar combines with the bacteria in the oral cavity, forming acid; acid barrages the teeth, causing a breakdown in the enamel and the beginning of the decay process.

FORMS AND CLASSIFICATION OF CAVITIES ▬

I. Dental lesions are classified according to the G.V. Black Cavity Classification, which is based on

---

G.V. BLACK CAVITY CLASSIFICATION

Class I
- Caries on occlusal surfaces of premolars (bicuspids) and molars
- Caries on buccal and lingual pits of molars and the lingual surface of anterior teeth

Class II
- Caries on proximal surfaces of premolars and molars

Class III
- Caries on the proximal surface of canines (cuspids) and incisors that do not involve the incisal edge

Class IV
- Caries on the proximal surface, including the incisal angle or edge of canines (cuspids) and incisors

Class V
- Caries on the facial and lingual gingival third of any tooth

Class VI
- Abraded incisal edges and occlusal tooth surface

Modification
- Caries on both mesial and distal proximal surfaces of premolars that will be connected as one restoration

Class I **Class II** **Class III**

Class IV **Class V** **Class VI**

---

the clinical location of the carious lesions (box above).

II. Cavity preparation is the process of mechanically removing tooth tissue to expose the carious lesion, remove the diseased tissue, and shape the remaining dentin and enamel so that the tooth can mechanically and biologically retain a restoration.

A. The objectives of cavity preparation of the tooth are as follows:
1. Provide margin placement in accessible areas
2. Provide adequate resistance in the tooth and restoration to withstand the future stresses of normal mastication
3. Provide adequate retention of the restoration
4. Protect the vital pulp

B. The system of cavity preparation includes a sequential pattern (box on page 94) as follows:
1. Open the tooth.
2. Provide **outline form.**
3. Obtain **retention** and **resistance forms.**
4. Establish **convenience form.**
5. Remove any remaining carious dentin.
6. Finish the enamel walls.
7. Provide extension for prevention.
8. Medicate the cavity.
9. Place the restoration.

C. Terms basic to most cavity designs include walls, floors, **line angles,** and **point angles.**
1. **Cavity walls** are generally vertical and superior to the pulp.
2. The floor is horizontal to the pulp.

G.V. BLACK ORDER OF PROCEDURE IN CAVITY PREPARATION
OUTLINE FORM
The form of the cavity preparation as it meets the tooth surface when it has been expanded to include all carious areas
RESISTANCE FORM
A shape that is given to a cavity to provide a filling that has the ability to withstand the stress brought on it in mastication
RETENTION FORM
The shaping of the cavity preparation to prevent the filling from being displaced; a large part of this is provided by the resistance form; in most cavities the retention form is made by shaping certain of the opposing walls so that they will be parallel or slightly undercut
CONVENIENCE FORM
The changes that are made in the basic outline form to facilitate visibility and placement of the restorative material
REMOVAL OF CARIES
The actual removal of carious or decalcified tissue from the tooth
FINISHING OF ENAMEL WALLS AND MARGINS
The placement of angles and bevels in the cavity preparation and the final smoothing of the cavity walls
EXTENSION FOR PREVENTION
The extension of the original cavity preparation to include pits and fissures that could become carious at a later time; to apply this principle to a carious lesion on the proximal surface will generally require the inclusion of the occlusal surface; even though the occlusal surface is not carious, it is the only feasible access to the proximal surface

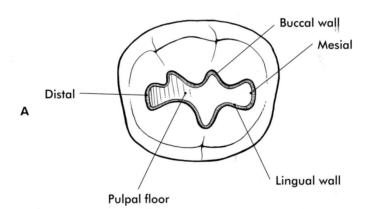

Fig. 6-2   A, Class I preparation illustrating various cavity walls.

3. The meeting of two walls of a cavity preparation is referred to as a *line angle*.
4. Where three walls unite, a point angle is created.
5. Walls, floors, and angles are named for the surfaces they approximate (Fig. 6-2).
6. See illustrations in Chapter 6.

Questions

Diseases of the Oral Cavity

1 A mesial occlusal cavity preparation is an example of a
a. Class I cavity preparation
b. Class II cavity preparation

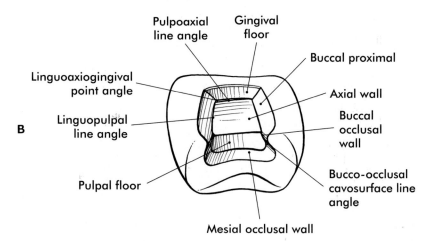

B, Class II preparation illustrating various line and point angles, cavity floors, and walls.

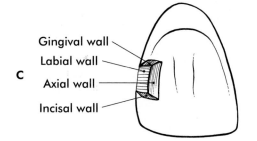

C, Class III preparation illustrating various cavity walls. (Courtesy William Sorenson, DDS, MS, Ann Arbor, Michigan.)

c. Class III cavity preparation
d. Class IV cavity preparation

2 A cavity preparation that includes the mesial incisal angle of a maxillary central incisor is classified as
  a. Class I
  b. Class II
  c. Class III
  d. Class IV

3 Another name for Vincent's disease is
  a. Acute necrotizing ulcerative gingivitis
  b. Acute ear infection
  c. Aphthous ulcer
  d. Herpetic lesions

In questions 4 through 7, match the term in column A with the description in column B.

Column A	Column B
_____ **4** Unilateral cleft	a. Absence of tissue in the center of the lip
_____ **5** Bilateral cleft	b. Defect on one side
_____ **6** Cleft lip	c. Open area between uvula and raphe
_____ **7** Cleft palate	d. Defect on two sides
	e. Open surface posterior to uvula

8 A cavity preparation that involves two proximal walls and the occlusal surface is a _____ and is most likely found on _____ .
  1. Class II
  2. Class III
  3. Class IV
  4. Class VI
  5. Anterior teeth
  6. Posterior teeth
  a. 1 and 5
  b. 1 and 6
  c. 2, 3, and 5
  d. 2, 3, and 6
  e. 4 and 6

9 A cavity preparation that involves one proximal wall and the occlusal surface is a _____ and is most likely found on _____ .
  1. Class II
  2. Class III
  3. Class IV
  4. Class VI
  5. Anterior teeth
  6. Posterior teeth
  a. 1 and 5
  b. 1 and 6
  c. 2 and 6
  d. 2, 3, and 5
  e. 2, 3, and 6

10 The physiologic wearing away of tooth structure is known as
  a. Atrophy
  b. Attrition
  c. Abrasion
  d. Erosion

11 Green stains found on children's teeth are often the result of
  a. Fluorosis
  b. Tetracycline
  c. Poor oral hygiene
  d. Pyrexia

12 The cardinal signs of inflammation include all but
a. Heat
b. Redness
c. Swelling
d. Pain
e. Petechiae

13 Which of the following are not external sources or genetic changes that may cause pathologic changes in tissues?
a. Mumps
b. Tetanus
c. Drugs
d. Tic douloureux
e. All of the above

14 A neoplasm refers to
a. an innocuous condition
b. an idiopathic situation
c. excessive tissue growth
d. malignant cells

15 When a lesion is examined, which step listed below is not followed?
a. History of lesion is recorded.
b. Conditions that appear abnormal on both sides are not evaluated.
c. Affected side is compared with unaffected side.
d. Conditions that appear abnormal on both sides are always evaluated.

16 Which is a common oral complication of radiation exposure?
a. Xerostomia
b. Pyogenic granuloma
c. Mucocele

17 All of the following are considered flat lesions except
a. Tumors
b. Pustules
c. Nodules
d. Granulomas

18 A red, noncoated, glossy area near the midline of the tongue that causes no pain is probably
a. Fissured tongue
b. Geographic tongue
c. Median rhomboid glossitis
d. Hairy tongue

19 Which of the following is the advised course of action of a suspected malignant lesion?
a. Chemotherapy
b. Complete surgical excisional removal
c. Biopsy
d. Radiation therapy

20 A condition defined as a white patch of the mucosa, for which a biopsy is necessary for confirmation of diagnosis, and that will not wipe away is referred to as
a. Candidiasis
b. Leukoplakia
c. Erythroplakia
d. Squamous cell carcinoma

21 The most common malignancy of the skin, which appears as painless crusted lesion with rolled borders, is
a. Epulis fissuratum

b. Squamous cell carcinoma
c. Basal cell carcinoma
d. Leukoplakia

22 Known as the most common and earliest oral manifestation of HIV, which appears as a white membrane and can be wiped away to remove a portion of the membrane, is
a. Candidiasis
b. Hairy leukoplakia
c. Kaposi's sarcoma
d. Pleomorphic adenoma

23 Small ulcers with necrotic centers and surrounded by areas of inflammation may be found in the oral cavity. These areas are commonly known as
a. Herpes simplex
b. Lichen planus
c. Gum boils
d. Canker sores

24 The spreading of cancer to various sites in the body is known as
a. Toxemia
b. Carcinoma
c. Metastasis
d. Articulation

25 A patient with a history of convulsive seizures has been treated with phenytoin (dilantin) for the past 3 years. A resultant condition that may be manifested in the oral cavity is
a. Rampant dental caries
b. Squamous cell carcinoma
c. Enamel hypoplasia
d. Gingival hyperplasia

Rationales

Diseases of the Oral Structures

1 B A Class II cavity classification includes an interproximal surface and the occlusal surface. In some areas of the country this cavity classification may denote the involvement of both proximal surfaces and the occlusal surface.

2 D The Class IV classification involves either the mesial or distal surface and the incisal edge. This classification is used in anterior preparations only.

3 A Vincent's disease, also known by the acronym ANUG, is an acute periodontal disease usually involving the interdental papillae. Necrosis and ulceration of the gingiva and throat may be accompanied by enlarged lymph nodes.

4 B The prefix *uni-* refers to one and lateral refers to the side. A cleft is a divide or split.

5 D The prefix *bi-* refers to two and lateral refers to the side. Refer to No. 4.

6 A A cleft lip is a congenital separation of the maxillary lip.

7 C A cleft palate is a congenital fissure in the roof of the mouth forming a communicating passageway between the mouth and nasal cavities.

8 E A modification of G.V. Black's cavity classification recognizes a Class VI cavity classification on posterior teeth involving both proximal surfaces and the occlusal surface.

9 B G.V. Black's cavity classification recognizes a single proximal and the occlusal surface of a posterior tooth as a Class II preparation.

10 C Atrophy is the shrinking of a structure; attrition is a wearing away through friction; erosion is a wearing away from trauma or inflammation; while abrasion is a wearing through normal mastication.

11 C Green stains usually result from poor oral hygiene resulting from deposits on the teeth that may be removed by the use of a dentifrice or may need a professional prophylaxis.

12 E Petechiae are small red or purple spots on skin from small hemorrhages. All of the other answers are cardinal signs of an inflammatory condition.

13 E Mumps and tetanus are systemic diseases that are troublesome to a patient but do not cause pathologic changes to tissue. Tic douloureux is a disease that causes neuralgia of the trigeminal nerve. Drugs do not manifest changes in pathology. Inflammation in oral tissues may cause pathologic changes.

14 C An abnormal growth of new tissue is known as a neoplasm.

15 D If a condition is observed on both sides of the mouth, it may be considered in the realm of normal. Conditions, such as mandibular tori, considered within the realm of normal for that patient, would not be evaluated as out of the ordinary.

16 A Xerostomia is a dryness of the mouth caused by decreased salivary production and may be a side effect of radiation treatment.

17 B Tumors, nodules, and granulomas are usually large and more raised in appearance, while pustules are flatter.

18 C Median rhomboid glossitis does not migrate like geographic tongue. Hairy tongue has elongated and discolored papillae and a fissured tongue has deep furrows.

19 C Tissue is biopsied first, prior to chemotherapy or radiation therapy, to rule out the chance that a lesion is non-malignant. After determining malignancy, the lesion is removed by surgical excision. A non-malignant lesion may be removed for patient comfort.

20 B Wiping candidiasis with gauze will remove some of the membrane, leaving a red irritated surface. Erythroplakia appears as a velvety red lesion on the mucosa, and squamous cell carcinoma is usually white, red, or speckled ulcerated area.

21 C Epulis fissuratum appears as a red, rounded tissue growth near the gingival papilla. A squamous cell carcinoma is a white, red, or speckled ulcerated area and leukoplakia will appear as a white patch or the mucosa.

22 A Refer to No. 20.

23 D Herpes simplex I virus looks similar to canker sores but is usually found on mucosa bound to bone, such as gingiva. Lichen planus appears as lacy, white lines or in a circular pattern with ulcerated areas and is caused by an immunological disease. Canker sores or aphthous ulcers are usually shallow, circular ulcers with yellow necrotic centers where the epithelium has died.

24 C A metastasis is the spreading of tumor cells to distant parts of a body since malignant tumors have no encapsulating tissue.

25 D Dilantin therapy causes a reactive growth of gingival tissue. This growth covers an abnormal portion of the crowns of teeth.

To enhance your understanding of the material in this chapter, refer to the illustrations in Finkbeiner/Johnson: *Mosby's Comprehensive Dental Assisting: A Clinical Approach*, Chapter 6.

CHAPTER 7

Infection Control

OUTLINE

Routes of Transmission
Common Blood-Borne Pathogen
 Diseases
Infection Control in Dentistry
Governmental Regulations
Infection Control Techniques

Personal Protection
Sterilization
Monitoring of Sterilization
Hand-Piece Asepsis
Surface Disinfection

Equipment Asepsis
Disposables
Laboratory Asepsis
Educating Patients about Infection
 Control Programs

KEY TERMS

Antimicrobial

Antiseptic

Autogenous infection

Asepsis

Aseptic technique

Barriers

Bioburden

Blood-borne pathogens

Centers for Disease Control and
 Prevention

Cold disinfection

Contamination

Cross-infections

Direct contact

Disinfection

Environmental Protection Agency

Hepatitis B virus

Human immunodeficiency virus

Immunization

Indirect contact

Infection control

Inhalation

Material Safety Data Sheet

Occupational Safety and Health
 Agency/Act

Polynitrile gloves

Sanitization

Sterilization

Tuberculosis

Universal precautions

The realism of infection transmission is an important factor in providing dental care. Several sources of infectious diseases are present during dental treatment, including blood, saliva, nasal discharge, dust, hands, clothing, and hair. Any of these sources can potentially transfer microbial and viral infections.

When defining infections common to dental treatment, two categories must be considered: **autogenous infec-** **tions** and **cross-infections.** The patient is the source of autogenous infection. An example is a patient who receives dental treatment, specifically an extensive scaling and polishing of the teeth. Subsequently, endocarditis develops, which can result from the introduction of virulent organisms (such as staphylococci or pneumococci) that reside in the mouth and can be introduced into the bloodstream during prophylaxis. The patient is the source of the endocarditis. Cross-infections are transferred from one individual to another.

ROUTES OF TRANSMISSION

I. Microbial transmission by dentistry-related secretions and exudates occurs by three general routes:
  A. **Direct contact** with a lesion, organisms, or debris during performance of intraoral procedures
  B. **Indirect contact** via contaminated dental instruments, equipment, or supplies
  C. **Inhalation** of microorganisms aerosolized from a patient's blood or saliva during use of high-speed or ultrasonic equipment
II. Potential dangers are often missed because the **bioburden** (blood, saliva, exudate) may be transparent or translucent, drying as a clear film and contaminating surfaces.
III. By routinely adhering to an **infection control** program, the dental team can work to minimize infectious disease risk between patients and attending personnel.
IV. An effective program includes proper **sterilization,** destruction of all microbial life, **disinfection** (killing pathogenic organisms), and clinical aseptic procedures.

COMMON BLOOD-BORNE PATHOGEN DISEASES

I. **Blood-borne pathogens** are microorganisms that are found in human blood and can cause disease.
II. Several infectious diseases are of concern to health care workers, including the following:
  A. **Hepatitis B virus (HBV)**—It is well established that HBV remains the major occupational infection for health care professionals.
  B. **Human immunodeficiency virus (HIV)**—Features that are associated with HIV infection are listed in the box on this page and Table 7–1.
  C. **Tuberculosis**—This disease is a chronic bacterial infection of the lungs.
III. Infection control procedures must be used routinely to minimize the transmission of all occupational infectious diseases (box on page 100). Representative infections are presented in Table 7-2.

INFECTION CONTROL IN DENTISTRY

I. Infection control refers to all processes used to eliminate the transmission of disease.
II. **Universal precautions** include the following:
  A. Reducing the concentration of pathogens so that normal host resistance mechanisms (those immune systems in a person) can prevent infections
  B. Breaking the cycle of infection and eliminating cross-infection
  C. Treating every patient and instrument as potentially infectious
  D. Protecting patients and personnel from occupational infections
III. Basic principles that should be considered in minimizing infectious risk that patients present to attending personnel should include the following:
  A. Patient screening
  B. **Aseptic technique**
  C. Personal protection
  D. Instrument sterilization

FEATURES ASSOCIATED WITH HIV INFECTION

Pneumocystis carinii (pneumonia and respiratory failure)
  Fungal infections
  Candidiasis
  Angular cheilitis
  Hyperplastic candidiasis
  Pseudomembranous form
  Florid form
  Atrophic form
  Lingual candidiasis
  Candidal lesions
  Gingival and mucosal candidiasis
Viral infections
  Herpes simplex virus
  Epstein-Barr virus
  Leukoplakia
  Varicella virus (zoster, shingles)
  Cytomegalovirus
  Human papillomavirus
Bacterial infections
  Gingivitis
  Periodontosis
  Nonoral flora opportunists
HIV-associated malignancies
  Kaposi's sarcoma
  Lymphoma
  Carcinoma
Other HIV-associated manifestations
  Recurrent aphthous stomatitis
  Hypersensitivity, lichenoid reactions
  Thrombocytopenia
  Sialadenitis
  Xerostomia

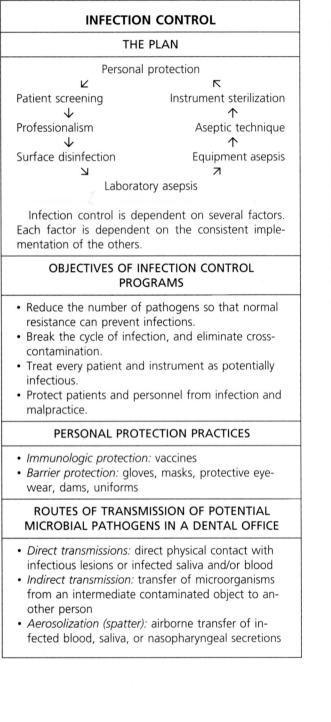

INFECTION CONTROL

THE PLAN

Personal protection

Patient screening ← → Instrument sterilization

↓ ↑

Professionalism Aseptic technique

↓ ↑

Surface disinfection Equipment asepsis

↘ ↗

Laboratory asepsis

Infection control is dependent on several factors. Each factor is dependent on the consistent implementation of the others.

OBJECTIVES OF INFECTION CONTROL PROGRAMS

- Reduce the number of pathogens so that normal resistance can prevent infections.
- Break the cycle of infection, and eliminate cross-contamination.
- Treat every patient and instrument as potentially infectious.
- Protect patients and personnel from infection and malpractice.

PERSONAL PROTECTION PRACTICES

- *Immunologic protection:* vaccines
- *Barrier protection:* gloves, masks, protective eyewear, dams, uniforms

ROUTES OF TRANSMISSION OF POTENTIAL MICROBIAL PATHOGENS IN A DENTAL OFFICE

- *Direct transmissions:* direct physical contact with infectious lesions or infected saliva and/or blood
- *Indirect transmission:* transfer of microorganisms from an intermediate contaminated object to another person
- *Aerosolization (spatter):* airborne transfer of infected blood, saliva, or nasopharyngeal secretions

Table 7-1 Comparison of HBV and HIV infection

Feature	HBV	HIV
Can prevent exposure/infection	Yes	Yes
Patient prevalence	Increased	Increased
Virus titer/ml	>1 million	100 to 1000
Infection risk (%)	10 to 35	<1
HCW prevalence (%)	10 to 50	<<0.01
Annual HCW deaths	200 to 300	0 to 5(?)
Infectivity markers	Yes (HB$_e$)	Yes
Infection outcome:		
Resolved	90% to 95%	0%
Death	2%	100%
Incubation period	2 to 6 months	>2 years
Postexposure prophylaxis	Yes	No
Infectivity	Variable	Life
Treatment	Interferon	No

Adapted from Hadley WK: Infection of a health care worker by HIV and other bloodborne viruses: risks, protection and education, *Am J Hosp Pharm* 46:54-57, 1989.

E. Disinfection procedures
F. Equipment **asepsis**
G. Dental laboratory asepsis

GOVERNMENTAL REGULATIONS ▬▬▬

I. Compliance with current guidelines and regulations for the implementation of policies regarding infection control, hazard communications, and medical waste disposal is expected from all dental professionals.

II. Several agencies are responsible for providing the dental professional with current information regarding the regulations governing these areas.

A. The **Occupational Safety and Health Agency (OSHA),** a federal regulatory agency, reacted to requests from health care employees to establish guidelines to protect workers from occupational exposure to blood-borne diseases (box at top of page 102). The rules were effective as of March 1992.

B. The **Environmental Protection Agency (EPA),** a federal regulatory agency, in response to the Medical Waste Tracking Act of 1988, developed a program overseeing the handling, tracking, transportation, and disposal of medical waste after it has left the dental office.

C. The **Centers for Disease Control and Prevention (CDC),** a division of the U.S. Public Health Service, is responsible for the investigation and control of various diseases, such as tuberculosis (which is occurring more frequently).

III. All infection control programs implemented in a health care provider setting should include a designation for task categorization in accordance with OSHA guidelines (box at bottom of page 102).

A. All individuals working in a health care pro-

Table 7-2 Representative infectious disease risks in dentistry

Disease	Etiologic agent	Incubation period
BACTERIAL		
Staphylococcal infections	*Staphylococcus aureus*	4 to 10 days
Tuberculosis	*Mycobacterium tuberculosis*	Up to 6 months
Streptococcal infections	*Streptococcus pyogenes*	1 to 3 days
Gonorrhea	*Neisseria gonorrhoeae*	1 to 7 days
Syphilis	*Treponema pallidum*	2 to 12 weeks
Tetanus	*Clostridium tetani*	7 to 10 days
VIRAL		
Recurrent herpetic lesion	Herpes simplex, types 1 and 2	Up to 2 weeks
Rubella	Rubella virus	9 to 11 days
Hepatitis A	Hepatitis A virus	2 to 7 weeks
Hepatitis B	Hepatitis B virus	6 weeks to 6 months
Delta hepatitis (hepatitis D)	Hepatitis D virus	Weeks to months
Infectious mononucleosis	Epstein-Barr virus	4 to 7 weeks
Hand-foot-mouth disease	Primarily coxsackievirus A16	<2 days to >3 weeks
Herpangina	Coxsackievirus group A	5 days
AIDS	HIV	Months to years
FUNGAL		
Dermatomycoses (superficial skin infections)	*Trichophyton, Microsporum, Epidermophyton,* and *Candida* genera	Days to weeks
Candidiasis	*Candida albicans*	Days to weeks
MISCELLANEOUS		
Infections of fingers, hands, and eyes from dental plaque and calculus	Variety of microorganisms	1 to 8 days

vider environment face the potential exposure to health risks.

B. These classifications are not rigid; crossovers may occur depending on the jobs performed.

C. For employees who fall within these categories, OSHA requires the following records to be maintained, including dates of occurrence:
1. Exposure determination
2. Infection control program
3. HBV vaccination availability/requirement/implementation
4. Postexposure evaluation and follow-up
5. Training
6. Record keeping

IV. OSHA's Hazard Communication Standards require that all dental professionals take steps to come into or to maintain compliance with the existing standard.

A. A program must be developed and implemented that instructs all individuals, compiles a list of hazardous chemicals, obtains and files **Material Safety Data Sheets (MSDSs),** and labels all chemicals properly.

B. This program must apply to all activities in which an individual may be exposed to hazardous chemicals under normal working conditions or during an emergency situation.

C. The hazard communication program coordinator is responsible for the following:
1. Disseminating information regarding the contents of the program
2. Recognizing the hazardous properties of the chemicals found within the workplace
3. Knowing safe handling procedures of chemicals
4. Implementing measures to ensure self-protection from hazardous chemicals

D. A list of all products in the facility that contain hazardous chemicals must be maintained.

E. An MSDS is a government-approved form or an equivalent form that provides specific in-

1992 OVERVIEW OF REQUIRED FEDERAL OSHA STANDARDS

- Employers must identify and train workers who are *reasonably anticipated* to be at risk of exposure, reduce or eliminate exposure, and offer medical care and counseling.
- Employers must have written exposure-control plans that will identify workers whose work requires them to be exposed to blood and other infectious materials and will identify the means to protect and train those workers.
- Employers must have a plan that includes a protocol for barrier techniques; sterilization; disinfection; hepatitis B vaccination; handling of office accidents, including postexposure to infectious materials; and plans to protect and train employees, with annual reviews and updates of the plan that are readily available to employees.
- Puncture-resistant containers must be used, hands must be washed as gloves are changed, and proper personal protective equipment must be worn.
- Laundering protective clothing at home is prohibited.
- Recapping of sharps must be accomplished using a one-handed technique or a mechanical recapping device.
- Employees are required to wear gowns and gloves when there is risk of exposure of skin to blood, body fluids, or saliva.
- General work clothes are not considered protection against exposure to blood, body fluids, or saliva.

- Employees must wear a mask, eyewear, or a face shield during exposure to splashes, spray, spatter, droplets of blood, body tissue, or saliva.
- Solid eyewear must have side shields.
- Employers must provide personal protective equipment to be worn by all employees, including gowns, gloves, masks, and eyewear, at no expense to employees.
- Sharps containers must be labeled and easily accessible to the area of sharps use.
- Vaccinations for HBV must be offered to employees at no cost after training is completed but within 10 days of placement in a position that involves occupational exposure. If a worker initially declines the hepatitis-B vaccination, access to the vaccination is still required if the employee has a change of mind.
- Employers must provide a training program during working hours to all employees in occupational exposure positions by June 4, 1992, and annually thereafter.
- Training records must be kept for 3 years after the training sessions.
- The standard requires that the following be handled as infectious waste by placement in special labeled containers: pathologic waste; sharps; blood and body fluids; items that release blood, body fluid, or saliva when compressed; items caked with dried blood, body fluid, or saliva if they can release these materials during handling.

TASK CATEGORIZATION

CATEGORY I

- These tasks require exposure to blood, body fluids, or tissues.
- Individuals in this category usually are dentists, hygienists, assistants, and laboratory technicians.

CATEGORY II

- These tasks involve no exposure to blood, body fluids, or tissues but may involve unplanned exposure to Category I tasks.
- Individuals in this category may include clerical or nonprofessional workers.

CATEGORY III

- These tasks involve no exposure to blood, body fluids, or tissues.
- Individuals in this category may include receptionists, bookkeepers, and insurance clerks.

formation on the chemicals purchased for use in a workplace.

F. Sheets for all products with hazardous potential are compiled, filed, and updated in a master list that is available to all individuals.

G. An MSDS for a hazardous chemical should include the following:
1. Manufacturer's name and address
2. Product name
3. Generic name if applicable
4. Potential routes of entry
5. Organs affected by the chemical
6. Means of protecting or reducing the effects of chemical exposure (e.g., eyewash)

H. Labels must be properly affixed to hazardous chemicals or substances.
1. Many products arrive with permanently affixed information regarding hazardous chemicals
2. Hazard-communication labels must be affixed to the container

I. Labels affixed to new containers must include the following:
   1. Indication that information for the MSDS was obtained
   2. Designation of the hazard class of the chemical included
   3. Outline of the routes of entry into the body
   4. List of organs that are affected after entry has occurred
J. Several chemicals not considered of potential concern contain hazardous materials and should be handled accordingly.

V. Certain equipment and devices should be available in a dental office in case a situation involving hazardous chemicals arises (box below).
   A. Spills of chemicals, gypsum products, and flammables require different reactions depending on the hazardous chemical.
   B. The following items will be helpful if a hazardous spill occurs:
      1. Fire extinguisher
      2. Eyewash stations
      3. Amalgam spill kit
      4. Masks (approved by the National Institute of Occupational Safety and Health)
      5. Protective clothing (long sleeves, high neck, fluid impervious material)
      6. Kitty litter, broom, and dustpan
      7. Protective heavy utility gloves (e.g., polynitral) and glasses

---

GENERAL PRECAUTIONS TO FOLLOW WHEN HANDLING HAZARDOUS CHEMICALS

Whenever employees work with hazardous chemicals, they should observe the following recommended general precautions:
- Handle chemicals properly in accordance with instructions from the manufacturer or supplier.
- Avoid skin contact with chemicals.
- Minimize chemical vapor in the air.
- Do not leave chemical bottles open.
- Do not use a flame near flammable chemicals.
- Do not eat or smoke in areas where chemicals are used.
- When appropriate, wear protective eyewear and mask.
- Dispose of all hazardous chemicals in accordance with MSDS instructions and applicable local, state, and federal regulations.

---

8. Bags to seal spilled materials and contaminated objects
9. Well-ventilated work areas, where ventilation can be turned off in the event of an accident
10. Scavenging system (when nitrous oxide is used)

INFECTION CONTROL TECHNIQUES

I. The goal of any infection control program must be to maintain sterile techniques and to avoid the potential of cross-infection through aseptic technique.

II. Aseptic technique, or asepsis, refers to the use of procedures that break the circle of infection and, ideally, eliminate cross-contamination.

III. The following techniques are examples of steps that can be taken to minimize contamination and cross-contamination during treatment procedures.
   A. The routine use of a pretreatment **antiseptic** mouth rinse that contains a substance to inhibit the growth of some microorganisms can lower the microbial load at a primary source for infection in the patient's mouth.
   B. An **antimicrobial** (inhibiting growth of microorganisms) hand-washing agent should be used regularly throughout the day, and hands must be washed thoroughly immediately before and after the treatment of each patient.
      1. The use of gloves does not serve as a substitute for routine hand washing with an effective liquid antiseptic because of the following reasons:
         a. Gloves may tear or perforate during patient treatment.
         b. Bacteria that remains on the skin after washing or enters through a compromised glove can multiply rapidly under the glove.
      2. An antimicrobial hand wash (using an antimicrobial substance to wash the hands) involves the following steps:
         a. Wet the hands with cold water to close the pores of the skin.
         b. Work the lathered soap completely over the hands and up onto the forearms.
         c. Clean the areas between the fingers thoroughly.
         d. Clean the nail area thoroughly.
   C. A comprehensive medical history should be obtained for each patient and reviewed and updated at subsequent appointments.
      1. This information can alert the dental team

to medical problems that could, in conjunction with dental treatment, adversely affect the patient.

2. Not all patients with infectious diseases can be identified by medical history, physical examination, or laboratory tests.

3. Health care professionals face many infectious diseases during contact with dental patients (box below).

4. The medical history is a poor indicator of prior infectious diseases; thus every patient must be considered infectious and subject to the same infection control procedures.

PERSONAL PROTECTION

I. Personal protection involves two basic considerations: Immunologic protection and barrier protection.

II. **Immunization** is the process by which resistance to an infectious disease is induced or augmented.

A. The human body can produce immunity to particular diseases or conditions; when no immunity exists for a disease, immunization is provided through vaccination.

B. Immunization to prevent and control cross-infection is an important aspect for dental health care providers.

C. Approved vaccines are available for a variety of infections (box below).

III. Dental care providers should use the following **barriers** to protect them from infectious disease.

A. Properly fitting latex gloves protect the dental care provider from exposure through cuts and abrasions on the hands.

1. Reusing gloves is not recommended because washing gloves with hand-washing antiseptics increases both the size and number of pinholes in the gloves and compromises the integrity of commercial gloves.

2. Dental personnel may need to change gloves while treating a single patient.

3. Medical-grade vinyl gloves are an alternative for latex gloves.

4. Manufactured gloves may come with talc or cornstarch on the inside surfaces.

5. Dental personnel should wear overgloves (thin, oversized, clear plastic gloves) when retrieving devices from the mobile cabinet, mixing dental materials, leaving the treatment room for a short time, and touching patient records; doing so reduces the need for disinfection of devices and surfaces.

6. Dental personnel are advised to wear polynitrile gloves when tearing a room down after treatment, cleaning high-velocity evacuation (suction) systems, and processing instruments. These gloves can be sterilized because they are resistant to the heat and chemicals used in sterilizing units.

7. To remove the gloves, grasp the end of the cuff and turn the glove inside out; grasp the second glove by the cuff and turn it inside out over the first glove.

INFECTIOUS DISEASES ENCOUNTERED BY HEALTH CARE PROFESSIONALS

Common cold
Pneumonia
Acute pharyngitis
Tuberculous infection
Tuberculosis
Herpangina
Chickenpox
Rubella
Hand-foot-mouth disease
Mumps
Rubeola
Herpetic infections
Cytomegalovirus
Acute herpetic gingivostomatitis
Herpes labialis
Recurrent intraoral infections
Herpetic whitlow
Chlamydia infections
Gonococcal infections
Syphilis
Trichomonal infections
Acquired immunodeficiency syndrome
Hepatitis
Acute and chronic sinusitis

IMMUNIZATION IS AVAILABLE FOR THE FOLLOWING DISEASES

- Hepatitis B virus
- Measles
- Rubella
- Influenza
- Mumps
- Certain other microbial infections
- Tuberculosis (testing is available to determine whether an individual has or has been exposed to tuberculosis)

B. Dental personnel should wear protective eyewear or an appropriate face shield during treatment procedures, in the dental laboratory, and in the sterilization/disinfection area when mixing and pouring chemicals.
1. Side shields can be affixed to prescription eyeglasses to provide protection.
2. Face shields are recommended if side shields are not used.
3. Protective eyewear with side shields is placed before patient treatment and removed with gloves in place after treatment is completed.
4. The eyewear can remain in place but should not be touched with ungloved hands.
5. Protective eyewear should be disinfected after use.
6. Protective eyewear should also be provided for each patient and disinfected after use.
C. The use of an approved face mask will protect the dentist, hygienist, assistant, and laboratory technician from microbe-laden aerosolized droplets.
1. The best masks are those that can filter at least 95% of droplet particles of 3.0 to 3.2 gm diameter.
2. A proper fit is required for both comfort and barrier efficiency.
3. Masks should be changed for each patient.
4. If a plastic face shield is worn, the appropriate face mask should also be worn.
5. The masks should be donned before gloves for ease of placement.
6. The mask is adjusted to facial configurations for proper adaptation.
7. A mask should not be allowed to hang below the clinician's chin after use; complete removal of the mask is recommended.
D. Dental personnel must wear the appropriate uniform or gown for all dental treatment, as follows:
1. Long-sleeved or short-sleeved uniforms or clinic jackets are used; each type has positive and negative features.
2. Changing the gown or uniform or wearing a protective cover over the uniform when an aerosol spray is being generated is recommended.
3. All clinical attire should be made of synthetic material so that contaminants are not easily absorbed into the material.
4. Seams, buttons, and buckles should be

kept to a minimum for the same reason as given in 3.
5. In oral or periodontal surgery and hospital dentistry, additional coverings may be considered.
6. Hair and shoe coverings offer additional protection to the health care provider.
7. Clinical attire should be removed each day when all clinical activities are completed.
8. Taking a shower and changing all clinical attire before leaving the facility is recommended.
9. Clinical attire should not be worn during food breaks or taken home to launder.
10. Clinical attire is not considered general clothing that is worn on a daily basis.
11. Wearing jewelry such as necklaces, bracelets, earrings, and rings should be eliminated or at least reduced.
E. Other barriers to consider include the following:
1. Rubber dam when performing restorative or endodontic procedures
2. High-speed evacuation device
3. Disposable covers or drapes on operatory surfaces

STERILIZATION

I. Disinfection is the inhibition or destruction of most pathogens—but not spores—on a given surface.
II. Sterilization is the destruction or removal of all forms of life, with particular reference to microorganisms.
A. The ultimate requirement for sterilization is the destruction of bacterial and fungal spores.
B. Sterilization methods applicable to dentistry include the following:
1. Prolonged dry heat
2. Unsaturated chemical vapor
3. Steam under pressure
4. Ethylene oxide
5. Certain chemical sterilants
C. Each method of sterilization has certain advantages and disadvantages (Table 7-3).
III. The CDC classifies instruments and devices into three categories, depending on the risk of transmitting infection and the need to sterilize (box on page 106).
IV. **Cold disinfection** refers to disinfecting instruments at room temperature by immersing them in a chemical solution.

Table 7-3 Features of sterilization methods

Method	Advantages	Disadvantages
Steam under pressure	Short cycle time Good penetration Wide range of material can be processed without destruction	Corrosion of unprotected carbon steel instruments Dulling of unprotected cutting edges Packages may remain wet at end of cycle May destroy heat-sensitive materials
Dry heat	Effective and safe for sterilization of metal instruments and mirrors Does not dull cutting edges Does not rust or corrode	Long cycle required for sterilization Poor penetration May discolor and char fabric Destroys heat-labile items
Unsaturated chemical vapor	Short cycle time Does not rust or corrode metal instruments, including carbon steel Does not dull cutting edges Suitable for orthodontic stainless wires	Instruments must be completely dried before processing Will destroy heat-sensitive plastics Chemical odor in poorly ventilated areas Slow-requires extended cycle times
Ethylene oxide	High capacity for penetration Does not damage heat-labile materials (including rubber and hand pieces) Evaporates without leaving a residue Suitable for materials that cannot be exposed to moisture	 Retained liquids and rubber materials for prolonged intervals Causes tissue irritation if not well aerated Requires special *spark-shield*—explosive in the presence of flame or sparks

---

CENTERS FOR DISEASE CONTROL AND PREVENTION: CATEGORIES FOR INSTRUMENTS AND DEVICES

Critical: Surgical and other instruments used to penetrate soft tissue or bone are classified as critical and should be sterilized after each use. These devices include forceps, scalpels, bone chisels, scalers, and burs.

Semicritical: Instruments such as mirrors and amalgam condensers, that do not penetrate soft tissues or bone but contact oral tissues, are classified as semicritical. These devices should be sterilized after each use. If, however, sterilization is not feasible because the instrument will be damaged by heat, the instrument should receive, at a minimum, high-level disinfection.

Noncritical: Instruments or medical devices such as external components of x-ray heads, that come into contact only with intact skin, are classified as noncritical. Because their noncritical surfaces have a relatively low risk of transmitting infection, these instruments and devices may be reprocessed among patients with intermediate- or low-level disinfection or detergent and water washing, depending on the nature of the surface and the degree and nature of the contamination involved.

A. Often referred to as *immersion disinfection,* this process represents an often abused aspect of office asepsis.

B. Solutions are often misused and thus destruction of all microbial forms cannot be guaranteed. Cold disinfection should not be confused with acceptable methods of sterilization.

V. **Sanitization,** a frequently used process, involves the use of agents to maintain the microbial flora at safe public health levels.

VI. Processing of dental instruments and armamentarium requires the use of utility gloves for protection.

A. Before sterilization the instruments can be placed in a holding or soaking tank to loosen hardened debris and then moved to an ultrasonic cleaner or placed directly into the ultrasonic cleaner to be cleansed of any debris.

B. Ultrasonic cleaning does not sterilize instruments but simply removes any debris that could compromise the sterilization process.

C. After instruments are removed from the ultrasonic cleaner, they must be rinsed thoroughly and tapped or blotted dry.

D. If the instruments are to be placed in cold disinfection because of their melting point, this should be done immediately after rinsing under water.

E. If the instruments are to be placed in dry heat or chemical sterilization, the instruments must be thoroughly dried; otherwise, corrosion of the metal may occur, resulting in dulled cutting edges and rusted joints.

F. Instruments to be sterilized in steam under pressure, especially metal instruments, those with sharp cutting edges or hinged parts, must be placed in a surgical milk or liquid emulsion to prevent corrosion. Certain instruments are not recommended for placement in the oil emulsion, such as mirrors, amalgam carriers, anesthetic syringes, and endodontic instruments.

G. Bagging instruments aids in verifying their sterility; color-coded indicators signify whether an instrument bag has reached sterilizing temperatures.

H. Instruments can be bagged as tray setups to enhance efficiency.

I. Care must be taken not to overload the bag or basket, which would prevent the sterilant from effectively reaching all the instruments.

J. Follow the steps listed for processing contaminated trays (box).

VII. Complete sterilization is achieved by the use of moist heat at high temperatures in the form of saturated steam under pressure in airtight vessels, such as an autoclave or omniclave. The technique is an efficient and effective method of sterilization.

VIII. Unsaturated chemical vapor is a system of sterilization that depends on a combination of heat, water, and chemicals in a pressurized system to be effective.

A. The chemicals include mixtures of alcohols, formaldehyde, ketone, acetone, and water.

B. The solution of premixed chemicals added to the jacket reservoir in the sterilizer must be purchased from the manufacturer because the ratio of each chemical in the preparation is critical.

C. When the apparatus is preheated, clean, and dry, place the loosely wrapped instruments in the chamber.

D. The major advantages of chemical vapor sterilization are as follows:
   1. A short cycle time compared with that of steam under pressure
   2. No rusting of instruments and burs in contrast to steam sterilization
   3. Dry instruments when cycle is complete
   4. Automatic cycle timing

STEPS TO FOLLOW WHEN PROCESSING CONTAMINATED TRAYS

- Determine whether the patient was at high-risk and handle appropriately.
- Discard disposables.
- Place instruments in a holding tank for the prescribed time.
- Clean instruments in an ultrasonic cleaner.
- Rinse instruments thoroughly and tap or blot dry.
- If appropriate, determine which method of sterilization or disinfection to use.
- If steam under pressure is used, dip sharp and hinged instruments in protective emulsion.
- If chemical vapor is used, dry instruments completely before processing.
- If a cold chemical is used, place instruments in the container and cover with solution. If the instruments are added after cycle timing has begun, restart the cycle.
- Before the sterilization process begins, instruments can be packaged for the appropriate sterilization method. Remove the instruments from the sterilizer or disinfection solution.
- Return the instruments to storage area.

E. Disadvantages of this system include the following:
   1. Requirement for adequate ventilation, which can constitute a problem
   2. Chemical vapors, particularly formaldehyde, that are released when the chamber door is opened at the end of the cycle, leaving a temporary unpleasant odor in the area
   3. The need for protective eye, hand, and face wear while depressurizing a chamber or handling the sterilant chemicals

IX. Dry heat sterilizes much less efficiently than moist heat.

A. High temperatures are required for a properly functioning hot-air oven.

B. Dry heat is suitable for sterilizing glassware and metal instruments that rust or dull in the presence of water vapor.

C. High temperatures destroy many rubber- and plastic-based materials, melt the solder of most impression trays, weaken some fabrics, and discolor some fabrics and paper materials.

X. Inadequate sterilization of instruments by various methods may be caused by problems (box on page 108).

XI. The sterilization time/temperature/pressure chart is given in Table 7-4.

XII. Preparation and sterilization procedures for a variety of instruments and materials are shown in Table 7-5.

MONITORING STERILIZATION

I. An integral component of office sterilization procedures is monitoring the efficiency of the system.

POTENTIAL STERILIZER PROBLEMS
STEAM UNDER PRESSURE
• Faulty preparation of materials • Improper loading • Faulty seals, heating coils, traps, exhaust lines • Air in the chamber • Wet steam
DRY HEAT
• Excessive temperature • Mistimed cycle • Interrupted cycle • Heat-sensitive materials • Packages not correctly spaced • Longer sterilization internal • Charred wrapping materials • Use of inappropriate equipment (e.g., toaster, conventional oven
UNSATURATED CHEMICAL VAPOR
• Wraps not designed or intended for chemical vapor units • Improper instrument wraps (e.g., sealed containers, foil, cloth) • Wraps not loose enough to allow vapor penetration • Inadequate spacing of packs • Faulty door gasket or seals (e.g., worn from exposure to chemical vapor) • Unit not located in well-ventilated area or prep room • Instruments not dry before being placed in the sterilizer

II. Factors that may diminish the effectiveness of a sterilizer include the following:
   A. Improper wrapping of instruments
   B. Human error in timing the cycle
   C. Defective control gauges
   D. Sterilizer malfunction

III. Chemically treated tapes that change color or biologic controls to check for the proper functioning of an office sterilizer can be used.
   A. Autoclave tape is not an effective monitoring material.
   B. The major use of specific chemical indicators to monitor sterilization seems to be a routine check for each load of items processed through the sterilizer.
   C. Gross malfunctions can usually be detected quickly by using indicator labels, strips, and steam pattern cards.
   D. The use of calibrated biologic controls remains the main guarantee of sterilization.
      1. A test strip with harmless active spores is placed in the sterilization chamber with a normal load of instruments.
      2. The test strip is returned to the manufacturer or monitoring agency to verify that sterilization has occurred.
      3. The office is provided with written documentation that is maintained as a record.

HANDPIECE ASEPSIS

I. Recommended methods for heat sterilization of hand pieces are use of an autoclave or an unsaturated chemical vapor sterilizer, although dry-heat units of a newer generation and with a shorter cycle also appear to be feasible.

II. For handpieces that cannot withstand heat, the CDC has outlined a compromise precleaning and disinfection protocol.

III. Handpieces should also be properly lubricated before they are wrapped for sterilization.

IV. Failure to maintain the hand piece properly in this manner can also diminish its efficiency.

V. These procedures and precautions apply to other

Table 7-4 Sterilization time/temperature/pressure chart

Types of sterilization	Time	Temperature (°F)	Pressure (lb)
Steam under pressure	15 to 20 min	250 to 270	15 to 20
Unsaturated chemical vapor	20 to 30 min*	270	Automatic
Dry heat	1 hr	320 to 350	0

*The cycle length or time is reduced in some machines.

Table 7-5   Preparation and sterilization process

List of instruments*	Sterilize before processing	Place in holding tank	Discard in biohazard bag	Discard in sharps container	Discard in trash receptacle	Discard in glycerine	Clean ultrasonically	Rinse in water and drain	Dip in emulsion and drain†	Dry instruments thoroughly‡	Immerse in disinfectant	Sterilize in steam under pressure§	Sterilize in dry heat
Mirrors		X					X	X				X	
Explorer		X					X	X	X			X	
Cotton pliers		X					X	X	X			X	
Spoon excavator		X					X	X	X			X	
Articulating paper					X								
Cotton pellets					X								
2 × 2 cotton gauze					X								
Glass dappen dish		X										X	
Prophylaxis polishing cup					X								
Prophylaxis polishing brush					X								
Patient napkin					X								
Operator's protective glasses		X					X	X			X	X	
Amalgam carrier		X					X	X				X	
Leftover amalgam						X							
Plastic saliva ejector					X								
Endodontic file		X					X	X		X		X	X
Anesthetic syringe		X					X	X				X	
Anesthetic needle				X									
Anesthetic syringe, HBV patient	X												
Extracted tooth with granuloma			X	X									
Burs		X					X	X	X			X	
Unused activated amalgam capsule						X							
Contra angle							X	X	X			X	
Diamond stone		X					X	X	X			X	
Composite finishing disk					X								
Scissors		X					X	X	X			X	
Rubber dam					X								
Rubber dam frame		X					X	X				X	
Metal air/water syringe tip		X					X	X				X	
Nu-tip a/w sheath					X						X		
Plastic impression tray		X					X	X				X	

*Contaminated instruments, not otherwise noted, have been used on patients when there is no indication of HIV or HBV noted in patient record.
†This step is used only with steam under pressure method of sterilization.
‡This step is used when dry heat or unsaturated chemical vapor sterilization is used.
§An alternative to steam under pressure is unsaturated chemical vapor, but instruments must be dried thoroughly.

items, such as A/W syringe tips and ultrasonic scalers.

VI. At all times, manufacturer's directions must be followed to preserve the integrity of the instruments.

SURFACE DISINFECTION

I. Surfaces that do not lend themselves to coverage must be cleaned and disinfected.

II. Disinfection of environmental surfaces is actually a two-step procedure.
  A. Initial mechanical removal of gross organic proteinaceous debris (precleaning) is required.
    1. The surfaces are sprayed with a disinfectant and/or detergent, followed by application of an appropriate disinfectant, with adequate time allowed for the chemical to achieve disinfection.
    2. This process is referred to as *spray/wipe/spray/wipe*.
    3. The first spray is to remove the bioburden.
    4. The second spray is to achieve disinfection after a time designated by the manufacturer.
  B. Table 7-6 lists representative disinfectants and the adverse effects involved with each.

III. Be aware of the instruments and equipment that are used during dental treatment and often become contaminated, such as cement bottles, varnish, paper pads, amalgamators, and light curing units.

A. The surfaces of these objects can also transmit disease from one patient to another.

B. These objects should be disinfected (just as other surfaces are) before they are used with another patient.

C. Using paper pads to mix and transfer dental cements and materials to the oral cavity allows contamination of the pad at chairside. Using glass or plastic slabs is an alternative.

EQUIPMENT ASEPSIS

I. Dental equipment that is small and heat resistant should be sterilized.

II. All other equipment must be covered or disinfected.

III. Office design, traffic flow, construction materials, and fixtures must be considered when implementing an asepsis regimen.
  A. The dental chair should be without cloth surfaces, seamless, and easily cleaned.
  B. Hoses on dental units should be smooth, be without ribs or grooves, and allow for easy disinfection.
  C. Other design features that minimize contact between hand and contaminated surfaces include the following:
    1. Dental chairs that are controlled by foot
    2. Sink faucets that are controlled by foot or forearm or are electronically controlled

Table 7-6 Representative chemical disinfectant types

Disinfectant*	Activity	Adverse features
Alcohol	Bactericidal and tuberculocidal; not sporicidal, limited virucidal activity	Denatures proteins, making it difficult to remove them from surfaces; denatured proteins protect bacteria from the effects of alcohol; rapid evaporation from treated surfaces
Chlorine dioxide	Rapid disinfection activity; can be used for sterilization with 6-hr exposure	Corrosive; activity greatly reduced in the presence of protein and organic debris; requires good ventilation
Glutaraldehyde	As 2.0%-3.2% immersion preparation, broad-spectrum antimicrobial activity; sporicidal after 10 hr exposure; long use life; surface disinfectant product available at 0.25% concentration	Very corrosive to skin and mucous membranes; allergenic with repeated exposures
Hypochlorite	Rapid-acting, broad-spectrum bactericidal, sporicidal, virucidal agent	Irritating to skin; corrosive; can degrade plastics
Iodophors	Rapid-acting, broad-spectrum disinfectant; residual antimicrobial activity remains on surface after drying	Corrosive to some metals; may discolor some surfaces; inactivated by hard water
Phenols	Broad-spectrum antimicrobial activity; effective in the presence of detergents	Can degrade plastics; irritating to skin and eyes; inactivated by hard water and organic debris
Quaternary amines	Effective against gram-positive bacteria; later generations, broader spectrum	May be inactivated by soaps and hard water; inactivated by organic debris

*Protective gloves should be worn when using disinfectant preparations.

3. Soap dispensers that are foot or forearm controlled

4. Towel dispensers (of disposable paper towels) that do not require touching a release mechanism

5. Plastic-lined waste containers that are recessed in cabinets beneath a countertop opening

6. Air-circulation exchange system or single-room air filtration unit that reduces the amount of airborne microbes

7. Floor covering, such as vinyl, that is constructed in a smooth and continuous manner, eliminating crevices that can trap debris

IV. Disposable barriers should be used whenever possible to avoid the necessity of excessive cleaning of both surfaces and equipment.

DISPOSABLES

I. Manufactured items identified for single use only, disposables (e.g., needles, saliva ejectors, prophylaxis cups, sealant), and composite brushes are not to be reused.

II. Disposables do not undergo recleaning and recycling but must be disposed of properly.

III. Needles and other sharps should be handled as follows:

A. Do not recap by hand.

B. Place in puncture-resistant containers for disposal.

LABORATORY ASEPSIS

I. Impressions, prosthetic devices, and the instrumentation used in their construction generally require handling by several individuals, in both the dental office and the commercial dental laboratories.

II. The American Dental Association and the CDC have recommended that impressions, appliances, and other items that are removed from a patient's mouth must be cleaned and disinfected before they are sent to the laboratory.

III. Items received from the laboratory for delivery to a patient must be cleaned and disinfected before placement in the patient's mouth.

IV. All items must be disinfected according to manufacturer's directions.

V. The materials and instruments used in constructing dental prostheses pose special problems in maintaining an aseptic environment.

A. Many of these items may be damaged by exposure to heat, or the chemicals may be used for disinfection.

B. The use of barriers to prevent contamination, of separate materials for new devices and those previously inserted in the mouth, and of unit doses of polishing materials will minimize cross-contamination in the dental laboratory setting.

C. Disinfection of dental impressions and prostheses must be undertaken with caution to avoid distorting impressions and damaging the metal, porcelain, or acrylic surfaces of prostheses.

D. Recommendations for the disinfection of impressions and prostheses based on the results of several research investigations include the following.

1. Immersion is preferable to spraying when possible because it ensures that all surfaces are adequately exposed to the disinfectant.

---

21 ITEMS FOR EVALUATING THE (MINIMUM) INFECTION CONTROL PROGRAM OF A DENTAL OFFICE

- Comprehensive medical history for each patient
- Hepatitis B vaccine
- Antiseptic mouth rinse
- Antiseptic hand rinse
- Disposable face mask
- Disposable latex gloves
- Protective eyewear
- Clinic attire
- Rubber dam
- Sharps disposable container
- Sterilizable hand pieces
- Ultrasonic cleaner
- Instrument packaging
- Heat sterilizer
- Sterilization monitoring
- Glutaraldehyde
- Surface cleaner
- Surface disinfectant
- Surface covers
- Waste disposal system
- OSHA poster

2. Thorough rinsing under running tap water is essential before disinfection to remove bioburden and after disinfection to remove any residual disinfectant.

PATIENT EDUCATION

I. Effective infection control must occur as a routine component of professional activity.
II. The use of universal precautions in the management of all patients greatly minimizes occupational exposure to microbial pathogens.
III. Procedures aimed at preventing the spread of infectious disease during dental treatment are continually evaluated by dental professionals and an increasingly inquisitive public.
IV. The following 21 items can be used to evaluate the (minimum) infection control program in a dental office (box on page 111).

Questions

Infection Control

1 *Bactericidal* refers to
a. Inhibiting bacterial growth
b. Bacteria in the bloodstream
c. Killing bacteria
d. Effect of bacteria on the body
2 What becomes contaminated in the dental treatment room with each procedure?
a. Floor
b. Patient record
c. Only intraoral instruments
d. All surfaces that come into contact with any microbes from the patient's mouth
3 Which materials are best sterilized by steam under pressure?
1. Tungsten carbide burs
2. Stainless steel hand instruments
3. Handpieces
4. Mouth mirror
5. Carbon steel instruments
6. Plastic head-rest covers
a. 1, 2, and 3
b. 1, 2, and 4
c. 2, 4, and 5
d. 1, 2, 3, 4, and 5
e. 1, 2, 3, 4, 5, and 6
4 Which microbes may be found in the oral cavity?
a. Bacteria
b. Fungi
c. Viruses
d. All of the above
5 Which diseases can be caused by contaminated dental instruments?

1. Traumatic bone cysts
2. Syphilis
3. ANUG
4. Thrush
5. Hepatitis
a. 1, 2, and 4
b. 1, 3, and 4
c. 2, 4, and 5
d. 3, 4, and 5
6 The effectiveness of an immersion disinfectant solution is altered by the
a. Number of instruments being processed
b. Dilution of water
c. Length of pressurization
d. Number of bacteria on the instruments
7 How long should an instrument be left in immersion disinfectant solutions before they are ready to be used again?
a. 30 minutes
b. 1 hour
c. 2 hours
d. 10 hours
8 An antibacterial solution that prevents multiplication of an organism but does not kill it is said to be
a. Hemolytic
b. Synergistic
c. Bactericidal
d. Bacteriostatic
9 Which error in the preparation of instruments for chemical disinfection is most likely to reduce the efficiency of the chemical?
a. Brief rinsing
b. Carryover of water
c. Failure to scrub instruments
d. Carryover of soap-containing water
e. Contamination of the instrument with dried blood
10 MSDS forms
1. Must be supplied by the manufacturer
2. Must be available to all employees
3. Are used to obtain information for labeling
4. May be necessary to obtain information after chemical exposure
a. 1 and 3
b. 2 and 4
c. 4 only
d. 1, 2, 3, and 4
11 A dental office manager whose responsibilities are only in the business office would be placed in which of the following OSHA task categories?
a. Category I
b. Category II
c. Category III
d. Category IV
12 Which of the following presents the greatest risk for the spread of infectious disease?
a. Patient to patient
b. DHCW to patient
c. DHCW to family member
d. Patient to DHCW

13 What is the preferred method of infection control for the x-ray machine control panel?
   a. Steam under pressure
   b. Disinfecting wipe
   c. Spray with aerosol disinfectant
   d. Barrier protection

14 What agency has established regulations regarding the rights of employees to know the potential dangers associated with hazardous chemicals in the workplace?
   a. ADDA
   b. ADA
   c. CDMIE
   d. OSHA
   e. EPA

15 How often should the high-speed handpiece be sterilized and lubricated?
   a. Each day
   b. Every third day
   c. Each week
   d. After each patient

16 Transferable diseases a person might encounter in the dental office include which of the following?
   1. HIV
   2. Strep throat
   3. Measles
   4. Rhinovirus
   5. Hepatitis B
   a. 1 and 5
   b. 1, 2, and 3
   c. 1, 3, 4, and 5
   d. 1, 2, 3, 4, and 5

17 Which categories of patients have a greater than average chance of harboring HIV?
   1. IV drug users
   2. Newborn children
   3. TB patients
   4. Organ transplant patients
   5. 40-year-old unmarried men
   a. 1 and 2
   b. 3 and 4
   c. 1 and 3
   d. 3, 4, and 5
   e. 1, 3, 4, and 5

18 Which of the following would have a task classification for personnel as outlined by OSHA standards for category I?
   1. Dental hygienist
   2. Custodian
   3. Phlebotomist
   4. Dental assistant
   5. Cosmetologist
   a. 1 and 3
   b. 2 and 5
   c. 1, 3, and 5
   d. 1, 3, and 4
   e. 1, 3, 4, and 5

19 Identify the diseases against which all dental personnel should be immunized.
   1. Tuberculosis
   2. HBV
   3. HIV
   4. Measles
   5. Mumps
   a. 1, 3, and 5
   b. 2, 4, and 5
   c. 2, 3, 4, and 5
   d. 1, 2, 3, 4, and 5

20 Rank infectious disease as one of the following conditions in order of greatest exposure to the DHCW
   a. Most common
   b. Less common
   c. Rare

21 Rank contamination as one of the following conditions in order of greatest exposure to the DHCW
   a. Most common
   b. Less common
   c. Rare

22 Which of the following would be the most ideal barrier techniques to protect the dental team?
   1. Use of only sterile instruments
   2. Patient rinse with mouthwash
   3. Complete patient history
   4. Use of HVE
   5. Use of rubber dam
   a. 1 and 3
   b. 2 and 4
   c. 1, 2, 3, and 4
   d. 1, 3, 4, and 5
   e. 1, 2, 3, 4, and 5

23 A health questionnaire completed by a patient indicates that the patient is HIV positive. The DHCW should
   a. Refuse treatment and refer the patient to a local dentist who treats patients with HIV.
   b. Treat the patient as any other patient would be treated.
   c. Delay treatment until the patient recovers.
   d. Tell the patient that the staff does not feel comfortable treating him or her.
   e. Refer the patient to a dentist who has HIV.

24 A health questionnaire completed by a patient indicates that the patient is HBV positive. The DHCW should do the following:
   a. Refuse treatment and refer the patient to a local dentist who treats patients with HBV.
   b. Treat the patient as any other patient would be treated.
   c. Delay treatment until the patient recovers.
   d. Tell the patient that the staff does not feel comfortable treating him or her.
   e. Refer the patient to a dentist who has HIV.

25 A health questionnaire completed by a patient indicates that the patient has tuberculosis. The DHCW should do the following:
   a. Delay treatment until the antibiotic regimen is underway.
   b. Treat the patient as any other patient would be treated.
   c. Refer the patient to a dentist who has tuberculosis.

Rationales

Infection Control

1 C Bacteria are small unicellular microorganisms of the class Schizomycetes. A bactericidal is an agent that is destructive to bacteria.

2 D Floors, patient records, intraoral instruments, or any other surface that is exposed to the microbes that exist in a patient's mouth are contaminated. Aerosols are commonly produced during dental treatment and may contaminate many areas not in direct contact with the oral cavity.

3 D Materials and instruments made of metal are more capable of withstanding the heat to which they are exposed during the sterilization process of steam under pressure. Devices made of plastic and glass may deteriorate since the temperature is in excess of 250 degrees F.

4 D Bacteria, fungi, and viruses can all be found in a patient's oral cavity.

5 C Traumatic bone cysts are caused by trauma to the tissue, and ANUG is a periodontal disease usually associated with poor oral hygiene. Syphilis and hepatitis are viral infections and thrush is a fungal infection that may be transmitted by contaminated dental instruments.

6 B Immersion disinfectant solution becomes less effective when excess water is introduced to the solution after the instruments are cleansed or if the solution is beyond its recommended reuse life.

7 D Most manufacturers recommend instruments be completely immersed in disinfectant solutions for approximately 10 hours to obtain maximum disinfectant ability.

8 D If a solution maintains growth of bacterial organisms, the solution does not kill the existing organisms as a bactericidal solution would, however it does not allow an increase in the number of organisms.

9 D Soap containing water diminishes the effectiveness of most chemical disinfectants.

10 D Although MSDS forms are being examined for change, currently they must be supplied by the manufacturer and made available to employees. This data is used to label other containers that are not originally from the manufacture. The form contains information to assist if an exposure occurs.

11 C There are three task categories:
- Category I for individuals who daily complete tasks that put them at risk for exposure such as the dentist or dental assistant
- Category II for individuals who may occasionally have the need to complete a task in which they might be at risk for exposure. An example may be a clerical staff member that may aid in tearing down a treatment room.
- Category III for a person such as the business office assistant, not in the treatment room area.
- Category IV is not a designated level.

12 D Although not always believed by the layperson, the greatest risk for the spread of infectious disease is from the patient to the DHCW.

13 D If possible, the best way to reduce transmission of disease with most dental equipment, if not sterilizable, is through the use of protective barriers.

14 D The Occupational Safety and Health Agency was originally formed and continues to be the agency primarily responsible for protecting employees through regulations of hazardous chemicals and other areas.

15 D It is recommended that handpieces be lubricated and sterilized after use with each patient to eliminate transmission of disease.

16 D Human immunodeficiency virus, strep throat, measles, rhinovirus (common cold), and hepatitis are all diseases seen in patients treated in a dental setting. Without the use of recommended infection control practices, transmission of any of these diseases is possible.

17 C Patients that are considered at greater risk of carrying and transferring HIV are IV drug users who share syringes and needles and patients with a form tuberculosis often associated with HIV.

18 A Refer to No. 11

19 B Currently immunizations are available for HBV, measles, and mumps but not for TB or HIV.

20 C The DHCW is rarely at risk of exposure to infectious disease due to the infection control protocol practiced.

21 A A DHCW may commonly be exposed to contaminates during the provision of treatment, but through the use of proper technique finds protection.

22 E Sterile instruments protect the DHCW from exposure prior to treatment; an oral rinse with antimicrobial mouthwash reduces microbes; complete health history determines whether the patient may be treated at this time, compared to if the patient has active TB; and the use of an HVE and rubber dam reduces contaminated aerosols.

23 B According to standard practice and the ADA law that protects against discrimination based on disability, the patient must be treated.

24 B Refer to No. 23

25 A The recommendation for the treatment of a patient with active TB is referral to the attending physician until the patient is deemed stable. A patient with nonactive TB may be seen as any other patient.

To enhance your understanding of the material in this chapter, refer to the illustrations in Finkbeiner/Johnson: *Mosby's Comprehensive Dental Assisting: A Clinical Approach,* Chapter 8.

Dental Radiography

OUTLINE

History of Ionizing Radiation
Radiation Physics
Dental Radiographic Equipment
Collimation and Filtration
Biologic Effects of Electromagnetic
 Radiation
ALARA Concept

Dental X-ray Film
Intraoral Film Packets
Patient Management
Intraoral Radiographic Techniques
Full-Mouth Radiographs
Procedure for Intraoral Dental
 Radiography

Extraoral Radiography
Common Errors in Intraoral
 Radiography
Processing Dental Radiographs
Mounting Radiographs
Duplicating Radiographs

KEY TERMS

Anode

ALARA concept

Atoms

Bisecting angle technique

Bitewing

Bremsstrahlung radiation

Cathode

Cephalometric

Characteristic radiation

Collimation

Electrons

Energy

Epilation

Erythema

Filtration

Gray

Kilovolt peak

Kinetic energy

Matter

Maximum permissible dose

Milliampere

Occlusal

Panoramic

Paralleling technique

Periapical

Position-indicating device

Rad

Radiation safety

Radiograph

Rem

Selective absorption

Sievert

Target

Temporomandibular joint

Tubehead

X-ray

Radiographs (visible images on a film) play such a vital role in diagnosing and managing care that it is difficult to imagine the practice of dentistry without them. Learning to safely operate and maintain radiographic equipment is essential. The quality of radiographic images directly contributes to the standard of care patients receive. For these reasons, federal law requires that states establish minimum educational and certification requirements for professionals who perform radiographic procedures.

HISTORY OF IONIZING RADIATION ▬▬▬▬

I. Crookes tube
   A. This tube was developed by William Crookes.
   B. It is also known as the cathode ray tube.
   C. It is an evacuated glass tube with two electrodes (**cathode** and **anode**) through which an electrical current is passed.

II. Wilhelm Conrad Roentgen
   A. Roentgen accidentally discovered **x-rays** on November 8, 1895.
   B. He discovered the following properties of cathode rays while investigating properties of the cathode ray:
      1. Consist of electrically negative particles
      2. Travel only a few centimeters in the air
      3. Can cause a fluorescent screen to glow
   C. Roentgen enclosed the Crookes tube with black paper and noticed that it glowed with fluorescent material on a workbench several feet away; he called the unknown ray *X*.
   D. The first radiograph (x-ray) made was of Roentgen's wife, Bertha; he placed her hand on a photographic plate and directed x-rays toward it; when the plate was developed, an image of the bones of her hand appeared.
   E. Edmund Kells, a significant contributor to the advancement of dental assistants, was the first dentist in the United States to use radiography. He conducted seminars and training programs in the application of radiography for dental diagnosis.

RADIATION PHYSICS ▬▬▬▬

I. All things in the world around us can be classified as either **matter** or **energy.**
   A. Albert Einstein discovered the interchangeability of matter and energy known as the *theory of relativity.*
   B. Einstein's mass equivalence equation, $E = mc^2$, describes the relationship of matter and energy where E is energy, m is mass, and c is the speed of light.

II. Matter is anything that occupies space and has form or shape.
   A. Matter is the substance of which all physical objects are made.
   B. Matter has many forms, including solids, liquids, and gases.
   C. Matter is composed of **atoms** grouped together in specific arrangements called *molecules.*

III. Energy is defined as the ability to do work.

A. There are seven fundamental forms of energy (Table 8-1).
B. Although energy can be neither created nor destroyed, it can change form, thus maintaining total energy within the universe constant.
C. Atoms contain energy.
   1. The energy holding the nucleus together is called *nuclear binding energy.*
   2. The energy holding **electrons** (negatively charged particles) in their shells is known as *electron binding energy.*
   3. Inner shell electrons have greater binding energy than outer shell electrons.
   4. Nuclear and electron binding energies are characteristic for a given atom; the magnitude of these energies increases as the atomic number increases.

IV. Ionizing radiation is energy released during ionization.
   A. Electrons can be removed from an atom in a process called *ionization.*
   B. Enough energy to overcome electron binding energy must be absorbed by the atom for ionization to occur.
   C. Ionization results in the formation of an ion pair—a negatively charged free electron and the remaining part of the atom, now positively charged.
   D. The amount of energy required to displace outer shell electrons is less than that required to displace inner shell electrons.
   E. Ionization most frequently occurs in the outer electron shells.
   F. X-rays can impart enough energy to an atom to displace inner shell electrons.
   G. When inner shell electrons are removed from an atom, the resulting ion is unstable.
   H. The remaining electrons in this unstable ion rearrange to fill the vacant inner shell, leaving the outer shell unfilled.
   I. **Characteristic radiation** is emitted from the atom when these electron rearrangements occur.
   J. The energy of the characteristic radiation emitted is approximately equal to the difference in the electron binding energy between the shells.

V. Particulate radiation consists of particles that have both mass and energy.
   A. Some particles may have a positive, negative, or neutral charge.

Table 8-1 Forms of energy

Energy form	Definition	Examples
Potential	Energy possessed by matter by virtue of position	A guillotine blade pulled to its maximum height
Kinetic	Energy possessed by matter	A moving automobile, a turning windmill
Chemical	Energy released when molecular bonds are broken	An explosion, the act of metabolizing food
Electrical	Energy produced by moving electrons	Household electricity; an alternating flow of electrons that drives motors, operates appliances, etc.
Thermal	Energy associated with molecular motion	Kinetic energy of atoms; heat—the faster molecules move, the higher thermal energy they possess
Nuclear	Energy contained in the atomic nucleus	Nuclear power plants and atomic bombs
Electromagnetic	Energy moving through space	Radiowaves, microwaves, light, x-rays

B. Particulate radiation cannot reach the speed of light

C. Examples include neutrons, protons, electrons, α-particles, and β-particles

VI. Electromagnetic radiation involves bundles of energy that have neither mass nor charge.

   A. Electric and magnetic fields are associated with the travel of the electromagnetic energy through space.

   B. Electromagnetic energies exist over a wide range of magnitudes, termed the *electromagnetic spectrum.*

   C. Interaction of electromagnetic radiation with matter may be described in terms of wave and particle behavior.

   D. The electromagnetic spectrum is measured according to frequency, energy, and wavelength.

   E. An important property of electromagnetic radiation is that substances selectively absorb, reflect, or transmit it, depending on their structure. **Selective absorption** (the ability of a substance to absorb or transmit x-rays) is used to create dental radiographs.

VII. The average annual effective dose of ionizing radiation to a U.S. resident is 3.63 millisieverts (mSv).

   A. Natural sources (e.g., cosmic, radon, terrestrial, and internal sources) account for 3.0 mSv or about 82%.

   B. Manufactured sources (e.g., medical, nuclear medicine, consumer product, and occupational sources) account for 0.63 mSv or 18%.

   C. Of manufactured sources, medical x-rays account for 0.39 mSv or 11%.

VIII. **Bremsstrahlung radiation** is the transformation of kinetic energy to electromagnetic energy in an x-ray tube.

   A. *Bremsstrahlung* is a German word that, roughly translated, means *braking radiation.* This term was coined because radiation produced in the diode tube occurs when electrons are decelerated.

   B. The production of Bremsstrahlung radiation within the diode tube is, however, an inefficient process.

   C. Only about 1% of the electron interactions at the target actually result in x-ray production.

   D. Bremsstrahlung radiation occurs only when electrons strike the target close to a tungsten nucleus; the positive nuclear charge places an electrostatic force on the electron, causing it to decelerate suddenly, releasing enough energy to produce an x-ray photon; most (99%) electrons striking the target dissipate acquired kinetic energy as heat; dissipation of kinetic energy as heat occurs when electrons transfer some energy to orbital electrons in the tungsten target atom but do not cause ionization.

   E. Some electrons interact with tungsten orbital electrons, imparting enough energy to ionize the tungsten target.

   F. When electrons displace inner shell electrons, characteristic radiation is produced; thus three major interactions of electrons with target atoms occur:
      1. Heat
      2. Bremsstrahlung radiation
      3. Characteristic radiation

DENTAL RADIOGRAPHIC EQUIPMENT ▰

I. Radiographic equipment or x-ray machines are devices that use moving charges (electrons) to produce electromagnetic radiation.

II. Laboratory electromagnetic radiation is designated as *x-rays.*

III. An x-ray machine contains the following components:
   A. Tubehead
   B. Suspension arm
   C. Control panel
   D. Power source

IV. The **tubehead** is the working part of the x-ray machine (Fig. 8-1).
   A. The *yoke* attaches the tubehead to a movable *suspension arm.*
   B. The tubehead rotates freely, allowing dental x-rays to be made from several directions and accommodating patients of different sizes and shapes.
   C. The tubehead is attached to the yoke by two *vertical connectors.*
      1. Vertical connectors allow adjustments in the vertical angle of the tubehead, whereas the yoke allows adjustments in the horizontal angle.

V. The suspension arm is used to adjust the height of the tubehead independent of its vertical or horizontal position.
   A. The **position-indicating device (PID),** the portion of the tubehead that emits the radiation, extends from the tubehead and directs radiation toward the patient. X-rays exit the machine from the PID only when the exposure switch is depressed.
   B. Within the tubehead housing is a *diode tube.* The diode tube is the most important part of the tubehead because x-rays originate within this tube.

VI. A wire in the suspension arm connects the tubehead to the control panel.

VII. Power is supplied to the system through an electrical outlet.

VIII. Components of the x-ray tube
   A. A schematic of the diode tube is shown in Fig. 8-2.
   B. The two main components of the diode tube are the cathode and the anode.
   C. The cathode provides a source of negatively charged particles (electrons).
      1. It contains a tungsten filament and a molybdenum *focusing cup.*
      2. When electrical current passes through the filament, electrons are given off by a process called *thermionic emission,* or *heat production.*
      3. The focusing cup further concentrates electrons into a cloud of charged particles.
      4. The **milliampere (mA)** setting on the control panel regulates the amount of electrical current passing through the filament.
      5. Increasing the mA increases the number of electrons emitted by the filament.
      6. In many dental x-ray machines the mA is

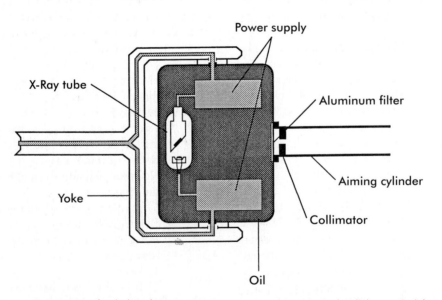

Fig. 8-1   Illustration of tubehead parts. (From Goaz PW, White SC: *Oral radiology, principles and interpretation,* ed 3, St Louis, 1994, Mosby.)

set by the manufacturer, usually between 7 and 10 mA.

7. In other dental x-ray machines the mA can be changed by the operator.

D. The anode contains a copper *stem* and a tungsten **target.**

1. When high voltage is applied to the tube, electrons are accelerated from the cathode toward the anode.

2. These accelerating electrons contain **kinetic energy,** the energy of motion.

3. When the electrons collide with the tungsten target, they stop suddenly, which transforms the electron's kinetic energy into electromagnetic energy, thus producing x-rays.

4. The electron does not become an x-ray, but rather its kinetic energy is transformed to x-ray energy.

5. The amount of kinetic energy acquired by electrons in the diode tube depends on the **kilovolt peak (kVp)**—the maximum amount of voltage that an x-ray machine is using—applied to the tube; when the kVp setting is high, the x-rays produced are more energetic and readily penetrate objects.

6. When the kVp setting is low, the x-rays produced are less energetic and more likely to be absorbed by objects.

7. Because soft tissues absorb more x-rays when the kVp setting is low, federal law requires dental x-ray machines to operate at 50 kVp or higher.

8. Dental x-ray machines are usually operated between 65 and 90 kVp.

IX. The control panel contains an on/off switch with an indicator light; an exposure button with an indicator light and audible signal, timer dial, and kVp and mA selectors.

A. Federal law requires the *exposure button* to be connected to an indicator light and audible signal.

1. The exposure button must be a switch that operates only with continuous pressure.

2. The *on/off switch* controls electrical current to the radiographic machine.

3. The *timer dial* controls the number of impulses generated by the radiographic machine.

4. The number of impulses produced is based on the cycle of electrical current available; if 60- or 70-cycle alternating currents are available, the number of impulses generated in 1 second would be 60 or 70 impulses; one impulse is equal to $\frac{1}{60}$ of a second.

5. The exposure switch or button is located on the control panel.

6. When the button is depressed, the circuit of electricity is completed, allowing the flow of electrons to occur and the x-ray process to continue.

B. The timer determines the length of time radiation is produced.

1. Like the mA, the timer also controls the number of x-rays produced, but not their energy.

2. When the kVp and mA are preset by the manufacturer, changing the timer is the only way to control x-ray output.

C. Federal laws also regulate the accuracy of x-ray machine timers.

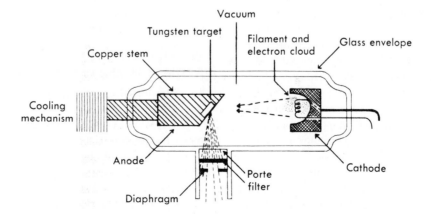

Fig. 8-2 The x-ray tubehead has two main components: the cathode and the anode. (From Frommer HH: *Radiology for dental auxiliaries,* ed 5, St Louis, 1992, Mosby.)

COLLIMATION AND FILTRATION

I. When electrons strike the anode, their kinetic energy is transformed into electromagnetic photons (x-rays).
   A. X-rays are produced in many directions and are of varying energies.
   B. To produce a useful beam of radiation, the x-rays must be collimated and filtered.

II. **Collimation** is the restriction in the size of the x-ray beam through the use of a lead shielding and diaphragms. The first step in constructing a useful beam of radiation is shielding the diode tube with a lead cylinder.
   A. The lead cylinder completely encases the tube except for a small opening—the *window,* or *aperture.*
   B. The lead cylinder completely absorbs x-rays, creating a beam of radiation at the window.
   C. The x-ray beam is further limited with an open-ended, lead-lined collimator.
   D. The collimator, also called the position-indicating device (PID), further restricts the diameter of the beam of radiation reaching the patient.
   E. The collimator is a major factor in minimizing exposure to a patient.
   F. The beam of radiation should be collimated so that it closely approximates the size of film used.
   G. Federal law requires that the dental x-ray beam be no more than 2.75 inches in diameter.
   H. With film holders it is possible to limit a dental x-ray beam even more than is required by law.

III. Filtration usually consists of a disk of aluminum placed at the window.
   A. X-rays are produced at the target not only in all directions but also at varying energies.
   B. Low energy x-rays can be preferentially removed from the beam with added **filtration.**
   C. Added filtration selectively removes low-energy x-rays from the primary beam, reducing patient dose.
   D. Federal law requires 1.5 mm of added aluminum filtration when operating at 50 to 70 kVp and at least 2.5 mm of aluminum when operating above 70 kVp.

IV. An important property of electromagnetic radiation is that substances selectively absorb, reflect, or transmit radiation, depending on their structure.
   A. Selective absorption of radiation is used to create x-ray images (dental radiographs).
   B. The amount of radiation absorbed by a substance depends on three aspects of its structure:
      1. Effective atomic number
      2. Physical density
      3. Thickness
   C. Structures with large atomic numbers, such as enamel and silver, absorb most of the x-rays in the primary beam.
   D. Structures with an intermediate atomic number, such as bones and dentin, absorb some x-rays, while many are transmitted.
   E. X-rays are readily transmitted through structures made up of material of low atomic number, such as soft tissue and the dental pulp.

V. Selective absorption is used to make radiographs. When x-rays are directed toward the jaw, the teeth, bones, and soft tissue selectively absorb them, creating a pattern of remnant radiation unique for that individual.

VI. In dental radiology x-ray film acts as a receptor to detect the photons that are transmitted through the patient.
   A. X-ray film is a clear polyester sheet coated with a silver-halide emulsion that is sensitive to radiation.
   B. When x-rays strike the emulsion, silver atoms are released, creating an area of blackness.
      1. Areas where many photons strike the film become black and are, called *radiolucent areas;* they represent structures penetrated by x-ray photons.
      2. Areas where the film remains light are called *radiopaque areas;* radiopacities correspond to tissues that have absorbed much of the radiation.
      3. Silver amalgam restorations absorb a lot of radiation and are radiopaque (white), whereas cavities caused by dental caries are radiolucent (black).

BIOLOGIC EFFECTS OF ELECTROMAGNETIC RADIATION

I. Factors determining the biologic effects of radiation
   A. Energy and amount of radiation absorbed
   B. Length of time over which exposure occurred
   C. Area of the body or type of tissue irradiated
   D. Environmental factors

II. High- and low-dose effects
   A. The most important determinant of biologic effect is the amount of radiation absorbed.

B. Biologic effects can be classified into two categories based on the amount of radiation absorbed: *high-dose* and *low-dose* effects.

C. High-dose effects occur when large amounts of radiation (>50 rem whole body) are absorbed.

D. Low-dose effects occur when radiation exposures are minimal.

III. High-dose effects

A. When tissues absorb high doses of radiation, biologic damage is predictable.

B. Radiation damage in a biologic system is not seen immediately; the time it takes to develop is called the *latent period.*

C. The latent period is the time between exposure to radiation and clinical evidence of a harmful effect.

D. When high doses of radiation are absorbed, harmful effects are seen after a short latent period (weeks or months).

E. It is easy to relate these detrimental effects to absorption of radiation.

F. High-dose effects are easily quantified and directly related to the amount of radiation absorbed.

G. The harmful effects produced by high doses of radiation also depend on cell type of tissue irradiated.

H. When only a part of the body is irradiated rather than the whole body, much larger doses of radiation are required to produce a response.

I. Cells and organ systems also differ in sensitivity to radiation; cells that are active and reproduce frequently are the most sensitive to radiation.

J. Organ systems in which cellular turnover is infrequent are usually resistant to the detrimental effects of radiation (Table 8-2).

K. Examples of high-dose radiation effects include the following:

1. **Epilation** (hair loss) and **erythema** (skin reddening) are examples of high-dose effects associated with therapeutic radiation.

2. Early radiation workers frequently suffered from the effects of high-dose radiation.

3. Nuclear weapons dropped on Hiroshima resulted in 90,000 casualties and the radiation-induced death of 45,000 people.

L. High-dose effects are not possible with modern dental x-ray machines using the amount of radiation required to produce a diagnostic radiograph.

IV. Low-dose effects

A. Low-dose effects are a concern in diagnostic radiology.

B. Detrimental effects associated with absorption of low doses of radiation include the following:

1. Radiation-induced malignancies

2. Local tissue damage

3. Genetic effects

C. Low-dose effects occur sporadically after a long latent period.

1. Any exposure to radiation is potentially harmful.

2. Exposure to low-dose radiation increases the incidence of diseases already present in a population.

3. The probability that low doses of radiation will be detrimental is small.

4. A small radiation-induced increase is difficult to notice when a naturally occurring incidence is large.

5. Latent periods are long (years or decades), making it difficult or impossible to associate a specific radiation exposure with a specific effect.

6. On an individual level, cause and effect cannot be measured because it is impossible to distinguish between radiation-induced and spontaneous disease.

7. Other environmental factors (cocarcinogens) may potentiate low-dose radiation, further confusing the relationship between low-dose radiation exposure and disease induction.

D. Certain facts relating to low-dose effects are accepted as true in light of current knowledge.

1. Certain tissues—those that make up *critical organs*—are particularity sensitive to low levels of ionizing radiation (Table 8-3).

2. **Radiation safety** procedures are directed toward minimizing exposure to these highly sensitive organs.

Table 8-2 Sensitivity of organs to high-dose radiation

High sensitivity	Intermediate sensitivity	Low sensitivity
Lymphoid organs	Endothelial cells	Salivary glands
Bone marrow	Fibroblasts	Lungs
Testes	Growing bone	Muscle
Intestines	Growing cartilage	Brain and spinal cord

Table 8-3 Critical organs

Tissue/organ	Low-dose effect
Hematopoietic	Leukemia
Thyroid gland	Neoplasia
Breast	Neoplasia
Salivary gland	Neoplasia
Gonads	Impaired fertility; mutations
Pregnancy	Fetal effects
Skin	Neoplasia
Lens of the eye	Cataracts

3. Low-dose radiation damage is cumulative over the lifetime of an individual.
4. Even though the risk from low-dose radiation is minimal, any reduction in exposure is believed to result in additional risk reduction.
5. It is believed that certain dental health benefits outweigh the potential risk of diagnostic radiation exposure.

V. Low-dose radiation risk
  A. *Risk estimates* are calculated because the harmful effects associated with dental x-rays cannot be proven or directly observed.
  B. Radiation-induced malignancy is one of the most important low-dose effects.
  C. Tissues at greatest risk of cancer induction after dental radiographs are obtained are the thyroid gland, salivary gland, female breast, brain, and bone marrow.
  D. The risk of radiation-induced cancer associated with dental x-rays is estimated as the number of excess cases per million persons irradiated per cSv (rem) per year.
  E. Patients must be reassured that radiographic procedures have been selected to provide important diagnostic information and that optimum techniques are used to reduce risk to acceptable levels.
  F. The patient must be informed of the necessity of radiographs to meet their specific dental health needs.

VI. Radiographs during pregnancy
  A. Dental radiographs are considered safe for patients who may be pregnant.
  B. Radiography for pregnant patients is avoided only when a fetus or embryo would be in or near the primary x-ray beam (such as lower abdominal or pelvic radiographs).
  C. In dental radiography the primary beam is limited to the head and neck region.
  D. The only radiation that a fetus or embryo is exposed to is secondary radiation.
  E. The final decision on radiographic exposure rests with the patient and her physician.
  F. Uterine doses for full-mouth intraoral radiography have been shown to be less than 1 mrem (even without a leaded apron in place).
  G. Uterine dose from naturally occurring background radiation during the 9 months of pregnancy is estimated to be about 75 mrem.
  H. There is no reason to postpone a properly justified dental radiographic examination because of pregnancy.

VII. Radiographs and radiation therapy
  A. Dental radiographs do not present an additional risk for individuals who have a history of radiation therapy to the head and neck region.
  B. Xerostomia frequently occurs after radiation therapy, resulting in a high risk for caries and other dental diseases in these individuals.
  C. Radiation therapy usually involves doses of more than 1000 rem, whereas diagnostic radiography results in doses of less than 1 rem.
  D. There is no reason to postpone necessary dental radiographic examination because of a history of radiation therapy.

ALARA CONCEPT

I. The National Council on Radiation Protection, a federal agency, establishes minimum radiation exposure limits.
II. The guiding principle for protection from radiation exposure is known as the **ALARA concept (*as low as reasonably achievable*).**
  A. When radiation is used, every available method for reducing exposure should be implemented to minimize potential risks and adverse consequences.
  B. When the ALARA concept is applied to patient exposures, it means that the maximum diagnostic benefit is provided with minimum exposure.
  C. When applied to occupational exposures, it means that diagnostic exposures should be completed without exposure to the operator.
  D. The greatest amount of radiation to which an individual can be exposed in the work environment is called the **maximum permissible dose (MPD).**
    1. Currently the MPD is 2.5 cSv (rem) per year.

2. Although a person can continue to work if exposed to less than 2.5 cSv (rem) in a year, the goal should be no exposure.

III. The ALARA concept is the guiding principle in dental radiography

A. Collimation

1. The beam of radiation should be restricted so that the smallest possible volume of tissue is irradiated.

2. Federal laws require that the beam diameter be no more than 2.75 inches at the patient's face.

3. Long, open-ended collimators (12 to 16 inches) are preferred because a smaller volume of the patient's face is irradiated than when shorter (8-inch) collimators are used.

4. Pointed plastic cones should never be used because they increase the volume of tissue irradiated and the amount of scattered radiation absorbed in the patient's head and neck.

B. Added filtration

1. Aluminum filtration reduces patient exposures by as much as 57%.

2. Federal laws require 2.5-mm aluminum filtration for operation voltages of 70 kVp or higher.

C. Equipment factors

1. X-ray machines that operate below 60 kVp are not recommended.

2. Low kVp x-ray machines result in absorbed doses almost twice as high as machines operating at 80 kVp.

3. Electronic timers are preferable to mechanical timers because they more accurately reproduce short exposure times.

4. Suspension arms should be stable and hold a position without movement or drift.

5. Routine checks and a preventive maintenance program ensure optimum equipment performance.

D. Film selection

1. X-ray film varies in the amount of radiation required to make a diagnostic image.

2. Film should be selected to give adequate diagnoses with the least amount of radiation and to provide quality images.

3. E-speed film is the most sensitive intraoral film commercially available, requiring about half the radiation of D-speed film.

E. Leaded apron and thyroid collar

1. Leaded aprons and thyroid collars reduce the possibility of radiation exposure to critical organs outside the radiographic examination area.

F. Optimum processing and darkroom conditions

1. Processing conditions should be monitored and checked before patient films are developed. Following these procedures decreases the number of retakes resulting from processing errors.

G. Film holders

1. Film holders assist in PID placement and minimize retakes resulting from projection errors.

2. Film holders also allow the use of a smaller beam diameter.

3. Examples of film-holding devices include bitewing tabs, hemostats, Stabes, XCP units, Snap-A-Ray, Intrax, and Precision paralleling devices.

H. Operator shielding

1. Dental professionals may be exposed to radiation from the primary beam or scattered radiation from the patient.

2. Standing behind a protective barrier is the best way to prevent unnecessary exposure.

3. If a barrier is not available, or it is not possible to be outside the treatment room, the operator should be at least 6 feet from the x-ray tube.

4. Never hold the film, hold or stabilize the tubehead, or stand in the path of the primary beam.

5. If a patient requires assistance during the exposure, a family member, protected with a lead apron and gloves, should be asked to help.

I. Office design

1. Primary barriers are those walls intended to absorb radiation from the primary beam.

2. Secondary barriers are intended to absorb secondary and leakage radiation.

3. Appropriate barrier thickness is determined when x-ray machines are installed.

4. Barrier requirements are determined for each x-ray unit and depend on maximum kVp, distance to the person to be protected, and occupancy factor of the areas adjacent to the x-ray machine.

J. Patient health history

1. Information regarding other radiographic exposures, recent dental radiographic exposures, and current medical conditions are important factors to evaluate when the need for radiographic exposure is assessed.

IV. Radiation is quantified in SI (Systeme Internationale) units (Table 8-4).
   A. Exposure (coulomb/kg; roentgens)
      1. X-rays cause the formation of ions in air.
      2. Exposure is defined as the number of ions produced by x-rays in a specific volume of air.
      3. Exposure is measured in units of coulombs per kilogram, or roentgens; 1 roentgen is approximately 2.58×10^{-4} coulomb/kg.
      4. Not all of the x-rays emitted from the tube are absorbed by the patient; thus exposure is always greater than the absorbed dose.
      5. Exposure and absorbed dose are directly related; when exposure dose is high, the amount of radiation absorbed is also greater.
      6. Exposure is the most frequently used measurement in radiation biology.
   B. Absorbed dose (gray, rad)
      1. Absorbed dose depends on individual characteristics of the irradiated tissue.
      2. Absorbed dose is a measure of the energy imparted to a mass of tissue.
      3. An absorbed dose of 1 **gray (Gy)** is defined as the absorption of 1 joule/kg; the traditional unit is the **rad** (*r*adiation *a*bsorbed *d*ose).
      4. One gray is equal to 100 rad.
   C. Equivalent dose (sievert, rem)
      1. The unit used in radiation protection is dose equivalent, or *sievert (Sv)*.
      2. This unit incorporates the quality factor (QF), which allows comparison of doses of different types of radiation.
      3. One sievert is equal to 1 Gy multiplied by the quality factor (1 Sv = Gy $\times$ QF); the traditional unit of dose equivalent is the **rem** (*r*ad *e*quivalent *m*an).
      4. One sievert is equal to 100 rem.

DENTAL X-RAY FILM

I. Radiographic film consists of a transparent plastic sheet, called the *base,* which is coated on both sides with a chemical emulsion.
   A. The emulsion contains silver halide crystals dispersed with gelatin.
   B. The exact composition of the emulsion silver halide crystals determines the sensitivity of the film to radiation or light.
II. Three types of film are used in dentistry:
   A. Intraoral (direct exposure)
      1. This film is sensitive to radiation.

Table 8-4 Summary of radiation units of measure

Quantity measured	Traditional unit	SI unit
Exposure	Roentgen	Coulomb/kg
Absorbed dose	rad	Gray
Equivalent dose	rem	Sievert

      2. It is used for periapical, bitewing, and occlusal exposures in the oral cavity.
   B. Extraoral (screen)
      1. This film is sensitive to a particular wavelength of light emitted by an intensifying screen.
      2. It is used for **panoramic, cephalometric, and temporomandibular joint (TMJ)** radiographs.
   C. Duplicating
      1. This film is sensitive to light emitted by a duplicating machine.
      2. It is never used for patient exposures but rather to copy existing radiographs using special darkroom equipment.
III. Film speed specifies how responsive the film is to radiation; high-speed film requires little radiation, whereas low-speed film requires more radiation.
IV. **Bitewing** projections are radiographs depicting the crowns of maxillary and mandibular teeth and the interdental alveolar crest.
V. **Periapical** projections are radiographs depicting most of the crown, the apical portion of specific teeth, and the surrounding alveolar bone.
VI. **Occlusal** projections are radiographs depicting larger areas of an arch in one film compared with that seen in other intraoral films.
VII. Radiographs are applied to various treatment procedures (box on page 125).
VIII. Film should be stored so that it is protected from light, exposure to radiation, moisture, and extreme temperature changes.
   A. Radiographic film has a shelf life.
   B. Film should be rotated so that the oldest film is used first.
   C. Radiographs should never be obtained with film after its expiration date.

INTRAORAL FILM PACKETS

I. Intraoral dental film is wrapped in layered, light-tight paper or plastic packets.
II. The back of the film packet provides important information for the user.

APPLICATION OF RADIOGRAPHS
DENTAL TREATMENT PROCEDURE
Common operative
Fixed prosthetics, partial
Simple extractions
Multiple extractions
Additional maxillofacial procedures
Dentures
Endodontic treatment
Periodontal treatment
Orthodontic treatment
Temporomandibular joint treatment
COMMON RADIOGRAPHIC TECHNIQUE
Bitewings, periapicals
Periapicals, full-mouth series
Periapicals, panoramic
Full-mouth series, panoramic
Full-mouth series
Panograph, cephalometric
Cephalometric, articular disk survey

III. Inside the packet, the film is completely covered with black paper, and a thin lead foil is positioned on the side opposite the image.
   A. The lead foil absorbs any remaining x-ray photons and prevents exposure from stray or scattered radiation.
   B. The lead foil must always be placed away from the tooth being radiographed, while the front or white side of the film is placed toward the PID.
   C. The film packet should be placed in the patient's mouth with the dot toward the occlusal or incisal edge of the tooth.
   D. The film packet is assembled so that the convex portion of the dot faces the front or white surface.
   E. Placing the front surface of the film packet toward the primary beam also places the convex surface of the dot toward the primary beam; thus, when the processed radiograph is oriented with the convex surface of the dot up, the teeth are viewed from a facial orientation.
   F. In processed radiographs obtained with a facial orientation (dot convexity up), the teeth on the patient's right are seen on the left side of the radiographic image, and the teeth on the

patient's left are seen on the right side of the radiographic image.
   G. Two-film packets are used when consultation regarding the patient's treatment is anticipated. Remember to separate the two pieces of film before processing.
IV. Intraoral film is available in five sizes:
   A. Child #0
   B. Anterior #1
   C. Adult #2
   D. Large bitewing #3
   E. Occlusal #4
V. The size of film used depends on the radiographic projection selected and the size of the patient's mouth.

PATIENT MANAGEMENT

I. Approach the patient with a positive and confident attitude to gain trust and decrease the patient's apprehension regarding the radiographic procedure.
II. Consider the unique needs of each patient.
III. Difficulties may arise during the radiographic procedure with patients who gag, have a shallow or narrow palate, have tori, are tongue-tied, do not understand directions, or are uncooperative.
IV. Patient management techniques can be used to accommodate patients with special needs (box on page 126).

INTRAORAL RADIOGRAPHIC TECHNIQUES

I. The **bisecting angle technique** was introduced in 1907 and is based on the geometric principle of isometry.
   A. This geometric principle states that two triangles are equal if they have one side in common.
   B. When the angle formed by the long axis of the tooth and the plane of the film is bisected, two triangles with a common side are created.
   C. When the x-ray beam is directed perpendicular to the bisecting line, the length of the projected image is the same as its actual length; the resulting image has minimal distortion.
   D. The bisecting principle works well with single-rooted teeth but is not as successful with multirooted teeth.
   E. This method is technically difficult.
II. The **paralleling technique** was introduced in 1924 to minimize distortion in the radiographic image.
   A. A 36- to 42-inch source-to-object distance was recommended, and this radiographic method became known as the *long-cone* paralleling technique.

MANAGEMENT TECHNIQUES FOR HANDLING PATIENTS WITH SPECIAL NEEDS

GAGGING

- Start taking the radiographs in the maxilla from anterior to posterior because the posterior is the most responsive area to the gag reflex.
- Position the film in the maxillary, allowing the teeth to rest on the film holder; do not have the patient move the film upward into the maxillary as the mandible closes.
- Move most of the film holder toward the anterior so that less material is toward the posterior of the patient's mouth.
- Adjust the exposure settings and position the PID in the general area to be radiographed before the film is positioned.
- Direct the patient to breathe through the nose and not the mouth.
- Place a topical anesthetics in sensitive areas of the oral cavity, which may reduce gagging.
- Use the tube shift method or buccal object rule technique if necessary to obtain the third molar view.

SHALLOW OR NARROW PALATE

- Change the film size to accommodate the patient's mouth size.
- Place the film as parallel as possible to the teeth (but it may be necessary to increase the distance of the film from the teeth).

  The bisecting technique instead of the paralleling technique may be required to achieve the required results.

TORI

Maxillary torus is not usually a problem, but if it is present, use an occlusal projection.

Mandibular tori/torus requires that the film be moved away from the lingual aspect of the teeth for patient comfort.

The film size may have to be changed.

DISABILITIES

If the patient cannot remain still, a second person may need to be in the treatment room to assist the patient. A protective apron must be worn by this person, also.

The patient who is confined to a wheelchair may need to be radiographed while in the wheelchair.

The patient who cannot tolerate the procedure at all may need to receive sedation to accomplish this procedure.

INABILITY TO UNDERSTAND DIRECTIONS

The assistant must determine why the patient is unable to understand directions. Is the person's hearing impaired? Is the patient able to speak?

If the patient is hearing-impaired but can read lips, be sure to pull your protective mask down to allow your lips to be seen.

Always talk to the patient while standing in front of him or her.

- Provide a paper and pencil for communication if the patient is unable to speak but can hear.

TONGUE-TIED

- Switch to the bisecting technique to obtain a diagnostic radiograph if necessary, if the paralleling technique is the technique of choice.

SPECIAL MANAGEMENT TECHNIQUES

- Explain the procedure and the importance of obtaining diagnostic radiographs if the patient presents a management problem
- Use a firm and directive tone of voice and approach.

  Explain the procedure in terms that the patient can understand if the lack of cooperation stems from fear, especially when the patient is a child. Describe the x-ray unit as a camera and show examples of radiographs as pictures of the teeth; answer any questions that might arise.

B. The film is placed parallel to the long axis of the tooth, and the x-ray beam is directed at a right angle to the film.

C. To place the film parallel to the tooth, it is necessary to move it a slight distance away from the crown.

D. Using film holders and smaller film packets in the anterior regions facilitates proper paralleling film placement.

E. Radiographic images produced by the paralleling technique have optimum image characteristics and minimum distortion.

FULL-MOUTH RADIOGRAPHS

I. The dentist orders the radiographs necessary to make an appropriate diagnosis for an individual patient.

II. When the patient has extensive dental needs, a full-mouth series of radiographs is ordered.

A. This series includes periapical radiographs to cover the apical area of all of the teeth or edentulous alveolar segments and bitewing radiographs to demonstrate the crowns and alveolar bone level, usually of the posterior region.

B. Panoramic, third molar, and occlusal projections are included when diagnostic criteria indicate the need for additional views.

C. Bitewing radiographs are made on a horizontal projection unless the patient has moderate bone loss, indicating a need for vertical interproximal projections.

III. When the patient has less extensive dental disease, the dentist usually orders *selected periapicals.*

IV. Bitewing radiographs are frequently ordered alone or together with selected periapicals.

V. All radiographs should demonstrate optimum quality, with consideration of quality control factors (box below).

VI. The teeth and anatomic structures visualized in the projection together with the direction of the x-ray beam are summarized in the box on pp. 128-130.

VII. Intraoral radiographs are usually required for the diagnostic evaluation of edentulous patients.

A. Intraosseous pathosis may develop at any time, even though the teeth have been extracted.

B. Pathologic entities affecting the edentulous alveolus, including odontogenic cysts, tumors, and neoplasms, are more common in older individuals.

C. The dentist usually prescribes 10 to 14 periapical projections for the evaluation of edentulous patients.

QUALITY CONTROL FACTORS

• The film should be placed so that it covers the prescribed area of interest for the specific projection.

• In periapical views the full length of the roots and at least 2 mm of periapical bone should be clearly visualized. When a pathologic entity is present, the entire lesion, including a border of normal bone, must be visualized (this may require supplemental projections).

• Interproximal contacts must be open and alveolar bone visualized in bitewing projections.

• Radiographs must demonstrate optimum density (blackness) and contrast (range of gray). A distinct visual difference in the density of enamel, dentin, and pulp and the presence of soft-tissue shadows in edentulous areas indicate optimum contrast.

• Radiographs must be free of distortion caused by errors in vertical or horizontal angles of projection, improper film placement, or bending the film.

• Radiographs must be free of processing errors.

D. Panoramic, occlusal, and lateral jaw radiographs are alternative projections used for edentulous patients.

E. Radiographic procedures for edentulous patients are similar to those used with dentate patients.

1. Exposure times should be reduced by approximately 5% to achieve an appropriate density.

2. All dental prostheses are removed before exposures are made.

3. Either bisecting or paralleling technique can be used for edentulous periapical projections.

4. Placing cotton rolls in the space normally occupied by the crowns of the teeth may be necessary.

5. Modification in techniques will be necessary.

VIII. Occlusal projections are used to obtain large areas of a single arch in one projection.

1. The size of the film allows for increased field projection.

2. An occlusal film packet is commonly 2 × 3 inches and may be a single- or double-film packet.

PROCEDURE FOR INTRAORAL DENTAL RADIOGRAPHY

I. Several steps are required to complete the radiographic examination.

A. The patient is examined, the dentist selects the necessary radiographs, and the exposure assignment is made to a qualified auxiliary.

B. Masks, gloves, and protective eyewear should be worn for all radiographic procedures; although aerosols are not produced during radiographic procedures, saliva can be ejected from the oral cavity as the patient opens the mouth.

C. Place all items unnecessary to the procedure (supplies, equipment, and charts) outside the treatment room.

1. Minimize surfaces touched by contaminated hands.

2. Cover all surfaces, including countertops, tubehead, exposure button, and control panel.

D. Practice film disinfection and safe handling of film as follows:

1. Place each film in a clear plastic sleeve before patient contact.

2. After exposure remove the film from the sleeve while avoiding its contamination.

FILM PLACEMENT CRITERIA AND STRUCTURES VISUALIZED IN INTRAORAL DENTAL RADIOGRAPHS

MAXILLARY CENTRAL-LATERAL INCISORS, PERIAPICAL PROJECTION

Teeth. The contact between the central and lateral incisors is centered on the film. The entire crown and root of the central lateral incisors, including apices, are fully depicted together with the interproximal alveolar crest of the adjacent central incisor and canine teeth.

Contacts open. The central ray is directed to open the contact between the central and lateral incisor.

Anatomic structures visualized. Floor of the nose, incisive fossa.

Film size. #1 or #2

MAXILLARY CANINE, PERIAPICAL PROJECTION

Teeth. The canine tooth is centered on the film. The entire crown and root of the canine, including the apex, is fully depicted together with the interproximal alveolar crest of the adjacent lateral incisor.

Contacts open. The central ray is directed to open the contact between the canine and lateral incisor.

Anatomic structures visualized. The *inverted Y* formed by the floor of the nose and the anterior wall of the maxillary sinus is often seen.

Film Size. # 1 or #2.

MAXILLARY PREMOLAR, PERIAPICAL PROJECTION

Teeth. The distal surface of the canine crown and the entire crown and root of the first and second premolar; including apices, are visualized together with the interproximal alveolar crest of the canine and first molar teeth.

Contacts open. The central ray should be directed to open the contact between the first and second premolar and contact between the canine and the first premolar.

Anatomic structures visualized. The floor and anterior wall of the maxillary sinus are visualized.

Film size. #1 or #2.

MAXILLARY MOLAR, PERIAPICAL PROJECTION

Teeth. The distal surface of the second premolar and the entire crown and root of the first, second, and third molars, including apices, are depicted together with the interproximal alveolar crest of the second premolar and the extent of the maxillary tuberosity.

Contacts open. The central ray should be directed to open the contact between the first and second molar. The contact between the distal aspect of the second premolar and the mesial of the first molar is usually open.

Anatomic structures visualized. The floor of the maxillary sinus, the maxillary tuberosity, and occasionally the hamular process of the sphenoid bone, and the coronoid process can be seen.

Film size: #2.

MAXILLARY DISTAL MOLAR, PERIAPICAL PROJECTION

Teeth. The distal portion of the first molar, the entire crown and root of the second and third molars, including the apices, are fully depicted, together with the full extent of the maxillary tuberosity.

Contacts open. The central ray should be directed perpendicular to the center of the film. Usually no contacts are open.

Anatomic structures visualized. The floor and posterior wall of the maxillary sinus, the maxillary tuberosity, often the malar eminence and the zygomatic arch, and occasionally the coronoid process and sigmoid process of the mandible can be seen.

Film size. # 2.

MANDIBULAR CENTRAL-LATERAL INCISORS, PERIAPICAL PROJECTION

Teeth. The contact between the central and lateral incisors is centered on the film. The entire crown and root of the central and lateral incisors, including apices, are fully depicted together with the interproximal alveolar crest of the adjacent central incisor and canine teeth.

Contacts open. The central ray is directed to open the contact between the central and lateral incisors.

Anatomic structures visualized. Occasionally the genial tubercles and/or the mental ridge or inferior border of the mandible can be seen.

Film size. #1 or #2.

FILM PLACEMENT CRITERIA AND STRUCTURES VISUALIZED IN INTRAORAL DENTAL RADIOGRAPHS—cont'd

MANDIBULAR CANINE, PERIAPICAL PROJECTION

Teeth. The canine tooth is centered on the film. The entire crown and root of the canine, including the apex, is depicted together with the interproximal alveolar crest of the adjacent lateral incisor.
Contacts open. The central ray is directed to open the contact between the canine and lateral incisor.
Anatomic structures visualized. The mental ridge and occasionally the lower border of the mandible are seen.
Film size. #1 or #2.

MANDIBULAR PREMOLAR PERIAPICAL PROJECTION

Teeth. The distal surface of the canine crown and the entire crown and root of the first and second premolar, including apices, are fully depicted together with the interproximal alveolar crest of the canine and first molar teeth.
Contacts open. The central ray should be directed to open the contact between the first and second premolar and the contact between the canine and the first premolar.
Anatomic structures visualized. The mental foramen and the mandibular canal are seen.
Film size. #1 or #2.

MANDIBULAR MOLAR PERIAPICAL PROJECTION

Teeth. The distal surface of the second premolar and the entire crown and root of the first, second, and third molars, including the apices, are fully depicted together with the interproximal alveolar crest distal to the third molar.
Contacts open. The central ray should be directed to open the contact between the first and second molar.
Anatomic structures visualized. The mandibular canal, the oblique ridge, the mylohyoid ridge, and the anterior border of the ascending ramus are seen.
Film size. #2.

MANDIBULAR DISTAL MOLAR, PERIAPICAL PROJECTION

Teeth. The distal portion of the first molar and the entire crown and root of the second and third molars, including the apices, are fully depicted together with the full extent of the maxillary tuberosity.
Contacts open. The central ray should be directed perpendicular to the center of the film. Usually no contacts are open.
Anatomic structures visualized. The mandibular canal, the oblique ridge, the mylohyoid ridge, and the anterior border of the ascending ramus can be seen.
Film size. #2.

HORIZONTAL PREMOLAR, INTERPROXIMAL PROJECTION (BITEWING)

Teeth. The distal coronal aspect of the canines and the crowns and crestal lamina of the first and second premolars are visualized as well as the interproximal alveolar crest distal to the canine and mesial to the first molar teeth.
Contacts open. The central ray should be directed perpendicular to the contact between the maxillary first and second premolars. The contacts open include the contacts between the first and second premolars. Usually the contact between the first molar and the second premolar is open.
Anatomic structures visualized. The distal portion of both the maxillary and mandibular canines, the entire coronal aspects of the premolar teeth, and the mesial coronal surfaces of the first molars are seen, as are the crestal lamina and a portion of the intraradicular alveolar bone distal to the canine, mesial to the first molar and surrounding the premolar teeth.
Film size. #2 or 3.

HORIZONTAL MOLAR, INTERPROXIMAL PROJECTION (BITEWING)

Teeth. The distal aspects of the second premolar crowns and the crowns of the first and second molars are visualized as well as the interproximal alveolar crest distal to the second premolar and second molar.
Contacts open. The central ray should be directed perpendicular to the contact between the maxillary first and second molars. The open contacts include those between the first and second molars and those between the second premolar and first molar.
Anatomic structures visualized. The distal portion of both the maxillary and mandibular second premolar, the entire coronal aspects of the first and second molar teeth, and the mesial coronal surfaces of the third molars, if present, can be seen. Also, the crestal lamina and a portion of the intraradicular molar and surrounding the molar teeth, are visualized.
Film size. #2 or #3.

Continued

FILM PLACEMENT CRITERIA AND STRUCTURES VISUALIZED IN INTRAORAL DENTAL RADIOGRAPHS—cont'd

VERTICAL PREMOLAR, INTERPROXIMAL PROJECTION (BITEWING)	VERTICAL MOLAR, INTERPROXIMAL PROJECTION (BITEWING)
Teeth. The distal coronal aspect of the canines and the crowns and crestal lamina of the first and second premolars, are visualized, as well as the interproximal alveolar crest distal to the canine and mesial to the first molar teeth. *Contacts open.* The central ray should be directed perpendicular to the contact between the maxillary first and second premolars. The open contacts include those between the canines and the first premolar and those between the first and second premolars. Usually the contact between the first molar and the second premolar is open. *Anatomic structures visualized.* The distal portion of both the maxillary and mandibular canines, the entire coronal aspects of the premolar teeth, and the mesial coronal surfaces of the first molar can be seen. The crestal lamina and a portion of the intraradicular alveolar bone distal to the canine, mesial to the first molar and surrounding the premolar teeth, can also be seen. *Film size.* #1 or #2.	*Teeth.* The distal aspects of the second premolar crowns and the crowns of the first and second molars are visualized as well as the interproximal alveolar crest distal to the second premolar and second molar. *Contacts open.* The central ray should be directed perpendicular to the contact between the maxillary first and second molars. The open contacts include those between the first and second molars and those between the second premolar and the first molar. *Anatomic structures visualized.* The distal portion of both the maxillary and mandibular second premolar, the entire coronal aspects of the first and second molar teeth, the crestal lamina, and a portion of the intraradicular alveolar bone distal to the second premolar and the alveolar bone surrounding the molar teeth, including the furcation, can be seen. *Film size.* #2.

3. Using care in opening the sleeve, allow the film packet to fall on a clean surface and dispose of the sleeves.
4. Remove gloves, wash hands, and reglove before touching each film.
5. Remove all saliva from the exposed film and spray/wipe/spray/wipe each film for the recommended time with an approved surface disinfectant.
6. Film packets must be completely dry before the outer cover is removed and the film is processed.
7. This method presents a potential for fluid contamination onto the unprocessed film.
8. Process films using an infection control technique for the daylight loader processing unit (box on page 131).

E. Set up the treatment area before exposing film.
1. Before the procedure, obtain mask, gloves, protective eyewear, and a paper cup together with sufficient radiographic film, cotton rolls, bitewing tabs, and film holders to complete the process for a single patient.
2. Assemble film holders and organize disposable supplies.

F. Maintain equipment asepsis after patient treatment.
1. If an uncovered equipment surface is touched, it must be disinfected.
2. Moisten a paper towel with disinfectant; starting with the least contaminated surfaces, wipe areas of possible contamination.
3. Do not spray the disinfectant directly on the tubehead or control panel.
4. Wipe the surface dry with a paper towel, then reclean the surface with a fresh disinfectant-moistened towel, allow it to remain on the surface as recommended by the manufacturer, and wipe dry. When disinfecting the tubehead and control panel and after using the second application of disinfectant, wipe the surface dry to protect the unit from excess moisture.
5. Allow all other environmental surfaces to dry by evaporation.
6. Wipe the lead apron clean and return it to the hanging rod. *Do not fold it.*

INFECTION CONTROL TECHNIQUE FOR USING DAYLIGHT LOADER

- Leave the treatment room with the exposed radiographs in a plastic cup.
- If you are wearing treatment gloves from the radiographic procedure area, avoid contact with other objects (e.g., door knobs).
- Place overgloves on the latex treatment gloves to avoid contamination of items. Another option is to remove the contaminated gloves, wash hands, and hold the plastic cup with the contaminated films, using a paper towel.
- Open safety glass of the daylight loader, and place the cup inside. At the same time, place the anterior film holder in the daylight loader with the films if it is needed.
- Close the safety glass of the daylight loader.
- If treatment gloves were removed or overgloves used, the safety glass will not require disinfection at a later time.
- Place a new pair of latex gloves on hands.
- Place both hands in the cuffs on both sides of the daylight loader, making sure your arms are securely covered by the cuffs to avoid light leakage.
- If overgloves are still on over contaminated treatment gloves, remove the overgloves inside the daylight loader and proceed with the process.
- Process all films; do not remove your hands from the daylight loader until all films are in the machine.
- If it is necessary to remove your hands during processing, protect the films from exposure and remove the contaminated gloves that were worn during processing inside the loader to avoid contamination.
- Place all contaminated film packets inside the plastic cup or other holder.
- Remove the treatment gloves inside out in the dayloader, and remove your hand from the cuffs.
- Open the safety glass with another pair of gloves or a protective towel, and remove the cup with opened film packets and used gloves.

7. Disinfect any surface touched or splashed during the procedure, including the headrest, adjustment levers, and arms (if they were not covered).
8. When disinfecting the x-ray unit, take care to prevent excess moisture from leaking into the inner surface of the machine.

9. Disinfect any uncovered surface that has been touched during the procedure, including the yoke, PID, tubehead, control panel, and exposure buttons.
10. Film-holding devices should be scrubbed free of debris, dried thoroughly, and sterilized.
11. Panoramic bite guides should be sterilized, disposed of, or covered with a suitable material.

II. Follow the steps of the procedure for exposing dental radiographs (box on page 132).

EXTRAORAL RADIOGRAPHY

I. Extraoral radiographs are used for the following purposes:
   A. To evaluate regions not covered by periapical films if necessary.
   B. To obtain radiographs when soft-tissue injury or edema contraindicates intraoral film placement
   C. To evaluate maxillofacial growth
   D. To determine the relationship between facial bones and the skeletal base.
   E. To assess the relationship between the mandible and the maxilla.
II. Common types of extraoral radiographs include panoramic, cephalometric, lateral jaw, and TMJ projections.
   A. Radiographs of the skull using a specialized head positioner are called *cephalometric projections.*
      1. Orthodontists use this projection to evaluate skeletal growth patterns, jaw relationships, and soft-tissue profiles.
      2. Lateral cephalometric radiographs are usually ordered for diagnosis, during therapy, and at the conclusion of orthodontic treatment.
      3. Lateral cephalometric radiographs may also be necessary to evaluate patients receiving implants or other extensive restorative dental treatment.
      4. Cephalometric analysis is the tracing of major anatomic landmarks depicted in the lateral cephalometric radiograph for diagnostic purposes.
   B. The lateral jaw projection provides a radiograph of the entire mandible and maxilla.
      1. This projection is often used for patients who are unable to tolerate intraoral film placement (e.g., children, older adults, or handicapped individuals).

PROCEDURE FOR EXPOSING DENTAL RADIOGRAPHS

PREPARING THE PATIENT

- Greet the patient in the reception area, check the patient's health history, and ask the date of the most recent dental radiographs. If previous radiographs were made at another facility, obtain the patient's permission to request them.
- Escort the patient to the treatment room. Seat the patient; adjust the occipital support so that the patient's head is comfortable and the occlusal plane is parallel to the floor.
- Explain the x-ray procedure to the patient. If the patient is nervous, explain the safety precautions that are taken to prevent overexposure to radiation. Explain that radiographs are necessary to provide adequate, high-quality dental care.
- Ask the patient to remove eyeglasses, dentures, or any other large objects around the head or neck. Drape the patient with a lead apron to cover the thyroid, spine, thorax, and abdomen.
- Wash hands and put on gloves, mask, and protective eyewear.
- Set kVp, mA, and timer, following recommendations for the radiograph you are taking. Make sure the patient's head is in a comfortable position and is immobile. Patient movement during an exposure creates a blurred image.
- Place the film packet in the patient's mouth. Proper film placement is essential for successful radiographs. Visually verify that the film covers the intended area.
- Position the tubehead, following guidelines for the radiographic projection you are making. Stabilize the tubehead, ensuring that all movement has stopped. Any movement of the tubehead during an exposure may create a blurred image.
- Step behind the protective barrier, viewing the patient to verify position. Confirm exposure factors. Depress the exposure button, and continue to hold it until the audible signal has completely stopped. If the button is released too soon, the radiograph will be underexposed.
- Remove the film packet from the patient's mouth, and place it in a paper cup outside the cubicle. (Do not leave the film packets in the cubicle; they will be exposed to scatter radiation.) When the procedure is completed, wipe the contaminated film packets dry with a paper towel, place them in an envelope or paper cup, and take them to the processing area. Each packet may be wiped dry after the exposure and then placed in a holding device until they are processed.

---

2. This projection is used to evaluate fractures of the mandible.

C. Temporomandibular articulation survey is common to oral surgeons or other practitioners who specialize in TMJ disorders.
   1. This survey is difficult to obtain because it requires the patient to maintain a specific head position without any movement for an accurate image.
   2. Specialized imaging procedures, such as magnetic resonance, are required to clearly define the articular disk and are usually required for patients with severe TMJ disturbances.

D. Panoramic radiographs are becoming increasingly more common in all areas of dental practice.
   1. These radiographs provide an image of both maxillary and mandibular alveolar processes, paranasal sinuses, and the TMJ on a single extraoral film.
   2. They are usually prescribed when the diagnostic region of interest is extensive or falls outside the area normally covered by periapical projections.
   3. Oral surgeons find this type of radiograph extremely helpful.

E. Tomographic radiography is an image *slice* that is created by moving the x-ray source and film.
   1. The size, shape, and location of the image slice is determined by the path of movement.
   2. Dental tomography is used in TMJ and implant imaging.

PROCESSING DENTAL RADIOGRAPHS ▬▬▬

I.   After radiographs have been exposed, the image is processed in much the same way a photograph is developed.

II. There are five basic processing steps:
   A. Developing
   B. Rinsing
   C. Fixing
   D. Washing
   E. Drying

III. Consistent high-quality radiographs are produced only when processing is standardized.

IV. Dental radiographs are developed in manual tank processors or in automatic film processors.

V.   Processing solutions affect the quality of the radiograph.

A. Integrity, temperature, level, and age of the processing solution affect the contrast and definition of the processed radiograph.

B. The liquids involved in either manual or automatic processing of radiographs include a developer, water, and fixer solution.

VI. Developer solution is the first solution in which an exposed radiographic film is placed.

A. The basic solution has a pH factor of approximately 7.

B. Ingredients of developer solution and their effect on the exposed film include the following:

1. Developing agent: Elon or Metol and hydroquinone—reduces the exposed silver bromide crystals to silver

2. Activator: sodium carbonate—alkaline medium that softens gelatin

3. Preservative: sodium sulfite—prevents developer oxidation

C. When the film is placed in the developer, the solution causes the silver to precipitate on the film base by reducing the exposed silver halide crystals.

D. The silver on the film creates radiolucent images on the radiograph.

E. The more energized or exposed crystals allow greater silver precipitation and thus a darker image on the film.

F. A correlation follows:

1. Metallic restorations block passage of radiation—create few energized crystals—precipitate less silver = radiopaque image

2. Pulp tissue allows greater passage of radiation—creates greater number of energized crystals—precipitates greater amount of silver = radiolucent image

G. Time and temperature affect the chemical reaction that occurs during the precipitation.

1. When films are left in the developing solution too long, more silver can precipitate, resulting in less definition of the image.

2. When all the silver is precipitated, a black image results.

3. Less silver precipitates from film when silver halide crystals receive less radiation exposure, resulting in a gray image.

4. When films are left in the developer too long, more silver precipitates than intended through the exposure process, resulting in a darker image.

5. An increase in temperature requires a shorter processing time in the developing solution.

VII. Washing radiographs between placement in the developing and the fixer solution stops action in the processing procedure.

A. Washing films removes the developer, avoiding fixer contamination, and stops the developing action.

B. Films are removed from the developer and agitated in the water.

C. The films are then placed in the fixer solution.

VIII. Fixing the film prevents it from discoloring or fading.

A. Fixer solution is acidic compared with developer solution.

B. The solution removes silver halide crystals that have been exposed or that are unexposed to radiation.

C. The ingredients and effect of the fixer solution on the exposed film include the following:

1. Clearing solution: sodium thiosulfate—removes undeveloped or unexposed silver bromide crystals from the emulsion

2. Hardener: potassium aluminum sulfate—shrinks and hardens the gelatin

3. Acidifier: acetic acid—maintains the acid medium on the film

4. Preservative: sodium sulfite—Avoids the deterioration of the thiosulfate

D. The film emulsion softens during developing and begins to harden during the fixing procedure.

E. To obtain optimum fixing, the film must remain in the fixer solution for 10 minutes during manual processing.

F. A wet read of a radiographic film may be obtained in 3 to 4 minutes after placement in the fixer solution, but the film must be replaced for final fixing.

G. If a film is not properly fixed, it will be brown or may fade.

IX. Radiographic films must be thoroughly washed for 20 minutes during manual processing in a water bath or tank.

A. The water must be circulating for maximum effect in the removal of fixer solution from the film.

B. Films are hung to dry; care must be taken to prevent films from touching each other, which causes damage.

C. If an automatic processor is used in this proc-

MANUAL PROCESSING PROCEDURE

1. Close and lock the darkroom door. Check solution levels, and replace or replenish if low. Gently stir the developer and fixer solutions, using a different stirring rod for each (stirring rods should be made of glass, plastic, or stainless steel, never wood).
2. Check the thermometer and determine the film-developing time, following the manufacturer's recommendations. Developing time depends on the temperature of the developer.
3. If the films are moist, dry each film with a paper towel before opening the film packets.
4. Select a film hanger and place an identifying label on it. Turn off the room light, and verify that no outside or extraneous light is present in the darkroom. Illuminate the safe light.
5. Unwrap film packets, and remove the film slowly. Holding the film by the edges and attach the film to the hanger. Be sure to keep film dry, and avoid smudging it with your fingers.
6. Place the film hanger in the developer solution. Agitate the hanger slightly to release air bubbles on the film surface, allowing optimum contact with the developer. Verify that all films are immersed in the developer solution. The films should not contact another film or the walls of the tank. Start the timer and replace the tank cover.
7. When the timer sounds, lift the cover and remove the film hanger from the developer. Rinse the films by agitating them for about 20 seconds in the water tank. Rinsing stops the action of the developer and prevents contamination of the fixer.
8. Place the film hanger into the fixer solution. Replace the tank cover, and set the timer for at least 10 minutes. If necessary, a brief inspection of the film can be made after 2 minutes of fixing. Be certain to return for complete fixing following this *wet reading*.
9. When the timer sounds, remove the film hanger from the fixer, and place the hanger into the water. The final wash requires a minimum of 20 minutes. Incomplete washing will result in films that discolor with age.
10. Because the final step in film processing is drying, remove the film hanger from the water and hang it on a drying rack. It is important to make sure the films do not contact other objects because wet films are easily scratched. Follow the manufacturer's instructions when using an electrical fan or a heated drying cabinet; prevent damage to radiographs from overheating.

ess, the films feed through the unit on a transport from the developer to the fixer solution, the water bath, and finally the drying unit; this process takes approximately 4 to 7 minutes because automated temperatures are elevated.

X. Manual processing procedure described in the box above.

XI. Manual darkroom maintenance is described (box on the right).

XII. The automatic processing technique involves several steps (box on page 135).

XIII. Guidelines are provided for automatic processor maintenance (box on page 135, right column).

XIV. Rapid processing
   A. This is necessary when radiographs are made during endodontic or other operative procedures.
   B. Rapid processing systems use concentrated solutions, often at high temperatures.
   C. Film is agitated in the developer solution for 10 to 30 seconds and then is fixed for 1 to 2 minutes.
   D. Although the quality of radiographs developed

MANUAL DARKROOM MAINTENANCE

FILM PROCESSOR MAINTENANCE

1. Keep tanks covered when they are not in use.
2. Clean surfaces of the tanks and countertop with a damp sponge after each use.
3. Clean the tanks when solutions are replaced.
4. Change solutions regularly.
5. Clean tanks with a gentle soap and soft-bristle (nonmetallic) brush; mineral deposits can be removed using a sponge and vinegar.
6. Rinse the tanks thoroughly with clear water, removing all traces of soap.

FILM HANGERS

1. Clean hangers in a solution of 1 oz sodium bicarbonate mixed in 1 gallon of water.
2. Soak the hanger for 1 hour at 100° F to 125° F.
3. Rinse the hangers thoroughly and allow them to dry.

AUTOMATIC PROCESSING TECHNIQUE

1. Check the solution level in internal replenishing tanks. If low, refill the tanks to the levels recommended by the manufacturer. If the processor is not equipped with an automatic replenisher, add the recommended amount of replenisher to the developer and fixer tanks. Use separate cups for each solution. Add solution slowly, away from the drain and toward the center of the tank. Avoid splashing.
2. Turn the main water valve on. Check the drain hose to make sure it is not obstructed and that it is inserted into the drain.
3. Observe the solutions in the internal tanks. A churning action indicates that the circulating pumps are working properly. Depress the process switch to verify that the rollers are turning. Turn on the heating unit if it is available on the processor.
4. Replace the top cover of the processor and insert a cleaning film. Daily use of cleaning film helps maintain rollers free of deposits. Purchased cleaning film is recommended. Alternatively, tow processed clear panoramic, occlusal, or smaller films can be used.
5. When the processor ready light comes on, verify the accuracy of the temperature-control setting by measuring the solution temperature using a hand-held thermometer.
6. Depress the process switch to begin automatic processing. Feed film lengthwise into alternating tracks to prevent overlapping. Allow at least 15 seconds between films. If films are fed into the processor too quickly, they will overlap, fail to dry adequately, or cause the roller transport to malfunction. Insert large films lengthwise, one at a time. Do not turn on the lights or open the darkroom door for at least 15 seconds after the last film is placed in the processor. If #0 or #1 film is being processed, each film is placed in a slot in a film-carriage device. Do not bend the film in the carriage because it must fit in the tracks of the processor. If #2 or #3 size films are processed, each is carefully placed in a separate track. Once the films are positioned, pull the lever to release the films onto the roller.
7. If the processor is not equipped with automatic replenisher, activate the replenisher switch after processing 20 periapical and 5 panoramic films or 90 periapical films.
8. At the end of the day, turn the power switch off and shut off the water supply. On some processors the cover may have to be propped open for venting.

GUIDELINES FOR AUTOMATIC PROCESSOR MAINTENANCE

- Never turn the rollers in the transport assembly by hand. Do not tamper with the film transport assembly or any other internal part of the processor.
- Do not turn the processor on when the internal tanks are empty or when solutions are below the fill level.
- Do not allow the replenisher tanks to become empty during operations.
- Do not place heavy objects on top of the processor or use the top as a film-loading or storage area.
- Do not use steel wool or abrasive scouring powder when cleaning tanks or metal parts of the processor.
- Keep the outside cover clean; pay particular attention to keeping the vents near the dryer assembly free of dust and debris.
- Always follow the manufacturer's directions when cleaning and maintaining the equipment because each processor may be different and involve specific instructions.

in rapid processing solutions is adequate for endodontic working films, the quality for contrast and archive is limited.

MOUNTING RADIOGRAPHS

I. Various anatomic and restorative landmarks can assist in identification during the radiographic procedure.
II. Several steps are involved in mounting radiographs (box on page 136).

COMMON ERRORS IN INTRAORAL RADIOGRAPHY

I. Several errors can occur during the radiographic process (Table 8-5).
II. These errors involve exposure, processing, and mounting techniques.

DUPLICATING RADIOGRAPHS

I. Radiographs may be needed for purposes other than that for which they were originally exposed.
II. Other sources that may need these radiographs include the following:
   A. Insurance agencies
   B. Dental specialists
   C. Other general practitioners to which a patient may transfer

Table 8-5 Common errors in intraoral radiography

Error	Result	Correction
EXPOSURE ERRORS		
PID cutoff	Portion of the film is not exposed	Align the x-ray beam so the central ray is centered on the middle of the film
Film placement	Apex cutoff	Position film in film holder so ⅛ to ¼ inch of the film is positioned above the incisal or occlusal edge
	Necessary teeth are not visible on film	Move the film to the anterior or posterior to produce the correct image on the film
	Excessive space between occlusal planes of bitewing	Direct the patient to bite and hold the film in place
	Crown cutoff	Position the film in the film holder so that the incisal or occlusal edge of the film is not below the plane
Film reversal	Herringbone effect as radiation projects the image from the foil on the film	Always make sure the correct side of film is positioned near the image
Crescent marks or bent films	Black crescent-shaped marks or image is very distorted	Slightly roll film around finger to adapt the film for patient comfort
Overlapping	Interproximal contacts are not open	Bring horizontal angulation as needed to the anterior or posterior, so the central ray is perpendicular to the film and the focal point
Blurred image	Lack of clarity on film	Instruct the patient to remain completely still during the procedure
Double exposure	Two sets of images on one film	Always be sure exposed film is placed separate from unexposed film

MOUNTING RADIOGRAPHS

1. Arrange radiographs on a viewbox with the dots oriented in the same direction either up or out (convex) or down or in (concave).
2. Organize the radiographs according to anatomic areas—arrange in groups of maxillary, mandibular, anterior, and posterior regions.
3. Position maxillary posterior radiographs with the crowns of the teeth toward the bottom edge of the mount. Identify mesial or distal anatomic landmarks to distinguish right from left. Premolar projections are mounted toward the midline of the mount on the inside; the most posterior landmarks are mounted toward the outside of the mount.
4. Identify maxillary anterior radiographs and place them with the crowns of the teeth toward the bottom edge of the mount. Identify the right and left incisor projections and place them with the central incisor toward the middle of the film mount. Orient the right and left maxillary canine projections, with the mesial structure toward the center of the film mount.
5. Identify the mandibular posterior radiographs, and arrange them with the coronal edge of the radiograph toward the top edge of the film mount. Place the molar projections toward the outside of the mount and the premolar projections toward the inside.
6. Arrange the mandibular incisor radiographs with the incisal edges directed toward the top of the film mount. Place the right and left central incisors toward the middle of the film mount. Orient the right and left maxillary canine projections with the mesial toward the center of the film mount.
7. Because the remaining four radiographs are the bitewing projections, orient these radiographs with the curve of Spee (occlusal plane between the maxillary and mandibular teeth) directed upward toward the distal. If the occlusal plane is flat, try to identify characteristics of the respective crowns. Frequently the bifurcation of the mandibular molars can be used as an aid in distinguishing mandibular from maxillary teeth. When the left and right projections are identified, orient them with the most mesial structures toward the middle of the film mount.

Table 8-5 Common errors in intraoral radiography—*cont.*

Error	Result	Correction
Light film	Low density or light images on film from underexposure	Check mA, time, or kVp for correct settings
Dark film	Dark, black films, creating inability to read images	Check mA, time, or kVp for correct settings
Clear film	No image on film	Film was not exposed
Elongation	Images on fim are lengthened or elongated beyond actual size	Correct the vertical angulation so the central ray is perpendicular to the film and focal point during the paralleling technique
Foreshortening	Images on film are shortened beyond actual size	
Jewelry, dental appliance left in mouth	Superimposed or radiopaque images appear on the film	Always have the patient remove dental appliances and jewelry before procedure
PROCESSING ERRORS		
Fluoride artifacts	Black spots	Remove all remains of fluoride from hands before processing (if fluoride treatment and radiographs are planned for one appointment, expose radiographs first)
Reticulation	Cracked, crazed appearance on film	Film is placed in high temperature processing and then cold temperature solution, causing a shrinkage and crazing of emulsion
Torn or scratched emulsion	Film base removed on film, reducing diagnostic value	Before films are dry, the emulsion is disturbed through contact with other films or hangers
Stained films	Stained areas, blotches	Work surfaces were wet or dirty during processing, disturbing the chemicals on the film
Discolored film	Brown staining	Films have not been fixed an adequate length of time
Light film	Low density of light images on film from underdeveloping	Check and correct for weak developing solutions, low developing time, or temperature of developing solutions
Developer cutoff	Straight line on films, radiopaque	Always check processing solutions to ensure tanks are full; never place films on top clips of film hangers
Clear film	Film has no image; emulsion is washed off	Do not leave films in water for more than 24 hours after fixing
Fogged film	Gray, unclear image contrast	Check for light exposure or improper film storage
Static marks	Black streaks	Open film packets slowly to reduce static electricity
Air bubbles	Radiopaque	Agitate film hangers in the processing solutions during placement in tanks
AUTOMATIC PROCESSING ERRORS		
Overlapped films	Processing by the chemical is not complete	Films are fed into the machine too quickly and overlap during processing; more than one film is placed into the same slot
Dirty rollers	Radiolucent markings or bands	Clean rollers regularly to remove residue
Light leak	Dark or fogged film	Hands were moved in the daylight loader that allowed light leaks around cuffs; hands were removed from daylight loader and films were not in the machine or protected with a cover

D. Court activities/malpractice suits

E. Forensic dentists

III. When insurance companies or other professionals require the patient's radiographs, the dentist is advised to retain the original radiograph and provide the consultant with a duplicate.

IV. Duplication is completed in the darkroom, under safelight conditions, with a duplicating machine and a special type of duplication film.

V. Several steps are involved in the duplication of existing radiographs (box on page 138).

PROCEDURE FOR DUPLICATING RADIOGRAPHS

1. Place original radiographs and a sufficient number of duplicating film packets, corresponding in size to the original films, inside the daylight loader that houses the duplicating system.
2. Close the safety view glass.
3. Insert the hand through cuffs of daylight loader and open the duplicator door within the unit.
4. Separate and lift the retainer plate from the duplicator door and stabilize it.
5. Remove the duplicating film from the film packet and place each film inside a section of the grid, with the lighter side of the film—the emulsed side—facing up.
6. Place an original radiograph on each duplicating film. Close the retainer plate and squeeze it lightly to lock into the duplicating grid.
7. Close the duplicator door and push firmly with both hands to activate the light source. In some systems, if both door latches are not secure, the films may become blurry.
8. After the light source shuts off, open the duplicator door and separate the retainer plate from the duplicating grid.
9. Remove the original films from the duplicating grid, set them aside within the daylight loader, and process the duplicating film in the normal manner in the automatic processor.

Questions

Dental Radiography

1 Of the following combinations of structures, which includes structures that appear radiolucent in a radiograph?
a. Nares, median suture, and medullary spaces
b. Incisive canal, genial tubercles, and nasal fossa
c. Maxillary sinus, mylohyoid ridge, and mental foramen
d. Hamular process, nutrient canals, and nasal cartilage
e. Coronoid process, mandibular canal, and maxillary septum

2 The central ray of an x-ray beam is correctly described as follows:
1. It has the shortest wavelength of any photon in the beam.
2. Photons travel at the speed of light.
3. It is composed of photons traveling in the center of the cone of radiation.
4. It is used to fix or locate the position of the x-ray beam.
a. 1 and 2
b. 1 and 3
c. 1, 2, and 3
d. 3 only
e. 4 only

3 The density of a radiograph is decreased by increasing the
a. Milliamperes
b. Exposure time
c. Developing time
d. Washing time
e. Tube-to-patient distance

4 Which of the following units describes the amount of x-ray exposure in the air?
a. Rad
b. Rem
c. Roentgen
d. PID
e. MRI

5 A very light radiograph may be caused by
1. Exposure time too short
2. Wrong side of the film toward the tube
3. Developing solution too warm
4. Removing the film from the fixing bath too soon
5. White light leaking into the darkroom
a. 1 and 2
b. 2 and 3
c. 3 and 4
d. 4 and 5
e. 2 and 5

6 Which of the following structures appear radiolucent on a radiograph?
1. Median palatine suture
2. Anterior nasal spine
3. Mandibular canal
4. Genial tubercles
5. Hamular process
a. 1 and 3
b. 1, 3, and 5
c. 1 and 5
d. 2 and 3
e. 2 and 4

7 Which of the following statements about radiation are correct?
1. X-rays can affect all living biologic forms.
2. Developing, young, biologically active cells are more susceptible to x-rays.
3. In dental radiography, only the primary, direct beam of radiation is a potential hazard.
4. Changes in normal adult cells that may be caused by radiation are of short duration, and the effects are soon dissipated.

a. 1 and 2
b. 1 and 3
c. 2 and 3
d. 2, 3, and 4

8 The x-ray beam is collimated to
a. Remove the less penetrating x-rays
b. Avoid delivering unnecessary radiation to the patient
c. Reduce the size of the beam and facilitate easier visualization of the central ray
d. Reduce the exposure time

9 Which of the following is true when the mA on an x-ray machine is reduced from 15 mA to 10 mA?
a. Wavelength of the x-rays produced is decreased
b. Number of volts in the filament circuit is decreased
c. Shape of the electron beam is changed
d. Number of x-rays produced is increased
e. Number of x-rays produced is decreased

10 After a film is removed from the developer and before it is placed in the fixer, the film should be washed in running water to
a. Remove the developer
b. Harden the emulsion
c. Dilute the fixer
d. Neutralize the fixer

11 Lack of sharpness of the radiographic image is increased by
a. Using a larger focal spot
b. Increasing the tube-to-patient distance
c. Decreasing the object-to-film distance
d. Immobilizing the patient

12 Elongation of the image on maxillary radiographs may be caused by
1. Insufficient vertical angulation
2. Excessive vertical angulation
3. Poor patient position
4. Improper placement of film
5. Extended target-to-film distance
a. 1 or 3
b. 1, 2, or 3
c. 1, 3, or 4
d. 2 or 4
e. 2 or 5

13 The purpose of the fixing solution is to
a. Shorten the film processing time
b. Complete the development of the latent image
c. Remove the silver halide crystals not exposed by the x-rays
d. Remove the silver halide crystals exposed by the x-rays
e. Fix the developed silver to the gelatin

14 The embossed dot on the film envelope is always placed _____ the PID.
a. Away from
b. Toward

15 The term _____ is used to describe the blackness of a radiographic film.
a. Contrast
b. Definition
c. Density
d. Detail

16 Milliamperage determines the _____ of potential radiation by changing the amount of electrons in the central beam.
a. Quality
b. Quantity

17 A(n) _____ radiograph records the crown, roots, and supporting structures of a tooth or teeth.
a. Bitewing
b. Extraoral
c. Occlusal
d. Periapical

18 A(n) _____ _____ is worn by dental personnel to measure the amount and type of radiation to which the individual was exposed.
a. Dosimeter badge
b. Identification badge
c. Lead apron
d. Thyrocervical collar

19 The shorter the wavelength, the _____ the ability of radiant energy to penetrate matter.
a. Greater
b. Weaker

20 When the paralleling technique is used, the central beam is projected at a(n) _____ angle to the film packet.
a. Bisecting
b. Oblique
c. Obtuse
d. Right

21 _____ radiation is radiation that has been deflected from its path during the impact with matter.
a. ALARA
b. Compton
c. Primary
d. Scatter

22 When exposing radiographs, the operator must stand behind a _____.
a. Folding screen
b. Lead-lined barrier
c. Plastic barrier
d. Wooden door

23 The lead apron and thyrocervical collar are placed to cover the patient's _____.
a. Chest
b. Gonads
c. Throat
d. All of the above

24 When the raised dot is placed outward (convex), the left side of the mounted radiograph corresponds to the _____ side of the patient's oral cavity.
a. Left
b. Right

25 The _____ technique is used to produce extraoral radiographs of the entire dentition and related supportive structures of the lower half of the face.
a. Bitewing
b. Panoramic
c. Cephalometric
d. Xeroradiography

26 The _____ period is the time before the cumulative effects of radiation on tissues are manifested and become visible to the eye.
   a. Acute
   b. Latent
   c. Long-term
   d. Short-term

27 One full-mouth series of 18 radiographs exposes an adult patient to approximately _____ mR of radiation.
   a. 0.1
   b. 0.5
   c. 1.0
   d. 5.0

28 In the _____ technique the central beam is set at a 90-degree angle to an imaginary line dissecting the angle formed by the long axis of the tooth and the film packet.
   a. Bisecting angle
   b. Paralleling

29 The _____ angulation is placed to direct the central beam accurately through the proximal contact of two adjacent teeth.
   a. Horizontal
   b. Vertical

30 Cone cutting on a dental radiograph is caused by incorrect _____.
   a. Horizontal angulation
   b. Placement of the central beam
   c. Placement of the film packet
   d. Vertical angulation

MARK ''A'' FOR *TRUE* OR ''B'' FOR *FALSE* FOR QUESTIONS 31 THROUGH 36.

_____ 31 The anode is the negatively charged electrode during x-ray production.

_____ 32 Electrons are positively charged particles.

_____ 33 An electron cloud is produced by the cathode filament.

_____ 34 Placing the film in the fixer before the developer will fog the film.

_____ 35 The film emulsion is a mixture of sensitive crystals and gelatin.

_____ 36 A cassette is a light-proof container equipped with screens.

37 Automatic film processors require
   a. A controlled water supply and cold solution
   b. Daily and periodic maintenance
   c. A solution change every week
   d. An increase in processing speed when more films are to be processed

38 Reverse or ghost images are produced in panoramic radiographs by the following:
   a. Radiopaque objects in the path of the x-ray beam on the other side of the patient being examined
   b. Defective rollers in the automatic processor
   c. Static electricity discharges
   d. Tears in the film's emulsion

39 The focal trough in panoramic radiography is the
   a. Zone of sharpness
   b. Collimated beam area
   c. Slit in the scatter guard
   d. Location of the electrons in the x-ray tube

40 The purpose of using a vertical rather than horizontal bite-wing is to
   a. Obtain additional interproximal information
   b. Assess bone level
   c. View periapical abscesses
   d. Observe pathologic changes

41 If a patient transfers to another dental office and asks for his or her radiographs to be forwarded to that office, you should send
   a. The original radiographs as requested.
   b. A copy of the radiographs and keep the original as a part of the patient's permanent record.
   c. Neither the original nor a copy of the radiographs because the patient is no longer coming to your office for treatment.

42 An atom is composed of which of the following particles?
   1. Protons
   2. Neutrons
   3. Gamma rays
   4. Electrons
   a. 1, 2, and 3
   b. 1, 2, and 4
   c. 2, 3, and 4

43 On a radiographic film, contrast is the
   a. Magnification of the image on the film
   b. Amount of difference between the black and white areas of the film
   c. Amount of penumbra on the film
   d. Degree of blackening on the film

44 An amalgam restoration appears white on a dental radiographic film. This image is referred to as
   a. Radiolucent
   b. Radiopaque
   c. Contrast

45 When a dental film is exposed, the amount of enlargement of the image on the film is controlled by the
   a. Definition
   b. Milliamperage and exposure time
   c. Source-to-film and film-to-object distance

46 A patient is seen who has recently begun treatment for cancer and is receiving oral radiation therapy. Which of the following may be a side effect of the treatment?
   a. Ulcers in the mouth
   b. Cervical decay
   c. Difficulty in swallowing
   d. Leukemia
   e. Thyroid cancer

47 _____ -Film
   a. Patient moved
   b. Patient slouching
   c. Patient's head tilted down

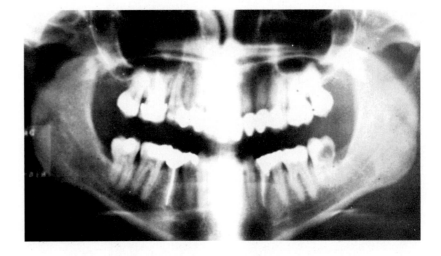

48 _____ - Film
   a. Patient moved
   b. Film cassette slowed after contact
   c. Lead apron placed too high on patient

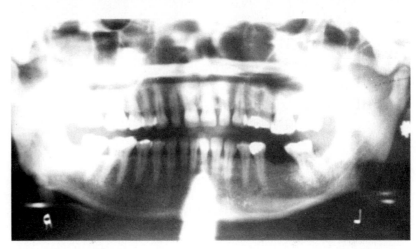

49 _____ -Film
   a. Improper film placement
   b. Foreshortened image
   c. Underexposed radiograph
   d. All of the above

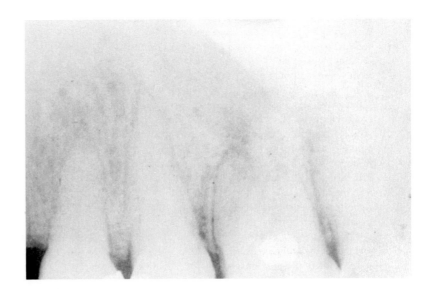

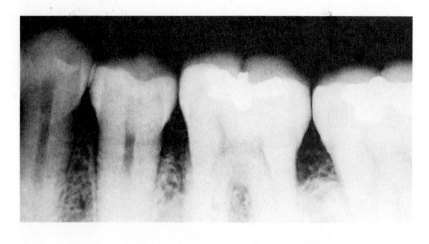

50 _____ - Film
a. Film placement
b. Wrong film size
c. Vertical angulation

Rationales

Dental Radiography

1 A Due to the lack of bony structure in the nares, median suture, and the medullary spaces, these structures appear darker or radiolucent on a film.

2 C Photons, other than those in the central beam, are longer in wavelength, have less ability to penetrate tissues, travel slower, and are outside the center of the electrified radiation.

3 E The further the central beam is from the patient, the lesser the ability to penetrate and provide adequate radiographic density. As wavelengths become further from the point of origination, the distance between the beginning and the end of the cycle is lengthened, decreasing penetration.

4 C The quantity or amount of radiation in the air is designated by the term roentgen. A rad is a designation for radiation absorbed dose; a rem is an abbreviation for roentgen equivalent man; PID is the position indicating device; and MRI is an abbreviation for magnetic resonance imaging.

5 A The only two factors listed that make a radiograph too light are short exposure time and reversing the film from the image being exposed, which forces the radiation to penetrate the lead liner. A warm developing solution will cause a radiograph to be darker; a film removed early from fixer may eventually brown; and a light leak will create a fogged image.

6 C The median palatine suture and the hamular notch are radiolucent, while the anterior nasal spine, mandibular canal, and genial tubercles are radiopaque.

7 A All radiation exposure may be harmful, and any changes in cells by exposure are cumulative and lifelong. Radiation does affect all biological life forms, and young active cells are more easily affected by radiation.

8 B Collimation of the radiation beam reduces waves that do not effectively penetrate a tissue to provide valuable images.

9 E A decreased mA reduces the number of x-rays produced as the radiation is created. This occurs because the amount of electricity and electrons is reduced.

10 A The developing process will continue to some degree until all the developing solution is removed from a film. This is most easily accomplished through rinsing with water to stop the chemical process.

11 A A larger focal spot does not allow for a greater penetrating radiation beam. This then creates an image with decreased clarity in the radiograph.

12 C Decreased vertical angulation, allowing for the central ray to be perpendicular to the film reduces elongation. The patient's head should be positioned to allow the jaws to be parallel with the floor. If the film is not positioned to correspond to the angle of the central ray, the image may be elongated.

13 C The acidic fixing solution allows for removal of the unexposed or undeveloped silver halide crystals, which then allows the softened film emulsion to reharden

14 B If the embossed dot is placed away from the PID, the lead film liner will block penetration of the radiation causing a herringbone effect on the image.

15 C Density is the amount of blackness on a radiographic film, while contrast is the difference in the degrees of blackness between adjacent areas. Detail is the visual quality of a radiograph that is affected by definition or sharpness.

16 B Milliamperage controls the number of electrons released, while kilovoltage controls the quality and affects the contrast of the film and the radiation dose.

17 D A bitewing radiograph might display the crown, and some of the surrounding bone and roots, but does not provide the complete view of areas that a periapical provides. An extraoral radiograph is taken with the film outside the patient's mouth and may not provide the quality or definition of an intraoral film. An occlusal film is an intraoral film that provides the reader with a third dimensional view of the structures.

18 A   Dosimeter badges are film badge devices that are worn to record one's exposure to ionizing radiation.

19 A   A shorter beam wavelength penetrates tissue easier and more quickly, decreasing the amount of scatter and unnecessary radiation to patients.

20 D   The PID should be positioned to allow the central ray/beam to contact the film in the mouth at a right angle. The central beam is perpendicular to the film. If the central beam is not, the film will be elongated or foreshortened.

21 D   Scatter radiation is radiation that does not have the ability to penetrate tissue to which it is directed. This could be from low kVp or from blockage from penetrating the tissue by another object.

22 B   A lead-lined barrier protects the operator while operating a radiographic unit from direct or scatter radiation. The radiographic wavelengths are blocked from penetrating the barrier and exposing the operator.

23 D   The lead apron provides protection to the patient's critical organs, including the chest, gonads, and throat/thyroid area. This protection for the patient equates to the lead-lined barrier that protects the operator of the unit.

24 B   When mounting radiographs, there are two accepted ways of mounting. One way is to mount as you would be looking at the patient. The other as if you were sitting on the patient's tongue and looking out of the mouth. To mount using the first method the convex area of the film would correspond to the right side.

25 B   The bite-wing film is an intraoral film basically showing the crowns of the teeth. The extraoral panoramic film depicts the teeth and surrounding structures. A cephalometric film is an extraoral lateral view of the skull and xeroradiography is a system that uses xerographic copying system recording images from a standard radiographic unit.

26 B   The time between exposure and any physical change manifested from the radiation is known as the latent period.

27 B   A 0.5 mR of radiation is the approximate exposure from a full-mouth series of radiographs using proper technique.

28 A   The bisecting technique uses isometric methods to bisect the angles of the object and film to produce an accurate image.

29 A   Properly placed horizontal angulation allows the central beam to open the contact of adjacent teeth.

30 B   The placement of the central beam affects exposure on the film. Incorrect placement may cause areas on the film not to be exposed to radiation.

31 B   The anode is the positive charge, and the cathode is the negative charge.

32 B   An electron is a negatively charged particle.

33 A   The filament is heated and produces an electron cloud necessary to obtain the radiation exposure.

34 B   The film will not be fogged, but will be black if placed in the fixer before the developer.

35 A   Film emulsion is a suspension of silver halide crystals in a gelatin.

36 A   A film cassette and screen are packaged so they are lightproof.

37 B   Regular maintenance is necessary to obtain maximum quality radiographs and to maintain functional equipment.

38 A   Items, such as jewelry, between the patient and the panoramic radiation beam cause ghost images.

39 A   The focal trough is the area of a panoramic radiograph where the plane of the object is not blurred and has greater sharpness of image.

40 B   Vertical bitewings are used to obtain information for diagnosis in suspected cases of bone loss or root caries.

41 B   A patient's radiographs are part of the legal patient record, which must be maintained for seven years after the last date of treatment. Only copies of the record, including radiographs, are forwarded to another office.

42 B   An atom is the basic unit of matter and is composed of postively charged protons, neutrons with no charge, and negatively charged electrons.

43 B   The difference in densities is viewed as contrast of the radiolucent and radiopaque areas of the radiograph.

44 B   Radiolucent images appear darker than radiopaque images that are lighter. See No. 43 for contrast.

45 C   An increased source of radiation distance to the film or the distance between the film and the object may distort the image on the film.

46 B   Radiation caries may result during cancer treatment due to xerostomia and reduced stimulation in the oral cavity.

47 C   The patient tilted the head down causing blurring of the incisors.

48 C   The lead apron was placed between the patient and the panoramic unit causing a radiopaque image.

49 D   The film is positioned improperly causing crown cut-off; the image is foreshortened by improper vertical angulation, and the film was underexposed causing a light image.

50 A   The film was improperly placed causing apical cutoff. The film should have been placed more towards the midline to have the first premolar completely in the exposure.

To enhance your understanding of the material in this chapter, refer to the illustrations in Chapter 9 of Finkbeiner/Johnson: *Mosby's Comprehensive Dental Assisting: A Clinical Approach.*

Pharmacology

OUTLINE

Introduction
Drug Actions, Interactions,
  Reactions, and Effects
Substance Abuse

Narcotics
Drugs Used in Dentistry
Drug History and Prescriptions
Emergencies

Responsibilities of the Dental
  Assistant
Patient Education

KEY TERMS

Allergic

Analgesics

Anaphylactic

Angioedema

Antagonistic

Antibiotics

Antibodies

Antigen

Antihistamines

Antiseptic

Barbiturates

Council on Dental Therapeutics

Drug Enforcement Agency

Food and Drug Administration

Generic name

Generic equivalent

Germicide

Hypnotic

Illegal drug

Legal drug

Narcotics

Pharmacology

Prescription

Sedative

Synergistic

Topical hemostatic agent

Trade name

Tranquilizers

Vasoconstrictor

The number of drugs used in dentistry is somewhat limited, but many patients seen by the dentist take drugs prescribed by a physician, as well as nonprescription drugs, on an occasional or regular basis. Prescriptions and nonprescription drugs have the potential to affect certain dental procedures and surgeries.

Many types of drugs are available for prevention or treatment of medical, surgical, and dental disorders. There is no one way to classify drugs. Different references may arbitrarily list the classes or types in different ways; Table 9-1 is an example.

INTRODUCTION

I. Definition
  A. **Pharmacology** is the study of drugs, including chemical formulas, uses, and positive and negative effects on all body structures.
  B. Facts about specific drugs include the following:
    1. How the drug is metabolized
    2. How the drug is excreted from the body and the organ of excretion

Table 9-1 Types of pharmacologic agents

Type	More common uses	Examples of drugs*
Adrenergic agents	Hypotension, cardiac arrest, asthma, allergic reactions, certain cardiac dysrhythmias (irregular heartbeats), control of superficial bleeding, nasal congestion	epinephrine, ephedrine, isoproterenol (Isuprel)
Adrenergic blocking agents	Hypertension, certain cardiac dysrhythmias, glaucoma, angina	atenolol (Tenormin), propranolol (Inderal), nadolol (Corgard)
Cholinergic agents	Myasthenia gravis, urinary retention	bethanecol (Urecholine), pyridostigmine (Mestinon)
Cholinergic blocking agents	Peptic ulcers, preanesthetic sedation	atropine, L-hyoscyamine (Levsin)
Narcotic analgesics	Relief of moderate to severe pain	codeine, meperidine (Demerol), morphine, pentazocaine (Talwin), propoxyphene (Darvon)
Narcotic antagonists	Narcotic overdose, reversal of the depressant effects of narcotics	naloxone (Narcan)
Nonnarcotic analgesics	Relief of mild to moderate pain	acetaminophen (Tylenol), aspirin, ibuprofen (Advil)
Barbiturate sedatives and hypnotics	Sedation, sleep induction	phenobarbital (Luminal), secobarbital (Seconal)
Nonbarbiturate sedatives and hypnotics	Sedation, sleep induction	flurazepam (Dalmane), triazolam (Halcion)
Cardiotonics	Congestive heart failure, certain cardiac dysrhythmias	digitalis, digoxin (Lanoxin)
Antiarrhythmic drugs	Cardiac dysrhythmias (irregular heartbeats)	procainamide (Pronestyl), propranolol (Inderal)
Anticoagulants	Prevention of thrombi (blood clots)	heparin, warfarin (Coumadin)
Thrombolytic drugs	To dissolve newly formed thrombi	altepase (Activase), streptokinase (Streptase)
Antianginal agents	Prevention and treatment of angina	diltiazem (Cardizem), isosorbide (Isordil), nitroglycerin
Peripheral vasodilating agents	Nocturnal leg cramps, peripheral vascular disease	cyclandelate (Cyclan)
Electrolytes and electrolyte salts	Replacement of lost electrolytes	calcium carbonate, potassium chloride (Kaon)
Diuretics	Heart failure, hypertension, edema	chlorothiazide (Diuril), furosemide (Lasix)
Antihypertensive agents	Hypertension	captopril (Capoten), guanethidine (Ismelin)
Central nervous system stimulants	Drug-induced respiratory depression, treatment of narcolepsy and attention deficit disorders (children)	doxapram (Dopram), methylphenidate (Ritalin)
Insulin	Diabetes mellitus	
Oral hypoglycemic drugs	Diabetes mellitus	glipizide (Glucotrol), tolbutamide (Orinase)
Sulfonamides	Infections	sulfamethizole, sulfisoxazole (Gantrisin)
Penicillin	Infections	amoxicillin (Amoxil), ampicillin (Amcill), carbenicillin (Geopen), penicillin G potassium (Pentids)
Cephalosporins	Infections	cefaclor (Ceclor), cephalexin (Keflex)
Broad-spectrum antibiotics	Infections	erythromycin (E-Mycin), kanamycin (Kantrex), minocycline (Minocin), tetracycline (Sumycin)
Antifungal drugs	Fungal infections	fluconazole (Diflucan), flucytosine (Ancobon)
Antitubercular agents	Tuberculosis	capreomycin (Capastat), streptomycin
Leprostatics	Leprosy	clofazimine (Lamprene), dapsone
Antimalarial agents	Prevention or treatment of malaria	quinacrine (Atabrine), quinine (Quine)
Anthelminthic drugs	Helminthiasis	mebendazole (Vermox), thiabendazole (Mintezol)
Amebicides	Amebiasis	chloroquine (Aralen), metronidazole (Flagyl)
Antiviral agents	Virus infections	acyclovir (Zovirax), amantadine (Symmetrel)
Urinary antiinfectives	Urinary tract infections	cinoxacin (Cinobac), nitrofurantoin (Furadantin)
Topical antiseptics and germicides		chlorohexidine (Peridex), povidone-iodine (Betadine)
Anterior pituitary hormones	Anterior pituitary hormone replacement (failure to grow, ovulatory failure)	clomiphene (Clomid), somatropin (Humatrope)
Posterior pituitary hormones	Posterior pituitary hormone replacement (induction of labor, diabetes insipidus)	oxytocin (Pitocin), vasopressin (Pitressin)

*The drugs listed in this column may not be used for all of the uses listed under "More Common Uses."

Continued.

Table 9-1 Types of pharmacologic agents—cont'd

Type	More common uses	Examples of drugs*
Glucocorticoids	Endocrine disorders, acute allergic states, skin diseases, asthma, rheumatic disorders	cortisone (Cortone), hydrocortisone (Cortef), prednisolone (Delta-Cortef), prednisone (Meticorten)
Mineralocorticoids	Partial replacement therapy for Addison's disease	fludrocortisone (Florinef)
Androgens	Male hormone replacement, inoperable breast cancer in females	fluoxymesterone (Halotestin), testosterone (Andro 100)
Anabolic steroids	Postmenopausal osteoporosis, metastatic breast cancer	nandrolone (Durabolin), oxymetholone (Androl)
Estrogens	Inoperable prostatic cancer, contraception, symptoms of menopause	chlorotrianisen (TACE), conjugated estrogens (Premarin), estradiol (Estrace)
Progestins	Amenorrhea, abnormal uterine bleeding, contraception	hydroxyprogesterone (Delalutin), norethindrone (Norlutin)
Oral contraceptives	Contraception	Ortho-Novum, Tri-Norinyl
Thyroid hormones	Hypothyroidism	levothyroxine (Levothroid), liotrix (Euthyroid)
Antithyroid agents	Hyperthyroidism	methimazole (Tapazole)
Oxytocic drugs	Initiation of labor, uterine atony	ergonovine (Ergotrate), oxytocin (Pitocin)
Uterine relaxants	Management of preterm labor	ritodrine (Yutopar)
Abortifacients	Abort or terminate a pregnancy	dinoprostone (Prostin E2)
Antineoplastic drugs	Malignant diseases	busulfan (Myleran), cisplatine (Platinol), doxorubicin (Adriamycin), lomustine (CeeNu)
Anticonvulsant drugs	Convulsive disorders	diazepam (Valium), mephobarbital (Mebaral), phenytoin (Dilantin)
Antiparkinsonism drugs	Parkinsonism	benztropine (Cogentin), levodopa (Larodopa)
Psychotherapeutic drugs	Mental illness	alprazolam (Xanax), chlordiazepoxide (Librium), diazepam (Valium), haloperidol (Haldol)
Antihistamines	Allergic disorders	astemizole (Hismanal), diphenhydramine (Benadryl)
Bronchodilators	Bronchospasm, asthma	albuterol (Efedron), phenylephrine (Neo-Synephrine)
Antitussives	Relief of coughing	benzonatate (Tessalon), dextromethorphan (Mediquell)
Antacids	Neutralize or reduce acidity of gastric contents	aluminum carbonate (Basaljel), magaldrate (Riopan)
Antidiarrheals	Diarrhea	loperamide (Imodium), paregoric
Antiflatulents	Intestinal gas	simethecone
Digestive enzymes	Replacement of pancreatic enzymes	pancreatin, pancrelipase (Cotazym)
Emetics	Induction of vomiting in certain types of poisoning	apomorphine, ipecac syrup
Histamine H_2 antagonists	Ulcers	cimetidine (Tagamet), ranitidine (Zantac)
Laxatives	Constipation	bisacodyl (Dulcolax), mineral oil, polycarbophil (FiberCon)
Antiemetic drugs	Nausea, vomiting	diphenidol (Vontrol), perphenazine (Phenergan)
Heavy metal compounds	Gold—rheumatoid arthritis	auranofin (Ridaura)
	Silver—burns, eye infections	silver nitrate, silver sulfadiazine (Silvadene)
Heavy metal antagonists	Heavy metal poisonings	deferoxamine (Desferal Mesylate), edetate calcium disodium (Calcium Disodium Versanate)
Vitamins/drugs used in treatment of anemias	Vitamin deficiency	vitamin B_{12}
	Various types of anemia	folic acid, iron
Immunologic agents	Immunity to specific communicable diseases	diphtheria and tetanus toxoids and pertussis vaccine (DPT), measles vaccine (Attenuvax)
Anesthetic agents	Anesthesia (local, general)	enflurane (Ethrane), bupivacaine (Marcaine), thiopental (Sodium Pentothal)
Skeletal muscle relaxants	Acute, painful musculoskeletal conditions	carisoprodol (Soma)
Drugs used in gout	Gout	allopurinol (Zyloprim)
Nonsteroidal antiinflammatory drugs	Mild to moderate pain	ibuprofen (Advil, Motrin), flurbiprofen (Ansaid)

3. Adverse effects
4. Appropriate dosages or dose ranges
5. Method(s) of administration
6. Contraindications for use
7. Warnings regarding serious and sometimes life-threatening adverse effects that may occur if the drug is administered
8. Improving methods of manufacture
9. Research
10. Continual updating of information

II. Drug Definitions
   A. A drug is a natural or synthetic, legal or illegal, prescription or nonprescription substance or chemical that has the potential to produce change in one or more functions of the body.
   B. A natural drug is obtained from plant, animal, or mineral sources; e.g., digitalis, which is obtained from a plant (purple foxglove) and is used to treat certain types of heart disease.
   C. A synthetic drug is created by chemical manufacture; e.g., glyburide (Micronase).
   D. A **legal drug** is one that is approved by the **Food and Drug Administration (FDA);** e.g., aspirin and penicillin.
   E. Sale and use of an **illegal drug** (e.g., heroin and cocaine) are against the law.
   F. A prescription drug requires a written form completed and signed by a licensed physician, dentist, or veterinarian.
      1. The prescription is then filled, or dispensed, by a licensed pharmacist.
      2. Prescription drugs also may be kept in a dental office for use before, during, or after dental procedures; e.g., diazepam (Valium), a tranquilizer, and mepivacaine (Carbocaine), a local anesthetic.
   F. A nonprescription or over-the-counter drug is any legal drug that can be purchased without a prescription.

III. Drug Legislation
   A. The *Pure Food and Drug Act* was passed in 1906.
      1. This was the first attempt by the government to regulate and control the manufacture, distribution, and sale of drugs.
   B. The *Harrison Narcotic Act* was passed in 1914.
      1. This act regulated the sale of narcotic drugs.
   C. The *Pure Food, Drug, and Cosmetic Act* was passed in 1938.

   1. This act gave the FDA control over the manufacture and sale of drugs, as well as over food and cosmetics.
   2. This law requires that these substances be safe for human use and that pharmaceutical companies perform toxicology tests before a new drug is submitted to the FDA for approval; following FDA review, approval may be given to market the drug.
   3. The Federal Trade Commission (FTC) controls and regulates the advertising of drugs.
   D. The *Comprehensive Drug Abuse Prevention and Control Act* was passed by Congress in 1970.
      1. This act was written because of the growing problem with drug abuse.
      2. It regulates the manufacture, distribution, and dispensing of drugs that have the potential for abuse.
      3. Title II of this law, the *Controlled Substance Act,* deals with control and enforcement.
      4. The **Drug Enforcement Agency (DEA)** within the U.S. Department of Justice is the leading federal agency responsible for the enforcement of this act.
      5. Drugs under the jurisdiction of the Controlled Substance Act are divided into five schedules based on their potential for abuse and physical and psychologic dependence (box on p. 148).
      6. Prescriptions for controlled substances must include the name and address of the patient and the DEA number of the licensed physician or dentist.
      7. Prescriptions for these drugs cannot be filled more than 6 months after the prescription was written or be filled more than five times.
      8. Under federal law, limited quantities of certain C-V (schedule V) drugs may be purchased without a prescription; the name of the purchaser and the drug(s) dispensed must be recorded by the pharmacist.
   E. Council on Dental Therapeutics
      1. The **Council on Dental Therapeutics** is one of the councils of the American Dental Association (ADA).
      2. The council's purpose is to study, evaluate, and distribute information regarding dental therapeutic and cosmetic products, such

---

DRUG SCHEDULES AS DETERMINED BY THE DRUG ENFORCEMENT AGENCY

SCHEDULE I (C-I)

High abuse potential and no accepted medical use (heroin, marijuana, LSD)

SCHEDULE II (C-II)

High abuse potential with severe dependence liability (narcotics, amphetamines, barbiturates)

SCHEDULE III (C-III)

Less abuse potential than schedule II drugs and moderate dependence liability (nonbarbiturate sedatives, nonamphetamine stimulants, limited amounts of certain narcotics)

SCHEDULE IV (C-IV)

Less abuse potential than schedule III drugs and limited dependence liability (some sedatives and anti-anxiety agents, nonnarcotic analgesics)

SCHEDULE V (C-V)

Limited abuse potential; primarily small amounts of narcotics (codeine) used as antitussives or antidiarrheals

---

as toothpaste, toothbrushes, and mouthwashes.
3. The council also supports contact with related regulatory, research, and professional organizations.
4. A product approved by the ADA council has a seal showing approval affixed on the product by the manufacturer.
5. Information regarding ADA approval is given to the public as well as to members of the dental profession.
6. Manufacturers may also mention ADA approval in advertising the product.

IV. Trade Names and Generic Names
  A. A **trade name** is the (brand) name a manufacturer gives to a product.
    1. When the trade name of a drug is printed or written, it is capitalized, for example, Lasix, the trade name for furosemide.
  B. A **generic name** is the nonproprietary chemical name of the drug.
    1. Generic names are not capitalized.
    2. All drugs have generic names.

3. The term *generic equivalent* is usually used to mean a drug that is no longer under patent rights and is available from more than one company; in some instances, references simply use the term *generic* to indicate a drug that is a generic equivalent.
4. Although most generic equivalents are basically the same as their trade-name counterparts, a few are known to meet a lower standard than the trade-name drug.

V. Sources of Drug Information
  A. *Physician's Desk Reference (PDR)*
    1. The *PDR* is published yearly and provides periodic updates.
    2. Front pages of the *PDR* contain color photographs of drugs for quick identification.
    3. The *PDR* contains an index of all products included in the book.
    4. The pink pages list drugs by brand and generic name.
    5. The blue pages list drugs by category; e.g., antibiotics, local anesthetics.
    6. Most drugs included in the *PDR* have a drug monograph (a complete listing of most known facts about the product).
    7. Subheadings in the drug monograph include the following:
      a. Chemical description of the product
      b. Clinical pharmacology
      c. Indications and use of the drug
      d. Contraindications to use of the drug
      e. Warnings and precautions related to use of the drug
      f. Adverse drug reactions
      g. Recommended drug dosages
      h. Form in which the drug is supplied (e.g., tablets, vials for injection, capsules)
  B. *Facts and Comparisons*
    1. This resource for drug information is published yearly as a bound volume and is available in a loose-leaf ring-binder edition that is updated monthly.
    2. Some dentists use this reference, especially oral surgeons.
  C. Drug Package Inserts
    1. Information contained in the drug insert is often, but not always, identical to the information contained in the *PDR*.
    2. Drug package inserts usually are not given to the patient when a prescription is dispensed.

3. Many pharmacists provide an information sheet containing information from the drug package insert.

D. *United States Pharmacopoeia (USP)* and the *National Formulary (NF)*
   1. These references are usually used by pharmacists or those involved in drug research.
   2. They include detailed information less pertinent to the patient and prescribing professional than to the dispensing pharmacist.

E. Textbooks
   1. Textbooks become outdated quickly and may not provide current drug information.
   2. Textbooks are an excellent resource for obtaining general information on how a specific class or type of drug works.

DRUG ACTIONS, INTERACTIONS, REACTIONS, AND EFFECTS

I. Drug Actions
   A. Several factors influence drug action and must be taken into account when a drug is prescribed by the dentist or used in the dental office.
      1. The age of the patient may influence the action of a drug.
         a. Children almost always require smaller doses of a drug than do adults.
         b. Older adult patients may also require smaller doses, although this depends on the type of drug that is administered.
      2. Drug dosages are often calculated on the basis of weight.
      3. The action of some drugs may be influenced by the patient's sex, weight, or body-fat ratio.
      4. The action of some drugs may cause defects in a developing fetus.
      5. The FDA has established five pregnancy categories indicating the potential of a drug for causing birth defects (box).
      6. Presence of disease may influence the action of some drugs; in some instances it may be an indication not to prescribe a drug or to reduce the dosage of a certain drug.
      7. Drugs may be given by the following routes:
         a. Oral
         b. Subcutaneous
         c. Intramuscular
         d. Intravenous
         e. Respiratory (inhalation)
         f. Intradermal
         g. Topical
         h. Parenteral

II. Drug Interactions
   A. Some drugs interact with or interfere with the actions of other drugs.
   B. Drug interactions can be **antagonistic** or **synergistic.**
      1. Antagonistic drugs may interact with food, chemicals, or other drugs and produce opposing effects.
      2. A synergistic drug effect may occur when a drug interacts with another drug (or drugs) and produces an effect that is greater than the sum of the separate actions of the two or more drugs.
   C. Some drugs must be taken on an empty stomach and some with food to achieve the best effect.

III. Drug Reactions
   A. An adverse drug reaction is a symptom that is usually not desired when a drug is introduced to the body; e.g., nausea, vomiting, difficulty breathing, diarrhea, dryness of mouth, constipation, and headache.

FDA PREGNANCY CATEGORIES

Pregnancy Category A: Studies have not demonstrated a risk to the fetus in the first trimester (up to the third month of pregnancy), and there is no evidence of risk in the second (the third to sixth month of pregnancy) or third trimesters (the sixth to ninth month of pregnancy).

Pregnancy Category B: This category includes two distinctions. One is that animal studies have not demonstrated a risk to the fetus, but no adequate studies on pregnant women are available. The other is that animal studies have demonstrated an adverse effect, but adequate studies on pregnant women have not demonstrated a risk to the human fetus during the first, second, or third trimester of pregnancy.

Pregnancy Category C: This category includes two distinctions. One is that animal studies have shown an adverse effect on the fetus, but adequate studies in humans are not available. The other is that there have been no animal reproduction studies, and no adequate studies have been performed in humans.

Pregnancy Category D: There is evidence of risk to the human fetus.

Pregnancy Category X: Studies in animals and humans demonstrate fetal abnormalities, and reports indicate evidence of fetal risk.

1. A drug allergy, or being **allergic** to a drug, is also called a *hypersensitivity reaction.*
   a. Allergy to a drug seems to occur after more than one dose of the drug is taken.
   b. When a drug allergy occurs, the individual has become *sensitized* to the drug. That is, the drug has become an **antigen**—any substance that stimulates the body to produce **antibodies,** which are specific protein substances manufactured by the body in response to contact with a specific antigen.
   c. If the patient takes the drug after the antigen/antibody response has occurred, an allergic reaction will result.
2. Allergic reactions may be manifested by various signs and symptoms, including the following:
   a. Itching
   b. Skin rashes (various types)
   c. Hives (raised, red blotches on the skin)
   d. Difficulty breathing
   e. Asthmalike symptoms
   f. Cyanosis
   g. Sudden loss of consciousness
   h. Swelling of the eyes, lips, or tongue
3. Another type of allergic drug reaction is an **anaphylactic** reaction, which usually occurs shortly after the administration of a drug. This type of allergic reaction is potentially life threatening and requires immediate medical attention.
4. Signs of an anaphylactic reaction include the following:
   a. Bronchospasm
   b. Extremely low blood pressure
   c. Cyanosis
   d. Dyspnea
   e. Loss of consciousness
   f. Convulsions
   g. Cardiac arrest
5. **Angioedema,** which is also known as *angioneurotic edema,* is another type of serious allergic drug reaction.
   a. Angioedema is manifested by the collection of fluid in subcutaneous tissues, which is evidenced by swelling.
   b. Areas that may be affected are the eyelids, lips, mouth, throat, hands, and feet, although other areas may also be affected.
   c. Angioedema can be life threatening when the mouth is affected because the swelling of tissues in this area may block the airway.
6. A drug idiosyncrasy is any unusual or abnormal reaction to a drug—any reaction that differs from the one normally expected with a specific drug and dose.

IV. Drug Effects
   A. **Drug tolerance** is a term used to describe a decreased response to the dose of a drug; usually an increase in dosage is required to obtain the desired effect.
      1. Drug tolerance may develop when certain drugs, such as narcotics and tranquilizers, are taken for a long time.
      2. It is often seen in persons who use illegal drugs such as heroin and cocaine.
   B. A *cumulative drug effect* may be seen in persons with liver or kidney disease because these organs are the major sites for the breakdown and excretion of most drugs.
      1. A cumulative drug effect occurs when the body is unable to metabolize and excrete one (normal) dose of a drug before the next dose is given.
      2. Because toxicity can occur with some drugs when too much of that drug is in the body, a cumulative drug effect may be seen.
      3. This effect may be serious, particularly with patients who have liver or kidney disease.

SUBSTANCE ABUSE

I. The social and economic impact of drug addiction and abuse directly or indirectly affects every member of society.
   A. The Commission on Dental Accreditation recommends that all accredited dental and dental-related programs provide enrolled students with information regarding substance use, misuse, and addiction by means of classroom lectures.
   B. Any patient seen by a member of the health team may be abusing drugs, including children and adults.
      1. Not limited to purchasing an illegal drug on the street.
      2. Includes both legal and illegal drugs and may be seen in all age groups and all socioeconomic levels.
      3. Often a hidden problem.
   C. Terminology
      1. *Substance abuse* is the use of a drug or chemical to produce a change in mood or

behavior in a way that departs from approved medical or social patterns.

2. *Compulsive substance abuse* is the need to use any drug or chemical substance repeatedly to produce the desired effect; the need to use a drug compulsively may be physical, psychologic, or both.

3. Physical dependency is a compulsive need to use a substance repeatedly to avoid mild to severe withdrawal symptoms and is the body's dependence on repeated administration of a drug.

4. Psychologic dependency is a compulsion to use a substance to obtain a pleasurable experience and is the mind's dependence on the repeated administration of a drug.

D. *Drug addiction* may be defined to include the following:
   1. Compulsive desire or craving to use a drug or chemical
   2. Involvement with the drug to the exclusion of all other activities, such as work, recreation, family, or school
   3. Strong tendency to return to the drug after withdrawal
   4. Physical dependence
   5. Abstinence syndrome that produces moderate to severe physical reactions
   6. Detriment to society in the drug and its use as well as in the user

E. *Drug habituation* may be defined to include the following:
   1. Desire to use a drug continually for the effects produced
   2. Little or no tendency to increase the dose
   3. No physical dependence but rather a psychologic dependence
   4. No true abstinence syndrome when the drug is withdrawn
   5. Detrimental effects that exist for the individual rather than society

NARCOTICS

I. Definition
   A. **Narcotics** are substances that produce insensibility or stupor.
   B. Narcotics are generally derived from opium.
   C. Narcotics can relieve pain by suppressing the central nervous system.

II. Heroin
   A. Heroin is a narcotic obtained from morphine, which is the principal alkaloid of raw opium; it is illegal in the United States.

B. Heroin is the strongest and most addicting of all the opium derivatives, or opiates; it is not used as an analgesic in the United States.

C. Physical addiction occurs rapidly, often within several weeks of frequent use; however, the time in which addiction occurs varies.

D. Addiction poses serious socioeconomic problems to individuals, families, and the community.

E. The cost of a heroin drug habit is high.

F. Continued use of heroin may result in other physical problems, such as malnutrition and physical neglect.

G. Those using the drug intravenously (mainlining) may develop serious medical disorders.

H. Heroin may be inhaled (sniffed) or injected subcutaneously (skin popping) or intravenously.

I. Abstinence syndrome consists of the signs and symptoms of heroin withdrawal (box).

J. Signs and symptoms of heroin overdose include the following:
   1. Stupor
   2. Pinpoint pupils
   3. Nausea
   4. Vomiting
   5. Decreased pulse and respiratory rate
   6. Signs of shock
   7. Possible coma

SIGNS AND SYMPTOMS OF HEROIN WITHDRAWAL (ABSTINENCE SYNDROME)*

Yawning
Perspiration
Tearing of the eyes
Increased nasal discharge
Gooseflesh
Abdominal cramps
Bone and muscle pain
Nausea
Vomiting
Diarrhea
Dilation of the pupils
Restlessness
Increase in body temperature
Increase in pulse and respiratory rate
Marked depression or despair
Intense desire for heroin

*The signs and symptoms of withdrawal usually begin when the next dose of heroin is due, reach a peak in 36 to 72 hours, and gradually diminish in 4 to 5 days.

III. Opiates
   A. Opiates are used for their narcotic and analgesic effects.
   B. Opiates, such as morphine, and other narcotics, such as meperidine (Demerol), are used less frequently than heroin as street drugs (i.e., drugs obtained from illegal sources).
IV. Narcotics and Terminally Ill Patients
   A. Terminally ill cancer patients who require repeated doses of a narcotic for pain eventually become addicted to the drug.
   B. Addiction in these patients is morally and legally acceptable.
   C. A terminally ill patient's health and drug history should be thoroughly examined before dental treatment is provided.
V. Cocaine
   A. Cocaine is an alkaloid obtained from coca leaves.
   B. Cocaine is highly addicting, and at the present time its use is the number one substance abuse problem.
   C. Use of cocaine has created serious and sometimes deadly consequences that affect individuals, families, and the community.
   D. Cocaine stimulates the central nervous system, producing marked euphoria and excitement.
   E. Dangers associated with the use of cocaine include the following:
      1. Physical and psychologic dependency
      2. Permanent damage to the nasal mucosa
      3. High cost financially
   F. Signs and symptoms of acute cocaine toxicity are listed (box below).

VI. Marijuana
   A. Marijuana is classified as a hallucinogen, a drug capable of producing a state of delirium characterized by visual and sensory disturbances that are bizarre and distorted.
   B. Marijuana belongs to the *Cannabis* genus of plants.
   C. Signs of chronic marijuana use are listed (box below).
   D. Marijuana is being used medically on a limited basis to lower intraocular pressure in persons with glaucoma and in terminally ill cancer patients.
   E. Specific guidelines in dispensing the drug are required.
   F. Legal use of marijuana is limited to research institutions or to physicians who have applied for government approval of marijuana use in certain patients.
VII. Psychotomimetic (Hallucinogenic) Drugs
   A. These drugs produce an acute change in the perception of reality.
   B. Drugs in this group include mescaline, lysergic acid diethylamide (LSD), 2,5-dimethoxy-4-methylamphetamine (DOM or STP), psilocybin, phencyclidine (PCP, or angel dust), and dimethyltryptamine (DMT).
   C. Use of these agents causes visual hallucinations and mood changes.
   D. Results are inconsistent and differ from person to person, and even within the same person, when the drug is taken under varying circumstances.
   E. Although physical dependence on these drugs does not occur, the user can develop a psychologic dependence.
   F. No physical withdrawal symptoms occur when use of the substance is discontinued.
VIII. Amphetamines
   A. Amphetamine, dextroamphetamine, and meth-

**SIGNS AND SYMPTOMS
OF COCAINE TOXICITY**

Irregular heartbeat
Hypertension
Memory impairment
Personality and behavior changes
Ulceration of the nasal mucosa
Perforation of the nasal septum (in those who inhale cocaine)
Needle marks along the pathways of veins (in those who use cocaine intravenously)
Loss of appetite with consequent weight loss
Psychosis
Hallucinations

SIGNS OF CHRONIC MARIJUANA USE

Lack of interest in school, work, and other people
Carelessness in personal hygiene and clothes
Preoccupied appearance
Lack of motivation
Memory difficulty
Passivity or apathy

amphetamine are intended for use as central nervous system stimulants and as anorexiants (drugs that suppress the appetite).

B. Because of the abuse potential of these drugs, their use in the medical treatment of obesity has declined.

C. Amphetamines have value in the treatment of some obese individuals and in those conditions or diseases requiring central nervous system stimulation.

D. When amphetamines are used, therapy is under the close supervision of a physician.

E. Amphetamines produce euphoria, alertness, and a sense of excitation. Users appear talkative, restless, and excitable. They may perspire freely, and their pupils may be dilated.

IX. Barbiturates and Nonbarbiturates

A. Barbiturate and nonbarbiturate drugs have their proper use in medicine but are also subject to abuse.

B. An overdose of these drugs can result in convulsions, delirium, coma, and, in some instances, death.

C. When these drugs are abused or are used under a physician's supervision for a long time, they must never be suddenly discontinued; the dose must be slowly tapered.

D. When a barbiturate is suddenly discontinued an abstinence syndrome develops, with the following characteristics:
1. Abdominal cramps
2. Nausea
3. Vomiting
4. Weakness
5. Tremors

X. Tranquilizers

A. Tranquilizers have been subject to widespread abuse by those involved in substance abuse as well as by persons who do not consider themselves *drug users.*

B. Addiction to tranquilizers appears to occur fairly rapidly, although the time required to produce addiction often depends on the type of tranquilizer, the individual, and the tendency to increase the dose required to produce the desired effect.

C. When withdrawal occurs, it resembles barbiturate withdrawal; the intensity of symptoms depends on the length of time that the drug was used and the dose that was most frequently used.

XI. Alcohol

A. For various reasons, alcohol is subject to widespread abuse among persons of all ages and socioeconomic levels.

B. Malnutrition, physical disease, broken marriages, crime, loss of employment, and accidents resulting in injury or death are associated with alcohol use.

C. The combination of alcohol and drugs can produce a synergistic effect.

D. Signs and symptoms of physical withdrawal from alcohol include the following:
1. Tremors
2. Weakness
3. Anxiety
4. Restlessness
5. Excessive perspiration
6. Nausea
7. Vomiting
8. Seizures
9. Hallucinations

XII. Methods of Treating Substance Abuse

A. Methods for treating substance abuse vary not only from drug to drug, but also in the methods that may be used for a specific drug.

B. Sometimes an individual addicted to one or more drugs or chemicals may need to try more than one treatment method to achieve results.

C. Success depends on the individual's desire to become drug free.

DRUGS USED IN DENTISTRY

I. The types of drugs used in any one dental practice may vary depending on the specialty of the dental practice.

II. Common Drugs Used in Dentistry

A. Analgesics
1. **Analgesics** relieve pain and/or discomfort.
2. Analgesics may be narcotic or nonnarcotic.

B. Antibiotics
1. **Antibiotics** are used to prevent or treat an infection.
2. Some antibiotics destroy specific microorganisms, whereas others slow or inhibit the multiplication of microorganisms.

C. Tranquilizers
1. **Tranquilizers** may be used to reduce anxiety and tension.
2. A tranquilizer may be given 30 to 45 minutes before a dental procedure.

D. Barbiturates

1. **Barbiturates** are usually used as hypnotics or sedatives.
   a. A **hypnotic** produces sleep and is normally taken at bedtime.
   b. A **sedative** produces sedation or relaxation and is usually taken during the day.
2. Intravenous barbiturates may be administered intravenously to produce unconsciousness during an oral surgery procedure.
3. An oral barbiturate may be prescribed to be taken at bedtime for 1 or more days after extensive oral surgery.

E. Nonbarbiturate hypnotics
1. These are sometimes preferred to the barbiturate hypnotics when the patient requires a drug to induce sleep after extensive oral surgery.
2. They appear to cause fewer problems with excessive sedation the following morning and are also considered somewhat safer for older individuals.

F. Antihistamines
1. **Antihistamines** oppose the action of histamine, a substance produced in response to injury or from coming in contact with antigens to which an individual is sensitive.
2. They are used to treat allergies.
3. In dental practice, they are usually used to treat an allergic reaction to a drug or substance used during a dental procedure.
4. The most commonly used antihistamine is diphenhydramine (Benadryl).
5. The injectable form of antihistamines is usually included in drug emergency kits.

G. Vasoconstrictors
1. A **vasoconstrictor** constricts blood vessels, primarily small arteries and capillaries.
2. Constriction of small blood vessels helps reduce or stop bleeding that may occur during or shortly after the dental procedure.
3. Local anesthetics containing a small amount of vasoconstrictor, such as epinephrine, may be used to control bleeding during a dental procedure.
4. Epinephrine also prolongs the action of the local anesthetic by decreasing its rate of absorption because the blood vessels are constricted and therefore absorb the drug more slowly.
5. Local anesthetic containing a vasoconstrictor is not recommended if the patient has

hypertension, high blood pressure, or a history of heart disease.

H. Topical hemostatic agents
1. A **topical hemostatic agent** controls bleeding by methods other than vasoconstriction.
2. Topical hemostatic agents that may be used in dentistry are listed (box).

I. Adrenocortical hormones
1. The adrenal gland manufactures the glucocorticoids and mineralocorticoids, which collectively are called *adrenocortical hormones*.
2. The glucocorticoids and mineralocorticoids are essential to life.
3. Glucocorticoids influence or regulate body functions, such as the immune response system; regulate glucose, carbohydrate, and fat metabolism; and control the antiinflammatory response.
4. Hydrocortisone and cortisone are the two major glucocorticoids produced by the adrenal gland.
5. Prednisone and prednisolone are synthetic glucocorticoids.
6. Hydrocortisone may be used to treat emergency allergic reactions.
7. Prednisone or prednisolone may be prescribed for a short time to reduce inflammation and swelling following certain types of oral surgeries.

J. Antiseptics and germicides
1. An **antiseptic** is an agent that stops, slows, or prevents the growth of microorganisms.
2. A **germicide** is an agent that kills bacteria.

DRUG HISTORY AND PRESCRIPTIONS ▄▄▄▄

I. History
A. The patient's complete drug history is an im-

TOPICAL HEMOSTATIC AGENTS

Absorbable gelatin sponge (Gelfoam): a gelatin-based sponge that can be cut to the desired size and placed on or in the bleeding area

Topical thrombin (Thrombinar): a substance that aids in the formation of a blood clot

Microfibrillar collagen hemostat (Avitene): aids in the clotting of blood; may be used in certain types of oral surgeries

Oxidized cellulose (Oxycel): aids in the formation of a blood clot; can be cut to the desired size before placement on or in the bleeding area

portant component of the general health history.

B. The health and drug history should include the following components:
1. Prescription drugs currently being taken or that were prescribed in the past 6 months
2. All nonprescription drugs that the patient takes on a regular or occasional basis
3. History of surgical procedures
4. History of past and present medical disorders
5. Pregnancy
6. Allergy history

II. Prescriptions
A. A **prescription** (Fig. 9-1) is a legal form written and signed by a licensed physician, dentist, or veterinarian for dispensing drugs that are required by law to be sold only by prescription.
B. Prescriptions contain several parts (box).
C. Various abbreviations used in writing prescriptions and in the patient's dental record (box on page 156).

III. Recording Drug Information
A. In addition to obtaining and updating the patient's health history, the dental assistant may be responsible for recording the following drug information:
1. All drugs used or administered before, during, and after a dental procedure; the name and dose of the drug and the route by which it is given are also noted on the dental record; when a local anesthetic is used, its name, percent, and amount are recorded.
2. Prescriptions written by the dentist are recorded.
a. Name and dosage of the prescribed or recommended drug

PARTS OF A PRESCRIPTION

- Heading
- Superscription
- Inscription
- Subscription
- Signature
- Physician, dentist, or veterinarian signature and Drug Enforcement Agency number
- Refill information
- Designation for filling with a generic equivalent

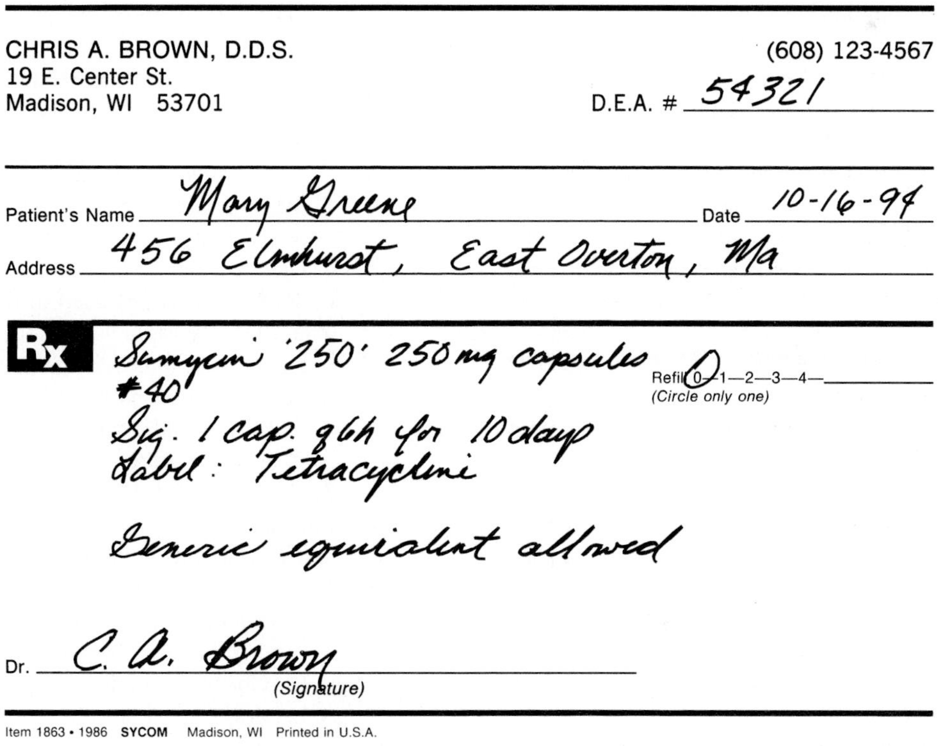

CHRIS A. BROWN, D.D.S.
19 E. Center St.
Madison, WI 53701

(608) 123-4567
D.E.A. # 54321

Patient's Name Mary Greene   Date 10-16-94
Address 456 Elmhurst, East Overton, Ma

Rx Sumycin '250' 250 mg capsules   Refill 0-1-2-3-4-
#40   (Circle only one)
Sig. 1 cap. q6h for 10 days
Label: Tetracycline

Generic equivalent allowed

Dr. C. A. Brown
(Signature)

Item 1863 • 1986 **SYCOM**   Madison, WI Printed in U.S.A.

Fig. 9-1 Example of a prescription.

ABBREVIATIONS COMMONLY USED IN WRITING PRESCRIPTIONS

qd	Daily
bid	Twice a day
tid	Three times a day
qid	Four times a day
qh	Every hour
q2h	Every 2 hours
q3h	Every 3 hours
q4h	Every 4 hours
q6h	Every 6 hours
q12h	Every 12 hours
stat	Immediately
ac	Before meals
pc	After meals
prn	Whenever necessary, as needed
tabs	Tablets
caps	Capsules
liq	Liquid
sig	Take
ml	Milliliter
tsp	Teaspoon

b. Number of capsules or tablets or the amount of the drug by volume

c. Directions for taking the prescribed or recommended drug

3. Names or types of nonprescription drugs recommended by the dentist for use after a dental procedure are recorded.

4. Drug samples given to the patient in the office to take immediately or at home are recorded.

5. Certain drugs administered, such as the short-acting general anesthetics and intravenous tranquilizers, are recorded.

EMERGENCIES

I. Adverse Reaction to a Drug or Product

A. A dental office should have an emergency kit that can be used to treat serious and even life-threatening allergic drug reactions.

B. Drugs contained in the emergency kit are usually in prefilled syringes, ready for immediate use.

C. Most kits contain some or all of the following items:

1. Epinephrine 1:1000
2. Ephedrine
3. Antihistamines
4. Diazepam (Valium)

5. Bronchodilating agent
6. Nitroglycerin
7. Hydrocortisone
8. Intravenous glucose
9. Ammonia inhalers
10. Additional equipment
   a. Tourniquets
   b. Sterile syringes
   c. Oxygen mask
   d. One or more oral airways
   e. Additional drugs

II. Responsibilities of the Dental Assistant

A. The dental assistant's most important responsibility is recognition of an adverse drug reaction, particularly allergic reactions that require emergency treatment.

B. Potential adverse drug reactions should be listed or described by the dentist to the dental staff.

C. The dentist is responsible for determining the type of emergency that occurred and the drugs and dosage to be used to treat the problem.

D. An emergency requires swift treatment.

E. The dental assistant should be prepared to take the following steps:

1. Bring the emergency kit to the room and open the kit.

2. Prepare the drug or drugs requested by the dentist by opening the package; some drugs must be mixed before a sterile syringe is filled with the dosage requested by the dentist; other drugs may be premixed in ampules, and a sterile syringe must be filled with the dosage requested by the dentist.

3. Prepare other materials, such as an oral airway or oxygen mask, by opening the package.

4. Record the drugs used in the emergency.

F. The contents of any kit should be checked monthly to ensure that the following requirements have been met:

1. All drugs and equipment are in place.
2. Drugs that were used have been replaced.
3. Any outdated drugs are discarded.

G. Periodically review the printed information and instructions contained in the kit.

H. Drugs

1. The dental assistant should assume responsibility for the following tasks:

a. Check expiration dates of the stock of drugs used in the office, and reorder drugs as needed.

b. Store all drugs in a cool, dry place unless directed otherwise by the manufacturer or dentist.

c. When drugs are restocked, place the new supply of drugs behind or underneath the present supply of drugs. Do not remove packaging until the drug is ready to be used.

d. Be aware of some of the more common adverse reactions of the drugs used in the office.

e. Follow recommended guidelines when handling needles and syringes during preparation for, during, and following administration of a drug.

f. Ask for clarification if there is any question regarding the drug requested by the dentist before or during a procedure.

g. When preparing a drug for administration by the dentist, check the label of the drug twice to ensure accuracy.

h. During a dental procedure, repeat the name of the drug when handing it to the dentist.

PATIENT EDUCATION ■■■■■■■

I. Information to Relate to the Patient
   A. An accurate health history, including a drug and allergy history, is an important part of dental care.
   B. Drugs are often administered or prescribed by the dentist.
   C. The dentist may decide to use a different drug or procedure because of information obtained from the health or allergy history.
   D. Certain medical conditions or diseases may require important changes in a dental procedure.
   E. Knowledge of all current prescription and nonprescription drug therapy helps the dentist treat the whole patient and may aid in the treatment of dental problems.
II. Instructions for the Patient Using Nonprescription Drugs
   A. Nonprescription drugs can be purchased without a prescription.
   B. Follow directions specifically.
   C. Do not place aspirin on soft tissues—it should be swallowed.
   D. Avoid substituting one drug for another.
   E. Topical application of certain nonprescription products for pain or discomfort should be used only as temporary measures.
IV. General Instructions Concerning All Drugs

A. When the dentist prescribes a drug, review with the patient the importance of the drug and the need to continue its use until the dentist advises otherwise.

B. Instruct the patient to read the drug label carefully and follow the dosage and recommendations for use that are printed on the container.

C. Advise the patient to notify the dentist as soon as possible if any of the following results occur:
   1. The drug fails to relieve the problem for which it was prescribed.
   2. The drug causes problems that were not present before the drug was taken.
   3. The problem for which the drug was prescribed or recommended becomes worse.

Questions

Pharmacology

1 Before prescribing any drug, which of the following data should be obtained?
a. Accurate medical history
b. Complete bacterial count
c. Complete blood cell count
d. Urinalysis study

2 Various methods of drug administration include
1. Intradermal
2. Retrodermal
3. Intraradicular
4. Intramuscular
5. Sublingual
a. 1, 2, and 4
b. 1, 4, and 5
c. 2, 3, and 4
d. 3, 4, and 5

3 Some drugs cannot be taken orally for which of the following reasons?
a. They are in liquid form.
b. Saliva will dilute them.
c. The enamel will corrode.
d. The digestive system will alter the drug.

4 Drugs may be derived from
1. Infusion
2. Animals
3. Plants
4. Sand
5. Synthetic materials
a. 1, 2, and 3
b. 2, 3, and 4
c. 2, 3, and 5
d. 3, 4, and 5

5 The abbreviation q4h means
  a. Every 4 days
  b. Four times a day
  c. Every 4 hours
  d. For 4 days

6 Analgesics used in dentistry include
  1. Aspirin
  2. Codeine
  3. Acetaminophen
  4. Phenobarbital
  a. 1 and 3
  b. 2 and 4
  c. 1, 2, and 3
  d. 1, 2, 3, and 4
  e. 4 only

7 The type of drug most commonly used to premedicate an anxious patient is a(n)
  a. Barbiturate
  b. Meperidine
  c. Antibiotic
  d. Anhistamine

8 Alcohol is a(n)
  a. Hormone
  b. Diuretic
  c. Central nervous system depressant
  d. Enzyme used in respiration

9 Narcotics used in dentistry include
  1. Codeine
  2. Tylenol
  3. Meperidine
  4. Morphine
  5. Aspirin
  a. 1, 2, and 3
  b. 1, 3, and 4
  c. 2, 4, and 5
  d. 3, 4, and 5

10 Some patients cannot take aspirin because of
  a. A previous heart attack
  b. Gastrointestinal irritation
  c. Production of gas pains
  d. The severe headaches it causes

11 Epinephrine in local anesthesia causes
  1. Constriction of the blood vessels
  2. Hyperventilation
  3. Prolonged effects of the anesthetic
  4. None of the above
  a. 1 and 3
  b. 2 only
  c. 1, 2, and 3
  d. 4 only

12 The antibiotic of choice for the treatment of oral infections is
  a. Penicillin
  b. Streptomycin
  c. Sulfa
  d. Tetracycline

13 The function of a hemostatic agent is to
  a. Thicken the blood
  b. Thin the blood
  c. Stop bleeding
  d. Increase the number of blood platelets in the circulating blood

14 Hydrogen peroxide can be used as a(n)
  a. Hemostatic agent
  b. Anodyne
  c. Oxidizing mouthwash
  d. Treatment for herpetic lesions

15 Which of the following drugs are applied topically?
  1. Fluoride
  2. Penicillin
  3. Anesthetic agents
  4. Iodine
  5. Tetracycline
  a. 1, 2, and 5
  b. 1, 3, and 4
  c. 2, 3, and 4
  d. 3, 4, and 5

16 Tachycardia is a _____ heartbeat; bradycardia is a _____ heart beat.
  a. Skipped, slow
  b. Rapid, slow
  c. Rapid, fast
  d. Slow, rapid

In items 17-20, match the term in column A with the description in column B.

Column A	Column B
_____ **17** Sedative	a. Organic compounds that depress the central nervous system
_____ **18** Subcutaneous	
_____ **19** Narcotic	
_____ **20** Intramuscular	b. Agent that soothes
	c. Drug derived from opium
	d. Within a muscle
	e. Within the skin

21 Modifications in dental therapy for the asthmatic patient may include
  a. Stress and anxiety reduction
  b. Requiring a patient to bring his or her bronchodilator to the dental appointment
  c. Use of nitrous oxide to relieve anxiety
  d. Both a and b
  e. None of the above

22 Examples of psychosedation before and during dental treatment include
  a. Use of calming medications
  b. Use of nitrous oxide before administration of local anesthetic possibly during treatment
  c. Administration of local anesthetic for pain control
  d. Both a and b
  e. All of the above

23 The following signa appears on a prescription: Amoxicillin 500 mg q12h Refill 0. The patient will
  1. Take the drug two times a day
  2. Take the drug four times a day
  3. Refill the prescription once

4. Be able to stop taking the medication when feeling better
5. Not be able to refill the prescription
a. 2 only
b. 1 and 5
c. 1, 4, and 5
d. 2 and 4
e. 2, 4, and 5

24 A patient visits the office when the dentist is not present and indicates concern about a drug that has been prescribed. To what source would you refer to obtain information for this patient?
a. *PDA*
b. *PDR*
c. Dictionary
d. Practice procedure policy

25 In reference to question 24, what information would you not be able to give the patient?
a. Importance of the drug
b. Direct the patient to speak to his or her physician
c. Stop taking the drug until the dentist directs otherwise
d. Certain changes in health or other medications may cause problems with the prescribed drug.

Rationales

Pharmacology

1 A An accurate medical history is extremely important prior to prescribing any drug. From appointment to appointment a patient's medical history may change. These changes may include diagnosis of a disease, addition or change in prescription and nonprescription drugs, or other factors may impact dental care.

2 B Intradermal, intramuscular, and sublingual are common methods of administration (i.e., under the skin, within the muscle or under the tongue). There are no such methods as retrodermal or intraradicular. Other methods that might be used to administer drugs include topical, subcutaneous, IV, and inhalation.

3 D The digestive system may alter the effect of a drug. When an antacid is taken orally at the same time as tetracycline, the antacid may chemically interact and impair absorption of the tetracycline into the bloodstream, reducing effectiveness.

4 C Currently drugs are manufactured through the use of animals, various plants, and synthetic materials.

5 C There is no abbreviation for every 4 days or to be taken for four days. The abbreviation for four times a day is qid and q4h is every four hours.

6 C Phenobarbital is not an analgesic used in dentistry, but a barbiturate sedative used in sleep induction. Aspirin, codeine, and acetaminophen are all used as analgesics.

7 A Barbiturates are used as hypnotics to produce sleep or as sedatives to produce relaxation. Barbiturates may be used intravenously for oral surgery to produce unconsciousness during the procedure.

8 C Alcohol is a central nervous system depressant that causes changes in the systems related to the CNS.

9 B Narcotics are used in dentistry to relieve pain by suppressing the central nervous system to reaction. Those narcotics commonly used for this purpose include codeine, meperidine, and morphine.

10 B Gastrointestinal irritation may be sensitive to the use of aspirin causing greater discomfort to the patient. Alternative drugs for such patients may include ibuprofen or acetaminophen.

11 A Epinephrine in local anesthetics is particularly helpful during dental treatment. This drug is a vasoconstrictor that reduces blood flow at the operative site and increases working time for the operator.

12 A Penicillin, or any of the drugs in this family are often used in the treatment of oral infections. Streptomycin is an antibiotic used in the treatment of TB. Sulfa drugs are bacteriostatic agents that inhibit folic acid. Tetracycline is a broad spectrum antibiotic used in treatment of bacterial infections and may cause stain of teeth in certain situations.

13 C A hemostatic agent is a procedure, device, or substance that arrests blood flow. In dentistry the hemostatic agent is usually in the form of a substance that is placed near blood flow to reduce or stop it for a short term procedure.

14 C Hydrogen peroxide is a topical antiinfective that may be used alone or with other substances to act as an oxidizing mouthwash to remove microbes.

15 B Penicillin and tetracycline may be taken orally, but not topically. Fluoride, anesthetic and iodine are drugs that can be applied topically.

16 B Tachycardia is a condition of increased heartbeat with myocardium contractions of greater than 100 beats per minute. Bradycardia is a condition in which the myocardium contracts at a rate slower than 60 beats per minute.

17 B A sedative depresses the central nervous system, causing relaxation.

18 E Cutaneous is something pertaining to the skin; subcutaneous pertains to below the skin.

19 A Most narcotics are derived from opium, which is a plant and is considered organic.

20 D If a drug is placed in the muscle it is considered to be administered intramuscular.

21 D If the patient is comfortable and knows what to expect he or she may feel more relaxed, reducing stress and anxiety. Anytime a patient is using a device such as a bronchodilator, it should be brought for dental appointments.

22 D The use of nitrous oxide before the administration of local anesthesia relieves patient anxiety. Nitrous oxide in conjunction with calming medications taken before a dental appointment reduces patient anxiety and potential emotional trauma.

23 B The abbreviation of q12h refers to taking a medication twice a day but every 12 hours, unlike bid which directs to take a prescription twice a day. The indication of 0 refills means the patient is unable to refill the prescription.

24 B The Physicians' Desk Reference is a reference text for drugs that is updated yearly. Included in the reference is a photo identification section, index of all products contained in the PDR, drug name by brand and generic name, drugs by category, and a drug monograph.

25 C A dental auxiliary is not delegated the responsibility of determining if a patient should or should not take a drug. This responsibility lies solely with the dentist of record.

To enhance your understanding of the material in this chapter refer to the illustrations in Chapter 10 of Finkbeiner/Johnson: *Mosby's Comprehensive Dental Assisting: A Clinical Approach.*

Dental Materials

KEY TERMS

Amalgam

Amalgamation

Base metals

Compressive stress

Corrosion

Council on Dental Materials,
  Instruments, and Equipment

Deformation

Dimensional change

Direct

Ductile

Electrical characteristics

Exothermic reaction

Flow

Force

Galvanic action

Hardness

Heavy-body material

Imbibition

Indirect

Light-body material

Luting

Malleable

Noble

Mechanical properties

Noble metals

Primary consistency

Retentive property

Secondary consistency

Shear stress

Solubility

Sorption

Strain

Stress

Syneresis

Tensile stress

Thermal conductivity

Viscosity

Wettability

Yield point

Virtually all phases of dentistry use dental materials during the course of treatment. The study of dental materials can present a complex experience that involves the basic concepts of chemistry and physics and requires following specific manipulation procedures outlined by the manufacturer. Dental materials are used for the following purposes:

- Replace or restore tooth structure lost through trauma or dental caries
- Prevent the invasion of caries
- Replace soft tissues
- Take impressions of existing conditions or teeth prepared for a prosthetic device
- Finish, polish, and cleanse a restoration or prosthesis

COUNCIL ON DENTAL MATERIALS, INSTRUMENTS, AND EQUIPMENT

I.   The **Council on Dental Materials, Instruments, and Equipment,** a subgroup of the American Dental Association (ADA) in partnership with federal organizations, the Federal Specifications and Standards, and the National Bureau of Standards, provides standards and specifications that all dental materials must meet.
  A.   The council performs the following functions:
    1.   Ensures the safety and effectiveness of the materials, instruments, and equipment
    2.   Encourages the development and improvement of materials, instruments, and equipment
    3.   Coordinates national and international standardization programs and the evaluation of materials, instruments, and equipment
    4.   Maintains a liaison with the Occupational Safety and Health Administration (OSHA) and other organizations to provide recommendations on materials, instruments, and equipment
    5.   Maintains a liaison with regulatory, research, and professional organizations.
  B.   The subjection of dental materials to these guidelines provides the dental practitioner with materials that meet quality control standards.
  C.   Through this council the ADA grants certification to certain dental materials and devices.
    1.   Certification indicates that the manufacturer has verified that a specific product has met ADA specifications and has followed ADA advertising and exhibition standards.
    2.   When a manufacturer's product conforms with these specifications, its name is on a list of all certified products.
    3.   An acceptance program for products rates each as acceptable, provisionally acceptable, or unacceptable as determined through testing for safety and usefulness.

PROPERTIES OF DENTAL MATERIALS

I.   The selection and manipulation of dental materials are affected by various chemical and physical factors, including the following:
  A.   **Dimensional change**—the amount of change in both length and volume that occurs during the chemical reaction of many dental materials
    1.   Definitions of common types of dimensional change (box).
  B.   **Thermal conductivity** is the rate of heat flow through a particular material.
    1.   Certain materials are poor thermal conductors, meaning that heat and cold are not transported through the material.
      a.   Enamel is a poor thermal conductor.
      b.   Amalgam and other metals conduct the thermal change through the material more easily.
  C.   Two **electrical characteristics** or properties important in dental materials are chemical and electrochemical.
    1.   **Corrosion** is a chemical reaction of non-metallic elements with metal, which may result in the formation of corrosive products.
      a.   An example of a corrosion product is rust that can develop on the surface of iron.
      b.   *Tarnish* is sometimes mistaken for corrosion, but it is only the surface discoloration or change in the finish of the metal.

TERMS THAT REFER TO TYPES OF DIMENSIONAL CHANGE

Percolation—the flow of liquids in and out of an area
Microleakage—microscopic openings at the point of contact or at the interface of a restoration
Shrinkage—loss of size or shape
Expansion—increase in size or shape
Syneresis—loss of fluid
Imbibition—absorption of fluid

2. Chemical corrosion involves the direct contact of the metal and the nonmetallic substance, which causes a reaction.
   a. A common example found in the mouth is silver sulfide.
   b. Certain foods, such as eggs, contain a large quantity of sulfur, which combines with other elements to corrode amalgam and other metallic restorations in the mouth.
   c. For sulfur to corrode amalgam, a chemical reaction creates silver sulfide, which attacks the amalgam surface.
3. Electrochemical corrosion is the result of an electrical current in the oral cavity.
   a. The fluids in the oral cavity must be good conductors of electricity or must be an electrolyte.
   b. Saliva, which contains salt, is an example of an electrolyte.
   c. Two metallic restorations of different composition must be present to act as batteries and carry an electrical current through the saliva.
   d. The electrical current contacting two dissimilar metals is known as galvanism or **galvanic action.**
   e. The galvanic action creates a roughness and pitting of the dental material.
   f. Galvanic action may also result in galvanic shock when a piece of aluminum foil or a fork comes in contact with a clasp of a retainer or partial denture or an existing metal restoration in the oral cavity.

MECHANICAL PROPERTIES

I. **Mechanical properties** that affect dental materials include the tensile, compressive, and shear forms of **stress** and **strain.**
   A. **Force** is an action against a material that will be exerted on the material when it is placed in the mouth.
      1. Force is measured in pounds.
      2. Biting force from the molars to the incisors decreases from approximately 130 pounds on molars to 40 pounds on the incisors.
      3. As teeth are lost and replaced by artificial ones, the force on the remaining natural teeth increases greatly.
   B. Force directed over a material creates resistance or stress within the material.

   C. Strain is another reaction to the push or pull of materials acted upon by force.
      1. Strain is seen on material when it deforms with stress.
      2. Stress and strain exist concurrently.
   D. There are three forms of stress:
      1. **Tensile stress** results when two forces are applied in opposite directions; the amount of force necessary to pull a material apart is known as *tensile strength.*
      2. **Compressive stress** is formed when materials are compressed; *Compressive strength* is the amount of pressure applied to cause a material to rupture.
      3. **Shear stress** occurs when equal or opposite forces are applied against opposite planes; the point at which a material is destroyed through the action of two portions sliding over each other is *shear strength.*
   E. The **deformation** point of a material is achieved when the material fails under stress and thus it is stated that the tensile, compressive, or shear strength of the material was inadequate.

HARDNESS, DUCTILITY, AND MALLEABILITY

I. **Hardness** tests are used to determine a material's resistance to scratching and denting.
   A. A test for hardness used in dentistry is Mohs scale, a test of scratch resistance (box).
   B. Other hardness tests include the following:
      1. Knoop hardness test (which assigns a Knoop hardness number)
      2. Brinell hardness number system
   C. When forces on a material exceed the proportional limit, or **yield point,** permanent deformation occurs, and the shape is permanently changed.

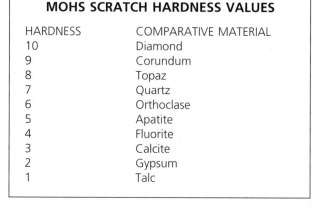

MOHS SCRATCH HARDNESS VALUES

HARDNESS	COMPARATIVE MATERIAL
10	Diamond
9	Corundum
8	Topaz
7	Quartz
6	Orthoclase
5	Apatite
4	Fluorite
3	Calcite
2	Gypsum
1	Talc

II. When reshaping or plastic deformation occurs, the material is **ductile, malleable,** or both.

III. A ductile material can undergo forces of tensile stress without failing.

IV. A material under compressive stress that does not fracture is malleable.

FLOW

I. **Flow, or slump and creep,** is a type of undesirable permanent deformation.
   A. When a force is maintained as a constant, certain materials continue to permanently deform.
   B. Compressive stress that can cause flow is created during biting.
   C. An example of flow is zinc phosphate cement mixed to a primary consistency.

SOLUBILITY AND SORPTION

I. **Solubility** is the rate at which a material dissolves in fluid.

II. **Sorption** includes *absorption,* the ability of the material to take in fluid as a solid, and *adsorption,* the concentration of molecules on the surface of a liquid or solid.
   A. The amount of both absorption and adsorption determines sorption.
   B. Certain dental materials are not selected for a purpose because of the solubility and sorption factors.
   C. An example of solubility is zinc oxide-eugenol dissolving in saliva; an example of sorption is irreversible hydrocolloid expanding when placed in water.

RETENTIVE PROPERTIES

I. An important factor in the placement of a dental material is its **retentive property** or the likelihood of the material to be retained in the tooth.
   A. This retention is also referred to as *adhesion.*
   B. Adhesion or retention may be achieved through the mechanical, physical, and/or chemical properties of the material.
      1. Physical adhesion must involve an electrostatic surface area between the tooth and the material and is not common in dentistry.
      2. A chemical adhesion is formed through a chemical bonding process whereby the material adheres to the enamel or dentin.
      3. Mechanical retention is created through three different processes: undercutting, luting, and bonding.

VISCOSITY AND WETTABILITY

I. **Viscosity** refers to the ability of a liquid material to flow.
   A. Viscosity is commonly determined by the consistency of the liquid.
      1. If a liquid is of low viscosity or flow when it is placed on a surface, it is more likely to have good wettability.
      2. A material of high viscosity tends not to flow well and is of lower wettability.
   B. Many dental cements are mixed as luting agents to cement cast restorations in a preparation.
      1. If a cement is mixed to a high viscosity, it does not adapt to the irregularities of the restoration and may not produce an acceptable seal or cementation of the cast restoration.
      2. Cements mixed to the appropriate viscosity in these cases would be mixed to film thickness, which is the viscosity appropriate for adhesion in the cementation of restorations

II. **Wettability** refers to the ability of a liquid to spread over a solid surface.

HAZARDOUS SUBSTANCES AS DENTAL MATERIALS

I. OSHA regulates activity in the workplace regarding employees' right to know about hazardous substances.
   A. The employer must provide employees with information about hazardous chemicals in the workplace.
   B. The employer must create a program that informs employees of hazardous materials that apply to the specific workplace.
   C. This program must include the following:
      1. Labeling of all materials
      2. Material safety data sheets
      3. Employee training
      4. Record maintenance

PREVENTIVE DENTAL MATERIALS

I. Preventive Materials
   A. Preventive materials are those used to prevent disease or to protect tissue.
   B. Preventive materials most commonly used in dentistry include the following:
      1. Fluoride
      2. Pit and fissure sealants
      3. Protective materials such as mouth guards, splints, and periodontal dressings

II. Fluoride
A. The element fluoride is found naturally in the environment.
B. It provides an anticarious effect when it is taken systemically during tooth formation or applied topically after eruption.
1. Fluoride changes the crystalline structure of enamel, making it less soluble.
2. Topically, it suppresses cariogenic bacteria in dental plaque and acts on the enamel to inhibit bacterial adhesion.
C. Fluoridated water consumed from birth can reduce caries formation by 50% to 65%.
D. Excess fluoride can cause mottled enamel.
E. Forms of fluoride include the following:
1. Oral rinses and dentrifices
2. Systemic form
3. Topical form
F. Forms of systemic fluoride include the following:
1. Water supply
2. Chewable or liquid drop supplements (if needed, should be given from birth to age 12 or 13)
G. Forms of topical fluoride include the following:
1. Acidulated phosphate fluoride (APF)
a. APF is available in a 1.23% gel in 1- or 4-minute formulas.
b. A four-minute single professional application twice a year provides adequate protection.
c. APF is a stable solution with a long shelf life.
d. Contraindications: APF is an irritant to inflamed tissues; on esthetic restorations, etching can occur.
2. Stannous fluoride
a. Stannous fluoride is an unstable solution; it must be mixed fresh for each patient.
b. From 8% to 10% liquid mixture every 6 months provides caries protection.
c. Contraindications: Stannous fluoride possesses a metallic flavor and cannot be flavored; it causes brown staining of decalcified teeth and esthetic restorations.
3. Sodium fluoride
a. Sodium fluoride requires four 3-minute applications scheduled 2 to 7 days apart.
b. It is scheduled for children at ages 3, 7, 10, and 13.
c. A single dose of sodium fluoride may be recommended at 6-month intervals for additional caries reduction.
d. It is compatible with tooth tissues and does not discolor.

III. Pit and Fissure Sealants
A. Pit and fissure sealants are a clear or shaded resin material placed on the pits and fissures of premolars and molars.
1. Material used as sealants offers a barrier between these vulnerable tooth surfaces and bacterial plaque.
2. For optimal protection the material should be placed soon after the tooth erupts.
3. When properly applied, sealants provide excellent caries protection.
B. Pit and fissure sealant materials are available in several forms, including self-cured and light-cured, tinted, or opaque and clear.
C. Avoid the use of pit and fissure sealants on teeth that exhibit the following characteristics:
1. Hypoplastic enamel
2. Amalgam restorations
3. Gold inlays or foils
4. Deep carious lesions
5. Synthetic porcelain restorations
D. Ideal teeth for successful sealant placement are the occlusal surfaces of premolars and molars.
1. Studies have shown that the retention rate (the duration that the sealant maintains margin integrity) on premolars is higher than on molars.
2. As treatment progresses toward the posterior in the oral cavity, the retention rate tends to lessen because of difficult access in placement.
3. Retention rate in mandibular teeth appears to be higher than in maxillary teeth, again attributed to access.
E. The rationale for sealant placement is as follows:
1. Sealants reduce the risk of dental decay on primary and permanent teeth.
2. Sealants have been shown to contain no toxic or carcinogenic agents that could have an adverse effect on the body.
3. The cost of placing sealants compared with the cost of placing a restoration that may have a life of 15 to 20 years is much less.
4. Though sealants have shorter life than a restoration does, the amount of tooth structure removed during the pit and fissure pro-

cedure is microscopic compared with the placement of a restoration.

5. If a sealant is lost or is defective, unlike a restoration, there appears to be no increase in caries incidence of these surfaces over teeth in which no sealants have been placed.

6. In certain circumstances, studies have shown that where decay is minimal on the occlusal surface, placement of pit and fissure sealants has arrested the dental decay.

F. Sealants are thin layers of resin material placed on the pits and fissures of the occlusal surfaces of posterior teeth.

1. The sealant creates a mechanical obstacle to any bacteria that attack the pits and fissures and try to break down the enamel, eventually resulting in a carious lesion.

2. Most sealants are composed of bisphenol A-glycidyl methacrylate (BIS-GMA), polymerized with a visible light source or via an organic amine, autocuring catalyst.

3. The advantage of a BIS-GMA photopolymerizing sealant system is that materials need no mixing.

4. The resin is polymerized with visible light.

5. BIS-GMA sealants that are polymerized by an organic amine accelerator are found in two-step systems, which require the mixing of a monomer and benzoyl peroxide initiator with a monomer and 5% organic amine accelerator.

6. The working time is much more limited when using a base/catalyst system.

IV. Mouth Guards

A. Mouth guards are designed to protect the teeth and other oral structures from injuries that result from contact sports.

B. Mouth guards are supplied in the following forms:

1. Preformed that are adapted to the mouth

2. Custom-made

C. Functions of a mouth guard are listed (box).

V. Other Preventive Devices

A. Occlusal bite splint

1. This is a device fabricated to aid in the treatment of patients with temporomandibular joint dysfunction or syndrome.

2. It is designed to open the patient's bite and to reduce attrition of the teeth.

3. Made of acrylic resin, it covers the occlusal surfaces and may or may not cover the incisal edges.

B. Periodontal dressing

1. This is placed over periodontal surgery sites to protect the tissue from trauma.

2. It may be made of zinc oxide and eugenol, noneugenol materials, and light-cured synthetic materials.

RESTORATIVE MATERIALS

I. Restorative Dental Materials

A. The process includes the following steps:

1. Remove diseased tissue.

2. Produce an esthetically pleasing condition.

3. Restore function to the oral cavity.

B. Restorative dental materials may be used in either **direct** or **indirect** restorative procedures.

1. A direct restorative material protects tissue, stimulates growth of tissue, or replaces missing structures directly in the mouth. For example, a medication is placed under a metallic restoration to protect the tooth from thermal reaction or to stimulate reparative growth in the tooth.

2. An indirect restorative material is manipulated outside of the mouth to aid in the production of a final restoration or appliance. For example, an impression material creates a negative of oral structures that can then be used to produce a model or positive reproduction of the structures. From this model, wax, gypsum, and gold can be used to create a restoration that is fabricated outside the mouth and then inserted in the oral cavity.

II. Factors That Affect Manipulation of Dental Materials

A. Manipulating time

1. This is the amount of time recommended

FUNCTIONS OF A MOUTH GUARD

1. Prevents tooth injury by absorbing and deflecting blows to the teeth
2. Prevents jaw fractures by creating a cushion between the teeth during the impact of a blow
3. Shields the lips, tongue, and gingival tissues from laceration
4. Reduces potential temporomandibular joint disorders by cushioning the lower jaw
5. Prevents potential concussions by absorbing the shock of a blow to the mandible

by the manufacturer to completely mix the material.

2. Excess manipulation time could reduce the amount of time needed to properly place the material, resulting in a less-than-desirable restoration, cement base, or impression.

B. Setting time
1. This is the amount of time it takes a material to harden.
2. Two time periods are involved in the setting of dental materials:
   a. *Initial setting time,* when the material has reached the point at which further manipulation is not possible or is difficult without distortion of the material.
   b. *Final setting time,* when the material has reached its complete hardness.
3. To increase a setting time means to lengthen or extend the amount of time it takes for the material to set.
4. To decrease the setting time means to lessen or shorten the amount of time required for the material to set.
5. Agents that increase or decrease setting time are called *retarders* and *accelerators,* respectively.

C. Moisture
1. The presence of moisture from the material being manipulated or from an external source may decrease the setting time of the material.
2. Moisture can come from high humidity in the atmosphere or from instruments and mixing surfaces not well dried.
3. **Syneresis** is the loss of water in a dental material, such as alginate or agar products that causes shrinkage in the material.
4. **Imbibition** occurs when the material is immersed in water and the absorption of water expands the material.
5. Both imbibition and syneresis cause distortion.

D. Temperature
1. Temperature also affects the setting time of certain materials.
2. An increase in temperature decreases the setting time of material and the time for manipulation and placement of the material before setting occurs.
3. Temperature can also affect the consistency of dental materials, such as waxes.

E. Consistency
1. Dental cements are prepared to different consistencies.
2. Cement of a **primary** or **luting consistency** is less viscous and flows easily.
   a. Primary consistency is used to cement or lute crowns, bridges, inlays, and orthodontic bands in place.
   b. Primary consistency results in the material being drawn into a 1-inch string when the cement spatula is laid in the mass of material and is lifted from the cement.
   c. Primary consistency has greater wettability and can flow to provide a thin film thickness.
3. Cement of a **secondary consistency** is more viscous; it is thicker or tackier and may even be rolled into a mass or rope.
   a. For a secondary consistency, extra powder is added to the mix.
   b. It is used as an insulating base under a restoration.
4. A secondary consistency or base consistency can withstand greater stress than one of primary consistency.
5. Other dental materials, such as impression materials, are mixed to different consistencies.
   a. **Light-body** material is thinner and is placed in and extruded from a syringe on a prepared tooth surface to reproduce minute details in the preparation.
   b. Light body impression material can be mixed as a wash impression.
   c. **Heavy-body** material is more viscous and is placed in a tray to be held in place.
   d. It does not provide the fine detail of oral structures but does achieve an accurate registration.
   e. A putty consistency, similar to the heavy body, is available and is thicker.

III. Armamentarium
A. Spatulas
1. Two types of spatulas are commonly used for mixing dental cements: a broad, nonflexible spatula to mix most zinc oxide-eugenol cements and a thin, flexible spatula to mix zinc phosphate and other cements.
2. A flexible plastic spatula supplied by the manufacturer is used for resin materials.
3. Larger spatulas are used to mix the catalyst

and base for impression materials; a thinner, more flexible spatula is used for mixing alginate materials.

B. Measuring devices: most manufacturers provide a scoop or similar device for measuring the powder liquid or paste to each dental material.

C. Mixing surfaces on which to manipulate materials
1. Mixing surfaces for most impression materials and cements may include a glass slab or paper pads made of treated, waxed, or plain material.
2. For mixing alginate impression and gypsum materials a flexible rubber bowl is commonly used.

IV. Dispensing Techniques
A. Suggestions for dispensing basic dental materials
1. Always fluff powder to avoid any settling of the chemical components.
2. Swirl liquid for homogeneity
3. Recap the powder and liquid after dispensing to avoid moisture contamination of each.
4. When dispensing liquid from an eyedropper or bottle, hold each in a vertical position to ensure that the correct proportion of liquid is dispensed.
5. Do not return unused liquid or powder to the bottle.

V. Cleaning Agents
A. Special substances designed for use with some dental materials include:
1. Bicarbonate of soda is recommended for cleaning materials that have debris from zinc phosphate cement.
2. Orange oil solution is recommended for zinc oxide-eugenol cements.
3. A solution of 10% sodium hydroxide assists in the removal of polycarboxylate cements.
4. All debris must be removed from working surfaces to avoid contamination of future mixes.

VI. Direct Restorative Materials
A. Direct materials are placed directly into the mouth to restore it to its natural anatomy.
B. Direct restorative dental materials are used to replace tooth structures lost to carious lesions or trauma, as sedative treatment, and for cosmetic procedures.
C. Common direct restorative dental materials include cements, amalgam, gold, and esthetic restorative materials.

D. Dental cements are used for several reasons and in several specialties of dentistry.
1. Luting agents for cementation of crowns, bridges, inlays, and orthodontics bands or brackets
2. Temporary luting agent for temporary restorations, or as a temporary itself
3. Thermal insulating bases or liners
4. Pulp capping
5. Pulp protection
6. Root canal therapy
7. Surgical tissue dressings

E. Dental cements function to protect the pulp in the following ways:
1. They reduce or eliminate the trauma of thermal conductivity by acting as a buffer between the pulp and a metallic restoration when electrical conductivity occurs.
2. They cover dentinal and enamel openings that are exposed during cavity preparation.

VII. Cavity liners and varnishes provide no thermal insulation but are often necessary to create a protective barrier between dentin and the restorative material (boxes below and pages 169-171).

CAVITY VARNISH
USE
Seal surfaces, particularly dentin tubules
COMPOSITION AND PROPERTIES
Solutions of resin in organic liquids Provides protection from chemical and electrical stimulation
FACTORS TO BE CONSIDERED
• It dries quickly (5 to 30 seconds) or may be light cured. • If left uncovered, liquid will evaporate. • Placing a small amount of varnish solvent reduces viscosity and lightens the varnish's color. • It is not compatible with monomers of resin or composite restorations. • Use it under a therapeutic base.
MANIPULATION
1. Place cotton pledget into cotton pliers. 2. Grip the pledget in the liquid and lightly dab it on a gauze sponge. 3. Apply soaked pledget to the cavity preparation, covering all cut surfaces. 4. If a second application is needed, use a second pledget and new cotton pliers.

CAVITY LINERS

Two types: zinc oxide-eugenol and calcium hydroxide—not used under composite resin
Available in two-paste or light-cured packaging systems.

MANIPULATION

1. Dispense approximately 1 to 2 mm of each catalyst and base.
2. Mix until homogeneous.
3. Apply with a clean instrument and allow to dry.
4. Place liner and clean instrument of debris.
5. If light cured, apply light to achieve set of the material.

ZINC OXIDE-EUGENOL CEMENTS

USE

Cementation of fixed prosthodontics
Sedative bases
Temporary restorations
Tissue packs
Root canal sealers

COMPOSITION AND PROPERTIES

Zinc oxide, rosin to reduce brittleness, zinc stearate to be a plasticizer, and zinc acetate for strength
Liquid consists of eugenol and olive oil as a plasticizer.
To increase strength, methyl methacrylate polymer or alumina is added to the powder and ethoxybenzoic acid to the liquid (improved or fortified zinc oxide-eugenol).
Many zinc oxide-eugenol cements are manufactured as two-paste systems.

FACTORS TO BE CONSIDERED

- Sedative or anodyne effects for tissues of the teeth

MANIPULATION

Follow manufacturer's directions for specific incorporation of increments, time, and final result, depending on desired use.
1. Swirl liquid and fluff powder.
2. Dispense the amounts of each according to the manufacturer's directions.
3. Incorporate powder and liquid in increments, or mix in mass together using a folding and packing motion.
4. To wet all the powder particles, maintain an exacting pressure on the spatula tip.
5. Mix powder and liquid to a homogeneous mass, whether for primary or secondary consistency.
6. With certain zinc oxide-eugenol cements, strop to achieve consistency.

ZINC PHOSPHATE CEMENTS

USE

For cementation of crowns, bridges, inlays, orthodontic bands and brackets
As insulating base
As temporary restorative material

COMPOSITION AND PROPERTIES

These cements are a combination of zinc oxide powder with magnesium oxide and pigments.
Liquid consists of phosphoric acid in water buffered with aluminum and zinc ions to delay setting reaction.
They can be prepared to primary or secondary consistency, depending on use.
As powder and liquid are incorporated, an exothermic (heat-producing) reaction occurs, created by the alkaline powder dissolving in the acidic liquid.

FACTORS TO BE CONSIDERED

- Extremely acidic and may irritate the pulp, a liner may have to be placed under it.
- Viscosity affected by time and temperature. For best results, follow these steps:
  1. Mix on cool glass slab.
  2. Incorporate optimum amounts of powder to achieve desired viscosity.
  3. During cementation of orthodontic bands, use frozen slab method.
- Setting time is also affected by use of higher powder-liquid ratio.

MANIPULATION OF CEMENT

Primary-consistency cement

1. Mix on a cool glass slab.
2. Swirl liquid and fluff powder.
3. Dispense powder and liquid in separate areas of slab.
4. Divide the powder into four to six increments.
5. Incorporate each increment of powder into the liquid using a rotating spatulation method over a broad area of the slab until luting consistency is achieved.

Secondary-consistency cement

1. Dispense a greater amount of powder at the beginning.
2. Follow the steps for primary consistency; place 1/5 of the mix in the corner of the slab.
3. Continue to incorporate the powder into the liquid mass using a folding and packing motion until you achieve a homogeneous mass that can be rolled.
4. If desired, cut the rope into small increments for placement.
5. Place cement with appropriate instrument.

POLYCARBOXYLATE CEMENT

USE

Luting agent for cementation of fixed prosthodontics
Insulating base

COMPOSITION AND PROPERTIES

Combination of zinc oxide powder and aqueous polyacrylic acid solution (used in place of phosphoric acid to reduce the acidity of the cement and the potential for pulpal irritation)

FACTORS TO BE CONSIDERED

- Usually mixed as quickly as possible
- May be mixed on a cooled glass surface to slow the chemical reaction
- Extremely adhesive to surfaces it contacts, so use of a paper pad may be preferred
- Typical working time 30 to 60 seconds; initial set reached in 3 minutes

MANIPULATION

Can be mixed to a luting or base consistency; the difference normally is obtained by increasing the amount of powder incorporated into the liquid.
1. Fluff powder; swirling liquid is difficult because of extreme viscosity.
2. Dispense appropriate powder and liquid ratio for consistency of cement needed.
3. Incorporate all the powder into the liquid using a folding and packing motion until all the powder is wetted.
4. Use broad stropping motion to develop primary consistency or more folding and packing for secondary consistency.
5. A cement mixed to primary consistency is shiny; as it becomes dull, dry, and stringy, its ability to flow is diminished, so it should not be used.

RESIN CEMENTS

USE

Primarily luting agents for cast porcelain restorations
Bonding agents with enamel
Cementation of orthodontic brackets

COMPOSITION AND PROPERTIES

BIS-GMA or BIS-GMA-like monomers without reinforced fillers
Low viscosity

FACTORS TO BE CONSIDERED

- Low viscosity of mix in early stages appears in some circumstances.
- It is recommended primarily for luting cast porcelain restorations.

MANIPULATION

The two components of this cement are in liquid form and are manipulated as follows:
1. Dispense equal drops from both bottles of liquid.
2. Mix the two liquids together completely; then either paint the cement on with a brush or place it in an application syringe and apply it via the syringe tip.

GLASS IONOMER CEMENT

USE

Supplied as types I and II
Type I: cementation of fixed prosthodontics, occasionally pit and fissure sealant
Type II: insulating bases, core buildup, and class III and V restorations

COMPOSITION AND PROPERTIES

This cement is a recent hybrid that combines the better qualities of other cements.
Glass ionomers are aluminosilicate-polyacrylate.
Powder is a silicate porcelain.
Viscous liquid is an aqueous solution of polyacrylic acid.
Cement releases fluoride ions.
Glass ionomer cements are not as strong as zinc phosphate cements, and, if contaminated by water early in the setting process, may fail.

FACTORS TO BE CONSIDERED

- Glass ionomer cements are bonded in place to aid in retention.
- Many manufacturers supply products in preproportioned capsules to reduce the possibility of moisture contamination.
- Because of moisture sensitivity, the cement must be mixed quickly.

MANIPULATION

If the glass ionomer cement is to be bonded, prepare tooth surfaces using an acid-etching technique. The acid etching is completed just before manipulation of the cement.
1. Dispense the manufacturer's directed proportions of powder and liquid on a paper pad.
2. Divide the powder into halves or thirds and incorporate each increment into the liquid until it is uniform.
3. Include increments within 40 seconds, giving a homogeneous mix of cement.
4. The cement appears shiny for the ideal luting consistency; when the gloss is lost, the consistency becomes heavier.
5. If the cement is in a precapsulated form, use a capsule activator to enmesh the liquid and powder in the capsule.
6. Place the capsule in an amalgamator to triturate the liquid and powder to reach proper consistency.
7. Place cement in a Teflon syringe or capsule applicator and apply it using either device, or remove it from the capsule and place it using a plastic instrument.

VIII. Dental **amalgam** is an alloy with mercury as one of the metals combined with a mixture of silver, tin, copper, and zinc. It is the most common restorative material placed in the oral cavity (box on page 172).

MERCURY HYGIENE

I. Contamination
   A. Mercury contamination may result from the following:
      1. Exposure to mercury through the skin
      2. Inhalation of mercury vapor
      3. Inhalation of airborne particles
   B. To avoid the possibility of mercury contamination, the ADA recommends specific guidelines (box on page 173).
II. Toxicity

A. Mercury level is measured by the amount and duration an individual is exposed to mercury vapors.
   1. The recommended safe mercury vapor level found in the air is 0.05 mg for a 40-hour week.
   2. An increase in this level could result in excess levels in the body.
   3. Early indications of excessive mercury exposure include tremors and decreased levels of nerve conduction, brain-wave activity, and verbal skills.
   4. Increased levels of toxicity could result in any of the following:
      a. Kidney dysfunction
      b. Irritability
      c. Depression

DENTAL AMALGAM

USE

Restore teeth to gain function and to relieve discomfort
Used most commonly in Class I, II, III restorations on molars and premolars
Used to restore the distal surfaces of cuspids, Class V, and modified Class VI preparations of teeth

FACTORS TO BE CONSIDERED

- A combination of alloy and mercury, which is a toxic element; therefore, great care must be taken in handling
- All OSHA and ADA recommendations followed to eliminate mercury contamination.
  NOTE: Since preproportioned amalgam capsules, with alloy and mercury in one capsule and separated by a thin diaphragm of plastic are recommended for use, only this type will be discussed in the manipulation step. Reusable capsules with removable metal pestles are still available, as are mercury dispensers or proportioners that allow for dispensing of a drop of mercury with a tablet of alloy.
- Amalgam mixed to different amounts, depending on what is needed to complete a restoration; a single spill or mix of 600 mg of alloy is used with smaller preparations and often during restoration of a primary tooth; a double spill of 800 mg of alloy is used in larger preparations
- With a mechanical amalgamator, alloy and mercury are triturated, mixed, for a specific time; amount of amalgam to be mixed and type of amalgamator are important factors
- Specific time and speed allotments are assigned for each type of alloy capsule with a particular amalgamator

ARMAMENTARIUM

Preproportioned amalgam capsule
Capsule activator
Mechanical amalgamator
Dappen dish or amalgam well
Amalgam carrier
Gun or syringe
Condenser

MANIPULATION

Place overgloves over examination gloves if they are contaminated to avoid contamination of the rest of the amalgam armamentarium.
1. Select a preporportioned capsule that is correct for the size of the preparation.
2. Activate the capsule by pressing hard on one end of the capsule on a hard surface or by using a capsule activator device.
3. Set the mechanical amalgamator for the correct time and speed for use with the particular capsule.
4. Place the capsule securely in the armature of the amalgamator to ensure that it will not be thrown from the unit.
5. Close the lid over the armature and capsule to ensure that no airborne particles will be propelled if the capsule is defective.
6. Set the timer for the correct time for the amalgam spill size.
7. Press the activation button on the amalgamator to start the trituration.
8. If the amalgamator is enclosed in a mobile cart, close the door to reduce noise next to the patient's head and to further reduce the possibility of airborne mercury particles.
9. Incorrect trituration times result in undermixed or overmixed masses of amalgam.
10. Remove the capsule from the amalgamator and, if suggested by the manufacturer, rap the end of the capsule on a hard surface to loosen the mass from the interior of the capsule.
11. Remove the overgloves.
12. Open the capsule and place the amalgamated mass in a dappen dish or an amalgam well.
13. Load the amalgam carrier, gun, or syringe with amalgam, and pass the instrument to the operator for placement in the preparation.
14. Exchange the carrier for a condenser of choice to condense or adapt the amalgam to the prepared surfaces of the tooth.
15. The goals of condensation are to apply equal pressure throughout the mass of material in the preparation to eliminate voids, compact the mass uniformly, and reduce excess mercury.
16. If the amalgam is of a type that can be polished at the placement appointment, then this may follow.

CLEANING DIRECTIONS

Removed easily from working surfaces of instruments while it is soft and pliable.

Once material has hardened, particularly in amalgam carrier, gun, or syringe, removal is difficult.

Regardless of the form of carrier that is used to transport the amalgam to the tooth, always check that all the amalgam is removed after the last increment is palced. If not, the instrument may be useless or need special attention to succeed in removing the hardened amalgam.

Place unused amalgam, silver alloy and mercury in manufacturer's scrap amalgam container or a container with fixer solution. Never place the unused amalgam in the trash, and never dispose of amalgam or mercury in any way other than through a licensed toxic waste contractor.

MERCURY HYGIENE RECOMMENDATIONS

1. Follow recommended safety procedures for cleaning spilled mercury or mercury-contaminated surfaces.
2. Make sure that treatment rooms and the entire office have proper ventilation.
3. Store amalgam scrap in sealed containers, and cover them with the appropriate solutions.
4. Avoid heating mercury or amalgam.
5. Avoid direct contact with mercury; do not handle it.
6. Dispose of mercury-contaminated items properly.
7. Use a precapsulated alloy to minimize the possibility of spilled mercury.
8. Use water spray and high-volume evacuation when removing amalgam to minimize vapors.
9. Enclose the capsule and amalgamator arms in a cover during trituration.
10. Monitor the office for atmospheric mercury on a yearly basis.
11. Monitor office personnel for mercury exposure on a yearly basis.

Table 10-1 Composition of amalgam alloys

Type of alloy	Component	Characteristic	Percent in alloy
Low copper	Silver	Luster, strength, durability, expansion	65 to 72
	Tin	Reduced expansion, strength, hardness; increased flow and workability	26 to 29
	Copper	High strength, low corrosion	2 to 7
High copper	Silver	Luster, strength, durability, expansion	40 to 70
	Tin	Reduced expansion, strength, hardness; increased flow and workability	0 to 30
	Copper	High strength, low corrosion	2 to 30

d. Memory loss
e. Minor tremors
f. Various nervous system disorders
g. Swollen gingiva
h. Pronounced tremors

COMPONENTS OF ALLOYS

I. The composition of alloys used for dental amalgam is regulated by ADA specifications.
A. Regulations state that the alloy is a combination of silver, tin, copper, zinc, gold, and mercury, with the last four in lesser amounts than the silver and tin.
B. The actual percentages of each metal vary.
C. Permission for use of other metals must be requested through the Council on Dental Materials and Devices.
D. The type and quantity of each component of an alloy provide specific characteristics that are desired in an amalgam restoration (Table 10-1).
E. Alloys are classified as *low-copper* or *high-copper alloys.*
   1. Low-copper alloys
      a. These are used less frequently than high-copper alloys.
      b. They are supplied as spherical or comminuted, with either pulverized or lathe-cut particles.

c. They are found in combination with silver-tin alloys, which, when combined with mercury, react to form a weak tin-mercury phase (a recognized area in the mass that is inferior to the rest).
   2. High-copper alloy
      a. The most commonly used high-copper alloys are spherical, comminuted, or admixed; they are sometimes referred to as combination particles.
      b. Comminuted high-copper alloys are supplied in various sizes, including fine cut and microcut.
      c. High-copper alloys do not have a tin-mercury phase as do the low-copper alloys but form a copper-tin phase that provides the alloy with superior properties.
II. Amalgamation is the reaction created by the introduction of mercury to the silver alloy.
A. This reaction causes a hardening of the amalgam through solution and crystallization.
   1. Mercury, a fluid, contacts the alloy and wets the particles of powder.
   2. Absorption of the mercury by the particles creates one of the following phases:
      a. Silver-tin (gamma phase)
      b. silver-mercury (gamma-1 phase)
      c. tin-mercury (gamma-2 phase)
   3. The silver-tin alloy is considered a gamma phase when the particles have not yet reacted with the mercury.

B. Amalgam displays many clinical properties.
  1. Amalgam undergoes dimensional change, specifically contraction and expansion, controlled by the techniques used during manipulation. Excess or incorrect trituration results in unwanted dimensional change.
     a. Contraction or expansion beyond the American National Standards Institute (ANSI)-ADA specifications may result in an amalgam restoration that pulls away from the margins of a cavity preparation, causing leakage to occur, or the amalgam may create sensitivity in a tooth.
     b. If expansion occurs, the amalgam may extend beyond the margins of the preparation.
  2. *Creep,* the change that takes place when the material is subjected to a constant load, may occur during normal mastication.
  3. The presence of voids due to inadequate condensation decreases the strength potential of the restoration.
C. Glass ionomers with silver alloys are used in restorative dentistry.
  1. Silver alloy combined with glass ionomer restorative material is often used in core buildups.
     a. A *core* is the buildup of tooth structure lost to carious activity or trauma to approximate the original tooth shape.
     b. The core is often covered by a cast restoration to maintain the integrity of the remaining tooth.

DIRECT ESTHETIC MATERIALS ▬▬▬▬

I. Plastic
  A. Plastic materials, such as composite, provide several benefits including the following:
    1. Esthetically pleasing
    2. Placed in a single appointment
    3. Less treatment time required than laminates or full-coverage restorations, which require multiple treatment appointments
II. Composite Materials
  A. Development of the smaller particle (microfilled) resins has increased the compressive strength of the material.
  B. Thermal conductivity of these materials is lower because of the organic matrix that provides a thermal insulator.
  C. More fillers in composite restorative materials increases hardness of the material, wear resistance, and abrasion.
  D. Polymerization shrinkage occurs because of the high density of polymer formed around the oligomer.
  E. Radiopacity exists in composites that contain elements such as barium, bromine, iodine, sirconium, strontium, zinc, and zirconium.
  F. Composites with other fillers will not attenuate radiation; thus not all composites appear radiopaque on dental radiographs.
  G. Composite with more organic matrix in the overall content exhibits a greater coefficient of thermal expansion.
III. Polymer Dimethacrylates
  A. Polymer dimethacrylates are composite or filled resin materials.
  B. The fillers are inorganic materials such as quartz, borosilicate glass, lithium aluminum silicate, barium aluminum silicate or barium fluoride, strontium, or zinc glasses.
  C. Each of these fillers is available in varying sizes: fine, irregularly shaped particles, microfine particles, and blends of the fine and microfine particle sizes.
  D. The filler material bonds with the matrix of an organic base, an oligomer, dimethacrylate or BIS-GMA, or urethane dimethacrylate, making viscous liquids.
  E. Various amounts and colors of inorganic pigments are added to provide diverse shade choice. Pigments range in shades and intensity from yellow to gray to white, opaque and translucent, to cover the spectrum of tooth colorings.
IV. Glass Ionomer Restorative Materials
  A. The use of ionomers has become more accepted and widespread as application has become more diverse.
  B. Ionomers are commonly used to restore, in particular, cervically eroded surfaces on teeth.
  C. Ionomers are manufactured as a selection of shades of powder with a liquid.
    1. The powder consists of an aluminosilicate glass combined with a liquid composed of water, polymers, and copolymers of acrylic acid.
    2. In certain products, silver particles and fluoride ions are added to this material.
  D. Glass ionomers have the following properties:
    1. They bond to enamel and dentin.
    2. They release fluoride ions into surrounding tooth structure.
    3. They are biologically compatible.
    4. They are radiopaque.

5. Surfaces can be etched so that composites can be mechanically bonded to them.
6. The retention of ionomers in cervical areas is greater than that of composites.
7. Their thermal coefficient of expansion is similar to that of dentin.

E. Glass ionomers require specific manipulation.
1. Adequate isolation techniques are important to protect the material from saliva contamination.
2. Manufacturers suggest delaying final finishing and polishing for 1 day to achieve the ideal restoration.

PACKAGING SYSTEMS

I. Two packaging systems are available: the *two-paste autopolymerizing* and the *single-paste, light-cure system.*

A. The two-paste system is contained in two jars, each of which includes 50% BIS-GMA and inorganic filler (box). One jar contains the catalyst, a benzoyl peroxide initiator, and the other contains an organic amine accelerator.

B. The single-paste system is photopolymerizing or photocuring.
1. It is packaged so that all the elements of

TWO-PASTE COMPOSITE
USE
Aesthetic restoration for class I, III, IV, and certain class V cavity preparations
FACTORS TO BE CONSIDERED
• The paste in the two jars should be stirred before use, because settling of the material may occur. • When using disposable mixing sticks, take care to use the opposite ends in each jar so as not to introduce the materials together, which may result in a chemical reaction. • Avoid contact of metal instruments with composite material because they may discolor the material.
ARMAMENTARIUM
Two-paste system kit with material, disposable mixing stick, and plastic pad (if a paper pad is used, take care to avoid contamination of the pad) NOTE: Acid etching and bonding material may be used in this or in the one-paste system. Placement instrument (e.g., Teflon plastic instrument or composite syringe with tip and plunger)
MANIPULATION
1. Perform shade selection. 2. Open jar containing the initiator, stir with the mixing stick, and dispense approximately one half of the size of the restoration. 3. Open the other jar, mix the material with the opposite end of the mixing stick, and dispense the same amount of material on the pad. 4. If the universal shade needs to be adjusted for the patient, combine the tinted material with the universal shade before it is mixed with the initiator. 5. Mix both materials for approximately 20 to 30 seconds until the mix is homogeneous and the colors of the material are consistent. 6. The working time of the material is approximately 1 to 1 ½ minutes for mixing and insertion into the cavity preparation. 7. Place the material by hand either with an insertion instrument or with a composite syringe, which reduces the incidence of voids during insertion. 8. Dispense a small amount of the material to be held between your fingers to simulate the heat generated in the oral cavity. This provides the operator with a guide to indicate when the material has reached a final set. 9. The material is set in approximately 5 minutes from initial mix. At this time complete the finishing and polishing steps.
CLEANING DIRECTIONS
Easily remove the material from the instruments before reaching a final set by using 2 × 2 gauze.

the material are combined in a single dispensing device.
2. Syringe compules have colored tips that correspond to the color of the material.
3. Material in the syringes is identified on an outside label.

PLASTICS IN PROSTHETICS ▬▬▬▬

I. Acrylic and Rubber-Reinforced Acrylic
   A. Acrylics are commonly used in dentistry because of the diverse properties possible, from soft and flexible to harder and more brittle.
   B. Acrylics are used to fabricate a variety of prosthetic devices including the following:
      1. Denture bases and teeth
      2. Temporary crowns and bridges
      3. Custom acrylic impression trays
      4. Orthodontics appliances
   C. Plastic used for the construction of denture bases is heat cured.
      1. Placed under pressure with heat to initiate polymerization.
   D. Material used for the other applications is self-cured plastic.
      1. Self-cured, cold-cured, or chemically cured plastic begins to polymerize when the monomer and polymer are combined; as polymerization occurs, heat is released in an **exothermic reaction.**

II. Vinyl Plastics
   A. Vinyl plastic is used in the construction of protective mouth guards and is composed of copolymers of vinyl acetate and ethylene.
   B. Other applications include use as fluoride trays and other flexible appliances.

III. Denture-Base Acrylic Plastics
   A. Most denture-base acrylic plastics are heat accelerated; a few are chemically accelerated materials.
   B. These plastics are usually found in powder and liquid form, but they also are produced in gels, sheets, and blanks.
   C. The powder of this plastic comprises predominantly polymer with peroxide that assists in the polymerization; these are combined with other components that provide translucency and color to allow for a plastic that resembles the patient's natural tissue color for the denture base.
   D. Most of the liquid is monomer with hydroquinone, an inhibitor that retards any polymerization activity of the liquid during storage. Polymerization can occur from exposure to ul-

traviolet light, so the liquid must be packaged in light-resistant containers.

IV. Soft Liners
   A. Soft liners are used to aid the patient with residual alveolar ridge changes that cause ill-fitting dentures, resulting in discomfort and irritation to the tissue under the denture.
   B. Other uses include tissue treatment after surgery and obturators for defects in the palate.
   C. Soft liners are either acrylic copolymers with plasticizers or copolymers.

V. Denture Teeth
   A. Denture teeth may be made of plastic or porcelain; each material has advantages and disadvantages.
      1. Plastic teeth are more resistant to breakage, create less noise during occlusion, and are easily brought to a comfortable finish after the grinding and polishing needed for adjustment takes place.
      2. Plastic teeth are softer and more susceptible to abrasion.
      3. Porcelain teeth are less able to accommodate the stress involved during occlusion.
   B. Plastic teeth are most often used where denture teeth oppose natural teeth, for patients with less than adequate ridge mass, and in areas where only low stress forces are applied.
   C. Porcelain teeth are usually preferred in areas where less stress is placed. This type of denture tooth is not usually placed to oppose natural tooth structure.

VI. Temporary Crowns, Bridges, and Inlays/Onlays
   A. Acrylics are a common form of plastic used in the fabrication of temporary crowns, bridges, and inlays.
   B. Acrylic consists of a liquid and powder that are mixed into a homogeneous creamy mass that becomes rubbery in a few minutes.
   C. Acceleration of the polymerization can be accomplished by placing the material in warm water.

VII. Impression-Tray Plastic
   A. Acrylic with filler is necessary to fabricate rigid custom impression trays.
   B. Acrylic is manipulated in a manner similar to that of the acrylic used in temporary restorations.

INDIRECT RESTORATIVE DENTAL MATERIALS ▬

I. Indirect and adjunct restorative dental materials are used to fabricate a restoration or prosthesis outside the oral cavity.

A. This restoration or prosthesis is placed in the patient's mouth at a subsequent appointment.

B. The following materials are used:
1. Impression materials
2. Waxes
3. Gold
4. Model and die materials
5. Porcelain

II. Impression materials are used to reproduce, record, or register the relationship of the teeth and the oral conditions.

A. Impression material is usually placed in an impression tray and then into the mouth while in its plastic stage; after setting to a rubbery stage, the tray, with the material still in place, is removed from the mouth, providing a negative reproduction of the structure.

B. Impressions are poured with a gypsum product in fluid form and allowed to harden to a set cast or model.

C. Impression material is removed from the gypsum cast to expose a positive reproduction of the condition of the mouth.

D. From this cast, orthodontic appliances, complete and partial dentures, cast restorations, temporary restorations, and temporary appliances are fabricated.

III. Impression materials have several characteristics (box).

IV. Impression materials are available in two forms: rigid and elastic.

A. Rigid materials provide an accurate registration of oral anatomy but fracture easily under stress or in the presence of undercuts.
1. Rigid materials are supplied in the following forms:
    a. *Impression compound,* stick or cake
        (1) Compound is composed of 40% res-

ins, 7% waxes, 3% organic acids, 50% fillers, and various coloring pigments.
(2) Compound is thermoplastic; that is, it softens when heat is applied and rehardens as it cools.
(3) Compound flows at mouth temperature, which is approximately 37° C, but a temperature of 45° C is needed to obtain the flow that adequately records the tissues of the mouth.
(4) Compound is a poor thermal conductor that requires kneading during heating or cooling and adequate time to ensure that a uniform temperature is maintained throughout the material.

b. *Impression plaster*
(1) Impression plaster is extremely rigid and fractures easily; it cannot be used where undercuts exist.
(2) It is used primarily to mount dental casts on articulators because it sets quickly (3 to 5 minutes).

c. *Zinc oxide-eugenol* impression material
(1) This material is packaged as a two-paste system.
(2) It is used as a wash impression or bite registration.

B. Elastic impression materials provide accurate registration and register undercut areas without fracture. They are supplied in the following forms:
1. Alginate, irreversible hydrocolloid
2. Agar hydrocolloid, reversible hydrocolloid
3. Agar-alginate combination
4. Rubber, polysulfides, silicones, polysiloxanes, polyethers

C. Alginate impression materials are used for the following purposes:
1. Preliminary impression for diagnostic models
2. Fabrication of mouth guards
3. Construction of temporary restorations
4. Fabrication of orthodontic appliances
5. Fabrication of custom impression trays
6. Opposing models in fixed and removable prosthetics

D. Other elastic impression materials are used for the impressions of teeth and oral tissues to fabricate crowns, bridges, inlays, onlays, orthodontic and other prosthetic devices.

CHARACTERISTICS OF IMPRESSION MATERIALS

1. Accuracy in clinical application
2. Ease in manipulation
3. Not toxic or irritating
4. Pleasant odor, taste, and color
5. Economic
6. Dimensional stability
7. Maintain shelf life
8. Compatible with die and cast materials
9. Consistency in texture and wettability
10. Adequate mechanical strength to resist tearing

MODEL AND DIE MATERIALS ▆▆▆▆▆▆

I. Three types of devices can be created from a dental impression:
   A. *Model:* a reproduction of teeth and oral tissues that is generally used for case-study or diagnostic purposes
   B. *Cast:* a working model of a reproduction to be used in the fabrication of an appliance or restoration
   C. *Die:* a replica of one or more teeth that is usually a removable portion of the cast
II. The types of materials used to make reproductions from dental impressions are gypsum products, epoxy, and electroplated metal.
   A. Use of any of the reproduction materials is precluded by the impression material and the reason for making the replica.
   B. The material should be accurate and have extremely little or no dimensional change to ensure accuracy of the restorations and appliances made from the replicas.
   C. The type of cast or die material must be compatible and desirable with specific impression materials (Table 10-2).
III. Gypsum products can be used in all aspects of model, cast, and die fabrication because they are compatible with impression materials.
   A. Gypsum products may be model plaster, dental stone, or improved dental stone (also called *high-strength stone*).

Table 10-2 Selection of cast or die materials according to use of impression

Cast/die material	Impression material
Gypsum	Dental compound
	Agar hydrocolloid
	Alginate
	Zinc oxide-eugenol
	Polysulfide rubber base
	Silicone rubber base
	Polyether rubber base
	Impression plaster (if heavily coated with a separating solution)
Epoxy resin	Polysulfide rubber base (with separator)
	Polyether rubber base
	Silicones (separator as necessary)
Electroplated copper	Dental compound
	Silicone rubber base
Electroplated silver	Polysulfide rubber base
	Polyether rubber base
	Addition silicone rubber base

B. Application or use of a model or cast determines selection of a material.
C. All three materials are products of the gypsum mineral calcium sulfate dihydrate, which, during manufacturing, lose water and are converted to hemihydrates of calcium sulfate.
   1. The process of removing the water and producing the hemihydrate differs with each product, resulting in different chemical and physical characteristics.
   2. Model plaster is the least strong of the products, followed by orthodontic plaster (model plaster with a small amount of dental stone) dental stone, and improved stone.
D. Addition of water to any gypsum product produces a chemical reaction that causes the material to harden.
   1. The amount of water needed to mix these materials is greater than that needed for the chemical reaction to occur.
   2. Water aids in wetting the calcium sulfate hemihydrate particles and helps the material flow into the impression.
   3. Water evaporates as the gypsum product sets during the exothermic reaction.
   4. The amount of the water needed is determined by the size, shape, and porosity of the particles.
   5. The water/powder ratio for each is as follows:

   Model plaster $\dfrac{45 \text{ to } 50 \text{ ml water}}{100 \text{ powder}}$

   Dental stone $\dfrac{30 \text{ to } 32 \text{ ml water}}{100 \text{ powder}}$

   Improved dental stone $\dfrac{19 \text{ to } 24 \text{ ml water}}{100 \text{ powder}}$

E. Working with gypsum products involves the following factors:
   1. Setting times
   2. Detailed reproduction
   3. Compressive strength
   4. Tensile strength
   5. Resistance
   6. Dimensional accuracy
F. Characteristics of gypsum products are listed (box on page 179).
G. Types and uses of gypsum include the following:
   1. Type I: impression plaster; used as impression or wash
   2. Type II: model plaster; used for fabrication of study models

3. Type III: dental stone; used for working model

4. Type IV: improved stone; used as cast or die material

H. **Spatulation** is the technique of mixing materials together to form a homogeneous mass. Certain factors during spatulation can cause variations in setting time and the expansion of gypsum products.

1. If spatulation time or rate is increased, setting time is shortened.

2. The rate of spatulation may affect setting expansion.

3. Hand-driven or power-driven spatulators are often used to avoid increased setting time and expansion.

CHARACTERISTICS OF GYPSUM PRODUCTS

SETTING TIME

1. Initial setting time (includes mixing and manipulation of material)
   - Increase in viscosity, decrease in flow
   - Loss of gloss
   - Usually between 8 and 16 minutes
2. Final setting time (when material can be separated from the impression material without fracture)
   - Usually between 45 and 60 minutes after initial manipulation in the mouth
   - Cool and dry

DETAILED REPRODUCTION

1. Manipulation technique may improve reproduction quality and detail.
2. Vacuum mixing increases detail.
3. Detail of reproduction varies with the product; i.e., epoxy or electroplated die quality is greater than that of improved stone or plaster.

COMPRESSIVE STRENGTH/TENSILE STRENGTH

1. Strength increases with decreased water.
2. Improved stone is stronger than other gypsum products.

RESISTANCE

Abrasion resistance and hardness are related to the compressive strength of the material.

DIMENSIONAL ACCURACY

Improved stone is the most accurate, followed by dental stone and model plaster.

---

4. Vacuum mixing may be used to reduce air bubbles and the possibility of voids.

DIES

I. Dies are replicas of the prepared tooth or teeth on which wax patterns are fabricated.

II. Dies may be constructed from three types of materials.

A. *Stone*

1. Stone may be used for all types of final impressions.

2. Stone is a strong material for a die but may be susceptible to abrasion during instrumentation.

B. *Epoxy*

1. Epoxy may be made from polysulfide, polyether, and silicone rubber impression materials.

2. Epoxy is made from a resin and a hardener that produces a strong, abrasion-resistant die.

C. *Metal plating*

1. Production involves an electroforming or electroplating process with an electric current and an electrolyte to form indirect dies for inlay, crown, and bridge restorations.

2. Metal plating creates a strong, abrasion-resistant die.

INVESTMENT MATERIALS

I. Investment material is used in the process of obtaining a cast metal restoration during a lost-wax technique.

II. The investment is a ceramic material that can be molded into a form that withstands the procedure for producing an alloy cast.

III. Investment material is a combination of refractory material, such as quartz, tridymite, or cristobalite; a binder material of calcium sulfate or a similar material; and a possible combination of sodium chloride, boric acid, potassium sulfate, graphite copper powder, and magnesium oxide.

IV. Categories of investment materials appropriate for casting dental restorations include the following:

A. Type I: inlay, thermal

B. Type II: inlay, hygroscopic

C. Type III: partial denture, thermal

V. Investment materials undergo a certain amount of thermal expansion, which allows the shrinkage of the gold casting as it cools during the procedure.

A. Expansion occurs as the investment material

hardens after manipulation and during the heating of the material that is molded around the wax pattern.

B. Temperature that a material must withstand to achieve ideal thermal expansion is 482° to 650° C.

C. If the material is hygroscopic, it can be placed in contact with water to increase the expansion, thus reducing the need for higher temperatures during the burnout procedure (482° to 650° C).

DENTAL WAXES

I. Categories of Waxes
   A. Pattern
   B. Processing
   C. Impression
II. Components of Wax
   A. *Paraffin:* a combination of petroleum and hydrocarbons for a high melting point
   B. *Microcrystalline wax:* similar to paraffin but from a heavier oil, creating an even higher melting point
   C. **Other components**
      1. *Ceresin:* distillates from natural-mineral petroleum refining for greater hardness
      2. *Carnauba:* from esters, alcohols, acids, and hydrocarbons for hardness, brittleness, and high melting points
      3. *Candelilla:* combination of paraffin hydrocarbons, free alcohol, acids, esters, and lactones to harden paraffin
      4. *Beeswax:* insect wax of esters to create a wax that is brittle but plastic at body temperature
III. Important Characteristics of Waxes
   A. Ability to undergo thermal expansion when creating wax patterns
   B. Flow, which is increased as the wax reaches its melting point or as load is increased—important with respect to deformation
   C. Lack of wax residue in the mold space following burnout
   D. Low stress levels when manipulated through heating and carving
IV. Pattern Waxes
   A. Pattern waxes are used to create a desired reproduction in wax that will become the shape of a metal casting or denture through use of the lost-wax technique.
   B. Pattern waxes include *inlay, casting,* and *baseplate* waxes.
      1. Inlay wax
         a. Inlay wax is used in the fabrication of cast metal restorations through the creation of a wax pattern of the restoration.
         b. Inlay wax is classified as type I, which is used to form direct wax patterns in the mouth, and type II, which is used to prepare wax patterns on dies.
         c. It is supplied in small sticks or premade shapes, in tins, or as bulk wax chunks.
      2. Casting wax
         a. This is used in the fabrication of a wax pattern of the metal framework for removable partial and complete dentures or other dental appliances.
         b. It is used by many practitioners to establish the occlusal clearance between a prepared tooth and the opposing tooth.
         c. It is supplied in thin sheets and ready-made forms and shapes that are slightly tacky in texture to ensure the final position on a model.
      3. Baseplate wax
         a. This wax is named for its original application as a rim of wax that is set on a baseplate tray for the establishment of the vertical dimensions of a denture.
         b. Baseplate wax is classified as type I, a soft wax for creating contours; type II, a wax of medium hardness for patterns used in the medium zones of weather; and type III, a hard wax for patterns used in tropical regions.
   C. This wax is alternatively used to establish a bite registration on a patient to reflect the relationship of the teeth in one arch to those in the other.
V. Processing Waxes
   A. Utility or auxiliary wax is used as an aid in the construction of restorations and appliances.
      1. It is supplied in ropes, strips, and sheets.
      2. It is commonly used to customize a stock impression tray to capture the entire anatomy in an impression (particularly the peripheral border) or to fill the palatal area of an impression tray for a patient who has a vaulted palate.
   B. Boxing wax is used in boxing an impression to create a form in which to pour a gypsum product.
   C. Sticky wax, when heated, is extremely sticky; as it cools, it becomes firm, not tacky, and somewhat brittle. It is used to assist in keeping

two objects together, such as a denture that is fractured and is to be repaired with cold-cured acrylic.

VI. Impression Waxes

A. These waxes are used to produce an impression of oral tissues; they must exhibit high flow and ductility.

B. Corrective impression wax is used to obtain edentulous impressions in a patient with undercuts or to correct an edentulous impression.

C. Bite registration wax is used to reproduce the accurate articulation of the dental arches.

1. This wax is supplied in preformed shapes of the arch to assist in positioning the wax over the teeth and to minimize the amount of wax used.

2. It is susceptible to distortion and may be reinforced with metal between two sheets of the wax to assist in softening the wax and holding its shape when it has rehardened.

GOLD AND DENTAL ALLOYS

I. Facts about Gold

A. Gold has been used for restorative purposes for many years.

B. The high cost of gold stimulated the introduction of other alloys, such as palladium-silver, nickel, cobalt chromium, and nickel-chromium alloy, and lowered the content of gold alloy used in dentistry for restorative procedures.

C. 24-karat (K) gold is extremely soft, ductile, and malleable.

D. Both karat and fineness are used to measure the gold content of an alloy.

E. Pure gold is 24 K, 50% gold is denoted as 12 K.

F. Pure gold is rated as 1000 in fineness (F); thus, if a metal is 12 K, it would have a fineness rating of $1000 \times 0.50 = 500$ F.

II. Gold Foil

A. Gold foil is used as a direct filling material in the mouth; during the procedure, gold foil must be annealed. To remove surface gasses to make it cohesive, gold foil is condensed into the cavity preparation.

B. The gold-foil procedure is time-consuming and complex and thus not often done.

III. Noble Metals

A. **Noble metals** (*gold, platinum, palladium,* and *iridium*) are used predominantly for casting dental restorations.

B. Silver, though present in small amounts in some casting alloys, is not considered a noble metal because it tarnishes easily.

C. Noble metals contain a minimum of 75% gold; the remaining metal is derived from the platinum metal group.

1. Properties of the noble metals provide the characteristics of the alloys to meet their varied applications.

2. Platinum has a high fusing point and is resistant to the corrosive oral conditions; it provides hardness and elasticity when added to gold alloys.

3. Platinum in the form of foil is used for the framework in constructing porcelain-fused restorations.

4. Palladium is commonly a component of silver or gold alloys; it has properties similar to those of platinum but is less expensive. When combined with gold, it lightens the alloy; when used with silver, it reduces tarnish and corrosion.

5. Iridium is added to gold alloys to reduce the grain; the resulting fine-grained alloy is stronger and more ductile. Iridium itself is very hard and brittle and has a high melting point.

IV. Base Metals

A. **Base** or **nonprecious metals** are combined with gold to improve properties for individualized applications of the alloys.

1. *Indium* does not tarnish in water or air and has a low melting point; this base metal can be used in place of zinc, particularly with patients who have a sensitivity to zinc.

2. *Tin* is high in luster and does not tarnish easily; it is relatively soft and has a low melting point. Tin is usually applied in conjunction with gold solder and specialized alloys. Combining tin with palladium and platinum increases hardness and brittleness of the alloy; combining tin with copper creates bronze.

3. *Zinc* combined with gold and platinum increases hardness and brittleness of the alloy. It also is a deoxidizing agent during the melting and casting of alloys, thus creating an alloy that is easier to cast.

4. *Copper* is combined with metals to increase hardness and strength and to enhance the quality of color of the alloy. Copper also assists in the heat treatment of the alloy, using heat and cooling to harden or

soften the material. Combining copper with zinc creates brass.

    5. *Nickel* in small amounts combined with gold alloys increases the strength and hardness of the alloy.

V.   Gold Alloys

    A. Gold alloys are used for casting purposes.

    B. Gold alloys are classified by ANSI-ADA specifications as type I, II, III, or IV.

       1. Type I is soft and is usually used in the fabrication of inlays that will be subjected to limited stress through mastication.

       2. Type II is of medium hardness and is used in all types of cast inlays and for certain posterior bridge abutments.

       3. Type III is harder and can withstand greater stress than type I or II, making the alloy useful for full crowns, certain three-quarter crowns and bridge abutments, and construction of precision-fitting inlays.

       4. Type IV is extra hard and strong enough to be used for partial denture clasps, precision cast bridges, and three-quarter crowns.

VI.   Soldering

    A. Soldering is done when two metals are connected through a special low-fusing alloy.

    B. Solder selection depends on the type of metals that are to be fused.

    C. Content of solder varies, depending on the alloy; gold solder containing a lower gold content with zinc and tin may be used or a silver solder designed to work with stainless steel and other metals.

    D. Usually a *flux* (a paste or powdered material) is placed on heated metal to remove oxidized areas from the surfaces before soldering.

FINISHING, POLISHING, AND CLEANSING AGENTS

I.   Fabrication of restorations and appliances and maintenance of existing prosthetics all require the use of finishing, polishing, and cleansing materials to achieve the ideal end product.

    A. Some of these materials are used intraorally, others only extraorally.

    B. The materials may be in powder or stick form or may be mounted on a stone or mandrel, disk, point, strip, or wheel.

II.   Finishing agents remove excess material or structure from a prosthesis.

III.   Polishing materials are used to smooth roughened surfaces.

IV.   Cleansing materials are used to remove debris from the surface of an object and commonly include dentifrices and prophylactic pastes.

V.   Four elements affect the rate at which something is finished:

    A. *Particle size* of the abrasive

    B. *Rate* at which the abrasive moves over a surface

    C. *Pressure* applied on the abrasive to a surface

    D. *Hardness* of the abrasive surface being finished

VI.   Abrasives may be found in the following substances:

    A. Dentifrices that contain calcium carbonate, dibasic calcium phosphate dihydrate, anhydrous dibasic calcium phosphate, tricalcium phosphate, hydrated alumina, sodium metaphosphate, calcium pyrophosphate, and silica

    B. Calcite or calcium carbonate

    C. Kieselguhr or siliceous materials from aquatic plants

    D. Pumice or siliceous volcanic glass

    E. Rouge or iron oxide powder

    F. Tin oxide or white powder

    G. Tripoli from North African rock or made from silica

    H. Zirconium silicate or a hard abrasive of small particles

VII.   Other abrasives include the following:

    A. Aluminum oxide on paper or plastic disks in various grits; reddish brown

    B. Cuttle—originally from fish bones, now from quartz on paper or plastic disks in various grits; beige

    C. Sand—a quartz on paper or plastic disks in various grits; beige

    D. Garnet—a natural substance on paper or plastic disks in various grits; red

    E. Diamond chips embedded in a matrix to create diamond points, disks, and stones; silver in color and hardest of the abrasives

    F. Silicon carbide on paper or plastic disks in various grits; black

VIII.   The types of materials recommended for finishing, polishing, and cleansing to obtain the desired final result on various surfaces are summarized as follows:

    A. Tooth structure: Use a dentifrice to clean and polish the surfaces of the teeth with a toothbrush or, professionally, use a prophylactic brush, cup, and paste.

    B. Denture base: Remove soft debris with brush and dentifrice; remove hard deposits and stains through repolishing the denture with several alkaline substances, including perborates, hypochlorites, and peroxides, or dilute acids and abrasive powders and creams. Also, may soak the denture in a solution of 5% sodium hypochlorite and 3 parts water or 1 teaspoon of hypochlorite and 2 teaspoons of a glassy phosphate (such as Calgon) in water.

C. Composite: To minimize roughness and to reduce finishing and polishing, place Mylar matrix strips interproximally before inserting the material; professionally, remove composite through the use of various grits of abrasive materials, starting with the coarsest and finishing with the finest. Examples of the instruments used include diamond stones, finishing burs, abrasive strips and disks, abrasive points, and polishing paste.

D. Amalgam: Place the material against a metal matrix band interproximally, condense it, and carve it to the desired anatomic proportions; then burnish it to smooth the surfaces of the restoration. To remove excess or roughened amalgam, use green stones, finishing burs, disks of adalox, silicon carbide, and cuttle; soft-brush with silex or tin oxide and finishing strips.

E. Gold: Finishing and polishing of cast gold alloy restorations is accomplished on the die during an indirect restoration. First, pickle the cast to remove oxidation, then polish proximal surfaces with a variety of devices; including disks of sand, cuttle, crocus, burlew and cratex wheels, rag wheels with a slurry of pumice or radoff, sureshine, bendick, chamois, and rouge.

Questions

Dental Materials

1 The acid etch technique involves the use of 30% to 50% _____ acid.
a. Hydrochloric
b. Ortho-ethoxybenzoic
c. Phosphoric
d. Silicophosphate

2 _____ force pulls and stretches a material.
a. Compressive
b. Shearing
c. Tensile

3 As the state of matter is changed from solid to liquid to gas, molecular movement is

a. Decreased
b. Unchanged
c. Increased
d. Stopped

4 In the formation of plastic the reaction involves the combination of single molecules called _____ into chains of molecules called _____.
a. monomers, polymers
b. polymers, monomers

5 The reaction described through the process in item 4 is called _____.
a. Processing
b. Chemical reaction
c. Polymerization

6 Which of the following is a test for measuring hardness?
a. Resilience
b. Toughness
c. Thompson
d. Knoop

7 If a dimensional change occurs in an impression to be used to create a restoration, the following can happen; it can
1. Result in shrinkage of the impression material.
2. Result in the expansion of the impression material.
3. Affect the accuracy of the dental restoration.
4. Affect the thermal coefficient of expansion of the material.
a. 1 and 3
b. 2 and 4
c. 1, 2, and 3
d. 4 only

8 An increase in the water proportion of a gypsum product can
1. Decrease the compressive strength
2. Increase the compressive strength
3. Decrease the setting time
4. Increase the setting time
a. 1 and 3
b. 1 and 4
c. 2 and 4
d. 2 and 3

9 Which is the correct sequence of events for creating a gold alloy casting?
a. Making the wax pattern, creating the die, investing the pattern, spruing the pattern, burnout, casting, and pickling
b. Creating the die, making the wax pattern, spruing the pattern, investing the wax pattern, burnout, casting, and pickling
c. Creating the die, making the wax pattern, spruing the pattern, investing the wax pattern, casting, burnout, and pickling
d. Creating the wax pattern, spruing the die, investing the wax pattern, pickling, casting, and burnout

10 Which of the following statements describes the purpose of the specifications of the American National Standards Institute and the American Dental Association?
1. The specifications measure clinical properties of materials to establish minimum standards.

2. The specifications measure critical physical and mechanical properties of materials to establish minimum standards.
3. Lists of certified materials ensure clinical success.
4. Lists of certified materials ensure quality control and are helpful in selection of dental materials for a dental practice.
   a. 1 and 3
   b. 2 and 4
   c. 1 only
   d. 4 only

11 Which of the following are examples of galvanism in restorative dentistry?
1. A piece of plastic wrap becomes wedged between two teeth and contacts a gold restoration.
2. A temporary aluminum crown contacts a gold restoration.
3. A temporary plastic crown contacts a gold restoration.
4. A metallic taste is a frequent complaint of a patient.
   a. 1 and 3
   b. 2 and 4
   c. 1, 2, and 3
   d. 4 only

12 Linear coefficient of thermal expansion is a measure of the
   a. Amount of heat transferred through a material
   b. Biting force a material can withstand
   c. Change in size of a material resulting from changes in temperature
   d. pH of a material

13 Pit and fissure sealants are retained on the tooth surface by
   a. Mechanical lock
   b. Chemical bonding
   c. Adhesion
   d. Cohesion

14 Which of the following safety measures should be followed when working with mercury?
1. Mercury should not be handled by bare skin.
2. Spills should be vacuumed up immediately.
3. Mercury and amalgam scrap should be placed in the trash.
4. Spills should be cleaned up with a special spill kit.
5. Mercury and amalgam scrap should be stored in capped, unbreakable jars.
   a. 1, 2, and 5
   b. 2 and 3
   c. 1, 3, and 5
   d. 1, 4, and 5

15 Hygroscopic expansion results from
   a. Temperature increases
   b. Temperature decreases
   c. Addition of water
   d. Removal of water

16 The weakest of the gypsum products is
   a. Dental plaster
   b. Dental stone
   c. Improved dental stone

17 Which of the following statements are true about ZOE cements?
1. They should be used under composite restorations.
2. Increases in temperature and humidity shorten setting time.
3. They may be used under amalgam restorations.
4. They may be used during pulp-capping procedures.
5. They are the strongest for permanent cementation.
   a. 2 and 3
   b. 2, 3, and 4
   c. 1, 2, 3, and 4
   d. All are true

18 Which of the following are reasons for placing a cement base?
1. Strengthens the pulp
2. Serve as a thermal insulator
3. Serve as a thermal conductor
4. Replace missing dentin
5. Stimulate dentin formation
   a. 2 and 4
   b. 3 and 4
   c. 1, 2, and 4
   d. 2, 4, and 5

In items 19-22, place an A for *True* or a B for *False* next to each statement.

_____ 19 Cements are used for luting of restorations and as bases.

_____ 20 Low-strength bases provide thermal protection for the pulp.

_____ 21 *Luting* and *base* are synonymous terms.

_____ 22 Zinc-phosphate cements are used in near exposures because of their obtundent quality.

In items 23-25, match the description in column A with the term in column B.

Column A	*Column B*
_____ 23 Ability of a material to withstand permanent deformation under a compressive stress	a. Stress
	b. Galvanism
	c. Malleability
	d. Ultimate strength
_____ 24 Point at which a material will fracture or rupture at a certain stress	
_____ 25 Battery effect produced by two different metals	

Rationales

Dental Materials

1 C Phosphoric acid is the common solution used in the acid etch step in a bonding procedure. Citric acid had been used in the past for this purpose.

2 C Compressive force occurs when two materials are compressed causing strain. Shear force occurs when equal or opposite forces are applied against opposite planes. Tensile stress results when two forces are applied in opposite directions.

3 C As a substance changes from solid to liquid, molecular activity is increased. This continues and intensifies as the same material is transformed from liquid to gas.

4 A A molecule that repeats itself, or is a combination of monomers, becomes a polymer. A polymer may also be a combination of several types of monomers.

5 C Polymerization is the conversion of two or more monomers into polymers.

6 D The Knoop hardness test is a method of measuring surface hardness by resistance to the penetration of an indenting tool made of diamond.

7 C Shrinkage or expansion are examples of dimensional change that result in diminished accuracy of a dental material, particularly impression materials. This change affects the ability to produce a restoration that is able to be placed in a prepared tooth.

8 B Excess water, beyond manufacturers directions, decreases the quality of a gypsum product. The gypsum matrix is weakened and will fracture easier. It will also take the gypsum longer to obtain total hardness with extra water.

9 B When an impression is taken, it is poured with a gypsum product, electroplated, or used in conjunction with an epoxy to create a model and a die. A wax pattern is created on the die. It is attached to a sprue, invested, allowed to harden, and placed in an oven for burnout of the wax. The alloy is melted and then cast into the investment. The alloy cools and is pickled to remove impurities.

10 B The American National Standards Institute and the ADA establish standards to ensure the safety and effectiveness of dental materials, instruments, and equipment and encourages improvements and development of materials, instruments, and equipment. They also coordinate national and international standardization of the above and maintain liaisons to other organization like OSHA.

11 B Galvinism occurs when an electric current is established in solution, such as saliva, which contains salts and is a good electrical conductor. As two different metals meet in the oral cavity, an electrical current occurs.

12 C Temperature of a material may cause thermal expansion. This change in the material changes the size or shape through temperature variances.

13 A The process of acid etching the tooth surface removes microscopic layers of enamel. This enamel is roughened to allow the mechanical locking of the resin to the tooth surface.

14 D Mercury absorbed into the body is cumulative, so all body surfaces should be protected from contact with mercury. Mercury should be handled as directed by each supervisory health regulation. Commonly, mercury spills are cleaned with specialized kits that absorb the liquid while reducing aerosolization. Mercury and scrap should be handled as directed, but is commonly stored in capped, unbreakable jars in water before disposal.

15 C Hygroscopic expansion is the greater increase in volume of a gypsum product when it sets in contact with water.

16 A Dental plaster is weaker than dental stone or improved stone. The difference in strength of the material is created when water is removed from the gypsum product mechanically.

17 B Increased temperature and humidity shortens the setting time of ZOE cements. The cement may be placed under amalgam restorations but may not be as strong as a glass ionomer or a zinc phosphate. ZOE cements also are obtundants and have a sedative effect used in pulp capping.

18 D Cement bases replace tooth structure lost from decay or trauma. This structure under a metallic restoration, reduces the thickness of the metal, thus decreasing thermal conductivity.

19 A Certain cements can be mixed to a primary consistency, which can be used as luting agents, or to a secondary consistency, which can be used to rebuild tooth structure as a cement base.

20 A Low strength bases, such as ZOE and calcium hydroxide, are commonly used for pulpal protection.

21 B Luting refers to a thin layer of cement that flows over the restoration and the tooth surface offering a bonding between the two for the retention of the restoration. A base is a thicker layer of cement used to rebuild lost tooth structure, provide thermal and compressive protection, and have an anodyne effect.

22 B Zinc phosphate cements are acidic to the pulpal tissues and do not provide an anodyne effect to a tooth.

23 C If a material is malleable it can withstand deformation under stress. An example would be to roll a material into a sheet without fracture.

24 D The ultimate strength of a material is that at which it can be subjected to before it permanently deforms, not going back to its original shape.

25 B Galvinism, or galvanic shock, occurs when two different metals touch in the right solution of an electrolyte. An example of the materials would be amalgam and cast metal restoration bathed in saliva all contacting at the same time.

To enhance your understanding of the material in this chapter refer to the illustrations in Chapter 11 of Finkbeiner/Johnson: *Mosby's Comprehensive Dental Assisting: A Clinical Approach.*

The Business of Dentistry

OUTLINE

Human Relations	Patient Records	Dental Insurance
Dentistry as a Service Profession	Financial Records	Filing Systems
Communications	Written Communication	Computer Applications
Appointment-Book Management		

KEY TERMS

Accounts payable	Facsimile	Preferred provider organization
Accounts receivable	Fixed fee	Primary carrier
Appointment schedule list	Fraud	Recall system
Capitation	Hierarchy of needs	Receipt/charge slip
Claim form	Human relations	Registration/health questionnaire
Client-centered therapy	Informed-consent form	Subscriber
Clinical chart	Inventory control	Table of allowance
Clinical record	Laboratory requisition	Telecommunications
Closed panel	Ledger card	Treatment plan
Code system	Ledger card tray	Unit
Communication	Nonverbal cues	Update form
Coordination of benefits	Office policy	Usual, customary, and reasonable
Daily journal sheet		

Dentistry is a business as well as a health care service profession. Therefore, while it is necessary to provide treatment for patients in a caring manner, it is also necessary to maintain maximum efficiency and production in order to make a profit.

The dental business office is the center for all activity in the office. A myriad of activities take place in this area. In addition to being the communications center, the business office schedules appointments; processes insurance claim forms; and maintains clinical, recall, financial, employee, and governmental records.

HUMAN RELATIONS

I. Psychology of **Human Relations**
    A. Dental professionals must understand the needs of their patients and be concerned with each patient as an individual.
    B. Dental personnel must get to know the patient and identify the level of the hierarchy he or she has reached.
    C. Abraham H. Maslow described a **hierarchy of needs** that identifies five basic levels ranging from basic biologic needs to complex social or psychic drives.
        1. *Physiologic or biologic:* Physical needs such as food, water, and shelter must be satisfied first, or life won't last long enough to satisfy any of the social and psychologic needs.
        2. *Safety or security:* Once the basic biologic needs are met, a person can advance to the next level and explore the environment; at this level the person feels safe and free from danger, threats, and other deprivations.
        3. *Social or love:* At this level of the hierarchy, an individual needs to interact with others who share similar beliefs and provide positive reinforcement; love and social interaction give the individual confidence to advance to the next level of the hierarchy.
        4. *Esteem:* Interactions with others at the previous level help generate further goals, such as higher self-esteem, better reputation, or additional recognition of peers; the self-satisfaction realized from achieving goals provides the impetus to establish new goals.
        5. *Self-actualization:* Self-actualized individuals are motivated by the need to grow; they must have achieved self-esteem and gained self-confidence.
    D. Rogers' **client-centered therapy**
        1. Client-centered therapy is based on the concept that "it is the client who knows what hurts, what directions to go, what problems are crucial, what experiences have been deeply buried."
        2. Rogers also suggests that the patient or other individual must be accepted as a genuine person with a unique set of values and goals and that others must be treated with "unconditional positive regard."
        3. Applied to dentistry, this philosophy encourages the dental assistant to listen to the patient.
II. Dentistry as a Service Profession
    A. Society is service oriented, and dentistry is an important health care service.
    B. The patient seeks both dental care and service.
        1. Only a patient who is satisfied with the services rendered will remain with the dental practice.
        2. The basis for patient retention is generally **communication:** the ability to understand and to be understood.
III. Desirable Characteristics for Building Relationships
    A. Success depends on developing people skills as well as technical skills.
    B. Skills that lead to successful communication include the following:
        1. Self-confidence
        2. Genuineness
        3. Openness to experience
        4. Enthusiasm
        5. Assertiveness
        6. Integrity
        7. Honesty
        8. Acceptance of others
        9. Being a good listener
        10. Being a team player
        11. Recognizing the needs of others
        12. Sense of humor

COMMUNICATIONS

I. Communication: the Basis of Human Relations
    A. Communication among staff personnel is directly related to productivity.
    B. Two types of productivity on the dental team are individual and group productivity.
        1. Each member of the dental team has a basic level of productivity that he or she can accomplish alone.
            a. This level of productivity may vary from day to day depending on specific conditions.
            b. *Potential productivity* is a person's maximum productivity.
            c. *Productivity gap* is the difference between basic productivity and potential productivity.
        2. The same procedure can be followed for group productivity.

II. Barriers to Communication (box below).

III. Using Nonverbal and Verbal Communication
   A. **Nonverbal cues** are gestures that indicate a person's inner feelings without verbal communication.
   B. Nonverbal cues often indicate how a person is coping with these feelings.
   C. Different types of nonverbal cues may indicate different feelings.
      1. Raised eyebrows: pain or fear
      2. Clenched fists: pain or fear
      3. Crossed arms: disgust or anger
   D. Health professionals can improve their use of verbal images. They have an obligation to allay fears and comfort patients by using words or phrases that trigger positive thoughts.
   E. A *patients' bill of rights* can indicate the protection and courtesy for the patient (box in the next column).

IV. Staff Management
   A. Three forms of leadership exist in management:
      1. *Authoritative:* The dentist makes all decisions with little input from the staff.
      2. *Participatory:* The dentist seeks input on practice decisions and shares responsibility with the entire staff. This seems to be the most effective form of leadership in a dental practice.
      3. *Free rein:* The prevailing attitude is easygoing; no one is directly responsible for making specific decisions.

B. Staff meetings should be scheduled regularly.
   1. Follow basic rules to achieve an effective meeting as listed:
      a. Notify each staff person in advance of the time, day, date, and location of the meeting.
      b. Obtain suggestions for agenda items from each staff member.
      c. Determine the agenda and prioritize items accordingly.
      d. Review accomplishments.
      e. Determine goals and needs for change.
      f. Maintain control of the meeting; do not allow it to turn into a complaint session.
      g. Review the outcome of the meeting and provide minutes.
      h. Begin and end on time.
C. Professional etiquette should be practiced.
   1. Professional *etiquette* consists of the forms, manners, and ceremonies established by

---

BARRIERS TO COMMUNICATION

JUDGING

1. Criticizing
2. Name calling
3. Diagnosing
4. Praising evaluatively

SENDING SOLUTIONS

5. Ordering
6. Threatening
7. Excessive or inappropriate questioning
8. Advising
9. Moralizing

AVOIDING THE OTHER PERSON'S CONCERNS

10. Diverting
11. Arguing logically
12. Ignoring

PATIENTS' RIGHTS

1. Be treated with respect and consideration for personal, medical, and dental needs
2. Be informed of all aspects of treatment
3. Be informed of appointment and fee schedules
4. Review financial and clinical records
5. Obtain a thorough evaluation of needs
6. Be treated as a partner in care and decision making that is related to treatment planning
7. Receive current information and be assured of quality treatment
8. Expect confidentiality of all records pertinent to dental care
9. Be informed whether the dentist participates in different third-party payment plans
10. Request and expect appropriate referrals for consultation
11. Be taught how to maintain good oral health for a lifetime
12. Receive treatment that will prevent future dental or oral disease
13. Expect continuity of treatment
14. Be charged a fair and equitable fee
15. Have appointment schedules and times maintained
16. Be treated by a staff of professionals who maintain good health and hygiene
17. Be respected for requesting a second opinion
18. Be respected as a human being with feelings and needs

convention and required by society in professional or official life.

2. Professional etiquette is more than just manners; it also involves attitude.
3. Tips for practicing professional etiquette in the dental office are listed (box below).

V. Telecommunication Systems

   A. A variety of **telecommunication systems** are used in the dental office.

   1. The telephone is the most important instrument in the office.

      a. Suggestions for improving telephone personality (box in the next column)
      b. Rules for incoming and outgoing calls (box on page 190)

   2. Many offices use some form of answering machine, voice mail, E-mail, or professional answering service when the dentist and staff are not in.

      a. Recorded messages on answering machines and voice mail should be as caring and personable as possible.

   b. Specific instructions as to what the patient should do in case of emergency and when the office will be reopened should be provided.
   c. Answering services should provide courteous, helpful, and prompt service.
   d. Establish in advance the way messages will be received, and follow up on them as promptly as possible.

   3. A **facsimile** (fax) system is an electronic means of communicating information rapidly.

      a. The fax system operates like a photocopy machine that sends an image by wire.
      b. The sender inserts the document into the machine, and an image of the document is scanned over standard telephone lines.
      c. At the receiving end, a similar machine receives the transmitted copy.
      d. The message can be handwritten or typed, or it may be a visual image, such as a graph.
      e. The cost of transmitting a fax is similar to that of a long-distance telephone call.

VI. Reception Room Techniques

   A. The reception room is the gateway to the office.

   1. The dental assistant meets and greets patients.

TIPS FOR PROFESSIONAL ETIQUETTE IN THE DENTAL OFFICE

- Use correct grammar, pronounce words correctly, and expand your vocabulary.
- Do not interrupt another person during a conversation. If an emergency arises, excuse yourself before interrupting, state the message, and then close by apologizing for the interruption.
- Do not eat or drink in front of patients.
- Perform proper introductions for unacquainted people.
- Introduce yourself to patients; shake hands heartily to extend a warm welcome.
- If two people are engaged in a conversation, avoid standing within hearing range. If you wish to talk to one of them, leave the area and return later.
- Say "Thank you" when a person has been helpful, has cooperated during treatment, or has complimented you.
- Send thank-you notes for thoughtful acts or gifts.
- Respect your colleagues' space and do not interfere with their work.
- If the phone rings while you are talking with someone, excuse yourself to answer it. If you anticipate a lengthy conversation, ask the caller if you can return the call and complete the business with the person at hand.
- Avoid having friends drop in to talk.

SUGGESTIONS FOR IMPROVING YOUR TELEPHONE PERSONALITY

Be considerate.
Be attentive.
Be discreet.
Identify yourself.
Speak distinctly.
Use proper grammar.
Speak at a moderate rate.
Speak in a pleasant, normal voice.
Keep a smile in your voice.
Transfer calls pleasantly.
Take messages courteously and accurately.
Have writing implements accessible at all times.
Use a message pad to record complete information.
Ask questions tactfully.
Close the conversation politely.
Have emergency telephone numbers readily available.

RULES FOR INCOMING CALLS

Answer calls promptly.

Be certain you are answering the appropriate incoming line by depressing a flashing button.

Answer with a simple, cordial salutation.

Identify yourself.

Avoid placing a caller on hold for a long time.

Thank the caller for holding when necessary.

Record vital information on a message pad and confirm the message at the conclusion of the call.

End the call with a courteous closure.

Allow the caller to hang up first and then gently replace the receiver.

Take any message the dentist needs to receive immediately to the treatment area in written form, but do not discuss it in front of the patient.

RULES FOR OUTGOING CALLS

Make calls only during acceptable business hours.

Be certain the call is placed at an appropriate hour for a particular time zone.

Be certain the phone number is accurate.

If you do not know the number, consult the telephone directory.

Have appropriate information available before placing the call (e.g., patient's record, dentist's notes, appointment book).

Ascertain that the line to be used is available (depress only an unlighted button) before you place the call.

Listen for the dial tone before you place the call.

Press buttons firmly but not too quickly.

When the call is answered, identify yourself and the dentist for whom you are calling.

State the reason for calling.

Repeat or confirm vital information at the conclusion of the call.

End the call with a courteous closure.

Allow the other person to hang up first and then gently replace the receiver.

IDEAS FOR ENHANCING THE RECEPTION AREA

- Offer a wide range of reading material: books or magazines on sports, current events, homemaking, children, arts, architecture, health, gardening, or other topics of interest.
- Place magazine/book racks at two heights—one for adults and one for children.
- Place coat racks at two heights—one for adults and one for children.
- Install a rack with index cards (or note paper) and pens with a sign stating that they can be used to copy material from the reading matter.
- Include a cookbook from a local organization.
- Make available an Etch-a-Sketch, a coloring book, or other compact games for children.
- Post educational dental literature.
- Mount bulletin boards with special recognition of patients.
- Display name plates identifying staff members.
- Post a welcome sign or bulletin board announcing new patients/staff members.

2. The room should reflect the personality of the dentist and staff.
3. The patient should be acknowledged on arrival in the reception room.
4. The reception room must be kept neat and orderly and be maintained at a comfortable temperature.
5. The reception room should be kept free of odors.
6. Reading materials must be kept current.
7. Ideas to enhance the reception room are provided (box above).

APPOINTMENT-BOOK MANAGEMENT ◼

I. Selecting an Appointment Book
   A. The color of the appointment book may reflect individual use.
   B. The style of an appointment book may vary in the following ways:
      1. Pagination
         a. One day per page
         b. One week per page
         c. Other formats
      2. Columnation
         a. Each day may be divided into two to five columns for use by multiple staff members.
      3. Bindings
         a. From three to nine rings, loose leaf
         b. Spiral
      4. Time increments
         a. An increment of time is a **unit.**
            (1) 10-minute units
            (2) 15-minute units
            (3) others
      5. Notations/graphics
         a. Months, days, dates, and time sequencing
         b. Holidays

II. Appointment-Book Entries
   A. Only one person should be responsible for appointment-book entries.
   B. All entries in the appointment book should be made in pencil, and the entries must be legible, complete, and accurate.
   C. Data entered in the appointment book should include the following information:
      1. Patient's full name, with cross-reference in case of duplication of names
      2. Home and business phone numbers
      3. Treatment to be provided
      4. Length of the appointment
      5. Age of the patient (if a child)
      6. Special codes to denote a new patient, premedication, or laboratory status of a case
      7. Suggested codes to denote the special needs of patients (box)
III. Appointment cards
   A. An appointment card is given to the patient after the entry is made in the appointment book.
   B. The card is filled out in ink.
   C. The day, date, and time are clearly and accurately entered.
   D. Cards are made for single appointments or for a series of appointments.
   E. Cards are available in a variety of colors and shapes.
   F. The dentist's name, address, telephone number, and broken-appointment policy should be included.
IV. Appointment Schedule List
   A. An **appointment schedule list** is an outline of basic appointment sequencing and the amount of time required for each procedure.
   B. The list indicates the number of units for specific treatments.
V. Daily schedule
   A. Prepare a schedule each day.
   B. Distribute a copy to each treatment room, laboratory, private office, or other major area of activity.
   C. Include the patient's name, the treatment to be provided, and other specific data.
   D. Update the schedule during the day as changes occur, such as emergencies or cancellations.

PATIENT RECORDS

I. Uses of Well-Maintained Records
   A. Aid in patient treatment
   B. Verification of treatment for insurance

SUGGESTED CODES FOR USE IN APPOINTMENT BOOK	
N	New patient
*	Earlier appointment preferred
B	Business phone number
H	Home phone number
L	Case at laboratory
Ⓛ	Case returned from laboratory
PM	Premedicate before treatment
√	Confirmed appointment (in red)
↓	Length of appointment

   C. Verification of financial activity for the Internal Revenue Service (IRS)
   D. Evidence in malpractice suits
   E. Aid in identification of victims of crime or disaster
II. Clinical Records
   A. A **clinical record** is maintained for each patient and is a composite of items that are most frequently kept in a patient file folder.
      1. **Registration/health questionnaire**
         a. This may be two separate records or a combined form.
         b. It includes complete personal information about the patient and a thorough health history.
         c. Answers to questions on this form are kept in strict confidence.
         d. Complete information is obtained with no discriminatory questions.
         e. If the patient is a child, a special pediatric form must be completed by the parent or guardian, not by the child or baby-sitter.
      2. **Update form**
         a. Use this form for a patient's return visit after an absence from the office.
         b. Update the patient's address, insurance, and employment changes and obtain information about changes in health status.
      3. **Clinical chart**
         a. Personal information and health data are transferred to this record.
         b. Information is confidential.
         c. Each time a patient is treated, the treatment, medication, anesthesia, and other data are recorded on this chart along with the date of entry.

d. Initials of the treating dentist or auxiliary should be recorded.

e. Any information about conversations with a patient or recommendations for treatment should be recorded and dated.

f. This documentation will serve as legal evidence if needed.

4. **Laboratory requisition**

a. Most states require that written instructions accompany each case sent to a commercial laboratory.

b. Indicate instructions and special precautions that need to be taken when handling the case.

c. A copy is retained in the patient's record.

5. **Informed-consent form**

a. This form must be signed by a patient or by a parent of a minor child to grant permission for the administration of an anesthetic or of other specified procedures.

6. Letters

a. Copies of all letters sent to or concerning a patient are retained.

7. Radiographs

a. Radiographic films are stored in the patient's record.

b. Each set is labeled with the patient's name, the date of exposure, and the dentist's name.

c. If copies of the radiographs are transferred to another office, a notation is made on the record of the date of transfer and to whom the films were sent.

d. Requests for transfer must also be included in the record.

8. Postal receipts

a. Radiographs or copies of other information that are sent to another office should be sent by certified mail.

b. A receipt is kept in the record as proof of transfer of the materials.

III. Treatment Plan

A. A **treatment plan** outlines the needs of the patient and the recommended treatment.

B. An assortment of visual aids is used to present the plan to the patient.

IV. Preventing Disease Transmission in Records Management

A. The safest way to avoid disease transmission from the treatment room via patient records is to not take the records into the room.

B. Alternative methods for handling patient records might include the following:

1. Touch or write on the record only after removing treatment gloves.

2. Wear overgloves when touching the record.

3. Enter and review all data on a monitor and protected keyboard in the treatment room.

V. Records Transfer

A. Patient data can be transferred only by written consent of the patient or the patient's legal representative.

B. The original record is retained in the office.

C. A copy of only that part of the record specifically requested is transferred.

D. A duplicate set of radiographs may be sent.

E. When possible, the materials should be sent in a manner that will provide a return receipt for the sender.

F. A reasonable clerical fee, consistent with local practice, may be charged for furnishing these records.

FINANCIAL RECORDS

I. Accounts Receivable

A. **Accounts receivable** is used for patient transactions, including debits or charges for services and credits or payments on a patient account, resulting in the accounts receivable balance or the amount the patient owes the practice. This record is a **ledger card** or computer record that is kept separate from the clinical record; it is generally maintained for each family or responsible person.

B. All financial activity for each member of a family, both charges and payments, is maintained on one file or ledger card.

C. Exceptions to family records exist during divorce or other legal separations.

D. These records provide protection for the dentist and patient, information for insurance and tax purposes, and data for practice analysis audits.

E. The two most common bookkeeping systems used today are the following:

1. Pegboard (a write-it-once system)

2. Computer software

F. Components of both systems provide the same documentation.

1. The pegboard system includes ledger cards for each patient, and day sheets are produced every day.

2. Computer software systems store data on the computer disks or drives, and hard cop-

ies can be made as needed. Computer files must be backed up routinely.

  G. Both systems provide the following:

    1. A **code system** is used to denote specific treatment or payments in an abbreviated form; codes may appear on the ledger card, statement, and/or the patient receipt.

    2. A **daily journal sheet** provides a listing of all activity for the day, including patient treatment and receipts.

    3. A patient ledger card contains all financial information for each patient or family; most ledger cards are in the name of the person responsible for paying.

    4. At the end of the month a photocopy or computer printout of the ledger card is sent to the responsible person as a *statement* or *request for payment*.

    5. A **ledger card tray** is used to store ledger cards, which are filed in alphabetical order and generally divided into two categories: *active* (with debit or credit balances) and *inactive* (with no balance and/or currently not under treatment); in a computer system the records are stored on a hard drive.

    6. A **receipt/charge slip** is given to the patient at the end of the procedure to indicate charges and payments.

  H. Suggestions are listed for maintaining accurate financial records (box).

II. Accounts Payable

  A. **Accounts payable** is for recording all transactions the dentist pays out (e.g., salaries, supplies, rent, utilities).

  B. Banking responsibilities of the dental assistant may include the following:

    1. Check writing
    2. Endorsing and depositing checks
    3. Maintaining an accurate bank balance
    4. Endorsing and depositing monies
    5. Reconciling bank statements

  B. Various checks may be used, including the following:

    1. Personal
    2. Certified
    3. Cashier's
    4. Money order
    5. Traveler's
    6. Bank draft
    7. Voucher

  C. Checks may be produced manually or through a computer software package.

  D. After the check is written, an entry must be

RULES FOR ENTERING DATA ON FINANCIAL RECORDS

- Always use ink, not pencil; these records are permanent.
- Use good penmanship; do not attempt to use fancy letters.
- Keep columns of figures straight.
- Write well-formed figures.
- Place decimal points correctly.
- Do not erase; if you make an error, draw a straight line through it and write the correct figure above it.
- Enter all charges and payments as soon as the patient leaves the treatment room.
- Make certain that for each patient listed in the appointment book an entry has been made on the day sheet.
- Check math carefully.
- Store records in a fireproof file.
- Make a backup of the computer file.
- Retain backup computer files at an out-of-office site.

---

made manually in the checkbook or entered in the computer to indicate the check number, date, payee, amount of the check, purpose of the check, and new balance.

WRITTEN COMMUNICATION ■

I. Business Letters

  A. The most common letters produced in the office include the following:

    1. Welcome to the office
    2. Referral to another dentist
    3. Thank you
    4. Birthday or congratulatory
    5. Recall notice
    6. Request for information
    7. Collection of delinquent account

  B. Basic rules for writing letters include the following:

    1. Correct any grammatical and typing errors. Use a dictionary or spelling check function on the computer to correct spelling.

    2. Use language that the reader can understand, and make the letter *you*-oriented rather than *I*-oriented.

    3. Be brief and concise; do not use lengthy sentences that contain multiple ideas.

    4. Demonstrate consideration and courtesy to the reader; display the same manners in

the written message that you would in person.

5. Write the letter as if you were talking to the person.
6. Maintain patient confidentiality, and provide information only to authorized sources for whom you have written consent.
7. Be complete and accurate, and be certain that all information is included and none of the statements can be misinterpreted.
8. Be neat; avoid smudges, erasures, and unclear copies.

II. Office Procedures Manual
   A. The manual is a step-by-step description of common procedures used in the office.
   B. It is specifically designed for the office staff.
   C. It serves as a training manual for new staff and reference manual for the entire staff.

III. Office Policy
   A. The **office policy** is a written communication designed for the patient.
      1. It outlines the office procedures, philosophy of the dentist, and staff functions.
      2. It provides a mechanism for education.
      3. It is generally presented to new patients at their first office visit.

IV. Regulatory Compliance Manual (OSHA policies)
   A. This is a reference manual for all staff members.
   B. It provides information on all regulations relating to infection control, hazard communication, training procedures, and medical waste disposal.

V. Newsletter
   A. A newsletter is an excellent marketing tool.
   B. It should be sent to patients regularly.

C. It updates patients about activities in the practice.
D. It provides a format for dental education.
E. It serves as a form of professional advertising.

VI. Recall System
   A. A **recall system** is a preventive program used to recall patients to the office.
   B. Patients are recalled for various reasons, including the following:
      1. Denture check
      2. Orthodontic development evaluation
      3. Periodontal evaluation
      4. Endodontic treatment follow-up
      5. Oral prophylaxis
   C. Patients are placed on a recall system in accordance with their dental condition. Most common recall times are 3, 4, or 6 months after the last appointment.
   D. Types of recall systems include the following:
      1. Mail: Notices are sent to a patients to inform them of the need to make an appointment.
      2. Telephone: Every patient due for an appointment is called by the business staff to schedule one.
      3. Advanced appointment: The patient makes the next appointment when leaving the office, and a card is mailed several weeks before the appointment for confirmation.
      4. Each system has advantages and disadvantages (Table 11-1).
   E. Maintaining a recall system involves the following steps.
      1. Educate the patients regarding the value of routine recall.

Table 11-1 Comparison of Recall Systems

Type of system	Advantages	Disadvantages
MAIL	Places responsibility on the patient	Patient may ignore the notice
		Postage is costly
	Message will be waiting for patient at home	Not certain the message was received
		May not receive a response from patient
TELEPHONE	Immediate response, either positive or negative	May not receive an answer or will need to leave the message on the answering machine
	Personal contact can be a practice building tool	May disturb the person
		Time consuming for a large practice
ADVANCED APPOINTMENT	Minimal cost involved	Patient may not know future plans or schedule
	No time required to implement	Appointment book is filled months in advance
		May forget the appointment

Adapted from Finkbeiner B, Finkbeiner C: *Practice management for the dental team*, ed 4, St Louis, 1996, Mosby.

2. Notify patients of the need for an appointment.
3. Follow up on patients who are negligent in making appointments.
4. Schedule appointments in compliance with insurance coverage to avoid nonpayment by the insurance company.

VII. Inventory Control
   A. **Inventory control** refers to the method of keeping track of the number and amount of dental instruments and materials used in the practice.
   B. Records for inventory of supplies are maintained in the business office.
   C. Three types of supplies are used in an office:
      1. Capital items (large, costly)
      2. Expendable items (disposable or consumed with each use)
      3. Nonexpendable items (reusable but not high cost)
   D. A file for capital equipment is maintained separately and includes the following information:
      1. Date of purchase
      2. Model number
      3. Maintenance record
   E. An expendable supply inventory system requires the following information:
      1. Rate of use
      2. Amount that is needed at all times
      3. Available storage
      4. Amount of capital available for purchases
      5. Shelf life of the material
   F. Supply purchase involves the following sequence of events:
      1. Order list or purchase order is completed.
      2. Order is placed with the dental supplier.
      3. Materials are received.
         a. Verify package contents with packing slip or invoice.
         b. Cross-reference invoices with the supplier's statement before making payment.
      4. If a product is not available, it is placed on back order for later delivery.
      5. If a product is returned, a credit slip is sent to the office and the account is credited for the proper amount.

DENTAL INSURANCE ▄▄▄▄▄▄▄▄▄

I. Parties Involved in Dental Insurance
   A. *Patient:* the person receiving the treatment; may be the **subscriber** to the insurance, a spouse, or a dependent child
   B. *Group:* a union, or business, or other organization that has negotiated dental insurance as a benefit
   C. *Carrier:* the insurance company that distributes the money to the provider for services rendered
   D. *Dentist:* provider of the dental services

II. Types of Prepaid Dental Plans
   A. Three basic types of insurance programs common to dentistry
      1. **Usual, customary, and reasonable fee**
         a. This plan, used by many dental service corporations, is based on the usual, customary, and reasonable fees of the dentist.
         b. The *usual* fee is the fee that is usually charged for a specific service by an individual dentist.
         c. The *customary* fee is the fee that is usually charged by dentists of similar training and experience for the same service within a specific and limited geographic area or socioeconomic level of society.
         d. A fee is *reasonable* when it meets the above two criteria (usual and customary) or can be justified because of special circumstances that pertain to a particular case.
      2. **Fixed fee**
         a. A fixed fee is established for service rendered.
         b. Fixed-fee coverage is often federally supported.
         c. Participants in this type of program must accept the fees listed on a fee schedule from the responsible agency as the total fee and cannot charge the patient an additional amount.
      3. **Table of allowance**
         a. A table of allowance fixes a dollar amount as the benefit for each individual's dental service.
         b. The patient is responsible for any difference between the dentist's fee and the amount provided for in the table of allowance.
   B. Alternative dental delivery systems
      1. **Capitation:** The dentist assumes the risk in delivering dental care rather than a third party, such as the insurance carrier; the dentist is paid a fixed fee, per capita per month, which entitles members of a group to a specified set of services.

2. Two common capitation programs
   a. **Closed panel:** The group contracts with a clinic for the delivery of dental care to its members; covered individuals must receive dental care from a clinic dentist or pay for the services themselves. Dentists working in such a clinic are generally salaried.
   b. **Preferred provider organization:** An individual practitioner or clinic may contract with a group purchaser of benefits to provide dental service at a cost that is lower than usual; the dentist thus becomes a preferred provider.

III. Basic Procedures in Dental Insurance Management
   A. Basic insurance terminology (box)
   B. Working with claim forms
      1. An insurance **claim form** is a statement of services, including date of service and itemization of fees, and a request for payment from the carrier.
      2. An ADA-approved form is divided into two parts:

INSURANCE TERMINOLOGY

Approved services—All services covered under a dental plan

Audit of treatment—An administrative or professional review of a dentist's treatment plan or of the dentist's reimbursement claims for services performed

Birthday rule—This rule is implemented in the coordination of benefits when the patient is a dependent; dependents are covered as primary under the plan of the parent whose birthday (month and day) occurs earlier in the calendar year.

Certificate of eligibility—An identification card or document that verifies the individual is covered by a particular group, provided the eligibility requirements continue to be met

Claim form—A statement listing services rendered, date of the services, and itemization of the fees; the completed and signed form serves as a request by the dentist for payment of benefits by the carrier.

Commercial carrier—A corporation that contracts with groups of consumers to administer dental care plans; it is a profit-making organization with a group of stockholders.

Contract year—The period (usually, but not necessarily, a calendar year) for which a contract is written; it could also be a fiscal year.

Copayment—The amount or percentage of the total approved amount that the subscriber is obligated to pay; this is not to be confused with the deductible amount.

Deductible amount—This is the portion or percentage that the subscriber must pay before the plan's benefits begin; this may be a yearly or a one-time amount.

Dental service corporation—A legally constituted organization that contracts with groups of consumers to administer dental care plans on a prepaid basis; these groups are sponsored by state dental societies and are nonprofit organizations.

Dependents—Persons (generally a spouse and children) who receive benefits of a subscriber covered by a dental plan

Effective date—The date the contract goes into effect and from which benefits are afforded

Eligible individual—A person entitled to benefits under a dental plan

Exclusion—Dental services not provided for under a dental plan

Maximum benefit—The maximum dollar amount a dental plan will pay toward the cost of dental care incurred by an individual or family in a specified period, whether a calendar year or a contract year

Member—The employee who represents the family unit in relation to the prepayment plan

Nonparticipating dentist—A dentist who has not entered into an agreement with a service corporation or agency and has not agreed to the rules and regulations of the board of directors of the corporation

Participating dentist—A dentist who has agreement to render care to a member and dependents under the rules and regulations promulgated by a board of directors or agency

Predetermination/preauthorization—A proposed treatment plan submitted for verification of eligibility and identification of covered benefits and plan allowances, limitations, and exclusions

Primary carrier—The dental plan that covers the patient as the employee (1) when the patient is the male employee or his dependent children; or (2) when the patient is the female employee

Secondary carrier—The plan covering the patient as a dependent when the patient is the spouse or dependent child of the employee covered by the primary carrier

Subscriber—The employee who represents the family unit in relation to the prepayment plan

a. The top part is a request for general information about the patient and/or subscriber.

b. The bottom part of the form requests information about the dentist and includes a listing of services rendered for the patient.

3. The information must be thorough and accurate.

  a. Shortcuts and incomplete information result in rejection of the claim form by the insurance company.

  b. Errors in the claim form delay payment and make it necessary to resubmit the claim form with the correct information.

4. Before completing a claim form, review it thoroughly and be certain you understand the information required for each space provided.

C. Code on dental procedures and nomenclature

  1. This code is designed to identify standardized procedures and services.

  2. A service is given a five-digit number.

   a. The first digit, a zero throughout the series, denotes the service as dental rather than medical.

   b. The second digit denotes the category of service.

   c. The third digit designates the class of a specific procedure.

   d. The fourth digit denotes the subclass of the procedure.

   e. The fifth digit allows expansion of the code as necessary.

  3. All codes within a single category are in a specific number series; for example, all diagnostic procedures are listed in the series 00100-00999.

  4. The code for a patient having a complete series of radiographs would be 00210 and would be broken down as follows:

   First 0: dental service

   Second 0: diagnostic service

   2: radiographs

   10: intraoral—complete series

   Last 0: for extension of code

D. Coordination of benefits

  1. **Coordination of benefits (COB)** arises when patients are covered by more than one dental plan.

  2. These benefits must be coordinated.

  3. This situation, referred to as the *primary-secondary rule of payment*, requires the dental assistant to observe the following basic rules of coverage:

   a. The employee, retiree, or surviving spouse is covered as primary under his or her own dental program.

   b. Dependents are covered as primary under the plan of the parent whose birthday (month and day) occurs earlier in the calendar year. If the parents' birthdays are identical, the **primary carrier** (the carrier responsible for payment) is the one who has covered the child for the longer time.

   c. Dependents whose parents are divorced or legally separated are covered as follows:

    (1) The natural parent with custody (except in the case of item 5)

    (2) The spouse of the natural parent with custody

    (3) The natural parent without custody

    (4) The spouse of the natural parent without custody

    (5) If the divorce decree places financial responsibility on one parent, that parent's plan is primary over any other plan; the preceding is then used to determine the remaining order of payment.

   d. When a COB occurs between carriers in two different states, the birthday rule is often used, but individual plans should be reviewed to determine the primary-secondary rule in this situation.

E. Payment voucher and check

  1. Some insurance companies provide a payment voucher with the check.

  2. A voucher describes the payment in a detailed description that facilitates the posting to the patient account.

F. Helpful hints for preparing claim forms (box on page 198).

IV. Preventing Fraud in Insurance Payments

A. **Fraud** is defined as deceit, trickery, or double-dealing, but no matter how it is defined, fraud is cheating.

B. The following actions constitute fraud:

  1. Padding fees

  2. Billing before completion of treatment

  3. Predating or postdating claim forms

  4. Falsely listing treatment that was rendered

  5. Not working within the contract

HELPFUL HINTS FOR PREPARING CLAIM FORMS

1. Be accurate.
2. Keep an extra supply of claim forms on hand.
3. Type all data on an electric typewriter or use a computer software package to generate forms.
4. Answer all questions completely, providing details when required. If a question does not apply, insert NA for *not applicable.*
5. Obtain the most current information on each type of insurance that the patients carry and become familiar with the provisions of each policy. Regularly attend workshops sponsored by various carriers to update your knowledge of insurance procedures.
6. Establish a list of contact persons, phone numbers, and addresses for each carrier used in the office.
7. Maintain complete and current information on each patient and update regularly.
8. Be certain to send claim forms to the appropriate carrier and the correct branch office.
9. When necessary, obtain prior authorization before treatment is begun.
10. Be certain the dentist and patient have signed the form before you send it.
11. Retain a copy of the completed form for the office.
12. If required, include copies of radiographs or periodontal charts and be certain each is well identified with the names of both the patient and the dentist.
13. Set aside a specific time to work on claim forms and review the status of previously submitted forms.

FILING SYSTEMS

I. Five basic methods of filing are used in most dental offices:
   A. Alphabetic
   B. Geographic
   C. Numeric
   D. Subject
   E. Chronologic
II. The most common file system is the open-shelf style with a file folder index that has a color-code system.

COMPUTER APPLICATIONS

I. Software Packages Commonly Used in Dentistry
   A. Word processing
   B. Accounts receivable
   C. Accounts payable
   D. Recall
   E. Inventory control
   F. Practice analysis
II. Basic Operations Needed for the Dental Office Computer
   A. Input
   B. Processing
   C. Output
   D. Storage

Questions

The Business of Dentistry

1 A *maximum and minimum* list is a record of the
   a. Expendable items and the minimum and maximum amounts that a supply house will send prepaid
   b. Items to be ordered and an indication of which have minimum and maximum importance
   c. Minimum amount of each item that can be ordered with a discount and the maximum amount that can be ordered conveniently
   d. Expendable items and indication of the maximum number to be kept on hand and the minimum number to have in stock before ordering

2 Before the dentist consults with the patient's physician regarding a medical problem, it is necessary for the patient to sign an informed-consent form.
   a. True
   b. False

3 Which is not a component of a clinical record?
   a. Clinical chart
   b. Health history
   c. Ledger card
   d. Radiographs
   e. Informed-consent form

4 Which is not a function of a patient financial record?
   a. IRS reports
   b. Practice analysis information
   c. Provide clinical data
   d. Protect patient and dentist

5 Which of the following is not a rule for entering data on financial records?
   a. Decimal points are not necessary.
   b. Make a backup of the computer file.
   c. Always use ink when making entries.
   d. Check mathmetic computations.

6 Which of the following is not an activity that constitutes fraud in insurance management?
   a. Padding fees
   b. Predating claim forms

c. Assisting a patient with inaccurate treatment-date entries

d. Billing before completion of treatment

e. All are considered fraud.

7 Accounts-receivable records include

1. Patient charges
2. Patient payments
3. Total monies owed the practice
4. Total monies the dentist owes
5. Checkbook balance

a. 1 and 3
b. 2 and 4
c. 1, 2, and 3
d. 4 and 5
e. 5 only

8 Which of the following statements is (are) not true regarding patient financial records?

1. They are legal documents.
2. Each record requires neat penmanship, accuracy, and thoroughness in making entries.
3. If prepared by hand, financial records are always written in ink.
4. They are subject to review by the patient as well as the IRS.
5. Erasures may be made to the entries, if done neatly.

a. 1 and 3
b. 2 and 4
c. 1, 2, and 3
d. 4 and 5
e. 5 only

9 When transferring patient records from the office to another site, the business assistant must do all except which of the following?

a. Obtain consent from the patient or legal representative.
b. Retain the original record in the office.
c. Transfer the entire record.
d. Copy the radiographs and retain the originals.

10 To avoid contamination of business records from the clinical site to the business office, the dental staff should

1. Not place records in the treatment room or near exposure to aerosols
2. Use overgloves when making entries
3. Remove contaminated gloves and wash hands before making entries
4. Spray the record with an OSHA-acceptable disinfectant
5. Not worry because bacteria, viruses, and spores are nonevasive to paper

a. 1 and 3
b. 2 and 4
c. 1, 2, and 3
d. 1, 2, 3, and 4
e. 5 only

For items 11-17, match the term in column A with the definition in column B.

Column A

_____ **11** Usual, customary, and reasonable

_____ **12** Fixed fee

_____ **13** Table of allowance

_____ **14** Capitation

Column B

a. A predetermined amount is established for services rendered.

b. A chart fixes a dollar amount as the benefit for each individual's dental service.

c. This is based on the usual, customary, and reasonable fees of the dentist.

d. A dentist is paid a fixed fee per capita per month, which entitles members of a group to a specified set of services.

Column A

_____ **15** Nonparticipating dentist

_____ **16** Primary carrier

_____ **17** Copayment

Column B

a. A dentist who has not entered into an agreement with a service corporation or an agency and has not agreed to the rules and regulations of the board of directors of the corporation

b. A dentist who has an agreement to render care to a member and dependents under the rules and regulations promulgated by a board of directors or agency

c. Amount of percentage of the total amount that the subscriber is obligated to pay

d. Dental plan that covers the patient as the employee

e. Dental plan that covers the patient as a dependent

Column A

_____ **18** Anesthetic syringe

_____ **19** Computer

_____ **20** Enamel hatchet

_____ **21** Stationery

_____ **22** Reversible hydrocolloid impression material

Column B

a. Capital
b. Expendable
c. Nonexpendable

23 Which of the following statements should be avoided when carrying on a conversation with a patient?

1. I'd like to remind you of your appointment.
2. Hello, Mrs. Brown, this is Dr. Tibble's office.
3. I'm calling to confirm your appointment.
4. The dentist is out of town at a convention
5. Hello, Mrs. Johnson, this is Linda from Dr. Ross' office calling.

a. 1 and 3
b. 2 and 4
c. 1, 2, and 4
d. 1, 3, and 5
e. 5 only

24 Which of the following should be avoided during an interview?
 a. Being prepared to answer a variety of questions.
 b. Being too aggressive
 c. Neatness
 d. Accuracy

25 The highest level of Maslow's hierarchy is
 a. Physiologic
 b. Security
 c. Social
 d. Self-actualization

Rationales

The Business of Dentistry

1 D A "maximum and minimum" list is an inventory record of expendable items. It indicates the maximum quantity to be kept on hand and the minimum quantity to have in stock before ordering.

2 A Before the dentist consults with the patient's physician regarding a medical problem, it is necessary for the patient to sign a "Release of Information" consent form. Without a signed document the dentist is in violation of patient confidentiality.

3 C A ledger card is a financial record and should not be retained in a patient's clinical chart. All other documents are a part of the clinical record.

4 C A patient financial record can be used for IRS reports, practice analysis information, and can protect patient and dentist, but it should not be used for recording of clinical data.

5 A The rules for entering financial data include:
 —Making a backup of the computer file
 —Always using ink when making entries
 —Checking mathematic computations

6 E Padding fees, predating claim forms, assisting a patient with inaccurate treatment date entries, and billing before completion of treatment are considered fraudulent activities.

7 C Accounts receivable records include the total monies owed the practice. In other words, when all of the debit accounts are added together and the credits subtracted, the amount remaining is the sum of outstanding accounts owed to the practice.

8 E Financial records are legal documents that require neat penmanship, accuracy, and thoroughness when making entries. If prepared by hand, financial records are always written in ink.

These records are subject to review by the patient as well as the Internal Revenue Service. If an error occurs, erasures may not be made to the entries, but a line is drawn through the error and the correct entry is made in the next available space.

9 C Before a patient record can be transferred from the office to another site, the business assistant must obtain consent from the patient or legal representative. Only a copy of the specific information for which consent has been granted is transferred. The original record is retained in the office. If radiographs are requested, copies are sent and the originals are retained.

10 C To avoid contamination of business records from the clinical site to the business office, the dental staff should not place records in the treatment room or near exposure to aerosols, use overgloves when making entries, or remove contaminated gloves and wash hands before making entries.

11 C UCR refers to a type of prepaid dental program based on the usual, customary, and reasonable fees of the dentist.

12 A A fixed fee is a type of prepaid dental program that is based on a predetermined amount established for services rendered

13 B A Table of Allowance is a plan that provides a fixed dollar amount as the benefit for each individual's dental service. The patient is responsible for any difference between the dentist's fee and the table amount.

14 D A capitation system is based on the fact that the dentist, rather than the third-party administrator, assumes the risk of delivering the dental care. A dentist is paid a fixed fee per capita per month, which entitles members of a group to a specified set of services.

15 A A nonparticipating dentist has not entered into an agreement with a service corporation or an agency and has not agreed to the rules and regulations of the board of directors of the corporation.

16 D A primary carrier dental plan covers the patient as the employee.

17 C A deductible amount is the amount or percentage of the total amount that the subscriber is obligated to pay.

18-22 A capital item is an item of major expense for the dentist and includes such equipment as a sterilizer, the dental chair, or computer. It is an item that has a long life and often caries a warranty and service contracts.

An expendable item has a one time use such as anesthetic carpules or cotton products.

A non-expendable item has multiple use but eventually needs to be replaced after a period of use. Examples would include hand cutting instruments, anesthetic syringes, or impression trays.

23 C When communicating with patients, avoid using "red flag" phrases that might denote discomfort or a nonprofessional attitude. For instance, people don't like to be reminded of appointments, instead confirm an appointment. When calling patients, identify yourself by name; an office doesn't talk, a person does. Finally, words like convention denote fun rather than study; a seminar or lecture denote professional education and updating.

24 B During an interview you should be prepared to answer a variety of questions, present yourself in a professional manner, and complete all forms neatly and accurately. Being assertive and asking questions is expected, but being too aggressive may cost you a job opportunity.

25 D The base of Maslow's hierarchy begins with satisfying basic physiologic needs and rises to the peak or top with self-actualization.

To enhance your understanding of the material in this chapter refer to the illustrations in Chapter 14 of Finkbeiner/Johnson: *Mosby's Comprehensive Dental Assisting: A Clinical Approach.*

Four-Handed Dentistry

OUTLINE

Benefits of Four-Handed Dentistry
The Dental Suite

Seating the Patient and Dental
Team

Pretreatment Preparation

KEY TERMS

Air/water syringe
Assistant's zone
Business office
Classification of motion
Color coding
Cuspidor
Dental unit
Dental stool
Direct vision
Electrosurgery unit
Ergonomics
Fixed cabinetry

Foot control
Four-handed dentistry
Handpiece
High-velocity evacuation
Indirect vision
Laboratory
Mobile cabinetry
Motion economy
Operator's zone
Patient chair
Preset tray

Radiography processing area
Reception room
Recovery room
See ability
Six-handed dentistry
Static zone
Supine
Transfer zone
Treatment room
Ultrasonic scaler
Zones of activity

Four-handed dentistry is a chairside technique that involves four hands working simultaneously to provide treatment to the oral cavity. This concept evolved in the 1950s and dramatically changed the practice of dentistry. Earlier, dentists practiced standing at chairside, which added unnecessary physical stress to an already highly demanding profession. In the 1990s, **ergonomics**—the concept of adapting the environment to the worker—

became the term for increased efficiency by design.

Research done in the 1940s indicated that a dentist who used one dental chair and worked with a chairside assistant could provide treatment to 33% more patients than a dentist who worked alone. Furthermore, with additional dental chairs and two full-time, well-qualified chairside dental assistants, the dentist could provide care to approximately 75% more patients.

BENEFITS OF FOUR-HANDED DENTISTRY ▬▬

I. Three Basic Benefits
    A. Increased patient comfort
        1. The patient lies on the back (**supine**) with the face upward and the arms and body well supported.
        2. Use **high-velocity evacuation (HVE)** and fiberoptic **handpieces.**
    B. Reduction in operator and assistant fatigue
        1. The operator and assistant are seated with their bodies well supported.
        2. Unnecessary motions (bending and reaching) are eliminated.
        3. Visibility is improved.
        4. Productivity is increased.
            a. When fatigue is reduced, the physical and mental stamina of the dental team is maintained for a longer time, efficiency is increased, and more treatment is provided for more patients.

II. Advanced Functions
    A. An adjunct to four-handed dentistry is advanced or expanded functions.
    B. These intraoral duties are delegated to an assistant or a hygienist.
    C. The dental practice act in each state specifies which duties may be delegated and the conditions under which the duties may be performed.

III. Basic Concepts of Four-Handed Dentistry
    A. Delegation of duties
        1. The dentist must delegate to a qualified assistant all duties that are legally delegable in the state.
        2. The dentist should perform those duties that require the skills of a licensed dentist, such as making the diagnosis, administering anesthesia, and performing irreversible procedures such as cutting hard and soft tissue.
        3. Duties that do not require the skill of the dentist should be performed by a qualified dental auxiliary as delegated by the dental practice act.
    B. Advanced planning
        1. The patient must have a prophylaxis and complete oral and radiographic examinations.
        2. The dentist must review the patient's record and arrange for sequential appointments to complete the treatment.
        3. Treatment must be provided in a logical sequence.

    4. Duties must be delegated for effective use of the dental auxiliaries.
    C. Seating the dental team
        1. Both the dentist and the assistant should sit on well-designed stools.
        2. The patient is supine, with the nose and knees on the same plane and the maxillary arch perpendicular to the floor.
    D. **Motion economy**
        1. Motion economy eliminates or minimizes the number and length of motions used at chairside.
        2. The principles of motion economy are listed (box).
        3. Motion can be classified into five categories according to the length of the motion. This **classification of motion** is provided (box on page 204).
    E. Conserving motion
        1. Rearrange equipment and materials so that they are closer to you.
        2. Ensure that all materials are prepared in advance.
        3. Reorganize a procedure to eliminate unnecessary steps.

IV. Six-Handed Dentistry
    A. **Six-handed dentistry** involves a second assistant at chairside performing tasks to assist the dentist or the assistant (or both).

PRINCIPLES OF MOTION ECONOMY

- Minimize the number of instruments to be used for a procedure.
- On a preset tray, position the instruments in the sequence in which they will be used.
- Position instruments, materials, and equipment in advance whenever possible.
- Place instruments and materials on a mobile cart as close to the patient as possible.
- Place the patient in a supine position.
- Provide work areas that are 1 to 2 inches lower than the elbow.
- Use operating stools that provide good posture and body support.
- Minimize the number of eye movements.
- Reduce the length and number of motions.
- Use body motions that require the least amount of time.
- Use smooth, continuous motions; avoid distracting zigzag movement.

CLASSIFICATION OF MOTION

Class I   Movement of the fingers only, as when picking up a small cotton pellet
Class II Fingers and wrist motion, as when transferring an instrument to the dentist
Class III Fingers, wrist, and elbow, as when reaching for a handpiece
Class IV Entire arm and shoulder, as when reaching into the mobile cart
Class V   Entire torso, as when turning around to reach for equipment on the fixed cabinetry

---

NEGATIVE PHRASES OFTEN USED TO RESIST CHANGE

It costs too much!
We tried it and didn't like it.
It wouldn't work in this kind of practice.
No one in this area does that.
We do not have enough instruments.
We do not have enough space.
It takes too much equipment.
Our patients would not like it.
It sounds like a production line.
This practice is not big enough.

POSITIVE PHRASES THAT INSPIRE CHANGE

It sounds as if it has merit.
Let us start a new trend.
That is interesting . . .
That is a great ideal!
I have faith in you.
I am glad you brought that up.
We should try it.
Good work!
It just might create a better environment.
Things are beginning to improve.

B. Six-handed dentistry could apply to any of the following situations:
  1. Retracting oral tissues during a surgical procedure when the chairside assistant is busy
  2. Controlling a patient who may be medically or physically compromised
  3. Preparing dental materials during complex procedures

V. Use of Preset Trays
  A. A **preset tray** is a collection of instruments or an armamentarium (assorted materials and equipment) identified for a specific procedure.
  B. Instruments and materials are placed on a specially designed tray in their sequence of use.
  C. Trays are timesaving and are used for most of the common procedures in dentistry.
  D. **Color coding** the tray and/or instruments can be used (specially colored or marked with colored tape or rings) for a specific procedure.
  E. Trays come in various styles.
  F. Most trays satisfy the basic criteria for preset trays, which include the following:
    1. They can be sterilized (preferably with the cover on) and stored as a single unit.
    2. They can hold a minimum number of double-ended instruments and adjunct supplies for a specific procedure.
    3. They can be specifically colored for given procedures, or a color-code tape can be affixed to the tray.

VI. Color Coding for Location
  A. Color coding aids in identifying the storage location for instruments that are not part of a specific tray setup.
  B. Instruments may be color coded to ensure that they will be returned to the proper room and location within the room.

C. Color coding can range from simple (instruments are coded with a colored tape for a specific room location) to complex (multiple markings on an instrument to indicate room, drawer, and location within a drawer).

VII. Implementing Four-Handed Dentistry
  A. A good attitude is necessary to encourage the staff to undertake a change to incorporate the concepts of four-handed dentistry into the practice.
  B. It may take time to bring about the change.
  C. Phrases often used to resist change are listed (box above).
  D. Phrases used to encourage the staff and start the change process are also listed (box above).

THE DENTAL SUITE ▬▬▬▬

I. Effect on Patients
  A. A well-designed and well-maintained office has a direct effect on the credibility of the practice.

B. The patient forms an image of the practice from the environment.

C. The patient is concerned with the following aspects of the dental office:

    1. Comfort

    2. Cleanliness and neatness

    3. Style

II. Basic Concepts of Office Design

  A. What type of image is desired?

  B. Which office design is appropriate for the type of practice?

  C. Which equipment will be most efficient yet be cost-effective?

  D. How can an attractive, comfortable office be created for patients and staff?

  E. What is an efficient traffic flow?

  F. How can a budget be maintained?

  G. How often will it be necessary to redecorate?

III. The Dental Suite

  A. The dental suite is composed of rooms, offices, and hallways. Each has a specific purpose; yet they must interrelate to provide an efficient, comfortable working environment.

  B. The dental suite may include the following areas:

    1. **Reception room**

    2. **Business office**

    3. **Laboratory**

    4. Sterilization area

    5. Radiography rooms

    6. **Radiography processing area**/darkroom

    7. Dentist's private office

    8. Insurance room/area

    9. Patient education/oral hygiene area

    10. **Recovery rooms**

    11. Storage rooms

    12. Rest room

    13. Staff lounge

    14. **Treatment rooms**

  C. The dental treatment room can be described as follows:

    1. All clinical activity takes place in the dental treatment room.

    2. Variations in these rooms include the following:

      a. Type of practice

      b. Number of dentists

      c. Number of auxiliaries

      d. Full- or part-time practice

    3. The treatment room should not be smaller than 8 by 10 feet.

    4. When possible, two room entrances can help create an efficient traffic floor plan for patients and staff.

    5. To simplify procedures, all rooms used for hygiene or operative treatment should be arranged and equipped identically.

    6. The treatment room and the sterilization areas should not be carpeted because of potential contaminant hazard.

    7. The two basic types of treatment room arrangements are as follows:

      a. Rear delivery

      b. Transthorax/side delivery

IV. Basic Dental Equipment

  A. Regardless of the brand chosen, the selection and placement of dental equipment should follow these general guidelines (Fig. 12-1).

    1. Position equipment for the patient's easy access to the dental chair.

    2. Provide comfortable seating for patient, dentist, and assistant.

    3. Eliminate the need for the dental team to twist, turn, or reach.

    4. Use aseptic-style hoses that eliminate tension and pullback.

    5. Eliminate the need for the dentist's eyes and hands to leave the site of operation.

    6. Position handpieces so that the assistant can easily pass them to the dentist.

    7. Eliminate tubing that touches the patient.

    8. Transfer instruments only within the transfer zone.

    9. Provide for easy use of the HVE hose and **air/water (A/W) syringe** simultaneously.

  B. The basic equipment for four-handed dentistry includes the following:

    1. **Patient chair**

      a. The chair should have a thin, narrow back.

      b. It should provide complete body and arm support for the patient when it is placed in supine position.

      c. Separate controls for elevation, tilting of the seat, and lowering of the backrest should be available for both the dentist and the assistant.

      d. It should provide for rotation.

      e. Upholstery on the chair should be easy to clean and made of a nonporous material according to Occupational Safety and Health Administration (OSHA) standards.

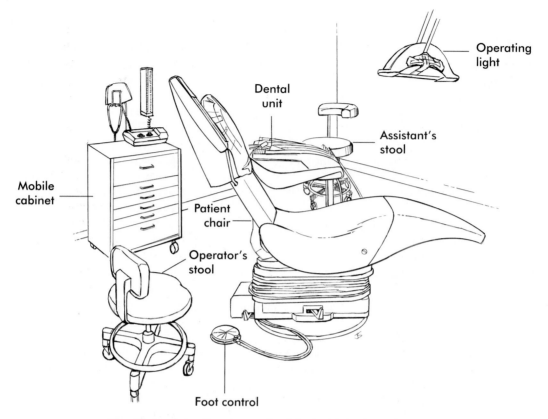

Fig. 12-1 A treatment room furnished with basic equipment.

f. Chair placement is primary to the location of other equipment in the room.

2. **Dental unit**
   a. The dental unit houses all the dynamic instruments the dentist uses during most operative procedures.
   b. It should adjust vertically but be independent of the vertical movement of the chair.
   c. Energy to the dental unit comes from electricity and from an air compressor stored outside the treatment rooms.
   d. Hosing for the handpieces should be smooth and should provide easy extension to any part of the room, with easy return to the permanent position on the unit.
   e. Each dental unit may house different equipment according to the needs of the dentist (Fig. 12-2).
   f. Other components of a dental unit might include an **ultrasonic scaler, electrosurgery unit,** or **cuspidor** (not recom-

mended for use in four-handed dentistry).
   g. The **foot control** is the device on the floor near the chair that is activated with foot pressure to operate all handpieces on the unit. It may include a chip blower option, which allows the dentist to provide bursts of air to the area being treated.

3. **Dental stool**
   a. The dental stool is required for the dentist and the assistant.
   b. The dentist's stool should have a broad, stable base; be well padded and may be flat or contoured; and should adjust from 14 to 21 inches in height and have a back support that adjusts vertically and horizontally.
   c. Both stools should have five casters for stability.
   d. The seat of the assistant's stool should adjust to a height of 27 inches and have an adjustable front and left-side body

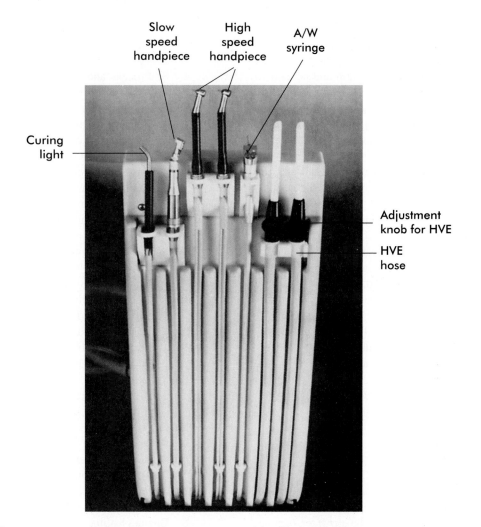

Slow speed handpiece

High speed handpiece

A/W syringe

Curing light

Adjustment knob for HVE

HVE hose

Fig. 12-2 Dental unit with various components identified. (Courtesy of Health Science Products.)

support to prevent unnecessary bending. Height adjustment by foot pressure is desirable.

4. Lighting
   a. Light should come from two sources: the general room light and the operating light.
   b. Room light should be diffused to avoid shadows and color balanced to simulate natural daylight as closely as possible.
   c. The operating light should be operable by either the assistant or the dentist and must provide an intensity that lights the patient's mouth adequately. Heat from the lamp should be directed away from the mouth.
   d. The operating light may be mounted on the ceiling, wall, or patient chair.

5. Cabinetry
   a. Two common types are **mobile** and **fixed cabinetry.**
   b. The mobile cabinet is the lifeline for supplies and materials used by the assistant during treatment.
   c. The mobile cabinet should provide easy access to all instruments and materials.
   d. Fixed cabinetry is generally used for the placement of sinks.
   e. Fixed cabinetry must be kept to a minimum.
   f. Wall-hung cabinets provide more floor space and make cleaning easier.
   g. Two sinks should be included in the treatment room—one for the assistant and one for the dentist.
   h. Knee or foot controls should be provided to turn faucets on and off.

i. Liquid soap dispensers and disposable towels should be placed near the sink.

j. A waste receptacle should be located nearby, be large enough, and be easy to empty without cross-contamination.

6. Emergency equipment/supplies

a. OSHA requires that an eyewash and emergency kit be available in the dental office.

b. A medical emergency kit and oxygen should be part of the emergency equipment.

c. Safety warning signs should be posted to indicate the location of the eyewash, oxygen, and emergency kit.

d. Oxygen tank and medical emergency kit must be examined regularly to ensure readiness and currency of drugs.

V. Equipment Maintenance

A. Equipment is maintained daily by the assistant; this routine care is distinct from disinfection, sterilization, and use of barrier techniques.

B. Daily maintenance includes the following:

1. Thoroughly cleaning the chair
2. Cleaning sinks
3. Restocking supplies
4. Flushing water lines

C. Periodic care is done by the assistant at weekly or monthly intervals and includes tasks such as cleaning the omniclave/autoclave, changing rubber rings in the air/water syringe, and changing solutions in a radiographic processor.

D. Periodic care also includes annual or biannual care provided by a service representative from a local dental supply company.

VI. Daily Office Preparation

A. Opening the office

1. Unlock all access areas, turn on lights, rearrange magazines, and dust all areas thoroughly.

2. Unlock all file cabinets, pull patient records and place in chronologic order, and post daily schedules in the appropriate rooms.

3. Turn on communication systems and other automated equipment, check answering machines or answering service, and organize work areas.

B. Radiographic processing area

1. Change water in the manual/automatic tanks and adjust to the correct temperature.

2. Turn on equipment.

3. Process and mount radiographs remaining from the previous day.

C. Treatment room

1. Perform routine housekeeping duties.
2. Change into clinical attire.
3. Perform the OSHA startup routine.
4. Turn on the equipment.
5. Position equipment for patient entry.
6. Prepare records outside the treatment area.
7. Remove perishable dental materials from the refrigerator.
8. Set up the armamentarium for the first patient.
9. Ensure the availability of appropriate trays and the readiness of any laboratory work that is needed for the day's patients.

D. Sterilization area

1. Preheat sterilizers as appropriate.
2. Prepare new ultrasonic and disinfectant solutions.
3. Remove instruments that may have been in solutions for disinfection overnight.

VI. Closing the Office

A. Reception room

1. Lock all access areas.
2. Turn off lights.
3. Pick up debris.
4. Rearrange magazines.

B. Business office

1. Send designated cases to the laboratory with a completed requisition.
2. Ascertain that laboratory work has been returned for the next day's patients.
3. Complete the daily bookkeeping entries.
4. Complete banking activities.
5. Confirm appointments, pull records, and prepare the daily schedule for the following day.
6. Turn off the automated equipment.
7. Turn on the answering machine/service.
8. Lock the files.

C. Radiographic processing area

1. Remove all radiographs from processing units or tanks.
2. Turn off the automatic processor.
3. If a manual tank is used, be certain to turn off the safe light and any water lines going to the tank.

D. Treatment room

1. Turn off all equipment.
2. Return all perishable dental materials to the refrigerator.
3. Remove all armamentarium from the room.
4. Perform the OSHA end-of-day procedures.
5. Remove clinical attire and, if possible, take a shower.
E. Sterilization area
   1. Sterilize all instruments.
   2. Arrange preset trays.
   3. Empty the solutions from the containers where possible.
   4. Pick up and organize the area for the next day.
F. Ongoing tasks include the following:
   1. Changing radiographic solutions
   2. Cleaning/defrosting the refrigerator
   3. Cleaning sterilizing units
   4. Changing disinfectant solutions
   5. Contacting a licensed waste removal service to transport hazardous wastes/sharps
   6. Sharpening instruments
   7. Restocking supplies
   8. Checking inventory
   9. Office evaluation

SEATING THE PATIENT AND DENTAL TEAM ▬

I. **See ability** (an ergonomic concept) means changing the environment to enhance the visibility of the dental team.
   A. From the suggested guidelines for see ability, several principles can be identified that will aid in positioning the dental team to provide maximum comfort and efficiency (Table 12-1).
   B. The area around the mouth is divided into four **zones of activity: operator's zone, assistant's zone, transfer zone,** and **static zone.** Figs. 12-3 and 12-4 illustrate these four zones with the patient's head as the face of a clock.
      1. The operator's zone extends from the 7 to 12 o'clock position for a right-handed operator and from 1 to 4 o'clock for a left-handed operator.
      2. The assistant's zone is from the 2 to 4 o'clock position for a right-handed operator and 8 to 10 o'clock for a left-handed operator.
      3. The transfer zone is the area around the patient's mouth where instrument transfer occurs; the transfer zone extends from the 5 to 8 o'clock position for a right-handed operator or 4 to 7 o'clock for the left-handed person.
      4. The static zone is the zone of least activity. It extends from the 12 to 2 o'clock position for a right-handed operator or 10 to 12 o'clock for a left-handed operator. Instruments or equipment that are used infrequently, such as a curing light or sphygmomanometer, and the assistant's cart when not in use, may be stored in this area.

II. Patient mobility is necessary in four-handed dentistry.
   A. The patient can change position to increase the visibility of the operating team for any operative site.
   B. The operator must use two forms of vision: direct and indirect.
      1. **Direct vision** occurs when the operator is looking directly into the cavity preparation or treatment site.
      2. **Indirect vision** requires the operator to look into a mirror to observe the area; the use of indirect vision eliminates the need for the operator to bend over to view the operative site.
   C. Patient positioning
      1. The patient is seated and placed in a supine position, with the knees and nose on the same plane.
      2. Once the patient is in the supine position, the operator can lower the chair until the patient's head is centered over the operator's lap.
      3. The operator should not have to reach up with the arms or bend over to work in the patient's mouth.
      4. Occasionally, lowering the chair base and raising the back of the chair enhances the operator's visibility; this is especially true when the operative site is the mandibular arch.
      5. Patients with special needs may require a more upright position, especially those with emphysema or other upper respiratory ailments.
   D. Operator positioning
      1. The operator's chair position changes in relation to the area of the mouth being treated.
      2. A change in the position of the operator within the zone of activity can greatly improve visibility and reduce back and neck

Table 12-1 General guidelines for effective four-handed dentistry

Area of operation	Vision	Operator's position*	Patient's chair position	Head position
MAXILLARY RIGHT POSTERIOR				
Buccal	Direct	9:00	Backrest horizontal	Straight, chin elevated slightly
Occlusal	Direct	9:00	Backrest horizontal	Chin elevated maximally, head straight
Occlusal	Indirect	11:00	Backrest horizontal	Straight, chin elevated slightly
Lingual	Direct	9:00	Backrest horizontal	Turned toward operator, chin elevated
MAXILLARY ANTERIOR				
Labial	Direct	11:00	Backrest horizontal	Straight, chin elevated slightly
Lingual	Indirect	11:00	Backrest horizontal	Straight, chin elevated slightly
MANDIBULAR ANTERIOR				
Labial	Direct	11:00	Backrest horizontal	Straight or turned slightly toward operator or assistant
Lingual	Direct and indirect	11:00	Chair seat lowered maximally, chair back elevated	Straight or turned slightly toward operator or assistant
MANDIBULAR RIGHT POSTERIOR				
Buccal	Direct	10:00	Seat lowered and backrest elevated slightly	Straight or turned slightly toward assistant
Occlusal	Direct	9:00	Seat lowered and backrest elevated slightly	Turned slightly toward operator, chin lowered slightly
Lingual	Direct	11:00	Backrest horizontal	Turned toward operator maximally, chin elevated slightly
MAXILLARY LEFT POSTERIOR				
Buccal	Direct	9:00	Backrest horizontal	Turned toward operator, chin elevated slightly
Occlusal	Direct	9:00	Backrest horizontal	Chin elevated maximally, head turned slightly toward operator
Occlusal	Indirect	11:00	Backrest horizontal	Turned toward operator
Lingual	Direct	9:00	Backrest horizontal	Turned toward assistant, chin elevated slightly
MANDIBULAR LEFT POSTERIOR				
Buccal	Direct	11:00	Backrest horizontal	Turned toward operator
Occlusal	Direct	10:00	Backrest horizontal	Straight, chin elevated
Lingual	Direct	9:00	Seat lowered and backrest elevated slightly	Turned slightly toward assistant

*The assistant's position remains the same (between 2 and 4 o'clock) in all situations.
Adapted from University of Alabama School of Dentistry, Birmingham, Alabama.

strain caused by bending and leaning (see Table 12-1).

E. Assistant positioning
1. The assistant's chair position remains the same regardless of the treatment site.
2. For better visibility of the mandibular arch, the stool can be raised slightly, but it seldom needs to be moved back and forth within the zone of activity.

PRETREATMENT PREPARATION

I. Typical Routine for Any Procedure
A. Prepare the treatment room.
1. Disinfect all exposed surfaces.

Retraction	Operator's fulcrum	High-veolcity evacuation tip parallel to tooth surface
MAXILLARY RIGHT POSTERIOR		
Left index finger	Hand piece head on left index finger	Lingual
Left index finger	Left index finger	Lingual
Right third finger	Buccal surfaces of right posterior teeth	Lingual
Left index finger	Left index finger	Lingual (distal tooth being treated)
MAXILLARY ANTERIOR		
Left index finger	Occlusal surfaces of right premolar teeth, or incisal surfaces of anterior teeth	Lingual (incisal edge)
Assistant retracts with left index finger	Occlusal surfaces of right premolar teeth	Lingual (incisal edge)
MANDIBULAR ANTERIOR		
Operator retracts lower lip with thumb and index finger	Buccal surfaces of lower right premolar teeth	Lingual
Operator retracts tongue with back of mirror	Buccal surfaces of lower right premolar teeth	Labial
MANDIBULAR RIGHT POSTERIOR		
Left index finger	Labial surfaces of lower anterior teeth	Lingual
Left index finger assistant retracts tongue with mirror	Labial surfaces and incisal edges of lower anterior teeth	Lingual
Operator retracts tongue with mirror	Labial surfaces of lower anterior teeth	Lingual (distal to tooth being treated)
MAXILLARY LEFT POSTERIOR		
Left index finger	Anterior incisal edges	Buccal (distal to tooth being treated)
Left index finger	Occlusal surfaces of right premolar teeth	Buccal
Assistant retracts with left index finger	Occlusal surfaces of right premolar teeth	Buccal
Assistant retracts with left index finger	Labial surfaces of lower anterior teeth left index finger stabilizes; handpiece head	Buccal
MANDIBULAR LEFT POSTERIOR		
Left index finger or mirror	Labila surfaces of lower anterior teeth	Buccal (distal to tooth being treated)
Operator retracts tongue with mirror Assistant retracts buccal tissues	Labial surfaces of lower anterior teeth	Buccal
Operator retracts tongue with mirror Assistant retracts buccal tissues	Labial surfaces of lower anterior teeth	Buccal

2. Arrange preset tray and armamentarium.
3. Set up records and radiographs.
4. Place barrier coverings.
5. Position equipment and armamentarium.
B. Provide an antimicrobial oral rinse for the patient.
C. Seat the patient (box on page 213).
D. Prepare barrier techniques for patient and operating team (box on page 213).
E. Seat the operating team (box on page 214).
F. Position the operating light.
G. Perform the clinical procedure.
H. Dismiss the patient.
   1. Turn off the operating light.

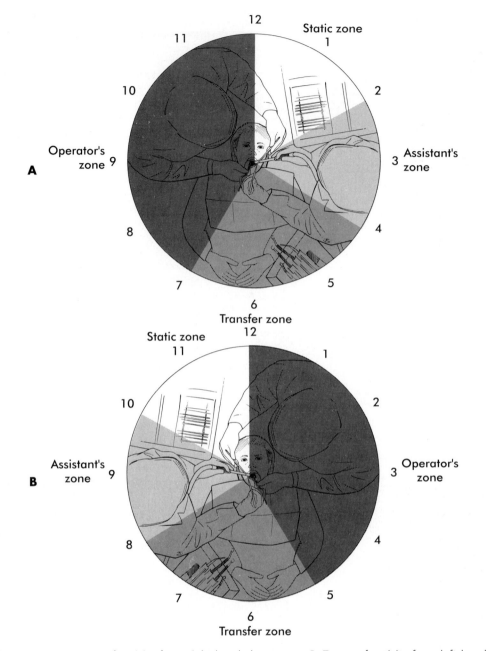

Fig. 12-3 *A,* Zones of activity for a right-handed operator. *B,* Zones of activity for a left-handed operator.

2. Move the unit out of the way.
3. Raise the backrest slowly in short increments to a comfortable sitting position.
4. Tilt the chair forward.
5. Lower the chair base.
6. Return personal items to the patient.
7. Allow the patient to remain seated to reestablish equilibrium.
8. Raise the arm of the chair.

9. Extend courtesy by directing the patient to the rest room to check appearance or freshen up, leading him or her back to the business office to make payments or future appointments, helping with coat, and extending thanks.

I. Return records to the business office.
J. Remove armamentarium and barrier coverings.

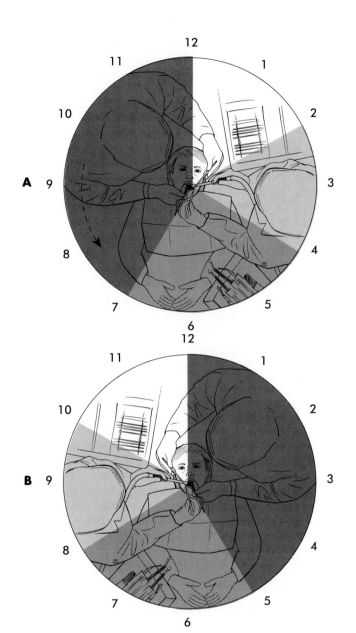

Fig. 12-4 *A,* The right-handed operator is at the 11 o'clock position for treatment on the maxillary anterior. *B,* The left-handed operator is at the 1 o'clock position for treatment in the same area.

SEATING THE DENTAL PATIENT

1. Lower the arm of the chair.
2. Offer to store personal items in a safe location nearby, out of the way.
3. Place the patient napkin and napkin clip.
4. Encourage the patient to move to the uppermost portion of the chair nearest the operator.
5. Position the patient's head in the head rest.
6. Raise the chair base about 10 to 12 inches.
7. Initially, tilt the chair back until the patient's calves are parallel to the floor.
8. Tilt the chair back an additional 45 degrees until the patient is supine.
9. Lower the operating light to a position the assistant can reach when seated.
10. Place the unit and mobile cabinet in position.

GLOVING AND UNGLOVING

1. Position major equipment and armamentarium.
2. Seat the patient.
3. Place mask and gloves.
4. Wash hands, dry thoroughly, and put on gloves.
5. Assist/perform the clinical procedure.
6. Prepare to dismiss the patient.
7. If the patient leaves treatment room alone or with another staff person, remain in the treatment room and perform cleanup according to OSHA guidelines.
8. When leaving the room with the patient, either place overgloves or remove mask, protective eyewear, and gloves and to wash hands.

     K. Clean and disinfect and/or sterilize the armamentarium and exposed surfaces.

II. Patients with Special Needs

    A. Older adults

       1. Older adults may need help getting to the treatment room.

       2. If their pace is slow, take time as you escort them to the treatment room.

       3. Help them as they get into or out of the chair, if needed.

       4. Place canes or walkers out of the way and inform patients about what you are doing so that they will not worry.

       5. Take care as you adjust the chair position because the patient may resist being placed in a supine position.

       6. Explain what you are doing to help reduce stress.

       7. At dismissal, allow them to remain in the chair longer to be certain that their equilibrium is well established.

       8. Aid them with their personal items and help them put on a coat or sweater, if necessary.

    B. Pregnant patients

       1. Pregnant patients may find it uncomforta-

POSITIONING THE OPERATING TEAM

OPERATOR

1. Adjust the stool to allow the operator's feet to rest firmly on the floor and to provide adequate support for the back.
2. The thighs should be parallel to the floor.
3. The patient's chair is lowered so that the chair back is nearly in the operator's lap over the thigh area.
4. The operator should be able to move freely in the operator's zone of activity.
5. The patient's head is positioned so that the mouth is as close as possible to the operator's elbow.
6. Elbows should be close to the side of the body.
7. Lower arms are nearly parallel to the floor.
8. Shoulders are parallel to the floor.
9. Back is straight.
10. Neck is not bent or strained.
11. Distance from the operator's eyes to the patient's mouth should be no less than 14 inches.

ASSISTANT

1. Position the stool as close to the patient's chair as possible.
2. The front edge of the stool should be nearly even with the patient's mouth to ensure that the assistant is in line with the patient's oral cavity.
3. Legs are parallel to the side of the chair and are facing the direction of the patient's head.
4. Feet rest on the rim of the stool and are parallel to the floor.
5. Position the body support to come around the left side and to support the assistant's torso when it is leaning forward, thereby reducing stress on the back and neck.
6. When seated, the assistant's eye level should be 4 to 6 inches higher than the operator's eye level. In general, the assistant's eye level should be just over the top of the operator's head (approximately 4 inches) when the work involves the maxillary arch; the eye level should be slightly higher for working on the mandibular arch.
7. Position the stool before positioning the mobile cabinet.
8. Position the mobile cabinet directly in front of the assistant's knees and as close to the chair as possible.
9. Avoid excessive bending or extending the arms to reach for materials or instruments.
10. Maintain a relatively straight back and neck.

ble to be supine or to sit for a long time without changing positions.
2. Tell the patient you plan to place her into a supine position and offer to modify this position to ensure her comfort.
C. Sensory-impaired patients
1. A patient who is blind or hearing impaired presents a different type of concern.
2. Frequently this person will be escorted to the office by a friend or family member who plans to help with communication.
3. Allow the patient to be as independent as possible.
4. Blind individuals communicate through other senses, such as touch, hearing, and taste. Therefore, explain what you are doing, let the patient feel the materials being used, and, if appropriate, explain that there might be an unpleasant taste from medicine being given.
5. A hearing-impaired patient sometimes has less obvious needs.
   a. The patient may smile or nod and appear to understand out of politeness.
   b. Establish the best communication possible: Stand directly in front of the patient, lower your mask, establish direct eye contact, and be sure that you have his or her attention. Speak slowly and distinctly.
   c. Do not overenunciate but speak normally because the patient may be lip-reading.
6. A physically impaired patient (especially one in a wheelchair) may require help getting into the dental chair.

Questions

Four-Handed Dentistry

1 Tray setups are beneficial because they
  1. Save preparation time
  2. Necessitate minimal monetary investment
  3. Eliminate delay in searching for instruments
  4. Are used only in restorative procedures
  5. Are adaptable to any procedure
  a. 1, 2, and 3
  b. 1, 3, and 5
  c. 2, 3, and 4
  d. 3, 4, and 5
2 Color coding preset trays permits
  a. Placement of more instruments on the trays

b. Easy identification of the procedure for which the tray is prepared

c. Quicker sterilization

d. More than one use for each tray

3 Hand instruments on preset trays are placed in

a. Order of use

b. Order of size

c. Random sequence

d. The order the assistant prefers

4 The best position for the instrument tray when assisting a dentist is in/on the

a. Static zone

b. Operator's zone

c. Assistant's zone

d. Fixed cabinetry

5 Indirect vision refers to

a. Looking at an object through protective glass

b. Looking at an object through a mirror

c. Looking directly at an object

d. Using fiberoptic lighting

6 Work surfaces should be located

a. 2 inches below the elbow

b. 4 inches below the elbow

c. 2 inches above the elbow

d. Even with elbow

7 When the assistant is seated in working position, the patient's calves should be

a. Parallel to the floor

b. Perpendicular to the floor

c. At an angle of 25 degrees from the floor

d. Varied according to the arch being worked on

8 If the operator is seated at the 11 o'clock position and the patient is seated upright, which of the following is/are true?

a. The labial surface of the anterior teeth will not be directly visible to the operator.

b. The lingual surface of mandibular anterior teeth will not be directly visible to the operator.

c. Both a and b are true.

d. Neither a nor b is true.

9 The classification of motion that involves movement of the entire arm and shoulder is

a. Class II

b. Class III

c. Class IV

d. Class V

10 Four-handed dentistry has which of the following objectives?

a. To increase productivity of the dental practice

b. To minimize stress and fatigue

c. To achieve high-quality dental service

d. All of the above

11 Which of the following is/are required to successfully practice four-handed dentistry?

1. Operating in a seated position

2. Employing skilled dental auxiliaries

3. Organization of the practice

4. Increasing the complexity of the procedure

a. 1 and 3

b. 1, 2, and 3

c. 1, 2, 3, and 4

d. 2 and 4

e. 4 only

In items 12-15, place an A for *True* or a B for *False* in the space provided as it relates to the statement.

_____ **12** A goal of four-handed dentistry should be to reduce the number of instruments to only those needed for the procedure at hand.

_____ **13** Preset trays are seldom used in four-handed dentistry because of the cost of instruments.

_____ **14** Class IV and V movements should be minimized in four-handed dentistry.

_____ **15** Work simplification often results in rearranging, eliminating, or combining and simplifying a procedure.

In questions 16-19, match the term in column A with the correct description in column B.

Column A	*Column B*
_____ **16** Operator's stool	a. Thin, narrow back
	b. Five castors
_____ **17** Assistant's stool	c. Four castors
	d. Accessible to right- or left-handed operator
_____ **18** Dental chair	
_____ **19** Dental unit	e. Adjustable intensity

20 Fiberoptic capabilities are available with

a. Intercom systems

b. Operating system

c. Handpieces

d. High-velocity evacuation systems

21 Which of the following is *not* a zone of activity?

a. Static

b. Transfer

c. Vision

d. Operator

In items 22-25, place an A for *True* or a B for *False* in the space provided.

_____ **22** The assistant's stool is placed as close to the patient chair as possible.

_____ **23** The assistant's legs are at a right angle to the patient's chair when the assistant is properly seated.

_____ **24** When seated, the assistant should be 4 to 6 inches higher than the operator.

_____ **25** If the operator is unable to see the field, he/she should adapt rather than moving the patient.

Rationales

Four-handed Dentistry

1 B Preset trays eliminate time and motion during patient preparation. They are used in all aspects of dentistry and can be adapted to any procedure. The initial purchase of instruments and trays will require a substantial investment, but the increased productivity will generally outweigh this cost.

2 B Color coding is used simply for identification purposes; to identify a procedure, a location, different operators, or a category of instruments.

3 A To maximize efficiency, hand instruments are placed in the sequence of use on a preset tray. This allows for quicker retrieval of instruments and eliminates disorganization.

4 C The instrument tray must be placed as close to the patient as possible and at the finger tips of the assistant. Therefore, it must be in the assistant's zone for maximum access. The mobile cabinet when not in use and other infrequently used instruments are stored in the static zone. The operator's zone is reserved for the operator to move about and should not house any instruments because they are not easily accessible to the assistant.

5 B Indirect vision is looking at a structure indirectly through the use of a mirror. The use of indirect vision allows the operator to observe an area in hard-to-access regions that would otherwise require imbalanced posture, causing undue stress or strain on the operator.

6 A Work surfaces that are slightly below elbow height are naturally comfortable and allow a person to reduce arm, neck, and back stress. If a working surface is too low or too high, stress is created. If it is not possible to lower the work area approximately 2 inches, then even with the elbow would be an alternative choice.

7 A The patient will be positioned in a supine position, which means that the patient is lying on the back, with the body parallel to the floor.

8 C With the operator at the 11 o'clock position and the patient seated upright, the operator would be directly observing the back of the patient's head. It is not possible for the operator to directly observe the anterior teeth in this position. It would be necessary to use a mirror for indirect vision or reposition the patient to provide direct vision of these sites.

9 C Classification of motion begins with class I as the motion requiring the least amount of movement. The classifications progress to higher levels as increased motion is required; class II, fingers and wrist; class III, fingers, wrist, and elbow; class IV, fingers, wrist, arm, and shoulder; class V, movement of the entire torso.

10 D Four-handed dentistry was designed to increase productivity while reducing stress and strain on the patient and operating team and maintaining quality care.

11 B Operating in a seated position ensures reduced potential stress for the operating team, thus increasing productivity. Employing skilled dental auxiliaries results in delivering dental care in a safe, efficient manner. An organized practice reduces the potential for errors and ensures an efficient productive environment. Increasing the complexity of a procedure only leads to increased time and motion and may result in additional stress and strain on the operating team.

12 A One of the objectives of motion economy is to reduce the number of instruments on a preset tray to those needed for a given procedure. Extra instruments require extra motion and reduce cost effectiveness.

13 B Preset trays are widely used in all phases of dentistry. The initial cost of the instruments and trays can be justified in the reduction in time and motion during the patient preparation phase of treatment.

14 A Class IV and V motions require the greatest number of movements to execute.

15 A Work simplification requires the dental team to examine the work process and determine how to minimize the amount of time and motion necessary to execute a given task. By rearranging equipment or materials, eliminating steps or procedures, or combining two steps into one the dental team is able to simplify their work.

16 C An operator's stool should have four castors and an assistant's five. The extra castors on the assistant's stool allow for increased stability since the chair needs to be raised to a higher level.

17 B See #16.

18 A One of the requisites of the patient chair is a thin, narrow back. This eliminates any obstruction to lowering the chair into the operator's lap and allows it to be adjusted to the lowest possible level.

19 D A transthorax unit is most desirable for four-handed dentistry. However, regardless of the type of unit, it should be able to be adapted to a left- or right-handed operator to avoid undue stress and easy access.

20 C Modern dental handpieces are supplied with fiberoptics that allow increased visibility for the dentist during intraoral procedures.

21 C The four zones of activity include the operator, assistant, transfer, and static zones.

22 A The assistant should be positioned as close to the patient as possible for increased intraoral visibility and ease of instrument transfer to the operator.

23 B The assistant's legs should be parallel to the patient chair. This enables the assistant to be positioned closer to the chair. Positioned at a right angle to the chair, the assistant will be further from the oral cavity, and this position will increase stress on the neck and back.

24 A Being 4 to 6 inches higher than the operator improves the assistant's visibility in the oral cavity. Positioned too low, it will not be possible to observe the site of the procedure and anticipate the needs of the operator. Such positioning can create stress and strain on the body and result in ineffectiveness.

25 B If you cannot see clearly, you cannot operate effectively. The environment, including the patient, should be altered. The patient will need to adjust for only a short time, whereas the operator will be working with many patients throughout the day and should be free of undue stress.

To enhance your understanding of the material in this chapter refer to the illustrations in Chapter 17 of Finkbeiner/Johnson: *Mosby's Comprehensive Dental Assisting: A Clinical Approach.*

CHAPTER 13

Dental Instruments and Instrumentation

KEY TERMS

Binangle	Handle	Palm grasp
Blade	Handpiece	Pen grasp
Bur	Hidden transfer	Rotary
Chuck	High-speed handpieces	Shaft
Cone socket handle	Instrument formula	Shank
Contra-angle	Instrument number	Single ended
Cutting edge	Instrument exchange	Single-handed exchange
Disk	Low-speed handpieces	Stone
Double ended	Mandrel	Torque
Fiberoptics	Modified pen grasp	Triple angle
Flutes	Monangle	Two-handed exchange
Fulcrum	Palm-thumb grasp	

Instruments are the primary domain of the chairside dental assistant, who is responsible for assembling and maintaining the sequence of instruments on the preset tray; exchanging instruments during treatment procedures; and sterilizing, ordering, maintaining, and sharpening instruments. Most dental instruments used in treatment today are either hand instruments, which require manual effort to operate, or rotary instruments, which are placed in some type of electronic handpiece.

The term **rotary,** when applied to cutting instruments used in dentistry, refers to a large group of devices—such as burs, stones, or disks—that rotate on an axis to cut, polish, abrade, and burnish tooth tissues and restorative materials in and out of the oral cavity. A **bur** is made of metal and fabricated into a variety of shapes. A **stone** is made of abrasive materials impregnated in a matrix and formed into various shapes. A **disk** is a flat paper, plastic, or metal surface impregnated with different abrasives.

This chapter emphasizes dental instruments used in

basic clinical dental procedures, common hand-cutting and rotary instruments, and the maintenance of these instruments. In each specialty chapter, such as oral surgery and endodontics, instruments unique to those specialties are described in detail.

HAND INSTRUMENTS

I. General Information about Instrument Design
  A. Dental instruments may be made of stainless steel, Teflon, or plastic.
  B. Hand instruments are supplied as **single ended (SE),** with one working end, or as **double ended (DE),** with two working ends.
  C. The working end of the instrument may be designed to provide a right or left end.
  D. Some instruments are designed to be used on the mesial or distal surfaces of the teeth.
  E. Some instruments may be designed to provide two distinct cutting or carving shapes.

II. Instrument Components
  A. **Handle** or **shaft**
    1. This is the portion by which the instrument is held.
    2. It may be smooth, ribbed or knurled, wide or narrow, round or square, cut into shapes like an octagon, or covered with plastic.
    3. Most handles are mounted to the shank of the instrument.
    4. Some instruments are designed with a **cone socket handle** that allows for the working end to be replaced; this handle is most commonly found in dental mirrors and scalers.
    5. Some instruments, such as the mirror, have a ruler calibration within the handle to check measurements of devices being used in the mouth during treatment.
  B. **Shank**
    1. This extends from the handle to the working end of the instrument.
    2. It is often angled to provide access to various areas of the mouth.
    3. The final angle of the shank is the actual working end.
    4. In hand-cutting instruments, the last angle is called the **blade;** it terminates in a **cutting edge.**
    5. In other instruments, the final angle of the shank may be a specialized shape.
    6. Shanks may be straight, with no angles; **monangle,** with one angle; **binangle,** with two angles; or **triple angle,** with three angles.

  C. **Blade**
    1. This is the final angle off the shank of the instrument.
    2. The terminal end of the blade is the cutting edge or working end of the instrument.
    3. In a hand-cutting instrument, such as a chisel or hatchet, a bevel extends at an angle off the end of the blade and terminates in a sharp cutting edge.
    4. Some instruments, such as cotton pliers and hemostats, have beaks that extend from the handle and do not have a blade.
    5. Instruments not used for cutting have working ends, referred to as *tips, nibs,* or *points.*
    6. Working ends may be smooth, serrated, or sharp and are designed in various shapes.

III. Instrument Nomenclature
  A. Most dental instruments have a name, formula, and manufacturer's number.
  B. Instruments are named according to their function.
  C. G. V. Black's **instrument formula** describes the dimension and angulation of a hand instrument.
    1. The formula is applied to all hand-cutting instruments that have cutting edges.
    2. The formula consists of three units, each with a measurement based on the metric system.
    3. The instrument formula is stamped on the handle by the manufacturer for each basic cutting instrument.
    4. An instrument with the formula 10 6 12 would have the following measurements:
      a. 10—the width of the blade in tenths of a millimeter; thus the width of this blade is 1 mm.
      b. 6—the length of the blade in millimeters; thus the length of this blade is 6 mm.
      c. 12—the angle of the blade in relation to the long axis of the handle or shaft in degrees centigrade; thus the angle of this blade is 12 degrees.
    5. In an instrument with a four-numbered formula, the second figure designates the angle of the cutting edge in relation to the blade.
  D. The dental manufacturer provides an **instrument number** on each dental instrument identifying the instrument for that manufacturer.
    1. The number correlates with the formula.

2. The higher the number, the larger the instrument size.

3. In hand-cutting instruments, a correlation exists between the instrument number and the instrument formula.

4. Manufacturers frequently use letter abbreviations in the instrument number to indicate the name of the instrument, as follows:
   a. B—burnisher
   b. BB—ball burnisher
   c. CP—cavity preparation (some form of hand-cutting instrument)
   d. GF—gold foil
   e. H—enamel hatchet
   f. C or CHI—chisel
   g. T—gingival margin trimmer
   h. PLG—plugger

IV. Categories of Instruments According to their Function
   A. Examination
   B. Cutting (hand and rotary)
   C. Insertion/condensing
   D. Finishing and polishing (hand and rotary)
   E. Adjunct
   F. A classification of hand instruments commonly used in operative dentistry is provided (box).
   G. A classification of the basic operative instruments is provided (Table 13-1).

V. Instrument Sharpening
   A. Using a dull instrument in the oral cavity can damage tissues and cause an avoidable accident.
   B. Chisels, hatchets, spoon excavators, gingival margin trimmers, and scalers should be sharpened routinely.
   C. Various devices are available for sharpening instruments, including the following:
      1. Electric oscillating instrument sharpener
      2. Assorted flat, conical, or cylindric stones in various grits
      3. Various mounted stones for use in a handpiece
   D. Sharpening oil is applied to the surface of most of these stones to prevent frictional heat, which could temper the metal and wash away metal particles
   E. Suggestions for sharpening instruments are listed (box on page 222).
   F. The oscillating instrument sharpener has preset guides for various cutting angles (box on page 222).
   G. Free-hand sharpening with mounted stones is frequently used to sharpen scalers.

CLASSIFICATION OF HAND INSTRUMENTS

EXAMINATION

Explorer
Mirror
Cotton pliers
Articulating paper forceps
Probes

CUTTING

Angle former
Chisel
Excavator
Gingival marginal trimmer
Hatchet
Hoe

INSERTION/CONDENSING

Plastic instrument
Placement instrument
Amalgam carrier
Condenser
Gingival cord packer

CARVING

Anatomic
Smooth surface

FINISHING AND POLISHING

Burnishers
Orangewood stick
Finishing strips
Amalgam files
Knives

ADJUNCT

Thumb forceps
Scissors
Dappen dishes
Napkin chains
Pliers
Spatulas
Matrices

ROTARY INSTRUMENTS

I. The **handpiece** is the electronic device that provides rotary action when used in conjunction with various attachments.
   A. The handpiece enables the operator to cut, polish, and abrade tooth tissue; cut bone; and polish and burnish all types of preventive and restorative materials.

Table 13-1 Classification of instruments

Instrument/device	Physical characteristics	Function
EXAMINATION INSTRUMENTS		
Explorer	Double ended (DE) or single ended (SE): sharp, pointed working end; common shapes are cowhorn, right angle, and shepherd's hook; graphite tips available	Detects tooth anomalies; checks margins or restorations; detects calculus
Mirror	SE: disposable or nondisposable; regular or cone socket handle; single or double sided; flat or concave face; width 7/8 to 2 inches; ruler calibration on handle available	Indirect vision; indirect illumination; retraction of cheek, lips, tongue
Tissue/cotton/pliers	SE: serrated or smooth beaks, pointed beaks; locking or nonlocking; angled beaks; groove in center of beak for grasping endodontic points	Grasp oral tissues; transfer materials into and out of oral cavity
Articulating-paper forceps	SE: locking pliers; beak parallel to handle	Grasps and holds articulating paper for insertion into oral cavity
Probe	DE or SE: pointed working end; calibrated in millimeters; various combinations; may have color-coded millimeter markings; Expro is combination of explorer and periodontal probe	Measures depth of gingival sulcus
CUTTING INSTRUMENTS		
Angle former	DE or SE: modification of a chisel; supplied in right and left; cutting edge at angle to blade; commonly beveled on side and end of blade	Defines line angles; places retention in dentin and bevels on enamel margins in cavity preparation
Chisel	DE or SE: standard or reverse bevel; cutting edge is at right angle to plane of instrument; Wedelstaedt chisel has curved blade	Planes and cleaves enamel and dentin walls during cavity preparation
Excavator	DE or SE: spoon-shaped blade that is rounded; wide range of sizes; curved blade	Removes soft carious debris from cavity preparation; places cavity medication; inverts rubber dam into gingival sulcus
Gingival marginal trimmer	DE or SE: instrument supplied as mesial or distal; each has a right and left end; angled cutting edge; curved blade	Places bevel at mesial or distal cervical and pulpal margins
Hatchet	DE or SE: paired right and left; cutting edge in same plane as the instrument	Prepares retention, sharpens internal line angles, and smooths internal cavity walls during tooth preparation
Hoe	DE or SE: cutting edge at right angle to blade; blade at nearly right angle to handle; commonly triple angle shank	Creates retention form in dentin; used with pull action
CONDENSING/INSERTION INSTRUMENTS		
Plastic instruments	DE or SE: plastic or metal; tip ends have various shapes, e.g., round, flat, or paddlelike; special modifications	Place composite restorative material or dental cements into cavity preparation
Amalgam carrier	DE or SE: mini to large end; plastic or metal; metal or Teflon ends; carrier or gun style; retrograde for endodontic filling	Transports amalgam to cavity preparation
Condenser/plugger	DE: smooth or serrated ends; flat or concave; square or ovoid ends; plain or tapered ends; monangle, binangle or triple-angle shank	Condenses amalgam into compact mass; removes excess mercury; adapts amalgam to cavity walls
Gingival cord placement instruments	DE: thin blade; resembles condenser; plain or serrated tip end	Place gingival retraction cord into gingival sulcus
Placement instrument	SE: small ball burnisher-type working end; shorter handle than traditional instruments; delicate working end	Places cavity medications

Table 13-1 Classification of instruments—*cont'd*

Instrument/device	Physical characteristics	Function
CARVING INSTRUMENTS		
Anatomic	DE: disk or clawlike end; rounded or spoon shaped	Recreate anatomic form in occlusal surface of amalgam restoration
Smooth surface	DE: flat, elongated, knifelike blade	Contour buccal, lingual, and proximal surfaces of amalgam restoration
FINISHING AND POLISHING		
Burnishers	DE or SE: flat, pointed, or circular rounded ends	Burnish or polish hardened metallic surfaces and cavosurface margins; refine anatomy
Orangewood stick/ points	Sticks, pegs, or points; soft, splinter-proof wood	Sticks or pegs aid in seating restoration such as crowns, bridges, or inlays; soft points used to polish teeth
Finishing strips	Linen or metal; extra fine to coarse grit; narrow to wide	Polish or finish interproximal tooth or restorative surfaces
ADJUNCT INSTRUMENTS		
Thumb forceps	Straight beak	Aids in maintaining aseptic working area; transfers materials to operative site from clean area; used extraorally only
Scissors	Many variations: straight or curved; sharp or blunt tips; suture, surgical, tissue, bandage, crown, and collar	Cut tissue, sutures, and a variety of materials
Dappen dish	Metal or glass; single or double ended; concave ends	Holds medicaments and various dental materials
Napkin chain	Alligator-like beaks for holding; metal or plastic	Holds patient napkin in place; holds materials
Spatulas	Various shaped blades: flat, curved, or pointed; narrow or wide; flexible or rigid; all metal or combination metal blade with wooden or plastic handle	Mix plaster or cements; carve wax or porcelain
Matrix	Plastic, celluloid, or metal strips; various widths; curved or straight; modifications in shapes	Provides missing wall when placing restorative material

B. **Fiberoptics** in a handpiece increases the visibility of the operative field.

C. The belt-and-pulley engine is dedicated primarily to laboratory use.

D. Two speeds of handpieces are available in dentistry today:

1. **Low-speed** (conventional) **handpieces** operate under 30,000 rpm.
   a. Applications of low-speed handpieces are listed (box on page 223).
   b. They are available in a standard and shorty or mini, with a single speed of 0 to 10,000 rpm or with multiple speeds ranging from 0 to 30,000 rpm.
   c. They are equipped to operate in a forward or reverse mode.
   d. They are often referred to as *straight handpieces*.
   e. They may have attachments called an angle or **contra-angle** that hold a rotary device.

2. **High-speed** (ultra-speed) **handpieces** operate at 30,000 to 600,000 rpm.
   a. Applications of high-speed handpieces are listed (box on page 223).
   b. They are used for rapid cutting of hard tissues.
   c. They are ready to be used with only a bur added; they never require the addition of an angle.
   d. High-speed handpieces often lack **torque** (the force to rotate) when excess pressure is applied.
   e. They are designed with water coolant systems and optional features, including lasers and fiberoptics.
   f. Most manufacturers produce a standard and a pediatric style.

METHOD FOR HAND SHARPENING INSTRUMENTS

1. Instruments and sharpening stones must be sterile to avoid cross-contamination during sharpening. At the conclusion of the sharpening procedures, these devices are sterilized before they are returned to their appropriate storage areas.
2. Examine the blade contours. Hold the blade at eye level and observe the angle of the cutting edge from the side. The use of magnifying loupes helps in evaluating the condition of the cutting edge.
3. The cutting edge must have an angle acute enough to cut but not so acute that the blade is weakened and breaks. Cutting angles of most hand-cutting instruments are about 50 degrees, compared with instruments with more acute angles, such as razors or scalpel blades that are used to cut soft tissue.
4. A dull instrument is created if the thin cutting edge breaks away in tiny metallic fragments when it is used against rough enamel. After repeated use the cutting edge becomes rounded or flattened and is no longer efficient. A dull edge usually can be observed by holding the blade to reflect light. A dull instrument produces sharp lines or catches in the light.
5. To sharpen the instrument on a flat stone, place a couple of drops of sharpening oil on the stone. Spread the oil evenly over the surface (carefully, with your fingers or with a 2 × 2 gauze sponge) to create a light film.
6. To recreate the sharp edge on the cutting instrument, remove metal evenly from the beveled surface so that it remains flat and the angle of the cutting edge is maintained.
7. An instrument like a chisel is place on the stone. The bevel is placed flat against the stone and pressure is applied to the instrument to move it across the length of the stone. This is done in one direction. On the return stroke, no pressure is applied.
8. As the blade moves across the sharpening stone, the direction must be straight and steady, with even pressure applied to the beveled surface. Avoid rocking or tilting the blade back and forth. This will alter the contour and prevent obtaining a sharp cutting edge.
9. Test the blade for sharpness by placing the blade on a plastic test rod at about a 45-degree angle, with the cutting edge pressing into the rod. If the cutting edge pierces the rod, it is sharp; if it glides over the rod, it is still dull.
10. When the desired sharpness is achieved, wipe the instrument free of the oil and fragments with gauze that has been saturated in alcohol. Continue to sharpen other instruments. At the conclusion of all sharpening, wipe the stone free of debris and oil and sterilize the stone and instruments.

    E. Most handpieces are activated by air passing over a variety of gears and turbines.

II. Various symbols and terms related to the use of rotary instruments include the following:

    A. *L*—long cutting surface. A bur with the number #169L would provide a longer cutting surface, allowing the operator to cut a greater length of tissue.

    B. *S*—short shank. The cutting surface of this bur is the same size as standard burs, but the length of the shank, which is the part that attaches to the handpiece, is shortened to allow the bur to be used in areas that are difficult to access.

    C. *FG*—friction grip. These burs have shorter shanks and are used only in handpieces and contra-angles with some type of **chuck** that holds them in place by friction.

    D. *RA*—right angle. This style of rotary device, whether it is a bur, stone, or disk, has a small latch at the base of the shank; placed into a latch-type contra-angle, it will be at a right angle to the head of the angle.

OSCILLATING INSTRUMENT MACHINE SHARPENER

1. Place the hand-cutting instrument into the appropriate slotted guide, which aids in steadily supporting the blade end while the wheel oscillates.
2. Make sure the instrument contacts the wheel surface at the predetermined angle before turning the unit on.
3. Press only lightly to bring the instrument into contact with the wheel. Extended contact will result in heat generation, can reduce the length of the blade, and may shorten the working life of the instrument.
4. The instrument can be placed on a rotating felt wheel to remove any metallic burs that remain after the sharpening process.

APPLICATIONS OF LOW-SPEED HANDPIECES

- Polishing teeth during a prophylaxis procedure
- Removing stains from teeth
- Refining cavity preparations after the tooth has been opened and shaped with a high-speed handpiece
- Removing soft carious material from the tooth during cavity preparation
- Making an occlusal adjustment of natural tooth or a restoration
- Making a smooth cut on a tooth with a disk
- Smoothing or burnishing a tooth with a stone or disk
- Polishing a restoration
- Grinding and finishing acrylic or metal on a prosthesis

APPLICATIONS OF HIGH-SPEED HANDPIECES

- Cutting/preparing tooth tissue to receive some form of restoration, such as amalgam, composite, or gold casting
- Sectioning a tooth for surgical removal
- Removing faulty restorations
- Finishing restorations, using specialized burs

TRADITIONAL BURS

- Inverted cone (series 33½ to 39 or 43)
- Round (series ¼ to 10)
- Straight fissure—plain cut (series 55 to 64)
- Straight fissure—crosscut (series 555 to 564)
- Tapered fissure—plain cut (series 169 to 172)
- Tapered fissure—crosscut (series 699 to 708)

stones, disks, and rubber points and wheels, often in conjunction with a polishing agent.

   L. *Finish*—Finishing is not unlike burnishing and polishing; it means removing excess restorative material from the margins and contours of a restoration to ensure a smooth line of demarcation between the cavosurface margin of the preparation and the restoration.

III. Various attachments are used, including angles, burs, stones, disks, and mandrels.
   A. Common types of angles include the following:
     1. Prophylaxis angle or right angle
     2. Contra-angle
     3. Auto Klutch chuck angle
     4. Endodontic head contra-angle
   B. Burs are divided into two parts: shank and working end.
     1. Three types of shanks are friction grip, latch type or right angle, and straight handpiece.
     2. Bur series denotes common size range (box above).
     3. Traditional bur shapes are shown in Fig. 13-1; other bur shapes available include end cutting (series 956 to 957), straight dome (series 1156 to 1158), tapered dome (series 1169 to 1172), straight dome—crosscut (series 1156 to 1558), and tapered dome—crosscut (series 1700 to 1702).
     4. Burs are designed to cut tooth tissue and bone, remove soft carious material from the dentin, burnish margins of restorations, cut restorative materials, and polish and finish restorations.
     5. Burs are made of steel or tungsten carbide.
     6. The difference between a cutting bur and a finishing bur is the number of **flutes** (cutting surfaces) in the working end; the more flutes on a bur, the greater the polishing capability.
     7. Diamond rotary instruments can be categorized as stones or burs; their primary func-

   E. *HP*—handpiece. Burs with this designation have longer shanks and are used only in a straight handpiece.
   F. *Mounted* versus *unmounted*—on a mounted rotary, the **stone** or **disk** is permanently mounted to a shaft or mandrel; an unmounted stone or disk must be attached to a mandrel or a shaft for use.
   G. *T & F*—Trimming and finishing burs and stones are designed in a shape and style that can be used in finishing and trimming tooth surfaces or restorations.
   H. *FF*—fine finishing. These burs and stones are designed with a more delicate cutting edge or have a finer grit for use in fine finishing of margins and various types of restorations.
   I. *Abrade*—to wear or cut away a tooth or restorative material by friction.
   J. *Burnish*—Burnishing is a process related to polishing, smoothing, and abrading that is commonly accomplished during the polishing of gold.
   K. *Polish*—Polishing makes a tooth or restorative material smooth and glossy, giving luster to the surface. This is accomplished with brushes,

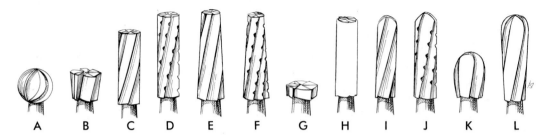

Fig. 13-1 Basic shapes of burs. Six traditional burs *A* through *F;* basic shapes of traditional cutting burs; round, inverted cone, straight fissure-plain cut, straight fissure-cross cut, tapered fissure-plain cut, tapered fissure-cross cut. Also illustrated are *G,* wheel shape, *H,* end cutting, *I,* round end fissure-plain cut, *J,* round end fissure-cross cut, *K,* round dome, and *L,* tapered dome burs.

tion is for tooth reduction in operative dentistry.

C. Abrasive points and disks
 1. A variety of points, disks, and wheels are available in assorted materials and shapes.
 2. A **mandrel** is a shaft onto which some type of disk, stone, or rubber device is placed.
 3. Disks are thin, flat circular objects made of metal, paper, or plastic that are used to polish, cut, or smooth teeth or restorative materials; supplied in a variety of sizes.

D. Acrylic stones and burs are large, bulky devices used to cut and polish acrylic denture base material. The stones can reduce the denture base while giving a smooth finish.

E. Supplemental components include the following:
 1. One component is a bur tool or device.
 2. A chuck is placed in the head of the handpiece as a retentive device for the bur.
 3. A hose connector gasket provides a tight seal between the handpiece and the hose.

IV. A checklist for using rotary devices is shown (box).

INSTRUMENT EXCHANGE

I. Instrument Exchange or Transfer
 A. **Instrument exchange** or transfer increases efficiency and reduces stress during routine dental treatment.
 B. Efficient instrument exchange can accomplish the following:
  1. It enables the operator to keep his or her eyes on the field of operation.
  2. It saves time and motion for the operating team.
  3. It reduces stress and strain on the operating team.
  4. When an instrument exchange is used in

CHECKLIST FOR USING ROTARY DEVICES

1. Are all of the rotary devices and attachments that are to be used for this procedure at chairside on the mobile cabinetry?
2. Were these devices sterilized before use on this patient?
3. Is the attachment, such as a contra-angle, bur, or stone, securely in place for use by the operator?
4. Has the appropriate handpiece been turned on and placed in position to be used?
5. After the procedure has been completed, were all of the rotary devices removed from the handpieces?
6. Are the chucks still secure in the handpieces?
7. Were the angles, burs, and handpieces properly sterilized after use on each patient?

---

conjunction with the oral evacuator and the air/water syringe, the operator can ensure that the operative site is always clean and the next instrument always ready for use.

C. The assistant's job at chairside is multifaceted and includes the following:
 1. Maintaining a clear, dry field of operation
 2. Retracting tissues that interfere with the operator's view of the treatment site
 3. Anticipating the operator's next need
 4. Passing the next instrument when needed
 5. Observing the patient's needs and vital signs
 6. Preparing materials or medicaments when needed
 7. Maintaining infection-control procedures

II. Common Instrument Grasps
 A. The **pen grasp** allows the instrument to be used the way a pen or pencil is used.

B. In the **modified pen grasp,** the operator uses the pad of the middle finger on the handle of the instrument.

C. The **palm grasp,** used for large bulky instruments, requires the operator to turn the hand back and open the palm to receive the instrument.

D. The **palm-thumb grasp** is used with instruments that require vertical movement, such as the Wedelstaedt chisel.

III. Common Methods for Instrument Exchange

A. The primary objective of instrument exchange is to ensure that four hands are always at work.

B. To accomplish an efficient exchange the following criteria must be met:

1. The instrument must be positioned for the arch that is being treated.

2. The operator must be able to grasp the instrument in a normal holding position without unnecessary hand movement.

3. The operator must keep his or her eyes on the field of operation.

4. If a double-ended instrument is being used, the appropriate end must be placed in the working position.

C. The basic instrument exchanges used in dentistry include the following:

1. **Two-handed exchange**

a. The assistant picks up the used instrument with one hand and delivers a new instrument with the opposite hand.

b. This exchange requires more movement than others and limits efficient use of the high-velocity evacuation and air/water syringe.

c. This is not the preferred exchange in operative procedures but may be used in oral surgery.

2. **Single-handed exchange**

a. Two areas of the assistant's passing hand are used: the *delivery* portion and the *pickup* portion.

(1) The delivery portion of the hand includes the thumb and first two fingers.

(2) The pickup portion includes the third and small fingers (Fig. 13-2).

b. The single-handed exchange allows the assistant to take the used instrument from the operator with the pickup portion of the hand and deliver the new instrument with the delivery portion of the same hand.

c. The assistant's opposite hand is free for retraction or oral evacuation.

d. This is the most common technique used in operative dentistry.

e. The procedure for instrument exchange is provided (box on page 226).

3. **Hidden transfer**

a. This technique is used to hide an instrument or a device (such as a local anesthetic syringe) from the patient.

b. A single-handed transfer can be used to exchange 2 × 2 gauze sponges, topical anesthetic, or an explorer.

c. During the transfer of the syringe, the two-handed transfer must be used while the operator receives the syringe in a palm grasp.

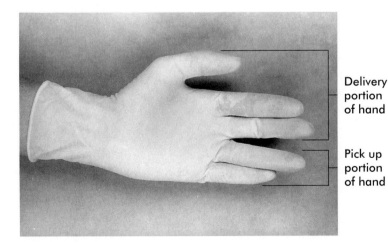

Delivery portion of hand

Pick up portion of hand

Fig. 13-2   The area of the exchange hand is divided into two parts—the delivery portion, which includes the thumb and first two fingers, and the pickup portion, which includes the third and small finger.

INSTRUMENT EXCHANGE: TEAM APPROACH	
OPERATOR	ASSISTANT
	Assemble instruments in sequence of use.
	Place on mobile cart.
	Place instrument tray as close to patient as possible.
	Using the left hand, pick up the explorer at the third of the instrument nearest you, and with the right hand pick up the mirror by the nonworking end of the handle.
	Position instruments in the delivery portion of the hands.
Bring both hands into the transfer zone.	Move hands with instruments into the transfer zone.
Position hands to receive mirror and explorer in a pen grasp.	Deliver both instruments with a firm motion.
Position in oral cavity.	
Signal for an exchange by lifting instrument from treatment site with right hand while maintaining fulcrum.	Pick up instrument to be transferred with left hand at the third of the instrument nearest you.
	Position instrument in delivery portion of hand.
	Move hand to transfer zone.
Bring instrument out of patient's mouth into transfer zone.	Parallel new instrument with used instrument.
	Pick up used instrument with the pickup portion of hand.
	Tuck instrument into palm.
	Deliver new instrument.
Grasp new instrument and return to treatment site.	Roll instrument back to end of fingertips and reposition in delivery portion of hand.
	Retain instrument in this position if to be used again.
	Return instrument to original position on tray if not to be used again.

   d. The syringe is hidden from the patient's view.
   e. This can be performed in the transfer zone or behind the patient's head to hide the syringe from the patient.
D. Team responsibilities in instrument exchange are as follows:
   1. For effective instrument exchange to take place, both clinicians must be committed to the concept of instrument exchange and be willing to assume specific responsibilities.
   2. Both the operator and the assistant must be concerned about safety and proper infection-control techniques during the exchange of all instruments and materials.
   3. Suggested responsibilities of the assistant and operator are listed (box on page 227).
   4. Safety precautions to follow for the protection of all concerned are listed (box on page 227).
E. Modifications for special instruments or situations are as follows:

   1. Dental mirror and explorer
      a. Initially, the mirror and explorer are passed simultaneously.
      b. Subsequent exchanges of the mirror are generally confined to the completion of the procedure or to times when it is not needed for retraction or indirect vision.
      c. Exchange of the explorer is the same as for other instruments.
   2. Scissors
      a. The operator must change finger position to receive scissors.
      b. The operator must turn the receiving hand outward and spread the fingers open to receive the scissors.
      c. The assistant picks up the scissors with the left hand and opens the handles slightly with the right hand.
      d. When the operator signals for the exchange, the assistant holds the scissors in the hinged area near the beak end and parallel with the operator's instrument,

RESPONSIBILITIES DURING INSTRUMENT EXCHANGE
OPERATOR
• Develop a standardized routine for basic dental procedures.   • Confine movements to the oral cavity and transfer zone.   • Maintain a fulcrum in the oral cavity.   • Avoid removing instruments from the preset tray.   • Develop a nonverbal signal denoting a need for instrument exchange.   • After giving the signal for an instrument exchange, place the used instrument in a position that will enable the assistant to easily parallel the new instrument without twisting the hand.   • When necessary, give advance distinct verbal direction to communicate a need for a different instrument. This should be done in plenty of time so as not to disrupt the flow of the procedure.   • Keep your eyes on the operative site.
ASSISTANT
• Develop a thorough understanding of the procedure.   • Maintain instruments in sequence of use.   • Anticipate the operator's need for the next instrument.   • Be alert to any change in the procedure and be ready to modify the sequence of instruments when necessary.   • Position the instrument for the proper arch—up for maxillary, down for mandibular.   • Have the next instrument ready and close to the transfer area before the operator gives the signal.   • Follow a safe standardized exchange procedure.   • Use positive pressure to ensure that the operator knows without looking up that the instrument has been delivered.   • Remove debris from the used instrument before returning it to the tray or the operator for use again.   • Keep preset tray and work area free of debris and disarray.

SAFETY PRECAUTIONS FOR THE OPERATOR AND ASSISTANT
• Limit movement that takes place outside the mouth to the transfer zone.   • Follow a safe, standardized exchange that allows secure pickup and delivery of the instrument.   • Firmly control the instrument at all times.   • Avoid tense movement.   • Deliver the instrument with positive pressure to the operator to ensure that it is in place.   • Observe patient movement, especially during transfer of a syringe or sharp instrument, to avoid contacting the patient with an instrument.   • Do not lay instruments or material on the patient napkin.

3. Tissue forceps (locking and nonlocking)
   a. Used forceps generally have some material between the beaks, such as a cotton pellet, articulating paper, or a wooden wedge.
   b. Locking pliers provide stability to the device being transferred.
   c. With nonlocking pliers, the material must be placed securely in the beaks before transfer.
   d. The assistant holds the forceps with the left hand, inserts the material to be transferred, and then grasps the forceps at the back end, firmly holding the beaks closed and positioning the instrument parallel with the instrument being exchanged; the transfer then takes place.
   e. During the return of the forceps, the assistant receives the working end of the forceps in the palm of the hand to prevent potential dropping of the contaminated contents from the forceps.
4. Dental handpieces
   a. Handpieces can be passed with the single-handed technique.
   b. After the handpiece is removed from the unit, it is paralleled; the finger signal is given for the exchange, the used instrument is picked up and tucked, and the handpiece is delivered.
   c. The return of the handpiece to the assistant's pickup portion of the hand is done in the same manner as with other instruments.

placing the curve according to the arch being treated. The assistant picks up the used instrument, and the operator places the thumb and first or second fingers into the finger rings of the scissors.
   e. The scissors are returned with the beaks toward the assistant and the normal exchange resumes.

d. During transfer of handpieces, care must be taken to avoid placing the cords on the patient's chest or face.

5. Air/water syringe
   a. The assistant grasps the tip of the a/w syringe in the delivery portion of the hand, positions the tip parallel (as closely as possible) to the used instrument, retrieves the instrument to be exchanged, and transfers the syringe so that the operator can grasp the handle.
   b. The assistant retrieves the air/water syringe by grasping the tip and then delivers the new instrument.
   c. Paralleling the new instrument is not easy during this exchange.

6. Dental cement
   a. The instrument used to insert the cement is passed in a single-handed transfer.
   b. The assistant holds the dental cement in its prepared state, on a pad or cement slab, under the patient's chin and in the transfer zone for the dentist to pick up with the packing instrument.
   c. The mixing slab with the material can be held in the right hand, and the left hand can be used to wipe the excess material from the instrument with a 2 × 2 gauze sponge.

7. Small items
   a. Items such as cotton rolls, 2 × 2 sponges, or cotton-tipped applicators, are treated just as any other hand instrument.
   b. Items are passed with the delivery portion of the hand and can be retrieved with the pickup portion.

F. Instruments for intraoral use are transferred as follows. This technique describes the process used with a right-handed operator:
   1. The grasps described earlier are used.
   2. Dental mirror
      a. Hold the dental mirror in the nonworking hand.
      b. Grasp the mirror with the thumb, middle finger, and index finger of the left hand using the pen grasp.
      c. To use the modified pen grasp, assume a comfortable working position, place the pad (instead of the side) of the middle finger against the shank of the mirror; the thumb and index finger should be opposite each other at the junction of the handle and the shank of the mirror. The handle will rest against the hand at any point beyond the first joint of the index finger, stabilizing the mirror.
      d. The operator must orient the mind and eye to using a dental mirror for indirect vision.
      e. Everything in the mirror is a reflection, and the hand instrument seen in the mirror's reflection must be coordinated with the image the eye sees.
      f. The mirror is placed in the patient's mouth while the small finger and ring finger retract the cheek.
      g. The mirror is placed and the light positioned for adequate illumination.
      h. The mirror is moved back and forth until a complete and clear image of the tooth or tissues is reflected in the mirror.
   3. Explorer
      a. Hold the explorer with a light but firm pen or modified pen grasp in the right hand for a right-handed operator and in the left hand for a left-handed operator.
      b. When an exploratory stroke is used, the instrument must be held lightly to ensure maximum tactile sensitivity.
      c. A **fulcrum** (finger rest) should be maintained on teeth that are close to the working area or site being explored.
      d. When the work area is on posterior maxillary teeth, it may be necessary to use an alternative rest, such as the mandibular teeth on the opposite arch.
      e. The dental assistant may use the explorer to check and mark the cervical margins of temporary crowns; check the hardness of a pit and fissure sealant; contour a periodontal dressing; or remove supragingival cement, an intraoral temporary, or a piece of rubber dam at the interproximal surface.
      f. During each of these tasks the explorer is used in three different positions: *vertical, oblique,* and *horizontal* (Fig. 13-3).
         (1) The margins of a temporary crown are examined with the vertical stroke to detect unnecessary bulk or roughness. If the tip gets caught on the cervical margin of the crown, this area will require modification or recontouring to prevent it from irritating the gingival tissues.
         (2) The horizontal and oblique strokes

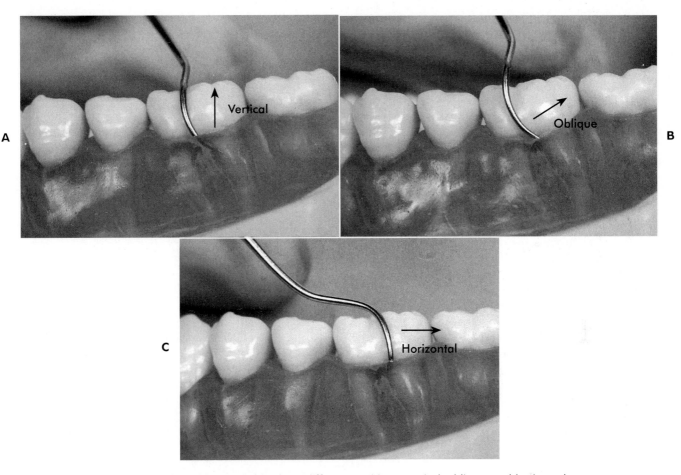

Fig. 13-3 The explorer used in three different positions: vertical, oblique, and horizontal.

aid in defining contours. The tip of the explorer can also be used to mark a metal crown that is too long and needs to be relieved at the cervical margin.

g. To use the explorer effectively, observe the following guidelines:

(1) Grasp the handle of the explorer in the operating hand in a modified pen grasp, with the middle finger on the shank of the instrument to increase tactile ability.

(2) Careful control of the explorer is necessary; this sharp instrument can puncture tissue.

(3) When the explorer is held properly, the operator has maximum tactile sense as well as complete control of patient and operator safety.

(4) Practice manipulating the explorer by grasping it between the thumb and

the opposing index and middle fingers and slowly rotating it clockwise.

(5) Continue this rotation until the instrument is turned approximately 180 degrees; then roll the handle counterclockwise to its original position.

4. Rotary instruments

a. Handpieces are bulky instruments, and—like the mirror and other hand instruments—dexterous use promotes safety.

b. Many of the legally delegable duties for auxiliaries that require the use of handpieces are performed outside the patient's mouth.

c. The differences between the use of a handpiece and a hand instrument include the following:

(1) Irreversible damage can be caused more commonly by misuse of a handpiece than a hand instrument.

(2) Maintaining a fulcrum when using a

handpiece is similar to that of hand instruments; however, the handpiece rotates and can cause damage to surrounding tissues or materials.

(3) The handpiece should not be activated until it is in the oral cavity.

(4) Handpieces are activated by energy through the use of another device, such as a foot control, and have varying speeds.

(5) For a handpiece to function, some type of attachment must be added to the working end, such as a bur, disk, or polishing cup.

(6) Because the handpiece is bulky, it must be held firmly to maintain control.

(7) Hold the handpiece in a palm-thumb or pen grasp, either of which allows the operator to maintain a fulcrum, intraorally or extraorally.

(8) Establish the fulcrum, turn on the handpiece, and place the working end on the surface that is to be treated.

(9) Exercise caution when using the handpiece to avoid exerting excess pressure.

Questions

Dental Instruments and Instrumentation

1 The assistant can help increase the dentist's visibility by
1. Using high-velocity evacuation
2. Eliminating the use of certain instruments
3. Using the air/water syringe
4. Retracting soft tissues
5. Using premixed materials
a. 1, 2, and 3
b. 1, 3, and 4
c. 2, 3, and 4
d. 3, 4, and 5

2 The assistant holds the hand instrument to be transferred between the
a. Thumb and first two fingers
b. Small finger and palm
c. Thumb and palm
d. Small finger and forefinger

3 A fulcrum is the
a. Amount of amalgam flow in 24 hours
b. Rest point on a prosthetic surveyor
c. Type of matrix retainer
d. Stationary point of a lever system

4 Hand-cutting instruments are used in restorative dentistry to
a. Remove deep carious lesions
b. Refine cavity preparations
c. Trim excess restorative material
d. All of the above

5 The operator wants to use a handpiece to remove the remaining carious dentin from the tooth. For this purpose a(n) _____ bur and a _____ handpiece would be used.
a. Inverted cone; low-speed
b. Inverted cone; high-speed
c. Tapered fissure; high-speed
d. Round; high-speed
e. Round; low-speed

6 The operator wants to open a cavity preparation on a premolar. For this purpose a _____ bur and a _____ handpiece would be used.
a. #34; low-speed
b. #34; high-speed
c. #2; low-speed
d. #57; low-speed
e. #57; high-speed

7 A cleoid-discoid instrument can be used as follows:
a. To carve the occlusal detail in a posterior restoration
b. To carve smooth surfaces of posterior amalgam restorations
c. To smooth and finish composite restorations
d. To finish the cavity preparation

In items 8-11, match each instrument in column A with a function in column B.

Column A	Column B
_____ **8** Ward's carver	a. Used in a push action to remove unsupported enamel
_____ **9** Hatchet	b. Retrieves devices from the mobile cart
_____ **10** Hoe	c. Carves anatomic grooves in amalgam
_____ **11** 5C carver	d. Used in a pull action to remove tooth structure
	e. Carves smooth surfaces of amalgam

12 Which instrument has a standard and reversed bevel?
a. Enamel hatchet
b. Wedelstaedt chisel
c. Spoon excavator
d. Gingival marginal trimmer

13 Which of the following instruments are considered a basic setup for most dental procedures?
1. Cotton pliers
2. Oral evacuator
3. Explorer
4. Dental floss
5. Mouth mirror
6. Thumb forceps
a. 1, 3, and 5
b. 1, 3, 5, and 6
c. 2 and 3
d. 2, 3, and 4

In items 14-16, place an A for *True* or a B for *False* in the space provided.

_____ **14** The larger the manufacturer's number on a hand-cutting instrument, the larger the instrument formula.

_____ **15** A DE spoon would supply both right and left working ends.

_____ **16** A DE gingival marginal trimmer would supply both mesial and distal working ends.

In items 17-20, select the appropriate device from column B that matches the function in column A.

Column A	Column B
_____ **17** Used in the laboratory to make gross cutting as in a denture alignment	a. Moore's mandrel
	b. Acrylic bur
	c. Craytex wheel
_____ **18** Tan-colored polishing device that is impregnated with pumice	d. Burlew disk
	e. Joe-Dandy disk
_____ **19** Made of carborundum	
_____ **20** Rubberlike device used to polish gold	

In items 21-25, place letters of the following steps in the spaces provided to indicate the sequence of steps used in exchanging an instrument. Begin by placing the letter of the first task on line 21 and continue to 25.

a. When the dentist signals, parallel the new instrument with the used instrument.

b. Roll the used instrument back into the delivery position.

c. Grasp the used instrument with the third finger and small finger and tuck the used instrument into the palm.

d. Deliver the new instrument into the dentist's hand.

e. If the instrument is not to be used, return the instrument to its original position on the tray.

_____ **21**
_____ **22**
_____ **23**
_____ **24**
_____ **25**

Rationales

Dental Instruments and Instrumentation

1 B To increase the dentist's visibility it is necessary to retract soft tissues and maintain a clear, dry field. The assistant needs to use the air/water syringe to maintain a clean mirror and a clear, dry operative field.

2 A The hand is divided into two parts—the delivery portion and the pickup portion. The delivery portion includes the thumb and first two fingers and is used to deliver the new instrument to the operator after the used instrument has been picked up with the third and small finger.

3 D A fulcrum is the point of support on which a lever turns. In dentistry, a fulcrum is the point of support where the operator places a finger or portion of the hand to maintain stability while using an instrument or handpiece.

4 D Hand-cutting instruments can be used to examine, cut, insert, condense, finish, or polish hard or soft tissues.

5 E A low-speed handpiece enables the operator to cut through soft, carious material. A high-speed handpiece would only spin and not cut soft debris. The round bur would be chosen because it cuts more effectively in this situation and would act as a scooping device.

6 B High speed is needed to cut through enamel effectively. Either a round or an inverted cone would commonly be used.

7 A A cleoid-discoid carver is an anatomic carver and can be used to create the pits and fissures found in the occlusal anatomy of amalgam restorations. These anatomic structures occur more commonly in the posterior teeth.

8 E This sharp, flat-bladed instrument is used to carve smooth surfaces, such as the buccal and lingual. Occasionally, it may be used to carve anatomic grooves, but the initial design was primarily for smooth surfaces.

9 A The enamel hatchet smooths the internal axial walls of a cavity preparation to remove unsupported enamel.

10 D The hoe performs basically the same action as the enamel hatchet, but it is used in a pull motion.

11 C This instrument is a small cleoid-discoid carver and is used to make fine anatomic grooves in an amalgam restoration on posterior teeth.

12 B Chisels and hoes have standard and reversed bevels. Enamel hatchets, gingival margin trimmers, and angle formers have right and left bevels, whereas a spoon has a rounded cutting edge.

13 A Basic to all dental procedures are the cotton pliers, explorer, and mirror. The cotton pliers is used to transfer materials into and out of the oral cavity, the explorer to probe and examine tissues, and the mirror to provide indirect vision. These activities are common to most dental procedures.

14 A The manufacturer provides an instrument number on each dental instrument that correlates to the instrument formula. Typically, the higher the number, the larger the instrument size.

15 A A DE spoon allows the operator to use the instrument twice without exchanging it. A DE spoon has one end that can be used on the right side of the tooth and the reverse end on the left side of the tooth.

16 B A DE gingival marginal trimmer is right on one end and left on the reverse. Both ends of the instrument are either mesial or distal.

17 B An acrylic bur is a larger cutting device that would be used extraorally on a device such as a denture.

18 D A Burlew disk is a rubber polishing device that can be used to polish intraorally or extraorally. It is impregnated with pumice to provide an abrasive feature.

19 E A Jo-Dandy disk is made of carborundum and is sometimes referred to as a *separating disk*. This brittle, inexpensive device is used extraorally to cut gold.

20 C A Craytex wheel comes in a variety of grits and shapes and is used to polish gold.

21 A

22 C

23 D

24 B

25 E Scenario for items 21-25:

When an instrument is to be exchanged, the dentist signals by bringing the used instrument into the transfer zone and turns the hand slightly. The assistant parallels the new instrument to be delivered with the used instrument. The used instrument is grasped with the third finger and small finger and tucked into the palm. The new instrument is delivered into the dentist's hand. Roll the used instrument back into the delivery position, or return the instrument to its original position on the tray if it is not to be used again.

To enhance your understanding of the material presented in this chapter, refer to the illustrations in Chapter 20 of Finkbeiner/Johnson: *Mosby's Comprehensive Dental Assisting: A Clinical Approach.*

Isolation Procedures

One of the primary duties of a clinical dental assistant is to maintain a dry field and improve visibility for the dentist during routine operative and surgical procedures. This can be done through the effective use of oral evacuation and isolation procedures.

ORAL EVACUATION

I. Description
    A. **Oral evacuation** is the process of removing fluids and materials from the mouth.
    B. It provides comfort to the patient and allows the operator to work in a clear operative field.
    C. Effective oral evacuation removes much of the

aerosol spray created by the handpiece, providing greater safety for the dental team.
D. Two devices used in dentistry for oral evacuation include the following:
    1. **High-velocity evacuation (HVE)** system or *oral evacuator*
        a. Used to remove large volumes of fluid and debris from the mouth.
        b. Does not need to be immersed in the fluids.
        c. Sometimes is referred to as **suction.**
    2. **Low-volume evacuation** system known as the **saliva ejector**
        a. Removes liquid slowly.

b. Does not pick up solid debris.
II. Saliva Ejector
  A. A saliva ejector is used in the following circumstances:
    1. During an oral prophylaxis
    2. When the operator is working alone
    3. When a patient resists the use of the suction
    4. When a patient salivates heavily under the rubber dam
  B. With the addition of an appropriate device, it retracts the tongue.
  C. Saliva ejectors are supplied in metal or plastic.
    1. Plastic is more common.
    2. Plastic is inexpensive and disposable.
III. High-Velocity Evacuation System
  A. The HVE system is a natural adjunct to sit-down, four-handed dentistry when the patient is placed in a supine position for treatment.
  B. Choosing an HVE tip involves the following considerations:
    1. Two basic types of tips
      a. Surgical
        (1) This is more site specific than the standard operative tip.
        (2) The narrow opening may clog frequently when evacuating blood and tissue; thus it is necessary to clear the tip with sterile water or saline solution.
      b. Operative
        (1) Used more frequently in general dentistry
        (2) Available in a variety of shapes
        (3) Made of metal or plastic
        (4) Supplied with an angled or a straight shaft
        (5) May be disposable or sterilizable
    2. Metal versus plastic tip
      a. A metal tip is more durable and can always be sterilized.
      b. Metal cannot be used during electrosurgery.
      c. Coldness created by air constantly running through the tip may cause discomfort in a tooth that is not anesthetized or to nearby soft tissues.
      d. Some plastic tips are not strong enough for use as a retraction device.
      e. Some plastic tips may be sterilized.
    3. Angled versus straight shaft—tips with a bend in the shaft seem to be more commonly used than straight tips.
IV. Auxiliary Evacuator Devices

  A. An adapter may be attached to the HVE hose, and a saliva ejector may be attached to the adapter.
  B. A svedopter can be used in the adapter or on the saliva ejector hose.
    1. It serves as a saliva ejector.
    2. It provides retraction of the tongue.
    3. It is supplied with three sizes of flange tips.
    4. A disposable version of this device is a *hygroformic,* which has limited retraction ability.

USING THE ORAL EVACUATOR TIP ■■■■■■■

I. Successful oral evacuation is dependent on a few simple rules (box below).
II. Suggested tips for oral evacuation are listed (box on page 235).

USING THE AIR/WATER SYRINGE ■■■■■■■

I. To supplement the effectiveness of oral evacuation it is necessary to use the air/water (a/w) syringe with maximum efficiency.
  A. The a/w syringe is used to rinse and dry the teeth and oral cavity.
  B. The a/w syringe provides three forms of spray: air only, air and water (aerated spray), or water only.
  C. When using the a/w syringe, turn the tip in the direction of the arch—up for the maxilla, down for the mandible.

RULES FOR ORAL EVACUATOR PLACEMENT

- Select the appropriate end.
- Use a thumb-to-nose or pen grasp (see Fig. 14-1).
- When working with a right-handed operator, the assistant operates the oral evacuator with the right hand and uses the left hand with a left-handed operator.
- Place the evacuator tip before the operator places the handpiece and/or mirror.
- Place the tip as close to the tooth as possible.
- Keep the edge of the evacuator tip even with or slightly above the occlusal or incisal edge of the tooth.
- Place the tip near the tooth surface closest to the assistant.
- When the handpiece is being used on the surface nearest the assistant, place the HVE tip slightly distal to the tooth being treated.

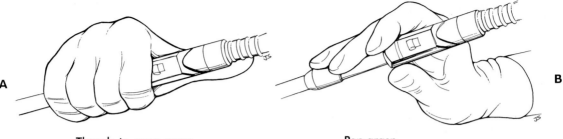

A Thumb-to-nose grasp   Pen grasp B

Fig. 14-1   A, Thumb-to-nose grasp B, Pen grasp.

SUGGESTIONS FOR ORAL EVACUATOR USE

1. Place the tip securely into the hose to avoid accidental dislodgement.
2. Minimize the noise of the HVE system by turning on the evacuator completely.
3. Turn the angle of the tip opening parallel to the buccal or lingual plane of the teeth to avoid contact with soft tissue.
4. Avoid contact with soft tissue when the tip is initially placed in the mouth by entering toward the midline where the opening is greater; then concentrate on specific placement.
5. Avoid cold-temperature discomfort to sensitive or nonanesthetized teeth by using a plastic HVE tip.
6. If a tip falls on the floor, replace it with a clean one and pick up the dropped tip at the end of the procedure.
7. Clean a surgical tip frequently by dipping the tip into a cup of sterile water or saline solution to avoid clogging.
8. Avoid quick and sudden movement of the tip. This can be distracting to the operator and potentially dangerous to the patient.
9. Avoid contact with the soft palate and pillar areas to eliminate potential gagging.
10. Remove the tip whenever possible to allow the patient to close and swallow. This prevents overdrying the mouth and gives the patient a break from the constant noise.
11. Observe fluids and debris collecting in other areas of the mouth and remove them intermittently.
12. When a complete mouth rinse is performed, turn the tip so that the back of the tip (the side opposite the tip opening) lies on the lateral surface of the tongue or cheek.
13. Keep the evacuator tip turned on at the end of the procedure for a short time to ensure that all fluids are drawn into the system and do not remain at the hose opening.
14. Avoid saying "oops" or "I'm sorry" or gasping when you grasp tissue with the HVE tip. Such reactions do not build patient confidence.
15. Avoid contact with sublingual tissues because they can be more susceptible to injury than other oral tissues.

D. When the operator stops the handpiece during a cavity preparation, rinse the tooth by using the aerated spray followed by a spurt of air to thoroughly clean and dry the tooth.

E. The a/w syringe can be used to clean and dry the mirror.

II. Follow the guidelines to maximize efficiency in placing the a/w syringe (box in right column).

PERFORMING A COMPLETE MOUTH RINSE ▬

I. At the end of any procedure, refresh the patient's mouth and ensure that no debris remains in the oral cavity.

MAXIMUM EFFICIENCY TIPS FOR USING THE AIR/WATER SYRINGE

1. Turn the tip in the direction of the arch—up for the maxilla, down for the mandible.
2. To thoroughly cleanse the site, place the tip directly over the opening of the preparation when a cavity preparation site is flushed.
3. Be assertive in cleansing a site. Don't hold the tip too far away. Place the tip within 1/4 inch and press firmly on the buttons to cleanse the area.
4. Quickly move the syringe tip into an area to be cleaned; flush, evacuate, and move the tip out of the area quickly.

II. A complete mouth rinse may be done by the assistant alone or as a four-handed procedure with the operator.
   A. The procedure for the two-handed method is described (box below).
   B. The team approach is described (box on page 237).

MAINTAINING THE HIGH-VELOCITY EVACUATION SYSTEM

I. Remove the evacuator tip after completion of each mouth rinse procedure and disinfect the hoses.
II. Keep the system turned on after treatment so that the fluids completely drain into the system.
III. At the end of the day, perform the following procedure:
   A. Always wear utility gloves, masks, and protective glasses when cleaning the system.
   B. Flush the system with a premixed, antimicrobial solution that is placed in a rubber bowl or other appropriate container.
   C. Flush thoroughly for 2 to 5 minutes using 1 or 2 quarts of solution.
   D. Remove and replace disposable traps in the evacuator trap cup.
   E. Remove and replace disposable screens in the saliva ejector hose.
   F. If heavy metals are found in the disposable trap, the materials are discarded in the heavy metals waste receptacle; if not, the debris is discarded in the biohazard waste receptacle following Environmental Protection Agency laws and recommendations in your state.

ISOLATION

I. **Isolation** means setting apart from others or placing something by itself. In dentistry, isolation is used during a treatment procedure to separate a specific tooth, a group of teeth, or a region in the mouth.
II. The following are the primary objectives of isolation:
   A. Maintain a dry field
   B. Retract soft tissue
   C. Prevent materials from falling into the oral cavity
   D. Aid in infection control techniques by decreasing aerosol sprays from the oral cavity
   E. Reduce potential contamination to the tooth
   F. Provide a visual contrast between tooth structure and rubber dam material
   G. Provide patient management

TWO-HANDED MOUTH RINSE PROCEDURE

A. Begin on the patient's right side at #8. Turn the a/w syringe tip toward the maxillary arch. Place the suction tip on the lingual surface near the incisal edge.
B. Spray an a/w combination to avoid splatter. (A solid spray of water will result in splash back.) Continue distally, using both devices simultaneously. When you reach the canine/cuspid area, move the evacuator tip completely to the lingual surface.
C. With the left hand, use the triplex syringe and retract the cheek.
D. Spray water on occlusal surfaces forcing water spray to wash the entire tooth. It may be necessary to spray toward the buccal or lingual surfaces when debris remains, especially when you are removing a substance such as polishing paste.
E. Observe the floor of the mouth and the posterior pillar areas to pick up any accumulation of fluids.
F. When all of the maxillary right quadrant has been completed, move to the mandibular arch and begin with tooth #25.
G. Turn the tip in the direction of the mandible. Repeat steps C through I in the same manner, but this time the evacuator tip can aid in retracting the tongue.
H. When the mandibular right quadrant has been rinsed thoroughly, ask the patient to turn toward you, and begin the maxillary left quadrant at #9.
I. Place the tip on the labial surface near the incisal edge and continue distally as was done for the opposite side.
J. On the left side, when the cuspid is reached, move the tip to the buccal surface, and use the oral evacuator to retract the cheek.
K. Continue to the molar region. Spray water on the occlusal to flush all tooth surface.
L. When the maxillary left side is rinsed thoroughly, turn the tip of the triplex syringe to the mandibular position.
M, N, and O. Begin at tooth #24 and progress distally following steps C through I again. At the conclusion of the complete mouth rinse, wipe any water spray from the patient's face with the napkin and thank the patient for cooperating during the procedure.

H. Increase patient comfort

I. Increase success of restorations by providing a dry operative field

III. Types of isolation materials include the following:

  A. Rubber dam

  B. Cotton rolls

  C. Cellulose wafers

  D. Svedopters

  E. Hygroformics

  F. Mouth props

IV. Rubber dam isolation is used in various specialty procedures.

  A. Endodontic procedures—Isolate a single tooth: the tooth receiving the treatment; with single-tooth isolation, contamination of the surgical site is reduced if not eliminated, which is important to successful endodontic treatment.

  B. Pediatric procedures—Isolate only the teeth that are involved in the operative treatment—usually two or three teeth; with young children the use of rubber dam can increase safety because youngsters may have active tongues or may move suddenly, thereby creating the potential for injury to soft tissue when high-speed handpieces or other instruments are used.

  C. Restorative procedures on anterior teeth—Isolate the anterior segment of the arch, incisors, cuspids, and first and second premolars.

  D. Restorative procedures on posterior teeth—Isolate the tooth being treated and one tooth posterior and two teeth anterior to that tooth; another option is to isolate the tooth that is being treated as well as the tooth posterior to it, and include all teeth anterior to the opposite central incisor or even the cuspid.

V. The rubber dam armamentarium is applied using the following materials and procedures:

  A. **Rubber dam material**

    1. Latex material into which holes are punched for teeth to be exposed during the treatment procedure

    2. Supplied in a roll from which pieces are cut, or in precut sheets of 4 × 4 inches, 5 × 5 inches, and 6 × 6 inches

    3. Manufactured in colors such as dark green (to provide contrast with oral structures), pastels, and light beige

    4. Has different weights or gauges including thin, medium, heavy, extra heavy, and special heavy

    5. Has a limited shelf life and tears more easily as it ages

    6. May create allergic reaction in patient; check the health history prior to using the material

  B. **Rubber dam stamp** and pad or **template**

    1. It provides a guide for punching holes in the rubber dam for teeth that are to be exposed or isolated.

TEAM APPROACH: FOUR-HANDED ORAL EVACUATION	
OPERATOR	ASSISTANT
Direct patient to turn toward operator. Retract cheek. Grasp a/w syringe. Begin at maxillary right central incisor. Direct water spray toward incisal edge. Continue toward distal, spraying the occlusal surface.	Pass a/w syringe with tip toward maxilla. Turn on HVE. Position HVE near incisal edge. Move HVE tip to lingual surface following movement of a/w syringe. Move HVE tip to pillar region to pick up excess water.
Turn a/w tip toward mandible. Continue to retract cheek. Begin at midline of mandible right central incisor. Spray water toward incisal edge. Continue toward distal, spraying the occlusal surface.	Position HVE on mandibular anterior lingual surface. Move HVE tip to lingual surface following movement of a/w syringe. Move HVE tip to pillar region to pick up excess water.
Direct patient to turn toward assistant. Repeat identical procedure for left side.	Repeat identical procedure for left side. Wipe off extraoral region around mouth (if moist) with napkin or 2 × 2 gauze.

2. A rubber stamp with images of a dental arch and tooth positions is placed on a standard ink pad with colored ink applied.

3. The stamp establishes markings on the dam for an ideal tooth configuration of the primary and permanent dentition.

4. The template is a 6 × 6-inch piece of plastic with holes, which can be placed over or under the rubber dam material to make markings with a pen.

C. **Rubber dam napkin**
1. This is placed between the rubber dam material and the patient's skin to prevent chafing, discomfort, or allergic reaction.
2. It absorbs saliva during and after the isolation procedure.

D. **Rubber dam frame**—used to hold and position the rubber dam material over the oral cavity.

E. **Rubber dam punch**
1. This is a forceps-like device that has a movable circular turntable at one end with holes of various sizes.
2. The size of the hole used depends on the size of the tooth to be exposed through the rubber dam.
3. Either five or six holes are on each turnplate, with the small holes intended for primary teeth and permanent mandibular incisors.
4. Opposite the turntable is a punch point that is forced through the rubber dam when the arms of the punch are brought together.

F. **Rubber dam clamps**
1. These are used to anchor the dam to the tooth to avoid movement and slippage of the rubber dam material during treatment.
2. They vary in size and shape to conform to the area where they will be placed.
3. Clamps are supplied with or without wings; (**winged** or **wingless clamps**) wings are projections at the clamp's jaw that attach to the rubber dam material to secure the clamp in the punched hole.
4. They are designed for use in specific areas, teeth, or procedures.
5. A **gingival retracting clamp** is designed to retract the gingiva.

G. **Rubber dam forceps**
1. This is used to place rubber dam clamps on the tooth/teeth to stabilize or anchor the rubber dam in the oral cavity.
2. Prongs on the beaks of the forceps fit in holes or grooves on the clamp to stretch the clamp to fit over a tooth.

H. **Ligatures**
1. These devices are used to ligate or anchor the portion of the rubber dam material that is not stabilized by the rubber dam clamp.
2. They may include the following:
   a. A piece of dental floss is tied around the circumference of the tooth that is exposed on the most anterior tooth.
   b. A piece of dental floss is doubled in thickness and placed interproximally on the surface farthest from the clamped tooth.
   c. A corner of the rubber dam is cut and placed interproximally next to the tooth that is exposed on the most anterior tooth.
   d. A premanufactured material, such as a Wedjet, is placed interproximally at the most anterior tooth that is isolated.
3. To prevent clamp aspiration, a piece of dental floss is tied to the rubber dam clamp and acts as a safety precaution.

I. Additional items needed for rubber dam application
1. Dental floss
2. Lubricant
3. Pen (if template is used)
4. Crown and collar scissors
5. Choice of instrument to invert the rubber dam material
   a. FP1
   b. Beavertail burnisher
   c. Spoon excavator
6. Saliva ejector and adapter hose if necessary
7. Alcohol or Bunsen burner (optional)
8. Stick impression compound (optional)
9. Matches (optional)

J. Rubber dam procedure
1. The procedure is described (box on pages 239 and 240).
2. Explain the procedure to the patient.
3. Four-handed rubber dam application is described (box on page 241).

K. Variations in rubber dam placement
1. Missing teeth require no holes to be punched.
2. Missing teeth replaced with a bridge require special adaptations (Fig. 14-2 on page 242).
3. Use of an anterior clamp may involve the placement of additional posterior clamps, additional ligatures, and application of dental compound for stability.

RUBBER DAM PROCEDURE

EXAMINATION OF THE TREATMENT AREA

1. Inspect the oral cavity for the alignment of the teeth.
2. Floss the patient's teeth to evaluate the contact areas before the rubber dam is applied.

PUNCHING THE RUBBER DAM

1. Punch the rubber dam once clearance to the interproximal areas is achieved.
2. Material left between the holes is the **septum,** the portion of the rubber dam that must slip between the teeth.
3. Punching the holes too close together stretches the holes, and the rubber dam does not cover all the gingival tissues.
4. The closeness of the holes does not allow for the inversion of the rubber dam.
5. If the rubber dam is punched so that the arch is too close together, the results are folds and stretching of the rubber dam toward the anterior of the mouth. If the rubber dam is punched so that the arch is farther apart and has less curve, the results are folds and stretching of the dam towards the lingual.
6. Observe the common rules for hole punching:
   a. For endodontic treatment only the tooth (teeth) being treated is (are) exposed.
   b. In operative treatment at least one tooth anterior and one tooth posterior to the tooth (teeth) being treated is exposed.
   c. An alternative method for punching the rubber dam is to expose more teeth—even an entire quadrant or segment.
   Note: The number of holes punched varies with the type of procedure and the personal preferences of the operator. If the hole is visible but a tag of the material remains in the opening, it must be removed by repositioning the punch over the hole and cutting the material again, or it can be pulled out with the fingers, leaving the hole intact and allowing the rubber dam to be inverted.

SELECTING AND PLACING THE CLAMP

1. Always place a ligature on the selected clamp as a safety measure before trying it in the oral cavity.
2. Place the clamp on the tooth posterior to the tooth being treated, unless the most posterior tooth in the quadrant is to be clamped.
3. Position the rubber dam forceps beaks in the hole openings of the rubber dam clamp. Grasp the forceps handles together, stretching the opening of the clamp wider.
4. If the operator positions the receiving hand with the palm down, pass the forceps and clamp with the beaks and cervical of the clamp face down.
5. If the operator's hand is positioned with the palm up to receive the forceps and clamp, pass the forceps with hands clear of the handles and the beaks of the forceps and the cervical of the clamp facing up.
6. Position the lingual points on the clamp first as a clamp is placed and then slide the buccal points down into place as is illustrated later during the placement of the rubber dam.
   a. The clamp should not impinge on the oral tissues or push the tissues down unless it is a gingival retracting clamp.
   b. The clamp should be stable and not rock back and forth or side to side.
   c. After repeated use, rubber dam clamps may lose tension.

ASSEMBLING THE RUBBER DAM

At this point the steps of assembly may vary, depending on the operator's preference to use winged or wingless clamps.
1. Assemble the frame and rubber dam material while the operator tests the clamp.
2. Lay the rubber dam material flat on a surface and position the Young's frame over or under the rubber dam material and assemble.
3. Remove the clamp from the rubber dam forceps and place it in the rubber dam material that is attached to the frame.
4. Position the projection of the jaws (the wing) on one side of the clamp in the most posterior tooth hole opening.
5. Place the beaks of the rubber dam forceps in the clamp forceps holes.
6. Choose one of several options when the operator has selected to use a wingless clamp, because the rubber dam procedure varies from the winged clamp procedure.
7. Position the clamp on the tooth first and pull the rubber dam, with or without the frame, over the clamp and tooth.

Continued

RUBBER DAM PROCEDURE—cont'd

PLACING THE RUBBER DAM ASSEMBLY

1. Evaluate access to the interproximal spaces after the rubber dam has been assembled.
2. Pass the assembly to the operator as a single unit.
3. Help guide the assembly into place and stabilize the frame to avoid injury to the patient.
4. The operator carefully sets the lingual jaw of the clamp onto the tooth first.
5. The operator widens the clamp opening and slides the clamp down as the buccal jaw of the clamp contacts the tooth surface.
6. The operator checks for stability of the clamp on the tooth by using a finger placed on the clamp.
7. The operator isolates the remainder of the teeth by stretching the material over each tooth.
8. Work the floss down the mesial surface of one tooth and the distal surface of the other.
   a. The floss is passed through the contact and then pulled off of the hand with the least amount of floss.
   b. The floss is then removed from the sulcus area by pulling free of the teeth.
   c. If the floss is pulled back up through the contact, the dam material may come with it and the placement of the floss into the sulcus must be repeated.
   d. As the septum of the rubber dam material is forced down between each consecutive tooth with the floss, the assembly becomes more stable.
9. Position the anterior ligature on the mesial surface once the most anterior tooth is isolated.
10. The operator removes the dam material from the wings of the clamp by hand or with the instrument of choice.
11. The operator positions the forceps in the clamp openings if any gingival tissue is exposed and slightly lifts the points of the clamp away from the tooth.
12. The operator uses an FP1, beavertail burnisher, spoon excavator, or other instrument to invert the rubber dam material.
13. Blow air with the a/w syringe on the surface where the instrument is positioned to help turn the material into the sulcus.
14. Place the rubber dam napkin under the dam material once the assembly is stable. If the rubber dam material blocks the patient's nose, it may be necessary to remove excess material by cutting an opening to breathe.
15. Place a saliva ejector under the dam in the mandibular arch as soon as the rubber dam assembly is completely in place.
16. See the Criteria for Clinically Acceptable Rubber Dam Placement (box on bottom of page 241).

REMOVING THE RUBBER DAM ASSEMBLY

Once the operative procedure is completed and debris (such as fluids and amalgam scrap) is evacuated from the dam surface, the rubber dam assembly is removed. The steps run almost in reverse of placement.
1. Remove the saliva ejector.
2. Remove the ligature, either by stretching it and pulling it through the contact or by using scissors to cut the buccal surface of the tied dental floss and pulling it from the buccal surface with cotton pliers.
3. Roll the dam over a finger and stretch the interseptal dam away from the teeth.
4. Use curved crown and collar scissors with the beaks pointed away from the tissues, and cut along the line or interseptal material that the operator has pulled away.
5. Pass a rubber dam clamp forceps to the operator and place the forceps in the holes of the clamp.
6. The operator lifts the frame and dam material as a unit from the oral cavity and passes it to the assistant.
7. Remove the rubber dam napkin and wipe any debris from the patient's face.
8. Place the rubber dam and frame on the top of the mobile cart and remove the frame to examine the dam for missing pieces.
9. Lay the material flat on the surface and reposition the cut pieces of rubber dam material.
   a. If a piece of material is missing, it might be in the patient's mouth.
   b. If, on inspection, the operator observes the piece of dam material in the mouth, it can be removed with an explorer or with floss.
   c. The piece of dam must be removed, or it will cause tissue trauma to the area.
The team completes a full mouth rinse on the patient. During rubber dam placement a patient's saliva may become viscous, and a refreshing rinse of the oral cavity is a courtesy to the patient. See Team Approach: Four-Handed Rubber Dam Application (box) for assistance in understanding how your actions will synchronize with the operator's actions.

TEAM APPROACH: FOUR-HANDED RUBBER DAM APPLICATION

OPERATOR	ASSISTANT
	Select clamp, and attach floss to ligature.
	Try in clamp.
	Assemble rubber dam.
	Floss interproximal contacts to determine clearance.
	Pick up entire assembly.
	Leave handle of forceps free for operator to grasp.
	Pass to operator.
Grasp handle and side of assembly.	
Position clamp over most posterior tooth.	Stabilize frame to avoid patient injury.
Open jaws of clamp.	
Position lingual jaw of clamp onto tooth.	
Position buccal jaw of clamp onto tooth.	
Lift forceps out of clamp holes.	
Return forceps.	Grasp forceps.
Using fingers, check stability of clamp.	Return forceps to mobile cart.
If not stable, retrieve forceps and reposition clamp.	
Begin to stretch punched holes over remaining teeth.	Wrap floss around one finger of each hand.*
	Assist in securing the remaining rubber dam between teeth.
	Work floss down the mesial of one tooth, then down the distal of adjacent tooth.
	Continue to floss between remaining exposed teeth until septum of dam is forced down between each tooth.
	Ligate mesial of most anterior tooth.
	Place napkin under dam.
	Pass spoon excavator or other instrument to invert dam.
Retrieve instrument to invert the rubber dam.	
Place instrument on dam at cervical buccal and turn edge of dam into sulcus.	Turn a/w tip to appropriate arch.
	Spray air at site of inversion.
Continue on buccal surface until all dam is inverted.	Follow operator to complete inversion on buccal, then move to lingual.
Move to lingual and repeat process.	Continue to spray air until all dam is inverted.
Ask patient to turn to improve vision as needed.	Cut excess dam from nose area if needed.
	Place saliva ejector if needed.

*If it is more convenient for the operator to floss the contacts and the assistant to hold the dam, the tasks can easily be reversed.

CRITERIA FOR CLINICALLY ACCEPTABLE RUBBER DAM PLACEMENT

Floss on the bow of the clamp is toward the buccal or facial side.
Clamp is stable on the tooth.
Holes are punched in the correct location.
Clamp is placed in the correct hole.
Orientation of the rubber dam assembly (no folds in material) is correct.

Rubber dam material is completely inverted.
Each tooth either has a seal through the inversion or is ligated.
No soft-tissue trauma is present.
Rubber dam napkin or other protection is placed.
Saliva ejector is in place.

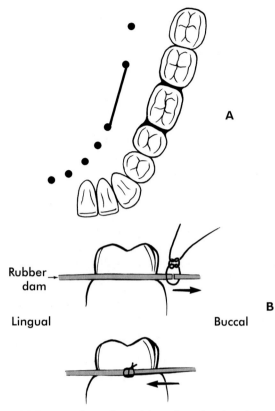

Rubber dam

Lingual

Buccal

A

B

Fig. 14-2 *A,* When the rubber dam is placed over a bridge, a hole is not punched for the pontic, but rather the holes adjacent to the pontic are punched, and a cut is made between those holes to fit the material over the pontic. *B,* The rubber dam is pulled under the pontic to the buccal area, sutured, and allowed to slide back into place.

VI. Other isolation materials include the following:
   A. Cotton rolls, alone or with cotton roll holders
   B. Cellulose wafers
   C. Svedopters
   D. Hygroformics
   E. Mouth prop

Questions

Isolation Procedures

1 High-velocity evacuation
   1. Increases the patient's desire to rinse
   2. Decreases the patient's desire to rinse
   3. Is used only with a rubber dam
   4. Decreases the amount of aerosol emanating from the patient's mouth
   5. Increases visibility
   a. 1, 3, and 5
   b. 2, 4, and 5
   c. 2, 3, and 4
   d. 2, 4, and 5

2 When the operator is working in the posterior area of the mouth, the HVE tip is placed
   1. Over the occlusal surface of the tooth being prepared
   2. Even with the occlusal height of the tooth being prepared
   3. Parallel to the buccal or lingual surface of the tooth being prepared
   4. After the operator places the mirror
   5. As close a possible to the tooth being prepared
   a. 1, 2, and 3
   b. 2, 3, and 4
   c. 2, 3, and 5
   d. 3, 4, and 5

3 When the operator is working in the anterior segment of the oral cavity, the HVE tip is held
   a. Near the incisal edge of the tooth being prepared
   b. On the opposite side of the tooth being prepared
   c. In the retromolar area
   d. In the vestibule

4 The use of a rubber dam provides the benefits of
   1. Controlling amounts of saliva through the dam
   2. Preventing aerosolization
   3. Providing a sterile environment
   4. Keeping debris out of the patient's mouth
   5. Helping retract the tongue and cheek
   a. 1, 2, and 4
   b. 2, 3, and 5
   c. 2, 4, and 5
   d. 3, 4, and 5

5 During the placement of a rubber dam, a spoon excavator can be used to
   a. Secure the rubber dam
   b. Invert the rubber dam
   c. Punch small holes in the rubber dam for the anterior teeth

6 The rubber dam napkin is used to
   a. Place the dam
   b. Secure the dam
   c. Prevent irritation around the patient's mouth
   d. Help the patient swallow

7 When a rubber dam is being applied, dental floss can be used to
   a. Help secure the dam
   b. Force the dam between the teeth being isolated
   c. Invert the dam around the teeth being treated
   d. All of the above

8 Which of the following is not a basic rule for placement of an oral evacuator?
   a. Keep the edge of the tip even with or slightly above the occlusal or incisal edge.
   b. Always allow the operator to place the handpiece first.
   c. Place the tip on the surface closest to the assistant.

9 The differences between the use of an HVE system and the use of a saliva ejector include which of the following?
   1. HVE only removes fluid.
   2. Saliva ejector only removes fluid.
   3. HVE removes fluid and debris.
   4. HVE must be immersed in the fluid to be effective.
   5. HVE does not need to be immersed to be effective.

6. Saliva ejector must be immersed to be effective.
7. Saliva ejector does not need to be immersed to be effective.
   a. 1, 2, 4, and 7
   b. 1, 2, 5, and 6
   c. 2, 3, 5, and 6
   d. 2, 3, 5, and 7

10 When assisting a right-handed operator in a procedure performed on the patient's left side, the dental assistant holds the HVE tip in the
   a. Right hand with a thumb-to-nose grip
   b. Left hand with a thumb-to-nose grip
   c. Right hand with a pen grasp
   d. Left hand with a pen grasp

11 When assisting a left-handed operator in a procedure performed on the patient's left side, the dental assistant holds the HVE tip in the
   a. Right hand with a thumb-to-nose grip
   b. Left hand with a thumb-to-nose grip
   c. Right hand with a pen grasp
   d. Left hand with a pen grasp

Answer the following questions using the diagram of a rubber dam clamp.

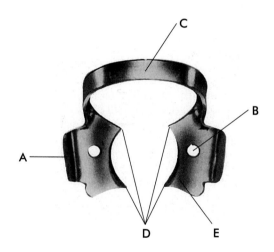

12 Which is used to secure the clamp to the tooth?
   a. A
   b. B
   c. C
   d. D
   e. E

13 Which secures the clamp in the rubber dam hole prior to placement?
   a. A
   b. B
   c. C
   d. D
   e. E

14 Which area provides gingival retraction?
   a. A
   b. B

c. C
d. D
e. E

15 Which assists in the placement of the clamp on the tooth?
   a. A
   b. B
   c. C
   d. D
   e. E

Identify the type of clamp to be used in each of the following situations. Choose the one best answer.
a. Molar
b. Premolar
c. Anterior

_____ **16** Endodontic treatment on #8
_____ **17** Operative treatment on #9
_____ **18** Operative treatment on #29
_____ **19** Operative treatment on #5
_____ **20** Operative treatment on #14

21 Rubber dam isolation provides which of the following?
1. A means of patient management
2. Reduced stress for the operator
3. Fluid control
4. Control over oral tissues
5. Reduction of microbial aerosols
   a. 1 and 4
   b. 2 and 3
   c. 3 and 5
   d. 2 only
   e. 1, 2, 3, 4, and 5

22 If a patient has a three-unit bridge in the mandibular right quadrant, which of the following is (are) true?
1. The rubber dam is placed normally.
2. The rubber dam is sewn under the pontic to reduce saliva control problems.
3. Rubber dam isolation cannot be used.
4. The rubber dam must be cut and pulled under the pontic.
5. Cotton roll isolation would be the ideal isolation.
   a. 1 and 4
   b. 2 and 4
   c. 1 only
   d. 3 only
   e. 5 only

Select from the following elements of armamentarium the isolation material or device that meets each of the descriptions listed below.
a. Young's frame
b. Dental compound
c. Stick wax
d. Rubber dam punch
e. Svedopter

_____ **23** Thermoplastic material used to stabilize a Ferrier #212 or another anterior clamp
_____ **24** Device made of metal or plastic, with projections on which the rubber dam is retained
_____ **25** Plierlike instrument with a rotating table that generally includes six holes of different sizes

Rationales

Isolation Procedures

1 B High-velocity evacuation removes fluids and debris from the patient's mouth rapidly, thus eliminating the desire to rinse the mouth. Because the evacuator tip is placed near the operative site, aerosols are quickly picked up and are not allowed to escape into the environment. Rapid removal of fluids increases the operator's visibility and eliminates fluids accumulating in the mouth.

2 C To efficiently remove fluids from the mouth with a high-velocity tip, the following rules should be followed:
Place the tip as close to the tooth as possible.
Place the tip on parallel to the surface of the tooth closest to the assistant, the buccal or lingual.
Place the edge of the tip even with the occlusal or incisal edge.
Place the tip before the operator places the handpiece.

3 B When the HVE is used in the anterior, the tip is placed on the lingual when the operator is working on the labial and the reverse when the operator is working on the lingual.

4 C The rubber dam isolates an individual tooth or a group of teeth. When in place, the rubber dam meets all of the objectives of isolation:
Maintaining a dry field
Retracting soft tissue
Preventing materials from falling into the oral cavity
Promoting infection control by eliminating aerosol sprays from the oral cavity
Reducing potential contamination to the tooth
Providing a visual contrast between tooth structure and rubber dam material
Providing patient management
Increasing patient comfort

5 B A spoon excavator with its curved blade enables the operator to cuff or invert the rubber dam into the gingival sulcus, eliminating potential seepage of saliva along the gingival margins.

6 C A rubber dam napkin made of a soft, absorbable material is able to absorb moisture around the patient's mouth, preventing chafing or irritation to the area.

7 D Dental floss functions in many ways during rubber dam application. It can help to secure the dam by being tied around a tooth as a ligature. It is used to force the dam down between the teeth to secure it in place, and it aids in inverting the dam around the tooth being treated.

8 B See answer No. 2 for the basic rules.

9 C The high-velocity evacuator rapidly removes fluids and debris from the mouth without being immersed in the fluids. The saliva ejector is a slow-speed method of removing fluids only. The saliva ejector does not have the capability of removing debris such as amalgam or dental cement from the oral cavity.

10 A The side of the patient's oral cavity being treated is not relevant. When assisting a right-handed operator, the assistant always holds the oral evacuator in the right hand and transfers instruments with the left hand. When assisting a left-handed operator, this position is reversed.

11 B See question 10.

12 D The parts of the clamp function to do the following:
The wings hold the dam prior to insertion and then help to secure it.
The bow aids in maintaining the clamp in position.
The forceps holes attach to the forceps to insertion.
The prongs secure the clamp to the tooth and may provide gingival retraction.

13 A See answer No. 12.

14 D See answer No. 12.

15 B The forceps holes retain the clamp in the clamp forceps, which in turn allows the clamp to be placed on the tooth.

16 C Because only one clamp is used in endodontics, it is the clamp that fits the tooth being treated, thus an anterior clamp.

17 B In operative treatment more teeth are isolated. In general, the tooth distal to the one being treated is clamped. Because a central incisor is being treated, and it is not common to place a clamp on the anterior tooth due to the bulkiness of the clamp, the next distal tooth to be clamped would be a premolar. This would ensure that a clamp would not interfere with the placement of the handpieces or other instrumentation.

18 A Generally, the clamp goes on the tooth distal to the tooth being treated. The tooth distal to this second premolar is a molar, thus the molar clamp would be used.

19 B The tooth distal to this first molar is a second premolar, thus the premolar clamp would be used.

20 A The tooth distal to this second molar is a third molar, thus a molar clamp would be selected. However, if the molar were missing, or if it were anatomically difficult to attach the clamp to the third molar, the clamp might be placed on the second molar or eliminated.

21 E See answer No. 4.

22 B To place a rubber dam with a fixed prothesis a cut must be made between the abutment teeth. This allows for the operator to slide the opened dam under the pontic and then suture it back together.

23 B Dental compound can be heated until it is soft and pliable. The compound is placed over the wing or bow of the clamp and allowed to harden in place. This hardened material helps to stabilize the anterior clamp.

24 A The Young's frame is designed to hold the rubber dam in place.

25 D A rubber dam punch is a forceps-like device that has a movable circular turntable at one end with holes of various sizes.

To enhance your understanding of the material in this chapter refer to the illustrations in Chapter 22 of Finkbeiner/Johnson: *Mosby's Comprehensive Dental Assisting: A Clinical Approach.*

Anesthesia

OUTLINE

Forms of Anesthesia
Local Anesthesia

Preparation for Anesthetic
  Procedure

Inhaled Gases

KEY TERMS

Amide

ASA Physical Status Classification
  System

Carpule

Cartridge

Conscious sedation

Ester

Field block

General anesthesia

Infiltration

Inhalation anesthesia

Local anesthesia

Lumen

Nerve block

Nitrous oxide

Pain

Paresthesia

Periodontal ligament injection

Topical anesthesia

Toxicity

The practice of dentistry can be an invasive process, and dental pain may result from a procedure. The dentist is responsible for providing the patient with comfortable dental treatment, which usually indicates the use of some form of anesthesia.

The International Association for the Study of Pain defines **pain** as "the sensory and emotional experience associated with actual or potential tissue damage." Pain can be a perception of uncomfortable stimuli and the response to that perception. An estimated 50% of individuals seek some form of medical care as a direct result of pain. Pain can be acute or chronic and can be treated with a form of analgesic.

Pain occurs when pain receptors, or nerve endings that warn of harmful changes in the body's environment, such as a rise in blood pressure or temperature, transmit impulses to the central nervous system (CNS), which interprets the signal and produces the perception of pain. Anesthesia eliminates pain by interrupting the transmitted impulse. Anesthesia is "the absence of normal sensation, especially sensitivity to pain." The goals in the relief of pain and anxiety are to control patient actions, maintain vital signs, and create a positive memory of dental care.

FORMS OF ANESTHESIA

I. In dentistry, anesthesia is provided in the following forms from the least invasive to the most invasive:
  A. **Topical anesthesia**—an application of a substance to the tissues that creates loss of feeling on the surface
  B. **Local anesthesia**—placement of a substance by

injection at a site that creates a loss of sensation to one part of the body

C. **Conscious sedation**—anesthetic agent used to produce a sedative effect while the patient remains conscious

D. **Inhalation anesthesia**—anesthesia produced by the respiration of an anesthetic agent without loss of consciousness

E. **General anesthesia**—an anesthetic agent that creates a state of unconsciousness with absence of sensation over the entire body

II. The indicators for the selection of relief for a patient are as follows:
A. Anxiety or fear
B. Medical history
C. Physical inability to receive dental treatment
D. Gagging
E. Pain threshold
F. Inability to sit for a long time
G. Level of invasive procedure to be performed

LOCAL ANESTHESIA ▬▬▬▬▬▬

I. **Local anesthesia** is the direct administration of an anesthetic agent to tissues—particularly oral mucosa—to block the sensation of pain.
A. Local anesthesia is also referred to as *regional anesthesia,* depending on the types of nerves that are affected by the anesthetic.
B. Two ways to administer local anesthesia are by topical application or by injection in tissue.
C. Various types of common local anesthetics, dosages, and contraindications are presented in Table 15-1.

II. Topical Anesthesia
A. The simplest local anesthetic is topical anesthetic.
1. It provides a surface analgesia by the application of a substance.
2. Several forms of topical anesthesia are applied with a cotton-tipped or other type of applicator.
a. Liquid or spray
b. Ointment
3. Application of topical anesthesia is an optional procedure in many dental offices.
4. Placement of topical anesthesia is a legally delegated responsibility of the dental assistant and/or hygienist in some states.
5. Topical anesthesia is placed on mucosal tissues and acts on particular nerve endings to relieve the sensation of pain and reduce the possibility of psychogenic response.

B. Two types of adverse reactions have been observed:
1. An allergic reaction to certain ingredients of the anesthesia that presents as *erythema*—a diffused redness of the tissues—or as *angioedema*—a swelling of the mucous membranes.
2. An overdose reaction that is caused by the quick absorption of the anesthesia through the mucous membranes, which eventually results in an increase in local anesthesia blood level.

III. Injectable Anesthetics
A. Local injectable anesthetics used in dental care are either **amides** or **esters,** which are types of compound chemicals used in anesthesia.
B. Common accepted amides include the following:
1. Lidocaine
2. Mepivacaine
3. Prilocaine
C. Common esters include the following:
1. Procaine
2. Tetracaine
3. Propoxycaine
D. If a sensitivity to a drug of one group exists, the other can be substituted.
E. Local anesthetics are supplied in liquid form in premeasured **carpules** or **cartridges** and in ampules.
1. The form selected depends on the operator's choice; the carpule form is most common.
2. Local anesthetics may contain a vasoconstrictor, which constricts blood flow at the site of injection.
a. This increases the duration of the anesthetic in the injection site.
b. It lowers the systemic toxicity of the drugs by slowing the absorption of anesthetic into the cardiovascular system.
c. It decreases the amount of blood at the injection site.
d. Common vasoconstrictors are Neo-Cobefrin and epinephrine, in a concentration of 1 part vasoconstrictor to 50,000 parts of anesthesia solution (1:50,000) or 1:100,000 or 1:200,000.
3. The American Society of Anesthesiologists (ASA) adopted a standard for referencing the physical classification of patients known as

Table 15-1   Pharmacology of dental anesthesia/analgesia*

Substance	Chemical composition	Primary function	Common dosages	Brand names	Duration	Contraindications	Hazards
Mepivacaine	d, 1-N-methyle-pipecolic Acid-2,6, dimeth-ylanilide	Local anesthesia	1:20,000	Carbocaine with Neo-Cobefrin	100 min	Patients with history of malignant hyper-pyrexia Heart patients	Biting of oral tis-sues
Lidocaine	Diethyl 1 to 2, 6 di-methylacetanilid	Local anesthesia	1:50,00 1:100,00	Xylocaine Octocaine	100 min	Same as above	Same as above
Benzocaine	Ethyl aminbenzoate	Topical anesthesia	As indicated	Hurricaine	15 to 30 min		Localized irritation; allergic reaction
Nitrous oxide		Conscious sedation	35% to 40%		10 to 15 min after delivery	Pregnancy (for re-peated exposure) Patient with mental or physical inability to communicate Patient with respira-tory problems	50% administration may cause gen-eral anesthesia
Barbiturate	Malonylurea	Conscious sedation, primary CNS de-pressant	50 to 100 mg	Nembutal	2-4 hr IV	Patients with cardio-vascular, renal, he-patic system impair-ment	Respiratory depres-sion resulting in death
Narcotic	Opiate	Conscious sedation, primary CNS de-pressant	8 to 16 mg	Morphine		No operating motor vehicles, tools or in-gesting alcohol and drugs	Bradycardia

*This chart is a sampling of available anesthesia agents. It is not all-inclusive for use, contraindications, or potential hazards. It is the dentist's responsibility to know the pharmacology of these and any other drugs that a patient may take.

the **ASA Physical Status Classification System** (box above).

a. This system provides the operator with a benchmark of categorizing patient medical risk.

b. If the ASA ratings are used, patients for whom dental treatment is contraindicated, such as those with an ASA IV rating, would be the least likely candidates for use of a vasoconstrictor.

4. If epinephrine is contraindicated, the drug of choice would then be a local anesthesia without a vasoconstrictor.

F. Three common forms of injections are performed in dentistry (Fig. 15-1 A-C).

1. **Infiltration**

a. This is the process of depositing anesthesia solution into tissues, allowing time for the absorption of the solution by the many terminal nerve endings at the site.

b. It is usually used when a single tooth is designated for treatment or when a biopsy, gingivectomy, or other tissue surgery is planned.

2. **Field block**

a. This is a deposit of anesthetic solution near a major terminal nerve.

b. It usually involves the deposit of anesthetic solution at the apex of a tooth; apex is completely encircled with anesthesia.

c. It anesthetizes the major terminal nerve branch or smaller terminal nerve endings that transmit pain to the brain.

d. It is occasionally used on the mandibular anterior teeth or even premolar areas of some patients depending on the anatomic structures.

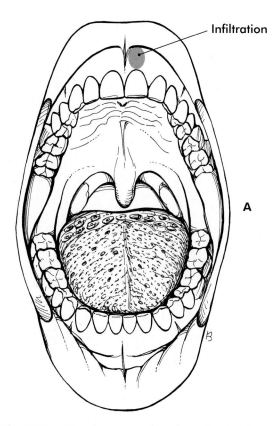

Fig. 15-1   Common examples of anesthesia injections. *A,* Infiltration.

3. **Nerve block**

a. This is most commonly used in the mandibular arch, with the deposit of anesthetic solution near the inferior alveolar nerve.

b. During innervation, the tongue, lip, cheek, gingiva, and teeth are anesthetized.

c. It is the only effective local anesthesia in the mandibular arch.

G. **Periodontal ligament injection** (intraligamentary injection)

1. This type of injection involves the injection of anesthetic solution under pressure into the periodontal membrane of a specific tooth.

2. It is a type of infiltration technique; an aspirating syringe or a periodontal ligament syringe is available for this technique.

IV. Special Concerns Regarding Administration of Local Anesthetic

A. The use of vasoconstrictor when contraindicated must be considered.

B. Injection of local anesthesia into a blood vessel can result in complications in vital organs, particularly the heart.

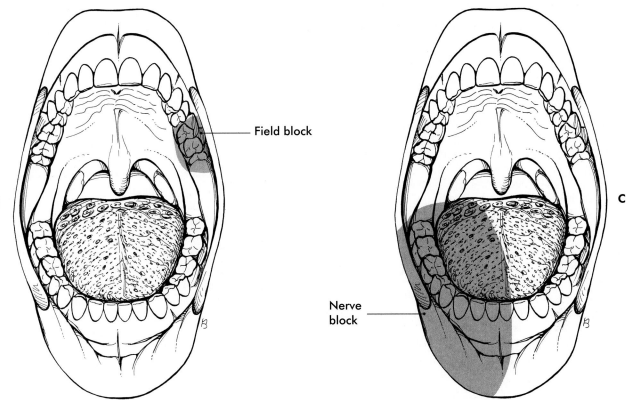

Fig. 15-1, cont'd   Common examples of anesthesia injections. *B,* Field block. *C,* Nerve block.

C. Duration must be explained to patient to avoid self-injury during this time from biting the tongue, lip, and cheek; once the anesthetic effect subsides, the pain will return.

D. When a child is treated, the parents or caregiver must be informed of this situation.

E. **Toxicity**—the degree to which an anesthetic solution can be poisonous—is a concern when working with dental anesthetics.
   1. Toxic reaction is related to the amount of drug in the blood that affects the CNS, the respiratory system, or the circulatory system.
   2. Reaction to toxicity depends on a number of factors, including the following:
      a. Compound of the solution used
      b. Amount of solution used
      c. Rate of injection
      d. Rate of absorption of the solution
      e. Age of patient
      f. Physical characteristics of patient

F. **Paresthesia**—numbness that occurs after the effect of the anesthesia is exhausted—must be considered.
   1. This is caused by trauma to nerve tissues,

hemorrhage near the nerve sheath, or contamination of the anesthetic solution.
   2. It usually resolves itself within 6 to 8 weeks after the onset, but damage can be permanent.

PREPARATION FOR ANESTHETIC PROCEDURE

I. Patient Health History Update
   A. Identify health contraindications to vasoconstrictors.
   B. Identify other health contraindications or reactions.

II. Selection of the Anesthesia Carpule
   A. Remove the carpule from the container and check the type of anesthesia, the concentration, and the expiration date.
   B. Inspect the carpule to determine whether it is safe to use (box on page 250).
   C. Review anesthetic selection checkpoints (box on page 250).

III. Selection of the Anesthetic Needle
   A. Select a disposable needle (box on page 250).
   B. Needles are supplied in two lengths: 1 inch and 1 ⅝ inches.

INSPECTION OF ANESTHETIC CARPULES

- Is the diaphragm or rubber plunger free of cracks or tears?
- Is the solution clear and free of discoloration?
- Are there cracks in the glass container?
- Is the carpule completely filled with solution?
- Is the type of solution selected the appropriate anesthesia based on the patient's medical history?
- Are there any air bubbles in the carpule?
- Has the expiration date passed?
- Have you rechecked the type of anesthetic to be used with this specific patient?

ANESTHETIC SELECTION CHECKPOINTS

Check point 1   When the patient record is examined
Check point 2   When the anesthetic solution is examined
Check point 3   Before assembly of the syringe

BENEFITS OF DISPOSABLE NEEDLES

- The presterilized needle is used only once for patient safety.
- The risk of needle punctures during a sterilization procedure is eliminated with disposal of the needle.
- Because the needle is for a single-use injection, a sharp needle is always used.

C. The needle selected depends on the operator's choice and the area to be anesthetized.
 1. Generally, a long needle (1 5/8 inches) is selected for use during a nerve block or for the mandibular injection.
 2. For an infiltration or field block the choice is usually a short needle (1 inch).
 3. An exception could be the selection of a needle for the maxillary premolar, cuspid, or incisor area, which may require a long needle to access the infraorbital nerve.
D. The diameter or gauge of the needle varies.
 1. The smaller the diameter of the needle, the larger the gauge number.
 2. The normal range of needle gauge used in dentistry is 25 to 30.
 3. A smaller-gauge needle is often used in the infiltration and field block.

4. For a nerve block, which requires a stronger and often longer needle, a 25- or 27-gauge, 1 5/8-inch needle might be used.
E. Parts of the disposable anesthetic needle are as follows:
 1. Anesthetic needle is manufactured with a plastic sheath cover that serves as a protective shield.
  a. One section of the protective cover is clear and the other may or may not be color coded to coordinate with the gauge of the syringe.
  b. Clear cover protects the hub end of the needle, which attaches to the hub of the syringe; other protective section of plastic covers the injection end of the needle.
 2. The needle itself has a hollow center called a **lumen,** which terminates in a beveled end.
F. The anesthetic syringe is described as follows:
 1. The most common form of syringe found in dentistry today is the metal or nonmetal aspirating syringe.
 2. The aspirating syringe provides the operator with several advantages:
  a. It allows the plunger of the syringe to be pulled back to determine where the needle has been positioned in the tissue; if it has been placed in a blood vessel, blood will be aspirated or drawn back into the carpule, and the operator can withdraw and reposition the needle.
  b. The needle and carpule used with this style of syringe can be discarded.
G. Assembly of the anesthetic syringe is described (box on page 251).
IV. Hidden Syringe Transfer Technique
A. This is an accepted method of instrument transfer during local anesthesia administration.
B. The technique reduces the patient stress and anxiety that frequently occur during the anesthetic procedure.
C. The procedure is described (box on page 252).

INHALED GASES

I. Conscious sedation
A. Inhaled gases are used for conscious sedation, an anesthetic procedure in which anesthesia and analgesia are accomplished without loss of consciousness, onset is rapid, and the patient recovers quickly.
B. Different drugs are used in the administration of conscious sedation.
C. Drug choice is predicated by the following:
 1. Patient's health history

ANESTHETIC SYRINGE ASSEMBLY

ASSEMBLING THE ANESTHETIC SYRINGE

1. Pick up the injection needle and break away the clear protective cover. Do not remove the opposing protective cover until the operator is ready to administer the anesthetic.
2. Hold the needle-end protective cover and carefully feed the hub end of the needle on a parallel plane into the hub end of the syringe.
3. Loosen the protective cover of the injection end of the needle, but do not remove it.
4. Always leave the cover on the injection end of the needle until you place the syringe into the operator's hand.
5. Increase the opening of the breech area to position the carpule in the breech-loading area of the syringe.
6. Place the preselected anesthetic carpule in the breech side of the syringe so that the metal diaphragm of the carpule is near the needle and the plunger end of the carpule is near the harpoon of the syringe.
7. Cup a hand around the breech of the syringe and firmly rap the opposing hand against the thumb ring to engage the harpoon in the carpule.
8. Check the forengagement of the harpoon in the plunger.
9. Remove any air bubbles.
10. Prepare the topical anesthetic before the injection if the operator is going to use it.

HIDDEN SYRINGE TRANSFER TECHNIQUES

1. Assume a caring role to allay any possible fears while the operator positions the patient's head to gain the best visibility at the injection site.
2. Pass a 2 × 2 gauze sponge to the operator to dry the oral mucosa at the site of injection.
3. Exchange the gauze sponge for the cotton tipped applicator that has been dipped in topical anesthetic.
4. The operator applies topical anesthetic to the site for 60 to 90 seconds.
5. Dispose of the applicator and pass the syringe to the operator.
6. Rest your hand under the operator's hand to steady the two together. With the right hand, carefully move the syringe below the patient's chin and place the thumb ring over the operator's thumb.
7. The barrel of the syringe is laid into the operator's palm and the breech side of the syringe is turned toward the operator.
8. Remove the protective cover on the needle and clear the hand from the site. The protective cover is laid in the lid of the tray, with the opening pointed toward the assistant; or the assistant can place the sheath in a manufactured recapping device.
9. Observe the patient's reactions during the injection—unusual flutters of the eyes, change in skin color, undue perspiration, or anguish.
10. The operator draws back on the plunger to ensure that the injection needle is not positioned in a blood vessel.
11. The operator completes the injection and removes the syringe from the patient's mouth.
12. Hold a 2 × 2 gauze between the thumb and index finger of the left hand. Retrieve the syringe from the operator; carefully clear the needle; grasp the barrel of the syringe, and pass the gauze sponge to the operator.
13. Do not recap the needle by using the two-handed technique. OSHA guidelines require that a recapping device or a single-handed technique be implemented.
14. The operator uses the 2 × 2 gauze and returns it to the assistant. As soon as the treatment is completed, an entry of services rendered is placed on the patient's permanent record. Pertinent information that involves the treatment is entered, including the type and amount of anesthesia administered.
15. After the treatment is completed, disassemble the syringe in the sterilization area.
16. Dispose of the needle and carpule in a sharps container.

 2. Physical examination
 3. Projected level of apprehension
II. Nitrous oxide
  A. **Nitrous oxide** is the most common anesthetic gas used in dentistry.
  B. It is one of the first anesthetics used to provide comfort to the patient.
  C. It can be used as an analgesic gas alone.
  D. It can be used in conjunction with other inhaled or injected agents.
  E. It is a sweet-smelling gas that affects patients within 2 to 5 minutes after breathing it, rather than the hour or more required by oral premedication.

FOUR-HANDED HIDDEN SYRINGE TECHNIQUE: TEAM APPROACH	
OPERATOR	ASSISTANT
	Assemble armamentarium.
	Place on mobile cart out of patient's view.
	Pass 2 × 2 gauze.
Dry site with gauze.	Pick up applicator with topical anesthetic.
Return 2 × 2 gauze, receive applicator.	Exchange applicator for 2 × 2 gauze.
Place topical anesthetic.	Discard 2 × 2 gauze.
Return applicator.	Receive and discard applicator.
Wait for topical anesthetic effectiveness.	Pick up syringe.
	Loosen protective cover slightly.
	Hold syringe in right hand.
Position right hand in transfer zone.	Stabilize operator's right hand with left hand.
	Position thumb ring over thumb and place barrel of syringe into palm of operator's hand.
Place thumb into thumb ring and place fingers on it to grip.	Turn breech opening so that operator can observe carpule.
	Withdraw protective covering.
	Release operator's right hand.
	Move hand out of position.
Move syringe to oral cavity.	
Make injection.	Place left arm over patient's torso area, if needed, to avoid patient making sudden movement (hold hand of young child if necessary).
	Observe vital signs, nonverbal cues.
	Grasp 2 × 2 gauze in receiving portion of hand (note reverse position in this transfer).
Return syringe (observe location of needle for safe transfer).	Observe location of needle for safe pickup.
	Grasp syringe by barrel.
	Pass 2 × 2 gauze.
Receive 2 × 2 gauze.	Return syringe to mobile cart.
Wipe injection site.	Recap with single hand or recapping device.
	Transfer setup to fixed cabinetry if desired.
Return 2 × 2 gauze.	Receive 2 × 2 gauze, discard.
	Pick up a/w syringe in left hand and HVE hose in right hand.
	Turn a/w nozzle to appropriate area, and turn on HVE.
Retract tissue.	Transfer a/w syringe.
Receive a/w syringe.	
Spray water at injection site.	Evacuate fluid from the mouth.
Return a/w syringe.	Receive a/w syringe.

F. It results in a pleasant, somewhat disoriented feeling that is often accompanied by numbness.

G. It can be titrated to a desired effect.
   1. *Titration* refers to the administration of small amounts of medication periodically until the patient is sufficiently relaxed.
   2. The oral surgeon or the delegated team member administers the gas until the patient reaches the desired state of relaxation and reduced anxiety, usually 3 to 5 minutes.
   3. The dosage is then adjusted to maintain that level.
   4. Unlike oral sedatives, the depth of sedation can rapidly be adjusted upward or downward to achieve the required result.

H. When the dental procedure is completed, the patient inhales 100% oxygen for approximately 5 minutes and quickly recovers.

I. Levels of nitrous oxide that can be administered and the patient's response are listed (box on page 253).

LEVELS OF NITROUS OXIDE AND PATIENT REACTIONS

10% to 15%—There is limited numbness in extremities, sedation, and tingling.

35% to 40%—Sedative effects are increased; the analgesic effect is that of 15 mg of administered morphine. Patient has sensation of heaviness or of floating, and room noises seem distant.

50%—Intensified analgesic symptoms occur; the patient becomes increasingly sleepy and may become unconscious. This is a dangerous state of general anesthesia.

K. A disadvantage of nitrous oxide is that the patient must be able to breathe through the nose for the gas to be effective because it is administered by a nasal mask. It doesn't work well with individuals who have a cold or are mouth breathers.

J. Some individuals may become nauseated by the gas, especially if it is administered at a high level or for a long period.

K. Administration of nitrous oxide is primarily the responsibility of the dentist, but in some states this duty is delegated to the hygienist. In certain states the dental assistant is delegated the responsibility of monitoring the administration of nitrous oxide to the patient.

L. Nitrous oxide is always administered with oxygen.

M. Normal room air contains about 20% oxygen; any anesthetic gas that is administered must have at least as much oxygen as room air. Because of this, many nitrous oxide machines are made to be *fail-safe*.

N. The system is manufactured so that it is impossible to administer more than 70% nitrous oxide or less than 30% oxygen. If for some reason the oxygen tank becomes empty and this circumstance is not recognized, the nitrous oxide machine turns off automatically so as not to deliver 100% nitrous oxide.

O. It is administered to the patient through a disposable or sterilizable mask that covers the nose only. A backup oxygen tank always should be available. Many offices have an alarm system that sounds when the level of the gases is too low, indicating that the tanks need to be replaced. In addition, the assistant is responsible for ensuring that the scavenging system is always functional.

P. Nitrous oxide can be classified as an analgesic rather than an anesthetic gas.

Q. It helps relieve mild pain, but a local anesthetic is required to ensure that the procedure is totally painless.

III. Other Inhaled Gases

A. Some oral surgeons use other anesthetic gases that render the patient unconscious; this is usually done in a hospital setting.

1. These agents are supplied to the oral surgeon in liquid form; however, when the liquid is introduced into the anesthesia machine, it is converted into a gas inside a vaporizer and then mixed with oxygen and possibly nitrous oxide.

2. The mixture of gases is then delivered to the patient through a flow meter, which carefully controls the ratio of gases and the rate of delivery.

B. Some of the general anesthetic gases are halothane (Fluothane), enflurane (Ethrane), and isoflurane (Forane).

1. These are usually administered in a slightly different mode than is the nitrous oxide.

2. With a general anesthetic gas an endotracheal tube is usually placed through the patient's nose or mouth and into the windpipe or trachea.

3. The anesthetic gases are administered through this tube in a controlled fashion.

4. Sometimes the anesthesia is light enough that the patient is still breathing on his or her own.

5. It may be necessary for the oral surgeon to help the patient breathe by squeezing a breathing bag.

6. This system holds less risk of exposure to exhaled gases for the dental team because the gases go directly from the patient's lungs into the anesthesia machine and are disposed of without being discharged into the treatment room.

7. Because the patient is unconscious and is using artificial respiration, the risk for the patient is significantly greater than when nitrous oxide is used and the patient is conscious and breathing on his or her own.

8. Because this system is so complex and the risk greater, a second individual (other than the treating surgeon) usually the anesthesiologist, administers the anesthesia.

IV. Intravenous Administration

A. Intravenous administration is used to inject anesthetic drugs into a vein.

1. The most common types of drugs used for this purpose are narcotics, such as Demerol; sedative-hypnotics, such as Versed; or ultra–short-acting barbiturates, such as Brevital.
2. These medications can be used in various ways to result in either conscious sedation (the patient has a rational response to commands with unassisted breathing) or general anesthesia (the patient is unconscious during the procedure).
3. General anesthesia is usually warranted when a patient is extremely anxious or the ailment is difficult to treat because of the patient's physical or mental condition.
4. This form of anesthesia depresses the CNS and alters the level of consciousness.
5. Depressed levels of consciousness can result in depression of vital functions or trigger cardiac arrhythmias.
B. Arthur E. Guedel, an American anesthesiologist, developed a system that describes the accepted stages of anesthesia; this system can help the operator observe signs the patient may exhibit during treatment (box).
C. Usually, a local anesthetic is administered in conjunction with conscious sedation or general anesthesia.
   1. This is mandatory with conscious sedation because the patient would still be able to feel pain without local anesthetic.
   2. With general anesthesia it reduces the depth of general anesthesia necessary to make the patient comfortable.
   3. Epinephrine in local anesthesia helps to control bleeding, and as the patient recovers from the procedure, there is no sudden burst of pain.
D. The techniques of intravenous conscious sedation and general anesthesia can be combined.
E. An advantage of using an intravenous anesthetic rather than oral medication is the rapid onset of action of most intravenous medications.
F. Another advantage of an intravenous anesthetic using either a sedative-hypnotic, such as Versed, or a general anesthetic is that the patient has amnesia and has no recollection of the procedure.
G. A disadvantage of intravenous anesthetics is that patients must be monitored much more carefully because they cannot communicate their state of health. They cannot protect their own airway, so extra precautions must be taken to make sure they do not choke.

GUEDEL'S SIGNS

Stage 1 (amnesia and analgesia)—begins with the administration of an anesthetic and continues until the patient has lost consciousness; respiration is quiet, sometimes irregular; reflexes are still present.

Stage 2 (delirium or excitement)—begins when the patient has lost consciousness and with the onset of total anesthesia; the patient may move the limbs, chatter incoherently, hold the breath, or become violent; vomiting, with possible danger of aspiration, may occur.

Stage 3 (surgical anesthesia)—begins with stable breathing patterns and total loss of consciousness; first signs of respiratory or cardiovascular failure appear.
   Plane 1—all movement ceases, and respiration is regular; eyeball movements are marked.
   Plane 2—eyeballs are fixed centrally; respiration remains regular.
   Plane 3—pupils no longer react to light; total muscle relaxation occurs; intercostal paralysis (paralysis between the ribs) is present.
   Plane 4—deep anesthesia occurs; no spontaneous respiration; sensation is absent.

Stage 4 (premortem)—signals danger; pupils are dilated to a maximum, and the skin is cold and ashen; blood pressure is extremely low; brachial pulse is feeble or absent; cardiac arrest is imminent.

Questions

Anesthesia

1 Nitrous oxide is an example of which of the following?
a. Local anesthetic
b. Topical anesthetic
c. Conscious sedation
d. General anesthetic

2 An intraligamentary injection would likely be used for which of the following types of treatment?
1. Tooth extraction
2. Subgingival curettage
3. Cavity preparation
4. Apicoectomy
5. Maxillectomy
a. 1 and 3
b. 2 and 4
c. 1, 2, and 3
d. 2, 4, and 5

3 A patient with no health contraindications or fear is to have an amalgam restoration placed. Which type of anesthesia will likely be used?

a. Local

b. General

c. Conscious sedation

4. Indications for selection of anesthesia include all of the following *except:*

   a. Anxiety or fear

   b. Medical history

   c. Level of invasive procedure

   d. Type of insurance coverage

   e. Physical inability to receive dental treatment

5 Which of the following are undesirable characteristics of a local anesthetic carpule?

   1. Clear solution

   2. Solution tan in color

   3. Free of bubbles

   4. Bubbles located only at hub end

   5. Carpule completely filled

   a. 1 and 3

   b. 2 and 4

   c. 1, 2, and 3

   d. 1, 3, and 5

6 All of the following are checkpoints for anesthetic selection *except:*

   a. When patient record is examined

   b. Before assembly of the syringe

   c. When the anesthetic solution is examined

   d. After administration of the anesthetic

7 After injection of local anesthetic, a hematoma appears at the injection site. This is an indication that the solution was

   1. Injected too rapidly

   2. Injected too slowly

   3. Injected into a blood vessel

   4. Not able to dissipate from the site

   5. The cause of bleeding beneath the mucosa

   a. 1 and 3

   b. 2 and 4

   c. 1, 3, and 5

   d. 1, 2, 3, and 4

   e. 2, 3, and 5

8 A week after a crown preparation on a mandibular molar was completed the patient contacted the office and complained about a tingling and lack of feeling on the lower lip. Which of the following statements might be true?

   a. Parasthesia might have occurred.

   b. This condition is normal following this type of treatment.

   c. This is a medical condition unrelated to dental care.

   d. The cervical margin of the temporary crown may be impinging on the mental foramen.

9 A local anesthetic is commonly administered in conjunction with conscious sedation or general anesthesia because

   1. It reduces the depth of general anesthesia necessary to make the patient comfortable.

   2. It reduces bleeding when a vasoconstrictor is used.

   3. As the patient recovers, there is no sudden burst of pain.

   4. It decreases duration when a vasoconstrictor is used.

   5. It eliminates the need to monitor vital signs

   a. 1 and 3

   b. 2 and 4

   c. 1, 2, and 3

   d. 1, 3, and 5

   e. 1, 2, 3, and 4

10 An endotracheal tube would be used in conjunction with which of the following?

   a. Mepivicaine

   b. Lidocaine

   c. Halothane

   d. N20

Match the parts of the syringe at the bottom of the page.

_____ **11** Harpoon

_____ **12** Thumb ring

_____ **13** Hub

_____ **14** Plunger

_____ **15** Thumb rest

16 The area between the dotted lines in Fig. 15-1 is known as the

   a. Barrel

   b. Breech opening

   c. Carpule opening

   d. All of the above

17 Which is the smallest gauge?

   a. 25 g

   b. 27 g

   c. 30 g.

18 Which of the following is (are) characteristic of a local anesthetic?

   1. Patient remains conscious.

   2. Patient becomes unconscious.

   3. Selected regions of the body lose sensation.

   4. Sensation in the entire body is lost.

   5. Patient becomes semiconscious.

   a. 1 and 3

   b. 1, 2, and 4

   c. 1, 3, and 3

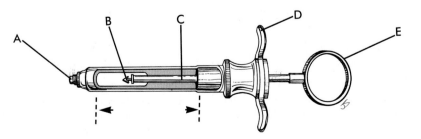

d. 1 only

e. 4 only

19 Which type of anesthetic provides anesthesia only to nerve endings located in the mucosa?

    a. Local

    b. Topical

    c. General

In items 20-23, match the terms in column A with the definitions in column B.

    Column A

a. Part of syringe used to force anesthetic into tissue

b. Area of syringe in which carpule is placed

c. Needle attached to it

d. Needle end of carpule

e. Used once and then disposed

    Column B

_____ **20** Breech

_____ **21** Diaphragm

_____ **22** Carpule

_____ **23** Thumb ring

24 Aspiration during the administration of a local anesthetic will

    a. Damage the mandibular artery

    b. Be extremely painful

    c. Determine whether the lumen of the needle is in a blood vessel

    d. Ensure profound anesthesia

25 Which of the following is a vasoconstrictor?

    1. Xylocaine

    2. Neo-Cobefrin

    3. Carbocaine

    4. Epinephrine

    a. 1 and 3

    b. 1, 2, and 3

    c. 2 and 4

    d. 4 only

Rationales

Anesthesia

1 C Conscious sedation, also known as *awake anesthesia,* is a procedure in which analgesia and anesthesia are accomplished without loss of consciousness. This type of anesthesia is not as complete as general anesthesia, and muscle relaxation is not required.

2 B An intraligamentary injection involves the injection of solution into the periodontal membrane of a tooth or teeth. This procedure is an infiltration technique that does not provide total innervation, which is necessary for tooth extraction, cavity preparations, and oral surgery.

3 A Local anesthesia is usually the choice during dental treatment because conscious sedation and general anesthesia place the patient at greater medical risk due to the effects on the body.

4 D If a patient is anxious about dental treatment, anesthesia to relieve anxiety may be necessary. No matter what type of treatment is provided, the medical history is always evaluated prior to administration. The type of dental care may predicate the anesthesia selected. If more invasive than normal, local anesthesia may not be used or may be used in conjunction with conscious sedation.

A patient with certain physical or emotional restrictions may direct the need for various types of anesthesia. Normally, dental insurance coverage is not a factor in the selection of anesthesia on the part of the dentist, but the patient may opt for local anesthesia if conscious sedation is not covered.

5 B If an anesthetic carpule is discolored—any color rather than clear—it should not be used. Bubbles in an anesthetic carpule should be expelled through the hub end of the needle prior to use on a patient.

6 D The patient record should always be examined prior to the patient's arrival, after the patient has updated the health history, and before setting up the anesthetic syringe. As the anesthetic carpule is placed in the syringe, it should again be checked to verify it as the correct anesthetic.

7 C A slower injection of anesthetic solution into the site reduces discomfort and the potential for damage to the tissue that may cause a hematoma. If the needle penetrates a vessel and is removed, there is a potential for bleeding into the surrounding tissues.

8 A Paresthesia (numbness after the effect of anesthesia has passed) is usually caused by trauma to nerve tissues, hemorrhage near the nerve sheath, or contamination of the anesthetic solution. This condition usually resolves itself in 6 to 8 weeks after the onset, but damage can be permanent.

9 C Local anesthesia reduces discomfort at the treatment site because the effectiveness is site specific and not a CNS suppressant as with conscious or general sedation. A local anesthetic with a vasoconstrictor reduces the amount of bleeding in the treatment site, thus making the procedure easier for the operator. A local anesthetic usually remains effective for some time after the procedure is completed, unlike the other types of anesthesia mentioned.

10 C Halothane is an inhaled anesthetic used in the general anesthesia procedure; the patient must be intubated with an endotracheal tube.

11 B The harpoon is the portion of an aspirating syringe that is impaled in the plunger of the anesthetic carpule.

12 E The thumb ring allows the operator to comfortably place the thumb so as to push the plunger and pull it back during the aspiration step.

13 A The hub of the syringe is the area where the needle is attached to the syringe. It is usually threaded to allow the needle to fit correctly.

14 C The plunger is connected to the thumb ring and the harpoon and assists in expelling the anesthetic solution at the injection site.

15 D The finger rest allows the operator to wrap fingers around it for increased stability during the injection.

16 D The barrel, breech, or carpule opening are known as the same area—the site where the anesthesia carpule is placed.

17 C The larger the number, the smaller the gauge. A 25-gauge needle is larger than a 30-gauge needle.

18 A The patient is always conscious during local anesthesia, and because the anesthetic remains effective in the injection site, only that area of the body loses sensation.

19 B A topical anesthetic is placed on the mucosal tissues to anesthetize the nerve endings. This type of anesthetic is usually used before local anesthetic administration to make the injection more comfortable for the patient.

20 B The carpule is placed in the breech opening of the barrel.

21 D The diaphragm is the metal-covered rubber area of the anesthetic carpule that the needle penetrates.

22 E Anesthetic carpules are a single-use anesthetic preparation.

23 A The thumb ring is the area where the operator places a thumb to help force the anesthetic from the carpule into the injection site.

24 C Aspiration (withdrawing blood into the syringe during an injection) allows the operator to know the lumen is in a blood vessel and should be repositioned to avoid injecting into the vessel.

25 C Xylocaine is a brand of local anesthetic with a vasoconstrictor, and epinephrine is a vasoconstrictor.

To enhance your understanding of the material in this chapter refer to Chapter 23 of Finkbeiner/Johnson: *Mosby's Comprehensive Dental Assisting: A Clinical Approach.*

Oral Diagnosis

A clinical record is an accumulation of data that is gathered from a clinical, radiographic, and photographic examination. From these data the dentist determines a diagnosis. A **diagnosis** is the translation of the data into an organized, classified definition of the conditions present. In some instances, treatment may be necessary before a final diagnosis is determined. The process of diagnosis is the legal responsibility of the dentist only, and though it may appear that the dentist makes a diagnosis quickly, it is arrived at through observation, logical and systematic thinking, and experience. To arrive at a diagnosis, the dentist must rely on the most complete and accurate data, including the patient's past and present history and existing symptoms and conditions.

Oral diagnosis is seldom just the identification of a single disease in the mouth; rather, it is a disclosure of oral or systemic conditions that will require treatment or management. The dentist should be concerned about the patient's total health, the relation of the oral cavity to the patient's general systemic health, the effect of systemic health on the management of the patient's oral conditions, and the patient's self-image. A diagnosis need not be negative. It can be a confirmation of good oral health, healthy tissues, and the absence of disease. Modern dentistry emphasizes not only the control of disease but also prevention of disease.

Patients are concerned for the future and what will occur with the conditions in their mouth when treated or the consequences of these conditions if they remain untreated. Therefore, the dentist makes a **prognosis**—the foretelling of the probable course of disease.

EXAMINATION PROCESS

I. Patient data collection is an ongoing process.

II. Initially, the patient visits the dental office as either a new patient or an emergency patient and then becomes a patient of record.

III. The phases of oral diagnosis focus on the following:
   A. Personal, medical, and dental history
   B. **Clinical examination**
   C. Radiographic examination
   D. Photographic examination
   E. Diagnostic models
   F. Laboratory tests
   G. Diagnosis

IV. The dental assistant plays an integral role in the collection of data for a **clinical record** by performing the following duties:
   A. Obtaining a patient history
   B. Exposing, processing, and mounting radiographs
   C. Obtaining and recording vital signs
   D. Obtaining preliminary impressions for study models
   E. Taking photographs
   F. Recording clinical data
   G. Charting oral conditions
   H. Completing laboratory requisitions
   I. Transferring the patient to a laboratory or physician for follow-up studies or care
   J. Obtaining laboratory results
   K. Preparing a clinical record for review
   L. Preparing materials for case presentation

PATIENT HISTORY

I. A **patient history** is a personal document containing specific information about the patient.
   A. This information is highly confidential.
   B. Thorough treatment requires complete and accurate information.
   C. Three parts of the patient history include the following:
      1. Personal history includes the following information:

NECESSARY DENTAL HISTORY INFORMATION

Frequency of dental visits and an oral prophylaxis
Past experience or reactions with local anesthetics and other intraoral agents
Dates, nature, and length of time of past specialty treatment, such as periodontal therapy and including subgingival curettage, gingival surgery, or occlusal adjustments; orthodontic treatment and any appliances still being worn; endodontic therapy, such as root-canal fillings or an apicoectomy; surgical procedures, such as extractions; other treatment that has been performed inside or around the oral cavity
Placement of fixed bridges, including the insertion dates and any complications that occurred
Use of removable dental prostheses, and when these appliances were adjusted or relined
Use of bite splints or other oral appliances; type and reason for use
Attitude of patient toward past dental treatment and experience

---

a. Complete legal name
b. Address
c. Business and home phone numbers
d. Place of employment
e. Social security number
f. Physician's name and address
g. Person responsible for payment
h. Spousal and other family information if applicable
i. Occupation
j. Insurance information
k. Person to contact in case of an emergency

2. **Medical history** is a collection of data provided by the patient about his or her general health; it is an important means of preventing medical emergencies.

3. **Dental history** provides information about previous treatment and dental experience and is often a component of the health questionnaire (box above).

CLINICAL EXAMINATION

I. Observe general diagnostic signs (box on page 260).

II. Obtain **vital signs**
   A. **Temperature** (box)
   B. **Pulse** (box on page 261)

GENERAL DIAGNOSTIC SIGNS

- Is there any facial asymmetry, such as a drooping eyelid, bulging eyes, or drooping lip?
- Is the skin color appropriate for the patient, or is there a grey pallor, yellowed skin or eyes, or redness on the skin? Is the skin drawn and glossy, or is it dry?
- Does the patient appear alert or withdrawn? Is the patient aware of the questions you are asking? Does the patient seem anxious?
- Are there obvious breath odors, and if so, can they be traced to a source?
- Is the patient ambulatory? Does he or she seem to be flexible when moving about?
- What is the reaction of the pupils? Are they dilated?
- What do the patient's nails look like? Are the nail beds discolored? Is there evidence of nail biting?
- Does the patient seem able to use his or her hands, or are they crippled? Do they appear arthritic?
- Does the patient react to stimuli?

  C. **Respiration** (box on page 261)
  D. **Blood pressure** (box on page 261)
  E. Factors to consider when obtaining blood pressure (box on page 262).
III. Changes in a patient's temperature, pulse, respiration (TPR), or blood pressure (BP) may be an indication of existing or future problems.
IV. Note normal versus abnormal vital signs.
  A. Temperature
    1. Normal is 98.6° F or 37° C.
    2. Exercise, excitement, the digestive process, infection, cold, shock, and drugs, may affect body temperature.
    3. It may vary with a patient's age and the time of day.
    4. An elevated temperature, commonly known as *fever* or ***pyrexia,*** is usually an indication of illness; *hyperpyrexia* is a high fever—usually above 105.8° F.
    5. A subnormal temperature, **hypothermia,** is often a result of trauma.
  B. Pulse rate
    1. Pulse rate fluctuates with age, weight, and size.
    2. The normal rate of an infant is 120 to 140 beats per minute.
    3. An adult's pulse rate is approximately 60 to 80 beats per minute.

OBTAINING BODY TEMPERATURE

ELECTRONIC THERMOMETER

- Wash and glove.
- Determine that the patient has not eaten, smoked, drunk, or rinsed or brushed the teeth within the last 15 minutes.
- Place a protective disposable sheath over the stem of thermometer.
- Hold the tip near the high graduated numbers of the thermometer.
- Turn on the electronic readout.
- Place the tip with the sheath under the patient's tongue and ask the patient to hold it in place for approximately 25 to 30 seconds.
- Listen for the sound of the electronic signal, which indicates that the temperature has registered on the electronic readout.
- Read the temperature with the plastic sheath in place.
- Turn off the thermometer probe.
- Remove the plastic sheath.
- Remove the protective gloves and wash your hands.
- Record the data in the patient's clinical record.

GLASS THERMOMETER

- Wash and glove.
- Wipe the thermometer with a disinfectant-saturated wipe.
- Shake down the mercury toward the bulb by holding the opposite end with the thumb and forefinger and snapping the wrist once or twice.
- Place the thermometer under the tongue, as with the electronic thermometer, and ask the patient to hold it stationary for approximately 3 to 4 minutes.
- Remove the thermometer and hold it parallel to the floor at eye level.
- Slowly turn the thermometer until you can see the exact point at which the mercury is registered.
- Wipe the thermometer with a disinfectant-saturated gauze.
- Remove the gloves, and wash your hands.
- Record the information on the clinical record.

Note: The registration is not in tenths of degrees other than 98.6° F.

    4. The pulse rate of females is usually slightly higher than that of males.
    5. It is usually slower when a person is at rest and at first waking.
    6. Pain, anger, fear, stress, and the element of surprise can elevate the pulse rate; physical

OBTAINING A PULSE RATE

Under normal conditions in a dental office, a patient's pulse rate is assessed in the radial artery of the wrist.
- Palpate the artery on the medial surface and thumb side of the wrist.
- Place the patient's arm in an extended position, with the palm up; provide support.
- Place two or three fingers on the radial artery and radius bone until you feel the pulsing blood. If you use excess force or use the thumb, you will not feel the contraction and expansion of the blood through the artery.
- Use a watch with a second hand or a digital second counter to count the pulse for 15 seconds.
- Multiply the number of pulses by 4 to determine the minute rate of pulsations. The pulse can also be counted for 30 seconds and multiplied by 2 for the minute rate.
- Record the patient's pulse rate in the clinical record. If you are uncertain of the rate, take a second reading.

OBTAINING A RESPIRATION RATE

The respiration rate fluctuates when body temperature increases with exercise, pain, or excitement or when diseases of the respiratory system are present.
- Continue to maintain the same position used to obtain the pulse rate.
- Try to obtain the measurement when the patient is unaware of your actions. Often a patient breathes abnormally when a breathing measurement is taken.
- Count the number of respirations with the rise and fall of the patient's chest as a single respiration.
- Count the respirations for 30 seconds; then multiply the number by 2 for the minute rate of respirations.
- If the rates are abnormal, count a second time to confirm the first number.
- Record the information in the patient's clinical record.

OBTAINING A BLOOD PRESSURE READING

- Describe the procedure to the patient; explain that the cuff may be tight around the arm for a short time.
- Have the patient remove or loosen any constricting clothing that might interfere with the reading.
- Seat the patient comfortably in a chair with the arm supported and the palm up, or have the patient lie down.
- Position yourself so that you are at eye level with the manometer.
- Remove all air from the cuff by opening the valve and forcing the air out.
- Wrap the cuff around the patient's arm over the brachial artery and slightly above the elbow; secure the cuff with the Velcro end. The width of the cuff should be roughly the diameter of the patient's arm. Cuff sizes vary for newborns, infants, children, adults, large adults, and the thigh. Incorrect sizes can distort readings.
- Place the stethoscope over the site where the pulse of the artery is felt.
- Pump the air bulb of the manometer to force air into the bladder of the cuff. The mercury should rise to approximately 20 mm Hg above an expected **systolic pressure** for the particular patient.
- Open the air valve of the manometer, allowing the air to escape slowly.
- Visually and mentally record the number at which the first heartbeat is heard (systolic pressure).
- Continue to release air through the cuff gradually, until the heartbeat can no longer be heard, and again make a visual and mental record of this number **(diastolic pressure).**
- Release the remaining air from the cuff and remove the stethoscope and cuff from the patient's arm.
- Record the information on the patient's clinical chart.

activity, increased heat, elevated body temperature, decreased BP, and disease that causes lowered oxygenation of the blood supply can cause changes in the pulse rate.
7. Terms related to pulse amplitude are described in Table 16-1.

C. Respiration rate
1. The normal respiration rate for an adult is 14 to 18 respirations per minute; respiration rate of females is faster than that of males.
2. An infant's respiration rate is approximately 40 counts per minute; a child's, 25 to 30 counts per minute.
3. Respiration patterns may vary from a slow, regular rate to a normal, fast, or patterned rate (Table 16-2).

FACTORS TO CONSIDER WHEN OBTAINING BLOOD PRESSURE

Several factors should be considered when obtaining an accurate BP reading, including the following:

Movement of stethoscope, operator, or patient will create inaccurate sounds.

Stethoscope and manometer should be maintained regularly to ensure that no breaks or leaks are present in the tubes, bag, or valves.

If stethoscopes are shared, be certain that the ear tips are cleaned and disinfected.

Make sure that the patient is seated comfortably and the operator is positioned to observe the manometer clearly.

The bladder of the cuff should be completely empty of air before use.

Repeated attempts to obtain a BP reading in the same limb may cause false readings.

Table 16-1 Terms related to pulse amplitudes

Pulse	Description
Normal	Pulse is easily felt and requires moderate pressure to disappear.
Absent	No pulse can be felt, even when extreme pressure is applied.
Thready	Pulse is difficult to feel; slight pressure causes it to disappear.
Weak	Stronger than thready pulse; when slight pressure is applied, it may disappear.
Strong	A pounding pulse that does not disappear with moderate pressure.

COMMON BREATHING SOUNDS

- Rales or crackles—intermittent sounds that are caused by moisture in the respiratory passage; these often sound like air-filled rice cereal after milk is poured over it.
- Rhonchi or gurgles—continuous, low-pitched sounds that occur when air moves through narrowed passageways in the lungs that contain an accumulation of secretions. These sounds may occur during inhalation but are commonly heard during expiration or during both. The sounds may change with coughing.
- Wheezing—high-pitched sound that occurs during respiration when air is forced through narrow respiratory passages; often heard in patients with asthma.
- Friction rub—grating noise that occurs when two structures rub across each other; occurs when membranes are dry and the pleura of the lungs rub against each other.

4. **Stridor** is a harsh, high-pitched sound heard on inspiration when the upper airway is narrow; it is common in children with croup.

5. **Dyspnea** describes difficulty in breathing, which may be a temporary condition in some persons, such as a runner who gasps for air at the end of a race or a person who may gasp for breath after quickly running up stairs.

6. **Adventitious sounds** are abnormal sounds, and (although they are often not heard) are evident with a stethoscope.

7. Common breathing sounds are described (box on the right).

8. Cardinal signs of breathing difficulties that indicate a patient's life is in jeopardy include the following:

   1. Cyanosis (blueness) is a cardinal sign.
   2. Cheyne-Stokes respiration occurs when the patient breathes deeply and rapidly for approximately 30 seconds, stops breathing for 10 to 30 seconds, and then repeats the cycle.

D. Blood pressure

   1. This varies according to age, gender, time of the day, exercise, stress, emotion, body position, and whether a meal has been ingested.

   2. The normal systolic measurement is up to 140 mm Hg; 140 to 159 mm Hg is considered borderline hypertensive; a higher reading is isolated systolic hypertensive.

   3. The normal diastolic reading is under 85; 85 to 89 mm Hg is the high end of normal, 90 to 104 mm Hg is mildly hypertensive, 105 to 114 mm Hg is moderately hypertensive, and 115 mm Hg and above is severe hypertension.

   4. **Hypertension** is elevated BP for a sustained period.

   5. **Hypotension** is below-normal BP.

Table 16-2 Types of breathing

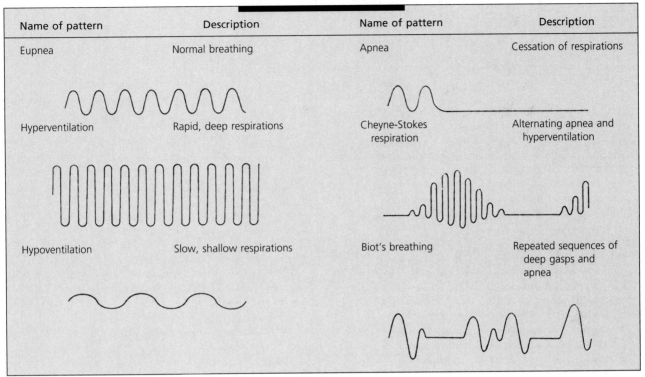

Name of pattern	Description	Name of pattern	Description
Eupnea	Normal breathing	Apnea	Cessation of respirations
Hyperventilation	Rapid, deep respirations	Cheyne-Stokes respiration	Alternating apnea and hyperventilation
Hypoventilation	Slow, shallow respirations	Biot's breathing	Repeated sequences of deep gasps and apnea

From Thibodeau GA, Patton KT: *Anatomy & physiology,* ed 2, St Louis, 1993, Mosby.

CHARTING ORAL CONDITIONS

I.   A variety of graphic symbols (Table 16-3) are used to indicate specific conditions that exist on the teeth and supporting structures of the mouth.

II.   The use of symbols makes it easy to look at a dental chart and to identify conditions in the mouth without reading a detailed narrative.

III. Table 16-4 lists alphabetic codes that are commonly used for a variety of oral conditions.

EXTRAORAL EXAMINATION

I.   This involves observing asymmetry, lesions, swellings, or discoloration.

II.   Data collection begins at this point.

III. This requires good listening skills, attention to detail, and a high degree of accuracy.

IV.   Portions of this examination may be performed by the dental assistant in some states.

V.   Data during this phase of the examination are obtained by observation or palpation.

VI.   The procedure for this examination is shown (box).

CONDUCTING AN EXTRAORAL EXAMINATION

1. Observe facial symmetry for irregularities (e.g., drooping eyelids or lips, prominence of the eyeballs, an enlargement in the neck, a cyst).

2. Inspect the skin of the face and neck for lesions, swellings, or discoloration; jaundice; or severe bruises about the head and face.

3. Inspect the nails for bluish color, pallor, rounded clubbing of the fingers, or lesions caused by nail-biting.

4. Observe the hands to note color and texture of skin and nails.

5. Examine the lymph nodes for size and shape, mobility, single versus multiple, and tenderness. Begin in the submental area and proceed to the submandibular and the carotid region. Examine the nodes in the jugular chain along the sterno-cleidomastoid muscle.

6. Examine the temporomandibular joint for tenderness, popping, clicking, or other abnormality in the opening, such as excessive lateral movement.

Table 16-3 Oral Conditions—Terms and Symbols

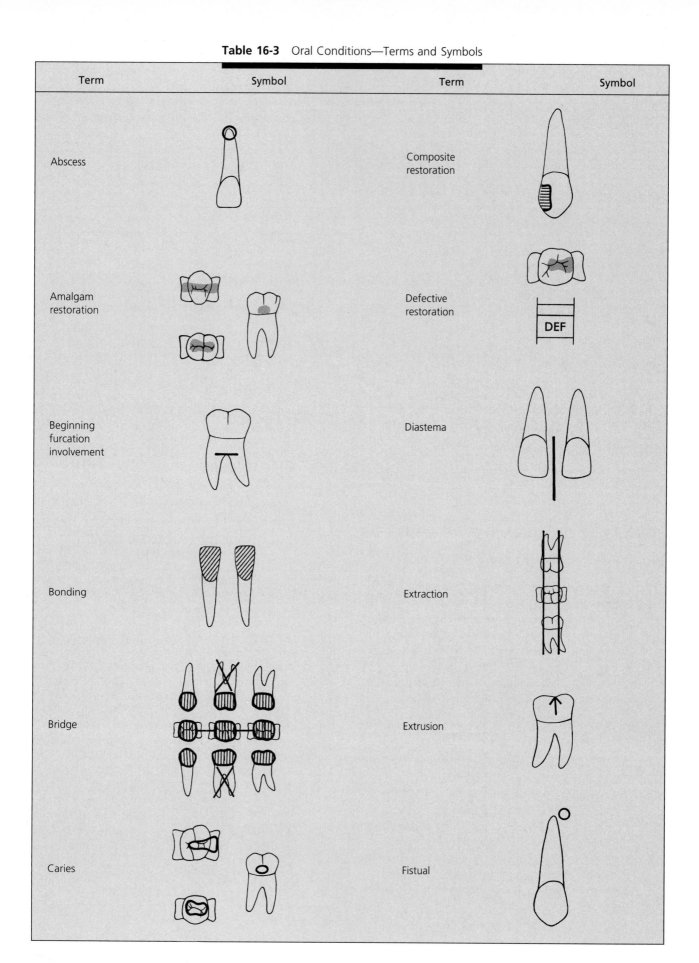

Term	Symbol	Term	Symbol
Abscess		Composite restoration	
Amalgam restoration		Defective restoration	
Beginning furcation involvement		Diastema	
Bonding		Extraction	
Bridge		Extrusion	
Caries		Fistual	

Table 16-3 Oral Conditions—Terms and Symbols—cont'd

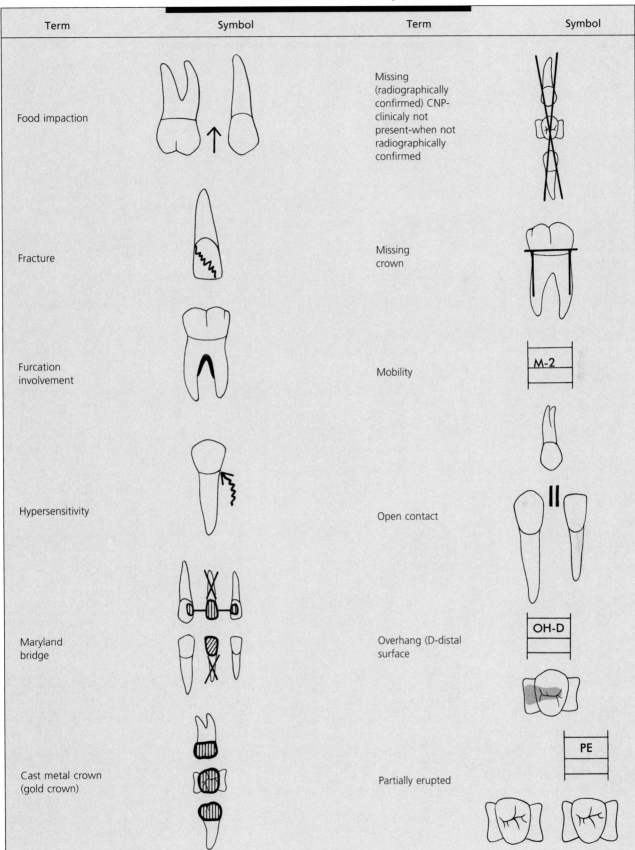

Term	Symbol	Term	Symbol
Food impaction		Missing (radiographically confirmed) CNP-clinicaly not present-when not radiographically confirmed	
Fracture		Missing crown	
Furcation involvement		Mobility	M-2
Hypersensitivity		Open contact	
Maryland bridge		Overhang (D-distal surface	OH-D
Cast metal crown (gold crown)		Partially erupted	PE

Continued

Table 16-3 Oral Conditions—Terms and Symbols—cont'd

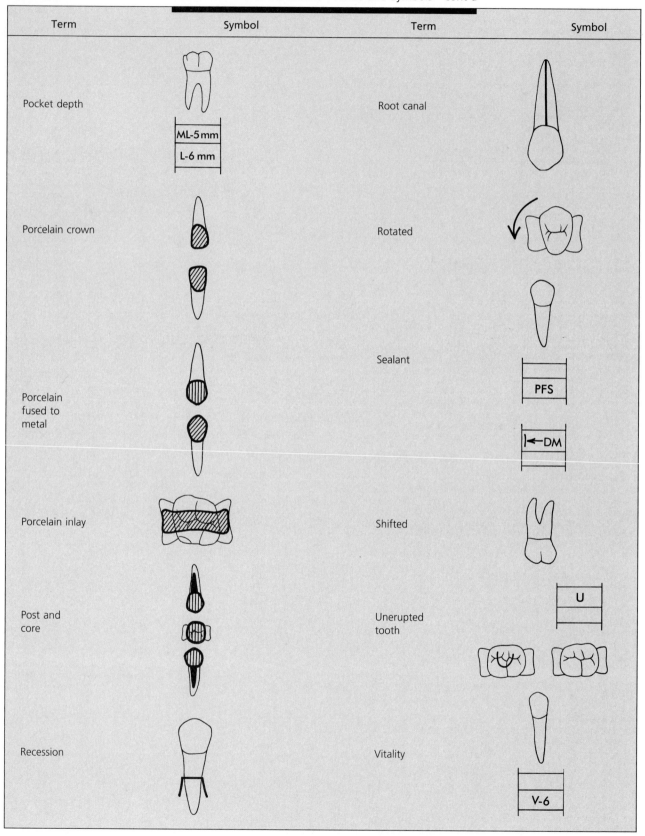

Term	Symbol	Term	Symbol
Pocket depth	ML-5 mm / L-6 mm	Root canal	
Porcelain crown		Rotated	
Porcelain fused to metal		Sealant	PFS / ←DM
Porcelain inlay		Shifted	
Post and core		Unerupted tooth	U
Recession		Vitality	V-6

Table 16-4 Suggested charting abbreviations

Abbreviation	Term	Abbreviation	Term
@	at	I & D	Incision and drainage
a, am, ag	Amalgam	IA	Incurred accidentally
amp	Ampule	IH	Infectious hepatitis
amt	Amount	IM	Intramuscular
anes	Anesthesia	imp	Impression
appl	Applicable, application, appliance	IMP	Impacted
		inj	Injection, injury
approx	Approximate	inop	Inoperable, inoperative
BF	Bone fragment	IV	Intravenous
BP	Blood pressure	lab	Laboratory
Br	Bridge	lac	Laceration
BW	Bitewing radiograph	lat	Lateral
Bx	Biopsy	ling	Lingual
C	Composite	liq	Liquid
carbo	Carbocaine	LLQ	Lower left quadrant
caps	Capsules	LN	Lymph node
cav	Cavity	LRQ	Lower right quadrant
CC	Chief complaint	M, mes	Mesial
CM	Cast metal	mand	Mandibular
cond	Condition	max	Maximum, maxillary
CSX	Complete series x-rays	MDR	Minimum daily requirement
cur	Curettage	med	Medicine, medical
CV	Cardiovascular	mg, mgm	Milligram
CVA	Cerebrovascular accident	MO	Mesioocclusal
D or DV	Devital	MOD	Mesioocclusodistal
dbl	Double	mo	Month
DEF	Defective	MS	Multiple sclerosis
Dg or Dx	Diagnosis	narc	Narcotic
DM	Diagnostic models	nc	No change, no charge
DMF	Decayed, missing, and filled	NCP	Not clinically present
DO	Distoocclusal	neg	Negative
DOB	Date of birth	norm	Normal
DR.	Doctor	occ, occl	Occlusal
EMT	Emergency medical treatment	OH	Oral hygiene
est	Estimate, estimation	OHI	Oral hygiene instructions
evac	Evacuate, evacuation	opp	Opposite
eval	Evaluate, evaluation	P	Pulse
ext	Extract, external	PA	Periapical
FBS	Fasting blood sugar	path	Pathology
FH	Family history	Ped	Pediatrics
FLD	Full lower denture	PO, postop	Postoperative
FMS	Full mouth series	preop	Preoperative
FMX	Full mouth x-ray	prep	Preparation, prepare for treatment
FR or frac	Fracture	prog	Prognosis
frag	Fragment	Px, Pro, Proph	Prophylaxis
frec	Frequent, frequency	R	Respiration
FUD	Full upper denture	R_x, RX	Take (thou) recipe
G	Gold	RC	Root canal
GF	Gold foil	req	Requisition
GI	Gold inlay	resp	Respiration
ging	Gingiva, gingivectomy	RHD	Rheumatic heart disease
HBP	High blood pressure	ROA	Received on account
Hx	History	SBE	Subacute bacterial endocarditis

Continued

Table 16-4 Suggested charting abbreviations—cont'd

Abbreviation	Term	Abbreviation	Term
Sig	Write on label I	TPR	Temperature, pulse, respiration
sol	Solution	TMJ	Temporomandibular joint
stat	Immediately	Tr.P	Treatment plan
stim	Stimulate, stimulator	URI	Upper respiratory infection
surg	Surgery, surgeon	ULQ	Upper left quadrant
Sx	Symptom	URQ	Upper right quadrant
T	Temperature	VD	Venereal disease
tab	Tablet	wh	White
TAT	Tetanus antitoxin	wnd	Wound
TB	Tuberculosis	x	Times (4x = 4 times); x-ray
TBI	Toothbrush instructions	xyl, xylo	Xylocaine
temp	Temperature	YOB	Year of birth
TLC	Tender loving care	yr	Year

INTRAORAL EXAMINATION

I. The intraoral examination is divided into the following three phases:
   A. Soft oral tissues
   B. Periodontium
   C. Teeth and their occlusal relationship
II. Visual inspection and palpation are used in this examination.
III. Visual emphasis should be on size, shape or contour, and color; palpation should be used to identify the consistency and the tenderness of tissue.
IV. Intraoral tissue examination is described (box).
V. Soft-tissue examination is described (box on page 269).

PERIODONTIUM EXAMINATION

I. This phase includes assessment of the tissues that support the teeth—the gingivae, cementum, periodontal ligament, and alveolar and supporting bone.
II. The alveolar and supporting bone evaluation requires the use of dental radiographs; the other tissues are evaluated visually and with the use of a periodontal probe and mirror.
III. Terms used to describe the conditions of the periodontium and accumulations of accretions are listed in Table 16-5.
IV. Fig. 16-1 depicts several shapes and forms of the periodontium.
V. During the periodontal examination the following findings are recorded in the patient's chart:
   A. General health of the gingivae and notation of any signs of inflammation
   B. Location and amount of plaque and calculus
   C. Lack of attached gingiva

INTRAORAL TISSUE EXAMINATION

- Note the tissue integrity of covering tissues; the epithelium over the surface should be intact.
- The degree of keratinization will vary in different parts of the oral cavity.
- Sense of touch will indicate consistency and whether tissue is soft, firm, hard, or nodular.
- Sense of touch will indicate tenderness; if a mass is found, determine whether it is mobile or fixed to surrounding tissue.
- Bilateral palpation can be used to compare one part with another.
- Note whether the anatomy differs from its bilateral counterpart or deviates from the normal.

   D. Presence and depth of periodontal pockets
   E. Presence of furcation involvement where pockets exist in multirooted teeth
   F. Mobility of teeth
   G. Position of teeth
   H. Effect of existing restorations on gingival health
VI. The periodontal probe and mouth mirror are the primary instruments used in this phase of the examination.
VII. To evaluate the gingival health the operator will do the following:
   A. Visually observe the buccal gingiva by retracting the cheek with the mirror; note changes in color, form, and texture throughout the segment.
   B. Use the periodontal probe to gently press against the attached gingiva, the gingival mar-

SOFT-TISSUE EXAMINATION

The first phase of the intraoral examination begins with the examination of soft tissues. The dental mirror may be used to improve vision or for retraction while the operator performs the following:

1. Examine the maxillary and mandibular lips. Lipstick should be removed. Look for a well-defined line of demarcation between the vermilion border and the skin; folds or lines of the lip should be evident at right angles to vermilion border. When the lip is palpated, it should feel supple, and the vermilion border should be a distinctive and uniform color.
2. Inspect the vestibular regions, frenum, and labial mucosa. Retract the mandibular lip and expose the mandibular labial mucosa. Similarly, raise the maxillary lip and examine the labial mucosa in this area.
3. Palpate the lips to determine consistency and the presence or absence of firmness. Any tissue discoloration, lesions, edema, lip or cheek habits, or undue stress on the frenum is noted. Any tenderness, swelling, or masses may be an indication of an infection or small tumors.
4. Examine the buccal mucosa on both sides of the oral cavity from the maxillary vestibule to the mandibular vestibule. Parotid papilla and nests of the labial salivary glands should be evident.
5. Palpate each cheek between the thumb and forefinger to determine the presence of tenderness or small tumors.
6. Palpate the parotid salivary glands for swelling or tenderness.
7. Progress to the posterior of the arches using a mouth mirror to examine the maxillary tuberosity and retromolar pad areas.
8. Inspect the hard palate, including anterior landmarks such as the rugae and incisive papillae. Palpate the entire hard and soft palate with the midfinger or forefinger to detect swellings that might indicate an infection in this area or small tumors of the minor salivary glands. Tori also may be evident in this region and may go unnoticed unless the region is palpated.
9. Continue to examine the soft palate posteriorly. When the soft palate is depressed with a finger, an underlying nodular-like area should be apparent. Depress the dorsum of the tongue to increase vision to the soft palate, uvula, and tonsils. Inflammation of the tonsils (if they are present) can be observed, and lesions such as a neoplasm or a papilloma may be evident on the tip of the uvula.
10. Examine the dorsum of the tongue. Ask the patient to stick out the tongue; grasp it with a 2 × 2 gauze. Inspect the dorsal surface and move the tongue laterally to inspect both sides for the presence of lesions. Ask the patient to raise the tongue to inspect the ventral surface for the presence of tumors.
11. Examine the floor of the mouth, viewing the lingual caruncle and sublingual folds.
12. Palpate the lingual aspect of the mandible, the submandibular glands, and the sublingual gland.
13. Check secretions of the salivary glands. Dry off the ductal openings of Wharton's duct, apply pressure under the anterior of the mandible, and look with a mirror at the lingual surface under the tongue.

A typical charting of the soft-tissue examination would be recorded on the patient's examination sheet.

gin, and the interdental papilla to determine the firmness of the tissue.

C. Probe the interdental papilla area to identify the presence of inflammation or bleeding.

D. At sites of gingival recession, measure the depth of the recession from the gingival margin to the cement-enamel junction.

E. Continue this process around other segments of the mouth.

VIII. Periodontium measurements are recorded at six points on each tooth (Fig. 16-2).

A. Measurements for each area are recorded in either numeric or graphic form.

B. This procedure is continued around the arch on the buccal aspect; then the operator transfers to the lingual aspect before proceeding to the opposite arch.

C. A healthy periodontium is one that can be probed at 2 to 3 mm.

D. An automated system may be used for this procedure.

IX. Examination of the furcation is necessary to determine the degree of involvement. A straight periodontal probe, a special furcation probe, or even a curet scaler can be used to determine whether bone still fills the area between the roots.

X. The operator determines the degree of mobility by exerting force in a buccal-lingual direction.

A. The operator tests each tooth systematically, generally beginning in the maxillary right quadrant, proceeding to the maxillary left quadrant, proceeding from there to the mandibular left, and concluding on the mandibular right.

Table 16-5 Terms commonly used
to describe conditions of the periodontium

Term	Meaning
Localized	The condition is confined to one area, to one tooth, or to a small segment of teeth
Generalized	Evident throughout most or all of the mouth
Slight	Beginning evidence or early stages of the condition
Moderate	Significant amount of progression, but not to the advanced stage
Severe	Most advanced stage
Bulbous	Enlarged, swollen, and rounded
Blunted	Receded, not sharp, rounded
Cratered	Crater-like depression in the center of the papillae
Normal, healthy	Tissues are dense and fibrous; in Caucasians the tissue will be uniformly pale pink; areas of pigmentation, from light to dark brown, may occur in various skin colors or races
Soft, spongy	Tissues are swollen and contain fluid
Stippled	Tissues contain many tiny indentations, a healthy condition
Bleeding	When gently probed, tissues bleed
Recession	Margin of gingiva located apical to the CEJ
Cleft	Narrow slit-like recession that occurs where margin tissue is destroyed
Red	This is erythema and indicates early or acute inflammation
Bluish purple	This is cyanosis and indicates an inflammation of chronic, well-established nature

B. Mobility may be classified as follows:

+ mobility — Movement that is barely discernible

I mobility — Movement from buccal to lingual totaling 1 mm

II mobility — Movement from buccal to lingual totaling 2 mm

III mobility — Movement from buccal to lingual totaling 3 mm

TEETH

I. The symbols shown in Table 16-3 are especially helpful in this phase of the examination.

II. All existing restorations, missing teeth, malpositioned teeth, dental caries, or other anomalies on the teeth are recorded at this time.

III. The operator may dictate the information while the assistant records it on an examination sheet.

Shape and Form of the Periodontium

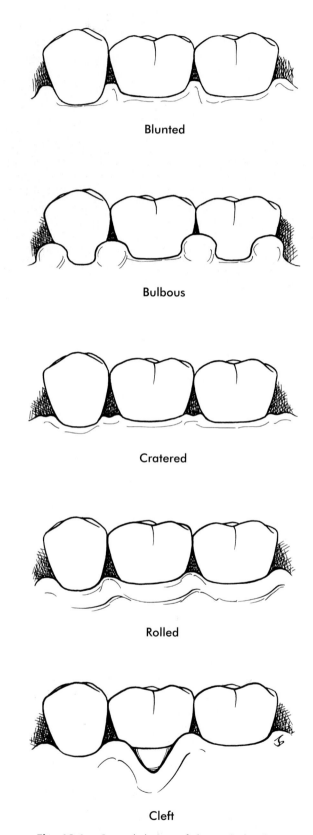

Blunted

Bulbous

Cratered

Rolled

Cleft

Fig. 16-1 Several shapes of the periodontium.

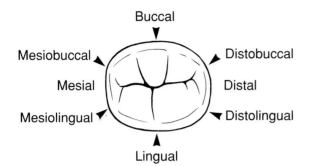

Fig. 16-2 Six points of periodontal measurement: disto-buccal, buccal, mesiobuccal and distolingual, and lingual and mesiolingual.

IV. The charts shown in Figs. 16-3 illustrate a variety of conditions.

OCCLUSION

I. Evaluating the relationship of the two arches in **occlusion** (closed together) is part of the oral examination.

II. The operator evaluates how the patient opens, closes, and laterally moves the arches to determine whether any abnormalities exist.

III. Factors that affect proper occlusion include the relationship and size of the arches; premature contact; teeth that are rotated, hypererupted, unerupted, or crowded; and occlusal relationships, including crossbite, overjet, and overbite.

IV. Examining the occlusion involves the following:
   A. The operator asks the patient to gently close the arches in a normal (centric) position.
   B. Articulating paper or marking paper is placed between the arches, and the patient is directed to bite down and slide the teeth from side to side.
   C. The operator determines whether the patient has normal, class I, class II (division 1 or 2), or class III occlusion.

RADIOGRAPHIC EXAMINATION

I. This is a reliable diagnostic aid for evaluating the tissues in a patient's mouth, especially those tissues not visible to the naked eye.

II. Bitewing radiographs aid in diagnosing interproximal caries and determining the level of the bone.

III. Periapical radiographs illustrate the entire tooth and its supporting tissues.

IV. Extraoral radiography provides a view of the teeth in relation to other head and neck anatomy.

V. Interpretation of radiographs for the purpose of diagnosing requires a thorough understanding of radiographic anatomy found on bitewing, periapical, occlusal, and extraoral radiographic films.

PHOTOGRAPHIC EXAMINATION

I. Clinical photography provides a visual image that illustrates color, shape, and texture of tissues and conditions in the oral cavity.

II. Before-and-after photographs are used to illustrate change that has taken place during the treatment period.

III. This can be used to differentiate between healthy and unhealthy tissue.

IV. A series of photographs can illustrate the process of constructing a prosthetic device.

V. Many dentists use photography to promote the practice.

VI. Forms of dental imaging and cosmetic imaging have proven successful as educational tools and practice builders.

VII. Photographic equipment can be categorized as traditional still photography, intraoral imaging, or cosmetic imaging.

OBTAINING DIAGNOSTIC IMPRESSIONS

I. **Diagnostic models** are three-dimensional positive reproductions of the patient's teeth and alveolar processes.

II. From diagnostic models, which are generally made of plaster, the dentist is able to do the following:
   A. Observe and analyze the position of the teeth
   B. Evaluate the occlusal relationships
   C. Examine the size and shape of the alveolar processes

III. The dental assistant is responsible for taking the impressions (where legally delegable), pouring them in plaster, and trimming the casts to specifications.

IV. A set of diagnostic models must be diagnostically acceptable and provide an esthetic and artistic exhibit for use during case presentation.

V. The steps in making the alginate impressions include the following:
   A. Assembling the armamentarium
   B. Selecting and preparing the appropriate sized trays
      1. Trays are supplied in small, medium, and large sizes; are solid or perforated; are made of plastic or metal; and are disposable or sterilizable.
      2. Look at the arch, select a tray, and try it in the patient's mouth until one tray fits.
      3. To obtain the best results, follow the guidelines listed (box on page 276).

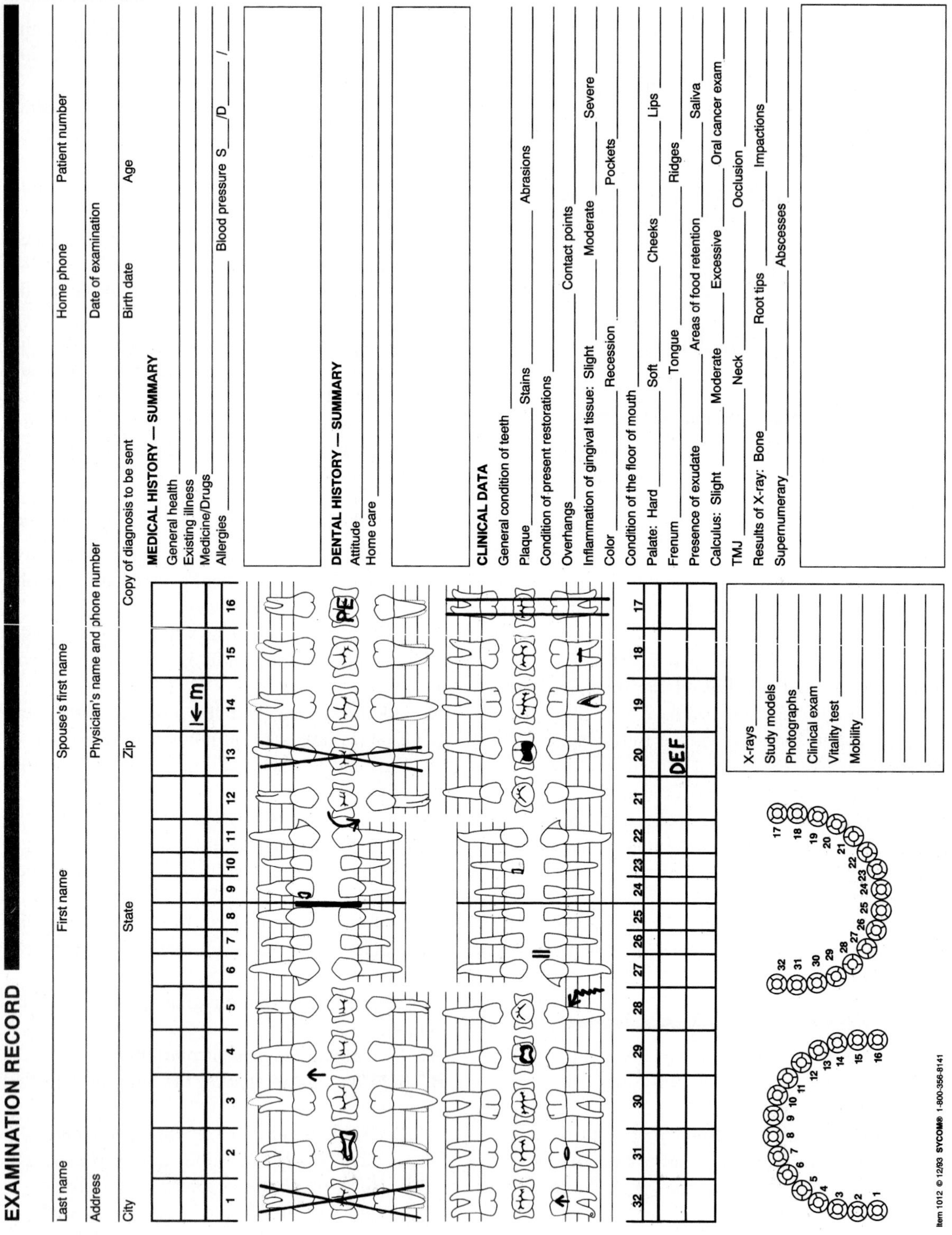

Fig. 16-3 Four separate charts completed for a variety of charting situations. A, #1 is missing; #2 has mesioocclusal caries; Food impaction between #3 and #4; Diastema between #8 and 9; #9 has mesial caries; #12 is rotated distally; #13 is missing; #14 is shifted mesially; #15 is partially erupted; #17 needs to be extracted; #18 has a beginning furcation; #19 has furcation involvement; #20 has a defective distoocclusal amalgam; #23 has mesiofacial caries; Open contact between #26 and #27; #28 is hypersensitive; #31 has cervical buccal caries; #32 is hypere-rupted

EXAMINATION RECORD

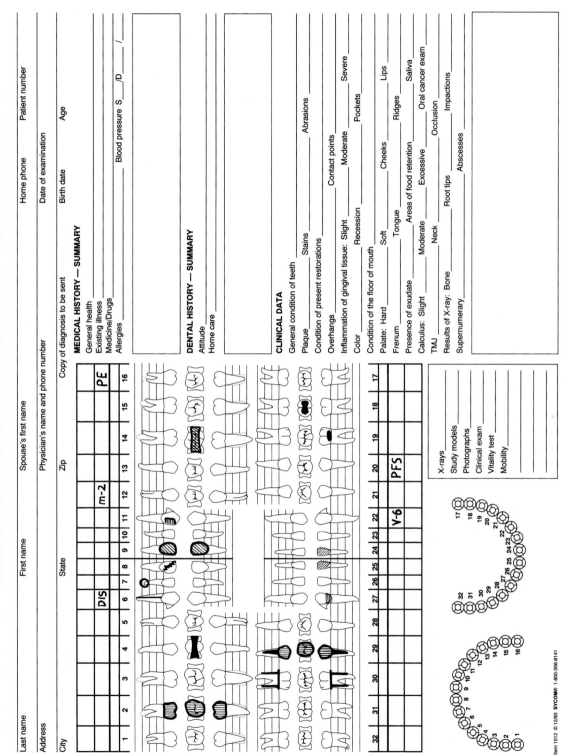

Fig. 16-3, cont'd. *B,* Tooth #2 has a full coverage gold crown; #4 has an MOD amalgam; #6 is discolored; #7 has a periapical abscess; #8 has a distal incisal fracture; #9 has a porcelain crown; #11 has a labial fistula; #12 has Class II mobility; #14 has a MOD porcelain inlay; #16 is partially erupted; #18 has an occlusal amalgam; #19 has a buccal cervical amalgam; #20 has a pit and fissure sealant; #22 has a vitality of six; #24 has a facial laminate; #25 has a facial laminate; #27 has a buccal cervical composite; #29 has a post and core, cast metal crown; #30 has a fractured crown.

Item 1012 © 12/93 **SYCOM**® 1-800-356-8141

EXAMINATION RECORD

Last name   First name   Spouse's first name   Home phone   Patient number

Address   Physician's name and phone number   Date of examination

City   State   Zip   Copy of diagnosis to be sent   Birth date   Age

MEDICAL HISTORY — SUMMARY

General health
Existing illness
Medicine/Drugs
Allergies   Blood pressure S____ /D____ /____

DENTAL HISTORY — SUMMARY

Attitude
Home care

CLINICAL DATA

General condition of teeth
Plaque _____ Stains _____ Abrasions _____
Condition of present restorations
Overhangs _____ Contact points _____
Inflammation of gingival tissue: Slight _____ Moderate _____ Severe _____
Color _____ Recession _____ Pockets _____
Condition of the floor of mouth
Palate: Hard _____ Soft _____ Cheeks _____ Lips _____
Frenum _____ Tongue _____ Ridges _____
Presence of exudate _____ Areas of food retention _____ Saliva _____
Calculus: Slight _____ Moderate _____ Excessive _____ Oral cancer exam _____
TMJ _____ Neck _____ Occlusion _____
Results of X-ray: Bone _____ Root tips _____ Impactions _____
Supernumerary _____ Abscesses _____

X-rays _____
Study models _____
Photographs _____
Clinical exam _____
Vitality test _____
Mobility _____

Item 1012 © 12/93 **SYCOM®** 1-800-356-8141

Fig. 16-3, cont'd. *C*, Tooth #4 has a DO amalgam with overhang; #6 has a porcelain fused to metal crown; #11 has a labial fistula; #16 is unerupted; #17 is unerupted; #18 is a distal abutment for 3 unit bridge, full coverage gold; #19 has a gold pontic; #20 has a mesial abutment, gold crown; #25 has a mesiolingual abutment for Maryland bridge; #26 has porcelain fused to metal pontic; #27 has a distolingual abutment for Maryland bridge; #28 has recession; #30 has a periodontal pocket mesiolingual 5 mm and lingual 6 mm

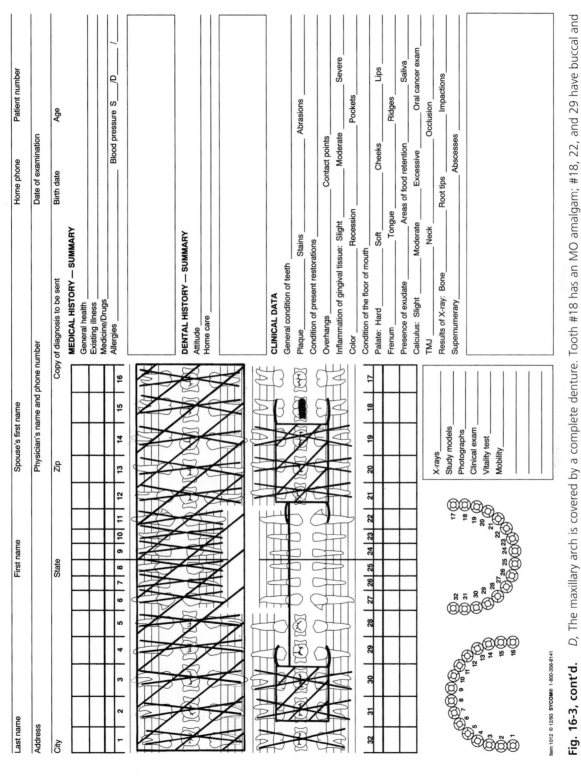

Item 1012 © 12/93 SYCOM® 1-800-356-8141

Fig. 16-3, cont'd. *D,* The maxillary arch is covered by a complete denture. Tooth #18 has an MO amalgam; #18, 22, and 29 have buccal and lingual partial clasps; the lingual bar extends from #21 through #29; partial denture replaces teeth #19 through #21 and #30 through 31; #32 is clinically not present.

GUIDELINES FOR SELECTING IMPRESSION TRAYS FOR DIAGNOSTIC MODELS
MAXILLARY ARCH
• Completely covers the maxillary tuberosity • Covers the anterior teeth so that the incisal edges are in contact with the flat arch portion of the tray at least 3 to 4 mm anterior to the raised palatal portion of the tray • Has enough width in the molar region to allow 4 to 5 mm distance between the widest and most apical portion of the alveolar process in the molar region
MANDIBULAR ARCH
• Covers all of the teeth and retromolar pad area • Allows for centering the teeth labially and lingually in the tray • Has a wax rope extension placed on the anterior labial flange to allow the alginate to flow deeply into the labial vestibule as the impression is seated in the mouth

	Small Powder:water	Medium Powder:water	Large Powder:water
Maxillary	2:2	2:2	3:3
Mandibular	2:2	2:2	3:3

3. Pour the measured water into the bowl, add the powder, and mix according to the manufacturer's directions.
4. To fill the mandibular tray, pick up the material with the spatula and load one side of the mandibular tray, bringing the top layer of the material around to the opposite side; force the material firmly into the tray to avoid creating bubbles.
5. When the tray is filled evenly, smooth the surface with a moist finger.
6. To load the maxillary tray, pick up all of the material with the spatula and place it on the tray with the bulk of the material in the anterior portion of the tray.
7. With a moist finger, smooth the surface of the material and, if desired, make a small indentation in the material at the site of the teeth.

E. Taking the impression
  1. The mandibular impression is taken first.
  2. Steps for obtaining alginate impressions are provided (box on page 277).

VI. Criteria for a clinically acceptable alginate impression include the following:
  A. The impression should be free of voids, air bubbles, and tears.
  B. All peripheral borders should be clearly defined.
  C. Anatomic areas should be clearly defined, including coronal portions of teeth, rugae, frena, retromolar pads, tuberosities, palate, and sublingual areas.
  D. Impression material should be uniformly thick without exposed tray surfaces.
  E. Disinfect wrapped impressions for 15 to 20 minutes before pouring with a gypsum product.

4. It is often advisable to add rope wax to the anterior flange area to help force some of the alginate into the deepest portion of the anterior vestibule.
5. If a patient has a high palatal vault, place a small amount of utility wax in the palatal region to eliminate potential voids.

C. Preparing the patient
  1. Briefly describe the procedure to the patient; explain the technique, the consistency of the material, and the duration of the process.
  2. During the procedure, demonstrate caring for the patient by positive reinforcement and thanking him or her for being cooperative.
  3. The patient is seated in an upright position with the eye-to-ear plane parallel to the floor.

D. Mixing the alginate
  1. Premeasured packets are supplied with the equivalent of three scoops of powder.
  2. If bulk material is used, follow the general rule for dispensing the material as shown.

SUPPLEMENTARY TESTS

I. Extensive medical laboratory tests are not used routinely in a dental office.
II. Occasionally such tests are ordered directly or through consultation with the patient's physician.
III. Test results that might be used in diagnosis or during a patient's dental treatment include the following:
  A. Vitality, thermal, or percussion tests are done in the dental office and may be used to indi-

OBTAINING ALGINATE IMPRESSIONS

MANDIBULAR

1. Stand in front of the patient.
2. Ask the patient to open the mouth slightly; too wide an opening will cause tension on the cheeks and make it difficult to insert the tray.
3. Slowly rotate the tray into the mouth.
4. With the free hand, grasp the mandibular lip and continue to insert the tray.
5. Seat the posterior of the tray first.
6. Be sure the teeth are centered in the tray; then seat the tray slowly but firmly in place.
7. Seat the tray until 1 to 2 mm of the alginate separates the teeth from the tray.
8. Hold the tray in place until the alginate is set.
9. When the alginate is set, break the peripheral seal gently, and remove the tray with a quick snap.
10. Examine the impression to ensure that all anatomy and associated structures have been imprinted in the impression.
11. If the impression is acceptable, rinse it under running water, shake off the excess water, spray it with an acceptable disinfectant, wrap it in a paper towel, and store it in a small plastic bag for 15 minutes.

MAXILLARY

1. Stand behind or to the side of the patient.
2. Slowly rotate the tray into position, making certain that the tray is centered in the mouth.
3. Seat the posterior of the tray first.
4. Grasp the maxillary lip with the free hand and pull it up and out of the way of the anterior portion of the tray.
5. Slowly but firmly seat the tray.
6. Seat the tray until 1 to 2 mm of space separates the incisal edges of the tray surface from the teeth.
7. When the impression has set, break the peripheral seal gently and then remove it with a quick snap.
8. Perform steps 10 and 11 above.

Note: To ensure complete and accurate registration of tooth anatomy, place a small amount of impression material on the occlusal surfaces by hand.

cate the physiologic condition of the pulp.
  B. Antibiotic sensitivity tests are used to determine the effectiveness of a specific antibiotic on a certain strain of bacteria that is causing a patient's illness.

  C. Caries activity tests are used to determine the potential effectiveness of a preventive program that has been recommended for a patient, particularly restriction of carbohydrate intake.
  D. A biopsy report or exfoliative cytology is used for the detection of disease.
  E. Blood tests are used to indicate glucose levels for diabetic patients, assess bleeding time for patients on blood-thinning medication, or provide white cell blood counts that may identify the presence of infection.

CASE PRESENTATION

I. When all the diagnostic data have been collected, the material is prepared for the dentist's evaluation and includes the following:
  A. Complete medical and dental history
  B. Thorough oral examination with current findings
  C. Mounted radiographs
  D. Summary of laboratory test results
  E. Trimmed set of diagnostic models
  F. Developed photographs
II. The dentist will interpret the clinical data, determine a diagnosis, and recommend a prescribed **treatment plan** (recommended course of care for a patient, including a sequence of appointments).
III. The dentist must carefully consider how the recommended treatment plan will be accepted by the patient.
IV. The dentist should consider the following:
  A. Does this treatment plan satisfy the needs for which the patient initially came to the office?
  B. Have priorities been established to provide for emergency care, prevention, and long-range dental care?
  C. What is the best method for presenting this diagnosis and treatment plan so that the patient has a thorough, accurate understanding of the needs and treatment procedure?
  D. Are alternative treatment plans available for the patient?
V. The conditions in a patient's mouth need to be explained in accurate and understandable terms.
VI. The patient needs to be informed of the risks involved and the consequences of not proceeding with the treatment.
VII. The process should take place in a nonthreatening environment that promotes discussion and allows the patient to ask questions.

VIII. When appropriate, informed consent forms should be completed.

IX. When the treatment plan has been accepted, appointments and payment arrangements are completed by the business office assistant.

Questions

Oral Diagnosis

1 Before treating any patient a(n)
   a. Complete bacterial count should be performed
   b. Accurate medical history must be taken
   c. Complete blood cell count should be obtained
   d. Urinalysis should be performed

2 Knowledge of the patient's medical and dental history can affect the
   a. Treatment plan
   b. Drugs prescribed
   c. Frequency of appointments
   d. All of the above

3 When a patient with a history of a prolapsed heart valve is receiving treatment, the patient should
   a. Receive treatment with antibiotics
   b. Receive treatment with the operator wearing surgical gloves
   c. Receive treatment with no special precautions
   d. Never be placed in a supine position

4 Chronic respiratory problems affect the
   a. Type of prosthesis a patient can wear
   b. Prognosis for root-canal therapy
   c. Positioning of the patient
   d. Design of cavity preparation

5 Which of the following is true of a thorough dental examination?
   a. Will prevent viral infections.
   b. Should be standardized so that nothing is overlooked.
   c. Is unnecessary in edentulous patients.
   d. Will decrease the rate of caries formation.

6 What aids are used to diagnose caries?
   1. Millimeter probe
   2. Periapical radiograph
   3. Sharp explorer
   4. Ball burnisher
   5. Bitewing radiographs
   a. 1, 3, and 4
   b. 2, 3, and 4
   c. 3 and 5
   d. 3, 4, and 5

7 The criteria for an acceptable alginate impression include which of the following?
   1. Registration of the mucobuccal attachment
   2. Reproduction of the mylohyoid ridge
   3. Reproduction of the retromolar area
   4. Reproduction of the tuberosity
   5. All tooth anatomy

   a. 1 and 3
   b. 2 and 4
   c. 1, 2, 3, and 4
   d. 1, 2, 3, 4, and 5

8 The normal respiration rate for a relaxed adult is _____ breaths per minute.
   a. 16 to 18
   b. 18 to 20
   c. 22 to 26
   d. 24 to 28

9 A foul breath odor may indicate _____.
   a. A lung or bronchial infection
   b. A peptic ulcer
   c. Diabetes mellitus
   d. Hypoglycemia

10 It is important to obtain a patient's vital signs before and at follow-up treatment because of which of the following?
   a. Changes may indicate illness.
   b. Fluctuations may be signs of future problems.
   c. Changes may indicate anxiety on the patient's part.
   d. All of the above are correct.

11 A normal body temperature for an adult is
   a. 96.8° F
   b. 99.8° F
   c. 98.6° F

12 The normal pulse rate for an adult is
   a. 60-80 beats per minute
   b. 70-90 beats per minute
   c. 120-140 beats per minute

13 Which is a normal respiration rate for an adult?
   a. 8-10 per minute
   b. 12-14 per minute
   c. 14-18 per minute
   d. 18-22 per minute

14 Under which of the following conditions might a patient not be referred for further evaluation of blood pressure to determine any abnormalities?
   a. The patient indicates he or she is on blood-pressure medication.
   b. After retaking the BP, it is normal.
   c. After retaking the BP, it is not normal.

In items 15-18, match each item in column A with the instrument or device that is used to check it during an intraoral examination (column B).

Column A		*Column B*
_____ **15**	Interproximal caries	a. Periapical radiograph
_____ **16**	Furcation involvement	b. Explorer
_____ **17**	Periodontal depth	c. Periodontal probe
_____ **18**	Tooth surface for caries	d. Bitewing radiograph
		e. Vitalometer

19 Which of the following would be considered implied consent?
   1. Use reasonable care in providing services in accordance with a set of community standards.
   2. Obtain an accurate health history for a patient before administering treatment.
   3. Employ competent personnel.

4. Make provisions for complete emergency care in a timely manner.

5. Explain the treatment and obtain signed consent.
   a. 1, 3, and 5
   b. 1, 2, 3, and 4
   c. 2 and 4
   d. 5 only

20 Inquiring about the drugs a patient is taking is necessary to

1. Prevent potentially harmful drug interaction
2. Develop an understanding of the total patient health profile
3. Be aware of potential emotional or physical reactions during dental care
4. Determine the need to interact with the patient's physician regarding patient care
   a. 1 and 3
   b. 2 and 4
   c. 1, 2, and 3
   d. 1, 2, 3, and 4
   e. 1 only

21 An elevated temperature is an indication of

1. Infection
2. Fatigue
3. Exercise
4. Korotkoff's disease
   a. 1 and 3
   b. 2 and 4
   c. 1, 2, and 3
   d. 1, 3, and 4
   e. 4 only

22 The assistant was unable to detect the systolic reading when taking a BP reading; in this case, it would be wise to do the following:

1. Have the patient remove any bulky clothing.
2. Remove the air from the manometer.
3. Reposition the stethoscope on the brachial artery.
4. Place the patient in a different position.
5. Ask a dentist to take the BP reading.
   a. 1 and 3
   b. 2 and 4
   c. 1, 2, and 3
   d. 5 only

In items 23-25, place an A for *True* or a B for *False* in the spaces provided.

_____ **23** Diagnosis and prognosis are synonymous terms.

_____ **24** When a patient has a history of hemophilia, it is necessary to perform a biopsy before treatment.

_____ **25** Each patient seen in the office must have a baseline periodontal chart completed.

Rationales

Oral Diagnosis

1 B The dentist has a moral, legal, and ethical responsibility to learn as much about the patient's medical history as possible prior to treatment. This history is a collection of data provided by the patient about his or her general health and will help prevent medical emergencies.

2 D This history includes information about the patient's past systemic diseases, injuries, operations, allergies, and dental treatment. It should also include a thorough drug history. When a patient confirms any of the questions on a health questionnaire, the patient must be queried to determine when a disease or change has occurred, the extent of the illness or change, the prescribed treatment or medication, and the present status of the condition.

3 A Any bacteria that invades the bloodstream during an invasive dental procedure will tend to lodge in the wall of the heart in the area of irregular blood flow. In most cases an infection can be prevented with the administration of an antibiotic.

4 C A patient who is susceptible to respiratory problems may find it difficult to be placed in a supine position. Therefore, it may be necessary for the patient to remain in an upright position, allowing for less difficulty during normal breathing.

5 B To be most effective, the dental team should establish a well-defined method of completing a dental examination. These steps should be standardized for all patients.

6 C The sharp point of the explorer can probe various surfaces of the tooth to manually and visually identify carious lesions. The bitewing is an intraoral radiograph depicting the crowns of maxillary and mandibular teeth and interdental bone crests. This radiograph readily depicts the presence of dental caries in interproximal locations.

7 D One of the criteria of a clinically acceptable alginate impression is that the anatomic areas should be clearly defined, including coronal portions of teeth, rugae, frena, retromolar pads, tuberosities, palate, and sublingual areas.

8 A Normal respiration for an adult is 14 to 18 respirations per minute; a female's respiration rate is faster than a male's. An infant's rate is approximately 40 counts per minute, and a child's rate is 25-30 counts per minute.

9 A The presence of a variety of organisms such as viruses, bacteria, rickettsiae, fungi, or parasites may produce toxins that give off an odor, which is then transmitted through the respiratory system.

10 D It is important to establish a baseline for a patient, which requires that during the initial examination the patient's vital signs are taken and recorded. During follow-up appointments the vital signs are retaken. Any significant changes may indicate a systemic illness, that future problems may be indicated, or that the patient is encountering undue stress or anxiety.

11 C A normal body temperature registers approximately 98.6° F. Various factors, such as exercise, excitement, the digestive process, infection, cold, shock and drugs may affect the level of body temperature.

12 A An adult's pulse rate is approximately 60-80 beats per minute. A female's pulse rate is usually slightly higher than that of a male. A infant's rate falls between 120 to 140 beats per minute.

13 C See No. 8.

14 B The initial BP may have been incorrectly registered, and the second reading is more accurate. If the BP was registered prior to treatment, the patient may have been anxious.

15 D See No. 6.

16 A A periapical radiograph illustrates the tooth apices and surrounding structure in a specific intraoral area. Thus any bone loss at the furcation area would be evident in this radiograph.

17 C A periodontal probe is calibrated in millimeters and is used to measure pocket depth, attachment width, and size of soft-tissue lesions.

18 B See No. 6.

19 B Implied consent refers to those implied duties that the dentist owes to the patient. When a dentist accepts a patient for treatment, this implies that the dentist agrees to accept certain responsibilities for that patient's dental care. These implied duties do not require a patient to sign a consent form but are considered the common duties that any responsible dentist would provide.

20 D See No. 2.

21 A One of the cardinal signs of infection is an elevated temperature. A patient who appears healthy and has no indication of an infection may have an elevated temperature due to recent strenuous physical exercise.

22 C If an assistant is unable to determine the systolic reading, it may relate to an obstruction of the brachial artery due to clothing. Therefore, bulky clothing should be removed. Before retaking the BP, remove the air from the manometer and reposition the stethoscope on the brachial artery.

23 B Diagnosis is the translation of data gathered by clinical and radiographic examination into an organized, classified definition of the conditions present. Prognosis is the foretelling of the probable course of a disease, a forecast of the outcome of a disease.

24 B Hemophilia is a blood-related disease and not a lesion that would require a biopsy.

25 A Prior to treatment a baseline periodontal examination should be done to denote the status of the periodontal tissues. At subsequent visits, the baseline can be used to identify any changes in the periodontal status of the patient.

To enhance your understanding of the material in this chapter refer to the illustrations in Chapter 24 of Finkbeiner/Johnson: *Mosby's Comprehensive Dental Assisting: A Clinical Approach.*

CHAPTER 17

Emergency Procedures

OUTLINE

Common Diseases That Affect
  Dental Care
Managing Dental Emergencies
Handling Specific Dental
  Emergencies

Managing Medical Emergencies
Emergency Action and
  Cardiopulmonary Resuscitation

Airway Obstruction
Medical Conditions
Older Adults

KEY TERMS

ABCs of emergency care
Abdominal thrust technique
Abscess
Advanced cardiac life support
  (ACLS)
Anaphylactic shock
Avulsed tooth

Cardiopulmonary resuscitation
  (CPR)
Emergency medical service (EMS)
Epilepsy
Grand mal seizure
Heimlich maneuver
Hyperglycemia

Hypoglycemia
Jacksonian epilepsy
Petit mal seizure
Psychomotor seizure
Stoma
Syncope

Each patient who visits the dental office for treatment brings a unique set of needs that may be compounded by systemic disease, recent changes in general health, prescribed medications, allergies, a disability, emotional stress, or an unknown health problem that can trigger an emergency.

This chapter reviews the relationship between a patient's medical health and dental care, learning to recognize symptoms that are common to dental and medical emergencies, and understanding the role of the dental assistant in managing life-threatening situations.

COMMON DISEASES THAT AFFECT DENTAL CARE (Table 17-1)

Managing Dental Emergencies

I.   The dental assistant assumes responsibility for screening calls to determine the nature of an emergency.
II. Display a caring attitude.
III. Obtain complete and accurate pertinent emergency information (box on page 283).
IV. Determine an office policy for handling medical or dental emergencies.

Table 17-1 Common diseases affecting dental care

Condition	Oral manifestation	Relation to dental treatment
Epilepsy	Gingival hyperplasia may result from drug therapy.	Seizures that are not controlled by drug therapy may occur during dental treatment.
Pregnancy	Poor nutrition may result in increased carious activity or in a periodontal condition.	Radiation (x-ray examination) or drugs may harm a fetus.
Sexually transmitted disease	Soft-tissue lesions, chancre, stomatitis, periodontal disease, hairy leukoplakia, lymphadenopathy, Kaposi's sarcoma, squamous cell carcinoma, xerostomia may be present.	Transmission of infectious disease during dental treatment may increase risk of infections and potential for bleeding.
Joint/artificial prosthesis	None are seen.	Dental treatment may introduce bacteria into body systems, causing secondary infections; bleeding might be excessive if anticoagulants have been taken.
Diabetes mellitus	Oral ulcerations, possible periodontal disease, and abscesses may be present.	Infection may increase; wound healing may be compromised in uncontrolled diabetic patients.
Murmur	Usually none are seen.	If functional, treatment is normal; if organic, premedication may be necessary to avoid infection or subacute bacterial endocarditis.
Tuberculosis	Ulcerations or lymph node involvement may be present.	Infection may be transmitted from patient to dental team member or from dental team member to patient.
Cardiac arrhythmia	Medical treatment may result in ulcerations, petechiae, xerostomia.	Use of epinephrine or increase in stress may cause arrhythmias; cardiac pacemaker patients may be at risk if interference occurs in the function from electric pulp testers or dental chairs.

V. Factors to be considered in establishing this policy include the following:
   A. Who determines whether the situation is life threatening?
   B. What is the chain of command when the person who usually makes this decision is absent from the office?
   C. What procedures are implemented to transfer a patient to another dental office or facility?
VI. Set aside some buffer time—approximately 15 minutes—each morning and afternoon for dental emergencies.
VII. Respect other patients' time.
   A. Be considerate of other patients when an emergency arises.
   B. If a major delay occurs, look ahead and determine whether appointments can be rescheduled.

HANDLING SPECIFIC DENTAL EMERGENCIES ▬

I. **Abscess**
   A. Two types of abscesses may occur in the oral cavity: *periapical* and *periodontal*.
   B. Each can cause significant discomfort to the patient.
   C. Symptoms frequently identified with the periapical abscess may include the following:
      1. Sensations of pressure
      2. Severe pain
      3. Severe reaction to hot temperatures but relief with cold temperatures
      4. Edema
      5. Redness
      6. Fistula on the oral mucosa near the apical end of the tooth
      7. Discomfort on biting
   D. Symptoms of the periapical abscess may also be identified by pain and may be accompanied by bleeding, redness, edema, and blunted gingival tissues.
   E. The patient must be seen by the dentist as soon as possible.
   F. Inform the patient that the dentist will be able to see him or her at a certain time to determine the nature of the problem and perhaps render some treatment; however, future appointments may need to be scheduled.

II. **Avulsed** (dislodged) **tooth**
   A. This frequently occurs in young children.
   B. Successful replantation requires quick action on the part of the parent or caregiver and the dental staff.
   C. The patient must be seen immediately.
   D. The success rate of replants is correlated with the time that has elapsed between the dislodging and the replant; replants done within 20 minutes have greater retention success than those performed an hour after the dislodging.
   E. Instruct the caregiver to wrap the tooth in a clean, moistened gauze or fabric (even immersing the tooth in milk is acceptable) and bring it and the patient to the dental office immediately.
   F. Instruct the caregiver to place a small piece of gauze or fabric over the tooth socket and direct the patient to bite on the gauze.

III. Fractured tooth/restoration or loosened crown
   A. When a patient has broken a tooth or has lost a crown or other type of restoration, the primary concerns include the following:
      1. Does the patient have the crown?
      2. Is there discomfort?
      3. Are sharp areas on the tooth irritating the tongue or cheek?
   B. If a crown or fixed prosthesis has loosened (and the crown is available), an appointment can be scheduled to determine whether the restoration can be recemented.
   C. If possible, the crown is recemented; if not, the crown may be used as a temporary, and new appointments need to be made to prepare the tooth for the new restoration.
   D. If the restoration is an intracoronal, the fractured material has no value.
   E. A fractured tooth or restoration is not unlike the situation described above; it is necessary to determine the type of restoration needed for patient comfort and whether this requires replacing the restoration or a more extensive restoration.

IV. Lost temporary restoration or interim dressing
   A. The temporary restoration is used to protect the tooth from discomfort, fracture, hypereruption, or potential drifting, and it is important that the temporary be replaced.
   B. A patient in pain needs to be seen immediately.
   C. If there is no discomfort and the dentist indicates that damage is not likely to occur, the patient may be seen for the regularly scheduled appointment.
   D. The same approach as described above may be used when a patient has fractured or lost a periodontal dressing.

V. Broken prosthesis
   A. When the patient calls about a broken denture or partial denture, he or she is usually concerned about esthetics.
   B. If the fracture can be treated in the office, the patient can wait for the repair.
   C. A more extensive repair may require the patient to return later that day or the next day.
   D. For prosthesis repair, check with the dental laboratory to determine the repair schedule for the patient.

VI. Displaced orthodontic band/bracket
    A. This is similar to a lost restoration but may require less time to replace.
    B. If the patient has the band/bracket, it should be brought along to the office, and an appointment should be scheduled for cementing it.
    C. Cement the new band/bracket.

MANAGING MEDICAL EMERGENCIES ▬▬▬▬

I. Establish a chain of command.
    A. All personnel must be aware of their own responsibilities during an emergency.
    B. All members of the team should be aware of the location of emergency equipment and be familiar with its maintenance and use.
    C. The assistant is usually responsible for organizing the emergency kit as directed by the dentist.
       1. All drugs in the kit must be replaced before the expiration date.
       2. Oxygen cylinders must be kept full and be maintained; all equipment should be easily accessible.
    D. Emergency telephone numbers must be current and posted at all telephone locations.
    E. Certification in a clinical course of basic life support and additional training of all office personnel in management of medical emergencies are recommended; some states require current certification of dental personnel in **cardiopulmonary resuscitation (CPR)** techniques for renewal of their individual dental licenses.

II. Emergency equipment must be available.
    A. The office must have complete and current emergency equipment.
    B. The emergency equipment should include an emergency drug kit with injectable and noninjectable drugs; other items include an oxygen delivery system, suction and suction devices, syringes, tourniquets, cricothyrotomy needle or scalpel, various sizes of artificial airways and airway adjuncts.
    C. All emergency drugs in the kit are available in unit doses or preloaded syringes.
    D. Use of drugs is not a recommended course of action until the ABC's (A=airway, B=breathing, C=circulation) of basic life support techniques have been tried without success.
    E. The use of oxygen or basic life support is the common course of care in most situations in dental offices.

III. Injectable drugs are an integral part of an emergency kit.

    A. Usually divided into three groups: essential, nonessential, and the **advanced cardiac life support (ACLS)** drugs.
    B. ACLS drugs are usually kept separate from the basic emergency kit.
    C. ACLS drugs are kept in dental offices that have personnel with advanced training in ACLS.
    D. Essential drugs are those deemed necessary to manage emergency situations and include the following:
       1. Epinephrine—selected to manage immediate allergic reactions.
       2. Antihistamine (chlorpheniramine)—used to treat allergic reactions that have a longer period (1 hour) of onset.
       3. Anticonvulsant (diazepam)—used to manage seizure disorders.
       4. Narcotic antagonist (naloxone)—used to act against narcotic and respiratory depression.
    E. Nonessential drugs are not always considered part of an emergency kit because clinical application requires additional clinician background in their use. These drugs include the following:
       1. Analgesics (morphine)—for use with pain, anxiety, and congestive heart failure.
       2. Vasopressors (methoxamine, Vasoxyl)—to raise blood pressure in unknown cardiac situations.
       3. Corticosteroids (hydrocortisone, Solu-Cortef)—for acute allergic reactions after use of epinephrine and antihistamines.
       4. Antihypoglycemics (50% dextrose solution)—to control seizures and unconsciousness with an unknown cause.
    F. ACLS drugs are administered by individuals with ACLS training for care of patients with emergency cardiac care situations. ACLS drugs include the following:
       1. Sodium bicarbonate—used during cardiopulmonary arrest.
       2. Atropine sulfate—for severe sinus bradycardia with hypotension.
       3. Lidocaine—for tachycardia and fibrillation.
       4. Calcium chloride—used during cardiac arrest.

IV. Noninjectable drugs should be included in the emergency kit.
    A. Contact with these drugs may be more common in the dental office.
    B. Noninjectable drugs include the following:

1. Oxygen—used at times in emergencies when respirations are difficult or do not exist.
2. Vasodilator (nitroglycerin)—particularly used with chest pain, often angina pectoris and acute myocardial infarction.
3. Respiratory stimulant (aromatic ammonia)—used to stimulate respiratory centers.
4. Antihypoglycemic (carbohydrate)—particularly used with diabetes mellitus or nondiabetic patients with hypoglycemia.
5. Bronchodilating agent (metaproterenol)—used for respiratory difficulty from asthma or allergic reactions.

V. A record of routine care and maintenance of emergency equipment should be maintained.

VI. Universal barriers should be maintained with the emergency equipment.

EMERGENCY ACTION AND CARDIOPULMONARY RESUSCITATION

I. Emergency action principles and CPR techniques are lifesaving skills that all individuals—especially health professionals—should be capable of performing when an emergency situation arises.

II. CPR skills are needed to assist individuals who have respiratory and cardiac emergencies.

III. Successful outcome of any emergency situation requires consistent repetition of steps.

IV. The repetition of steps ensures remembering the steps in an emergency situation.

V. When faced with an emergency situation in a dental office, the emergency action principles advocated by the American Red Cross and American Heart Association apply.
A. The patient should be comforted if conscious and should be assured that the professional is trained in first aid.
B. Assess the patient for responsiveness by positioning yourself near the patient, touching the patient, and shouting "Are you OK?"
C. If the patient does not respond, shout for help to draw attention if you are alone, so that someone will alert the **emergency medical services (EMS)** system.
D. At this point the patient must be placed on his or her back.
E. The rescuer should place personal protective barriers and then survey the patient's condition to determine the **ABCs of emergency care**—*airway, breathing,* and *circulation.*

VI. Rescue breathing
A. The next step in administering emergency aid to the patient is the A of the ABCs: opening the patient's airway.
1. Place your hand (the one closest to the patient's head) on the forehead and apply force backward, tilting the head back.
2. Bring the patient's chin forward until the teeth almost contact.
3. Lift the tongue away from the back of the throat and open the airway.
4. After the airway is opened, move on to B (breathing).
B. Check for maintenance by looking, listening, and feeling for any activity of breathing for 3 to 5 seconds.
C. If the chest moves and you can hear and feel air passage, the patient is breathing; however, if there is only chest movement, the patient may not be breathing.
D. If the patient is not breathing, place the patient's head in the head-tilt/chin-lift position and close the nose opening by pinching the nostrils.
E. Open your mouth, take a deep breath, and immediately seal your lips tightly over the patient's mouth.
F. Force two full breaths at 1 to 2 seconds per breath into the mouth, with pauses between to replenish your air supply and watch for the patient's chest to fall after you have removed your mouth.
G. At this point, repeat the techniques for listening and feeling the air being released from the patient's chest.
H. If any resistance is met when breath is released into the patient's lungs, the tongue may be blocking the airway and the head position may need to be adjusted.
I. Then move on to C (checking circulation) as you check the carotid pulse to determine whether the patient's heart is beating.
J. If EMS was not called before these steps were performed, they should be called at this point and informed as to whether the patient is conscious, is breathing, and has a pulse.
K. If the patient has a pulse but is not breathing, begin rescue breathing by maintaining the airway and administering a breath every 5 seconds and checking the rise and fall of the chest and the pulse.
L. Continue this procedure until EMS personnel arrive and relieve you.
M. During rescue breathing the rescuer may force air into the patient's stomach, which can cause

vomiting; the stomach contents can be aspirated into the lungs, which could lead to death.
N. Make sure the patient's head is tilted properly; do not breathe too fast into the lungs, and do not breathe into the lungs after the chest has risen to prevent the patient vomiting.

AIRWAY OBSTRUCTION

I. It is possible for a patient to aspirate a dental object during treatment when a rubber dam is not used for isolation.
II. An airway may become obstructed in a restaurant or in the home, and the person might need emergency first aid to assist in breathing.
III. When you are faced with this situation as a rescuer, ask the person, "Are you choking?"
   A. If the person has a partially obstructed airway with good air exchange, the person can cough or wheeze.
   B. In this circumstance you should stay with the person but do nothing else; allow the patient to cough up the object to clear the airway.
   C. If the patient has a poor air exchange (indicated by a weak cough and a high-pitched noise), provide assistance as if there were a complete airway obstruction that would not allow the person to breathe, cough, or speak.
   D. If choking is confirmed, EMS should be called and informed of the situation.
   E. The **Heimlich maneuver,** or **abdominal thrust technique,** requires the patient to be in a standing or sitting position.
      1. The rescuer stands behind the patient, wrapping both arms around the patient's waist.
      2. A fist is made with one hand, and the thumb of the fist is placed against the middle of the patient's abdomen, above the navel and below the lowest edge of the breastbone.
      3. The opposite hand grasps the fist, and with both elbows positioned out from the patient's sides, the fist is pressed into the abdomen on the midline with a quick upward thrust.
      4. The thrusts are repeated until the obstruction to the airway is released or until the person becomes unconsciousness.
      5. If the person becomes unconscious, he or she should be lowered to the floor, a finger sweep should be done to open the airway, and two breaths should be administered.
      6. If the air does not fill the lungs, six to ten abdominal thrusts should be given.

      7. This action is repeated until the obstruction is freed or until EMS arrives and assumes responsibility.
      8. When abdominal thrusts are difficult (e.g., with someone who is nearing term in pregnancy or is obese), chest thrusts are performed in place of the abdominal thrusts.
   F. After assistance has been provided for a person in an emergency, he or she should be taken to the nearest hospital for evaluation.
IV. Complete airway obstruction in an unconscious adult calls for the following actions:
   A. In this situation repeat the steps described above in III.
   B. If unable to breathe air into the patient, retilt the patient's head must be and provide two additional breaths.
   C. With the patient lying down, administer six to ten abdominal thrusts as you straddle the patient's thighs.
   D. Place the heel of one hand in the middle of the patient's abdomen in a similar position for the thrusts administered in the earlier description; position the second hand directly on top of the first, with the fingers of the second pointed upward.
   E. Press the abdomen quickly, with an upward thrust, six to 10 times.
   F. After performing the thrusts, perform a finger sweep of the mouth.
   G. If nothing is removed from the airway, repeat these steps until the airway is cleared or until EMS personnel take over.
V. CPR calls for the following actions (many of the steps mentioned in previously described emergency situations are repeated for the adult patient whose heart has stopped beating):
   A. First, check the ABCs; then determine the patient's level of responsiveness.
   B. If the patient is not responsive, shout for help and position the patient on his or her back.
   C. Open the airway; look, listen, and feel for breathing; then administer two full breaths if the patient is not breathing.
   D. Check the carotid pulse and have someone contact EMS for assistance.
   E. If the patient has no pulse after you check the carotid artery for 5 to 10 seconds, begin CPR.
   F. Kneel beside the patient and over the chest; position the hands on top of each other with the fingers interlaced and over the breastbone.
   G. Compress the chest by pushing the breastbone down approximately 1 to 2 inches in smooth, even strokes.

H. Administer 15 compressions followed by two full breaths; this constitutes a cycle.

I. The rate of compressions should be 80 to 100 per minute.

J. Recheck the patient's carotid pulse after completing four cycles of CPR.

K. If you feel no pulse, give two breaths and continue CPR.

L. CPR should be continued until the heart starts beating, until another CPR-trained rescuer arrives, until EMS takes over, or until you physically cannot continue CPR.

M. If you find a pulse, check for breathing; if the patient is breathing, maintain the open airway and observe the breathing and pulse closely.

N. If no one responds to your shouts for help, administer CPR for 1 minute, shouting for help as you are able.

O. If no one has answered the shouts for help, the patient must be left for the minimal time that is necessary to phone EMS; then return and continue CPR.

P. If a second trained rescuer is available during CPR, this person should notify EMS and then relieve you when you become exhausted.

Q. Then observe the rise and fall of the patient's chest and check the carotid for a pulse during compressions.

R. The second rescuer can also provide compressions as the first rescuer administers ventilation.

S. The first rescuer gives directions so that the team can work efficiently.

MEDICAL CONDITIONS

I. Heart conditions

A. Heart stopping as the result of heart attack, myocardial infarction, or heart failure

1. *Symptoms:* No pulse is evident.
2. *Treatment:* Administer CPR.

B. Angina pectoris

1. *Symptoms:* The patient has extreme substernal pain that may radiate to the arm, with swelling in the extremities; may also have shortness of breath and increased anxiety.
2. *Treatment:* Place the patient at a 45-degree angle; if the patient carries nitroglycerin tablets, place one under the tongue to be absorbed through the mucous membranes; a second tablet can be administered in approximately 20 minutes. If the patient wears a transdermal patch, the second tab-

let is not always recommended. The attack of angina usually subsides in 2 to 4 minutes after nitroglycerin is taken. The use of oxygen aids in relieving the attack. Oxygen usage during dental treatment may act as a preventive step for the angina patient.

C. **Syncope**

1. *Symptoms:* Temporary loss of consciousness occurs, which may not always provide the dental professional with warning. Problems may be found when vital signs are obtained. Symptoms that include a change in pallor and possible excess perspiration provide insight into potential medical needs.
2. *Treatment:* Place the patient in the dental chair, or, if necessary, on the floor, in a supine position. Position the feet higher than the head, allowing the blood to flow away from the stomach and to the brain. Break an ammonia inhalant and pass it by the nostrils, forcing the patient to inhale quickly, which in turn forces extra oxygen into the system. A record of this incident is made in the patient's file with the pulse and blood pressure.

II. **Anaphylactic shock**

A. *Symptoms:* Results are those from an extreme allergic reaction to an allergen, such as food, an insect bite, or a specific drug. The allergen causes a release of histamines, which in turn cause edema and decreased vascular movement. The swelling of the larynx and bronchi forms a blockage of the airway, resulting in cyanosis.

B. *Treatment:* Treatment is similar to that for syncope; it is administered immediately to ensure patient recovery, and an antihistamine is used to reduce edema. Epinephrine is usually the drug of choice, in a dose of 1:1000 of 0.5 ml, followed by contacting the patient's physician. The use of oxygen may make the patient more comfortable as long as breathing continues. An entry of the patient's allergen is made in the record.

III. **Hyperglycemia**

A. *Symptoms:* This may result in *hyperglycemic coma,* also known as *diabetic acidosis;* it might occur when the patient has an elevated blood sugar level (possibly caused by eating too much sugar), has an infection, or has not taken the appropriate dose of insulin. The patient may have a rapid or weak pulse, rapid breathing, and dry mouth with acetone breath.

The patient becomes less responsive or non-responsive and may lose consciousness.

B. *Treatment:* The hyperglycemic patient needs insulin or other medications that are normally taken immediately. Contact the physician of record. This emergency may require the care of an EMS team, followed by physician direction for care.

IV. **Hypoglycemia**

A. *Symptoms:* The patient may be diabetic or nondiabetic and have blood glucose levels that have dropped below 50 mg/100 ml from a high level of insulin. The onset of symptoms may lead to the loss of consciousness or insulin shock; this may include disorientation, fatigue, hunger, and/or pallor; during stressful situations, temperature changes, convulsions, tachycardia, and syncope may occur. Factors that cause hypoglycemia are not eating meals, excessive exercise before meals, or an overdose of insulin.

B. *Treatment:* If the patient is conscious, the ingestion of sugar increases the blood sugar level and results in the loss of symptoms. A cup of orange, apple, cranberry, or pineapple juice could be administered to increase the blood sugar level. Ten Lifesavers or other hard candy might also increase the blood sugar. If the patient is unconscious, it may be necessary to administer an injection of glucose.

V. Seizure disorders

A. Convulsive episodes are usually a result of transient alterations in brain function.

1. Onset of a convulsive episode in a patient is not usually life threatening, and action on the part of someone witnessing a seizure is usually not necessary.

2. If multiple seizures (or status epilepticus) occur, a medical emergency may result.

B. Seizures cause changes in the state of consciousness, motor activity, or sensory phenomena and often do not last long.

C. **Epilepsy** is a recurrent convulsion caused by various cerebral and noncerebral disorders; it manifests itself as a tonic state, with constant muscular contraction, and produces an appearance of stiffness or rigidity.

1. **Grand mal seizure** is a form of epilepsy in which the patient has a tonic-clonic form of seizure that usually lasts 2 to 5 minutes.

a. Tonic-clonic seizures involve muscle spasms and are followed by loss of consciousness, muscle rigidity, and uncoordinated movement of limbs.

b. Most people with epilepsy have grand mal seizures.

c. This form of epilepsy occurs in persons of all ages.

2. **Petit mal seizure** may be the only seizure disorder the patient has, or it may be combined with other forms of seizures.

a. A lapse of consciousness of approximately 5 to 10 seconds is normal; a 30-second lapse may occur in some cases.

b. The patient does not normally move, except for a possible blinking of the eyelids or dropping of the head; this absence of movement is sometimes combined with a blank stare.

c. This form of epilepsy usually develops in childhood and may decrease as the person ages; it is not often found in persons older than 30.

3. **Jacksonian epilepsy** is also referred to as a *simple partial seizure* because the patient does not always lose consciousness. This usually begins as a spasm in a limb or part of the face and then spreads.

4. **Psychomotor seizure** is usually combined with another form of seizure and is considered minor by comparison.

a. The patient loses contact with the environment for 1 to 2 minutes.

b. Symptoms of this seizure include smacking the lips, moving the eyes, incoherent speech, turning the head, and amnesia.

5. Treatment for epileptic seizures usually involves phenytoin (Dilantin), which has a side effect of hyperplasia of the gingival tissues; therefore, proper oral hygiene is important.

6. Treatment is not necessary for most epileptic seizures.

7. The patient should be allowed to let the seizure run its normal course.

8. To avoid injury, care should be taken to remove any objects the patient may hit or that might fall on him or her during the seizure.

VI. Cerebral palsy

A. This is a neural disorder that results in brain damage that occurred at birth or during the postnatal period before development of the central nervous system was complete.

1. Motor centers are affected by the disease; muscle weakness, paralysis, and other possible disorders occur.

2. The disease can manifest itself in two forms: *spasticity* (muscle tension) and *athetosis* (uncontrolled body movements).

B. The patient often has poor oral hygiene techniques because of lack of motor control.

C. The patient may need to be premedicated to relax him or her and to reduce unexpected movements during treatment.

VII. Older Adults

A. The aging process is not a medical condition.

B. In older adult patients a variety of complications often occur during dental treatment that involve the following:
1. Drug interaction
2. Physical mobility
3. Oral conditions

Questions

Emergency Procedures

In items 1-7, match the terms in column A with the definitions in column B:

Column A		Column B
_____	**1** Syncope	a. First step in preparing for an office emergency
_____	**2** Recognition	
_____	**3** Prevention	b. Trendelenburg position recommended
		c. Second step in preparing for an office emergency
		d. The basics for reviving a patient

Column A		Column B
_____	**4** CPR	a. Form of epilepsy
_____	**5** Petit mal	b. Worst type of seizure for a patient
_____	**6** ACLS	
_____	**7** Stoma	c. Opening in throat for an airway
		d. Advanced level from the ABCs
		e. The basics of reviving a patient

8 Patients with a history of cardiac disease should be given
a. Morning appointments
b. Afternoon appointments
c. Appointments at any time
d. Appointments at the end of the day when other patients will not be in the office

9 The site most commonly used in obtaining an accurate pulse rate is the
a. Brachial artery
b. Carotid artery
c. Radial artery
d. Temporal artery

10 While a patient is having a cast metal crown seated, the crown drops to the back of the throat. You should
a. Give the patient water and ask him or her to swallow.
b. Have the patient sit up with head over knees.
c. Allow the patient to cough up the crown.

11 The situation known as _____ is considered a compromised state of body function, and the means of assisting a patient with this condition is to place the patient in a position in which the _____.
1. Depression
2. Syncope
3. Neurotic
4. Head is flat and turned to the side
5. Head is lower than the body
6. Head and shoulders are higher than the rest of the body
a. 1 and 4
b. 2 and 5
c. 2 and 6
d. 3 and 5
e. 1 and 5

12 The recommended course of care for a patient going into insulin shock is to
a. Send the patient home to rest.
b. Administer an insulin injection.
c. Provide the patient with protein.
d. Provide the patient with sugar or a sweetened fruit drink.

For items 13 and 14: A patient arrives in your office for an early morning dental appointment before the dentist arrives. The patient complains of not feeling well and having clammy skin, racing pulse, and slight numbness in the arm.

13 What would you suspect is the possible problem?
a. Diabetic episode
b. Potential heart attack
c. Shock
d. Epileptic episode

14 What should you do under these circumstances?
a. Wait till the dentist arrives to consult.
b. Call the patient's spouse for information.
c. Call EMS.
d. Contact the patient's physician.

For items 15-19: From the list below, place in correct sequence the CPR techniques necessary to revive a patient. Begin with 15 as the first step and continue to the last step in 19.
a. Tilt head, close nose openings, and force two breaths of 1 to 1 1/2 seconds each.
b. Check circulation.
c. Ask, "Are you OK?", shout for help, or call EMS.
d. Check for breathing.
e. Open airway.
_____ **15**
_____ **16**
_____ **17**
_____ **18**
_____ **19**

20 When you have completed the steps in items 15 to 19, and the patient has a pulse but is not breathing, you must
a. Start chest compressions.
b. Continue rescue breathing.
c. Create a stoma.

21 If the patient continues with no breathing and an airway obstruction is possible, you must
a. Create a stoma.

b. Immediately begin CPR.

c. Administer abdominal thrusts.

For items 22-25: After administering the thrusts, you are unable to breath air into the patient. List the steps below in the correct sequence. Begin with 22 as the first step and continue to the last step in 25.

a. Administer 6 to 10 additional abdominal thrusts.

b. Administer breath.

c. Perform a finger sweep of the mouth.

d. Retilt the head and administer two additional breaths.

_____ 22   _____ 24

_____ 23   _____ 25

Rationales

Emergency Procedures

1 B Syncope is a brief lapse in consciousness that is usually preceded by a feeling of light-headedness. It often may be prevented by lying down or by sitting with the head between the knees. The Trendelenburg position is one in which the patient is lying down.

2 C Recognizing that a medical emergency is occuring is the second step in office preparation for emergencies.

3 A Using all the tools available before an emergency occurs is part of the preventive aspect of an emergency policy. An example of this is reviewing the patient health history and determining whether the patient has taken prescribed medication prior to any treatment.

4 E CPR techniques are the basic lifesaving skill needed to aid a patient in respiratory and cardiac emergencies.

5 A A petit mal seizure is an epileptic seizure characterized by a sudden, momentary loss of consciousness, sometimes accompanied with slight twitching of the face or loss of muscle tone.

6 D ACLS involves skills beyond those used in CPR. The primary care giver, such as the dentist or physician, usually has these skills.

7 C A stoma is an artificial opening of an internal organ on the surface of the body. An example of this is a tracheostomy (an opening made in the trachea to facilitate breathing).

8 A Early morning appointments are usually beneficial to patients with a history of cardiac disease. These patients usually require less stress, such as waiting for appointments, and often take medication in the morning when it is best regulated.

9 C The radial artery is usually the most accessible to the dental professional and provides an accurate pulse rate.

10 B While in a supine position the patient may swallow or aspirate the crown. If immediately seated upright, the patient may be able to bring the crown to the anterior aspect of the mouth.

11 B See No. 1.

12 D An oral or parenteral dose of sugar immediately provides the patient with some relief. Usually orange juice is recommended if the patient is conscious. If not conscious, the placement of a cake frosting type of gel under the tongue will accomplish the same effect.

13 B The patient should be placed at a 45-degree angle in the dental chair because there is the possibility of an angina attack or a myocardial infarction. Obtain as much information as possible before the dentist arrives. The patient health history should be reviewed. Determine whether anyone came to the office with the patient or if there is someone to contact.

14 C If the patient appears to be in great stress and cannot be placed in the dental chair, EMS should be contacted immediately.

15 C When a patient has a respiratory or cardiac emergency, the rescuer should first ask the patient if he/she is OK. If not, the rescuer should shout for someone to call EMS immediately or do so himself or herself if necessary.

16 E The patient's head should first be positioned to determine whether the airway is open, with the patient lying supine.

17 D The rescuer looks, listens, and feels for breathing.

18 A If it is determined the patient is not breathing, the head is tilted and the chin is lifted, the nose opening is closed, and two breaths are forced into the mouth.

19 B The rescuer checks for circulation by checking the pulse at the carotid artery.

20 B Continue rescue breathing, making sure the head is positioned correctly; check the pulse again.

21 C If an airway obstruction is determined, the Heimlich maneuver (abdominal thrust technique) is required. The patient must be seated or standing. If the patient is unconscious, the rescuer must straddle the patient to administer the thrusts.

For the conscious victim, the thrusts are administered between the navel and below the breastbone, with the rescuer's hand made into a fist and the other grasping it. The fists are pressed into the abdomen on the midline with a quick upward thrust. The thrusts are repeated until the obstruction is released or the person becomes unconscious.

22 D If the airway is not cleared and the patient is unconscious, position the patient on the floor. Perform the head tilt-chin lift to open the airway access and administer two breaths of air.

23 A Six to ten additional abdominal thrusts are completed with the rescuer straddling the patient and using the palm of the one hand positioned in the same area of the previous thrusts with the second hand laid over it.

24 C Check the mouth for the obstruction by performing a finger sweep.

25 B If an object is removed in the finger sweep, check for breathing. If nothing is removed, the breathing is checked again and breaths are administered in the cycle.

To enhance your understanding of the material in this chapter refer to the illustrations in Chapter 25 of Finkbeiner/Johnson: *Mosby's Comprehensive Dental Assisting: A Clinical Approach.*

CHAPTER 18

Preventive Dentistry

OUTLINE

Prevention in Dentistry
Motivation
Patient Education
Diet Analysis
Home Care
Flossing

Auxiliary Oral Hygiene Aids
Interdental Aids
Care of Prosthetic Devices
Oral Hygiene for Patients with
    Special Needs

Oral Prophylaxis
Coronal Polishing
Fluoride
Mouth Guards

KEY TERMS

Bass technique

Charters technique

Dentifrice

Diet analysis

Disclosing agent

Flossing

Fluoride

Fones technique

Interdental aids

Modified Stillman technique

Motivation

Oral hygiene aids

Oral hygiene score

Oral prophylaxis

Patient education

Pit and fissure sealant

Press-roll technique

Preventive dentistry

Scaler

According to the American Dental Association (ADA), preventive dentistry involves the ''Procedures in the practice of dentistry and community health programs which prevent the occurrence of oral diseases and abnormalities.'' The ADA also states that ''Optimum oral health is within the reach of every individual, but achievement requires the combined efforts of the practitioner, the patient, and the community.''

PREVENTIVE DENTISTRY

I. **Preventive dentistry** places responsibility on the patient and dental team.

II. A preventive program in a dental office must consider the following factors:
    A. Patient education
    B. Brushing and flossing the teeth to prevent periodontal disease and dental decay
    C. Routine dental care, including examinations, prophylaxis, radiographs, and other preventive and restorative procedures
    D. Provision of mouth guards

III. Other factors that influence a preventive program are the following:
    A. The relationship of a patient's dental needs to

his or her oral hygiene habits, eating habits, and socioeconomic conditions
  B. The need to motivate the patient to make changes in food selections and eating habits
  C. Educating the patient in the correct oral hygiene techniques
  D. The way the dental staff works as a team to provide optimal patient education programs
IV. The patient assumes responsibility for proper home care.
V. The dental professionals provide routine preventive procedures in the office.

MOTIVATION

I. **Motivation** is the incentive that triggers a particular behavior. A part of motivation is education.
II. Motivating a patient requires an understanding of the patient's needs, a positive attitude, encouragement, and good follow-up.

PATIENT EDUCATION

I. **Patient education** is the process of using a variety of teaching aids to inform the patient of dental needs; it becomes the first step in a successful prevention program.
II. Often the primary responsibility for preventive education is delegated to the dental hygienist, but every member of the dental health team must be skilled in patient education.
III. The dental professional must be able to do the following:
  A. Be a teacher, an effective listener, and a role model
  B. Recognize the patient as an individual who has priorities, ideas, needs, skills, and a lifestyle
  C. Consider all variables before making a final recommendation to the patient
  D. Begin a patient education program with information about healthy oral tissues
  E. Use visual aids, brochures, and patient education packets
  F. Encourage the patient to recognize abnormalities in his or her mouth
IV. When teaching oral hygiene procedures, the dental professional must do the following:
  A. Provide the patient with a toothbrush and mirror
  B. Have the patient demonstrate his or her toothbrushing technique and evaluate the patient's skills
  C. Give directions for improvement
  D. Demonstrate the technique to the patient
  E. Provide encouragement throughout
  F. Encourage questions; maintain eye contact; and provide an enthusiastic, positive attitude
  G. Reinforce instructions with written information about technique

DIET ANALYSIS

I. **Diet analysis** is the evaluation of a diet on the basis of caloric intake and dietary components. In dentistry, analysis is concerned with sugar intake, consumption pattern, and types of foods consumed.
II. The following suggestions will help the patient develop good dietary patterns:
  A. Ask the patient to complete a food analysis form/questionnaire (a history of food habits).
  B. Educate the patient about the relationship of diet to the development of dental caries and periodontal disease.
  C. Guide the patient in identifying adequate and inadequate nutritional patterns in the diet, such as the following:
    1. Physical form of sugar items
    2. Frequency of intake of sugar items
    3. Consumption pattern
  D. Provide guidance in developing a nutritious diet.
III. Food habits are usually behavior patterns that may not be recognized and are often difficult to change.
IV. To identify eating patterns, ask the patient to maintain a 5-day diet diary.
V. At a subsequent appointment, a dialogue with the patient regarding the diet diary is needed to accomplish the following:
  A. Review and identify nutritional adequacy and offer positive reinforcement on good food choices
  B. Identify food groups that may contribute to dental disease
  C. Describe various foods and critical nutrients of the food pyramids
  D. Analyze eating patterns and offer alternative suggestions for change
  E. Review the effect of systemic nutrition and local food factors on dental disease
VI. Provide suggestions for alternative food selections, including the following:
  A. A sugar substitute can be used in coffee instead of granulated sugar.
  B. A toasted English muffin or bagel can be eaten instead of a muffin or cinnamon roll.

C. Sugar-free gelatin can replace gelatin-containing sugar.

D. Eat cheese cubes and soda crackers instead of a chocolate candy bar.

E. Eat fresh fruit or fruit salad instead of a brownie.

F. Eat plain popcorn instead of caramel corn.

HOME CARE ■

I. Home care is the primary responsibility of the patient.

II. Home care includes the following:
   A. Toothbrushing
   B. Flossing techniques
   C. Use of dentifrices
   D. Use of other auxiliary aids

III. Toothbrushing
   A. The goal of toothbrushing is the mechanical removal of bacterial plaque and debris and the stimulation of soft tissues.
   B. The quality and not the quantity of brushing helps ensure healthy tissues.
   C. Toothbrush design variables include the following:
      1. The handle can be in the same plane as the head or offset at an angle.
      2. The total length varies with adult toothbrushes, which are longer than those recommended for children.
      3. Tufts can be in two to four rows, with 5 to 12 tufts per row.
      4. Brushing planes are even, flat, or uneven.
   D. Toothbrush bristles are either natural or nylon.
   E. Toothbrushes should be replaced at least every 3 months or as soon as the bristles appear bent.
   F. The size and style of the toothbrush are based on the patient's preference, skills, oral conditions, and mouth size.
   G. An automatic or electric toothbrush can be recommended for children or for patients who are disabled or bedridden or have a low level of manual dexterity.

IV. Toothbrushing Methods
   A. **Bass technique** or sulcular method—recommended for patients with periodontal disease, loss of gingival contour, or heavy cervical plaque.
      1. A soft-tufted toothbrush is recommended.
      2. The technique is described (box).
      3. Advantages include the following:
         (1) It disrupts plaque at and under the gingival margin.

BASS TECHNIQUE

1. Place the bristles at a 45-degree angle to the long axis of the tooth.
2. Position the bristles in the sulcus and contact the gingiva and tooth simultaneously.
3. Gently vibrate the brush in short back-and-forth strokes while the bristles remain in the sulcus.
4. Vibrate the brush in each area for a count of 5 to 10.
5. Clean the lingual areas in a similar manner, using the toe of the brush on the anterior teeth.

PRESS-ROLL TECHNIQUE

1. Place the side of the toothbrush bristles on the gingiva, with the tips of the bristles pointing apically.
2. Press the bristles against the tissue until it blanches slightly.
3. Roll the brush so that the bristles slowly point toward the facial surface of the tooth and continue to move the brush toward the crown.
4. Replace the bristles in the apical position and repeat the procedure.

---

         (2) It provides good gingival stimulation.
         (3) Moderate dexterity is required.
         (4) It is widely recognized as an effective plaque-control technique.
      4. Disadvantages include the following:
         (1) Too much motion or pressure can cause tissue trauma.
         (2) The process is time-consuming.
   B. **Press-roll technique**—used with patients who exhibit healthy gingivae and normal oral tissue contour.
      1. A soft- or medium-tufted toothbrush is recommended.
      2. The technique is described (box above).
      3. Advantages include the following:
         a. It is easy to learn.
         b. Moderate dexterity is needed.
         c. It provides good gingival stimulation.
      4. The disadvantage is that plaque at and under the gingival margin is not adequately destroyed.
   C. **Fones technique** (circular scrub)—uses gentle pressure on the bristles and rotates the brush in small circles; is useful for children and

---

FONES TECHNIQUE

1. Close the teeth and place the bristles at a 90-degree angle to the teeth in the maxillary molar area.
2. Using gentle pressure, rotate the brush in small circles, covering the teeth from the maxillary gingiva to the mandibular gingiva.
3. Count to 5 as you brush in each area.
4. To brush the anterior teeth, bring the teeth together in an end-to-end position and continue brushing in small circles.
5. To brush the lingual surfaces, follow the same steps but use the toe of the brush for the anterior areas.

MODIFIED STILLMAN TECHNIQUE

1. Place the toothbrush bristles at a 45-degree angle to the long axis of the tooth, pointing it apically. The bristles should contact the gingiva and the cervical area of the tooth. Do not position the bristles in the sulcus itself.
2. Press the bristles against the tissue until it blanches slightly.
3. Vibrate the brush in approximately 20 short back-and-forth strokes while gradually moving the toothbrush coronally.
4. Replace the bristles in the original position and repeat the procedure for each area of the mouth.

---

adults with healthy gingivae and normal tooth position.

1. A soft, multitufted toothbrush is recommended.
2. The technique is described (box above).
3. Advantages include the following:
    (1) It is easy to learn.
    (2) Minimal dexterity is needed.
    (3) It can be mastered by young children.
4. Disadvantages include the following:
    (1) It is too random.
    (2) It can traumatize soft tissues.
    (3) Bristles do not enter the sulcus.

D. **Modified Stillman technique**—used for cleaning the entire tooth; recommended for patients with gingival recession and/or puffy gingival tissue.
1. A soft- or medium-tufted toothbrush is recommended.
2. The technique is described (box).
3. Advantages include the following:
    a. It provides good gingival stimulation.
    b. Moderate dexterity is required.
4. The disadvantage is that bristles do not adequately disrupt plaque at the gingival margin area.

E. **Charters technique**—directs the bristles toward the incisal/occlusal surface with a vibrating action; recommended for gingival massage for patients with a loss of gingival contour, with single or abutment teeth, or after periodontal surgery.
1. A soft- or medium-tufted toothbrush is recommended.

CHARTERS TECHNIQUE

1. Direct the bristles toward the occlusal/incisal surface at a 45-degree angle to the long axis of the tooth.
2. Press the brush to flex the bristles between the teeth.
3. Move the brush to a count of 10 in short, vibrating strokes, keeping the bristles in place.
4. Repeat this procedure for each area of the mouth, making sure that the bristles reach each interproximal area.

---

2. The technique is described (box above).
3. Advantages include the following:
    a. It permits cleaning interdentally.
    b. It provides good stimulation.
4. Disadvantages include the following:
    a. It requires good manual dexterity.
    b. It requires considerable motivation.
    c. Bristles do not enter the gingival sulcus.
    d. Placement is difficult, especially on lingual surfaces.

F. All methods conclude with occlusal brushing and brushing of the tongue.

FLOSSING

I.   **Flossing** is done primarily to mechanically remove bacterial plaque and debris from the interdental surfaces of each tooth, where a brush cannot reach.

II. It is the most effective auxiliary aid for plaque removal.

III. Direct patients to floss once a day for cleansing

the teeth and for stimulating the interproximal tissues.

IV. Types of floss include the following:

A. Waxed versus unwaxed

1. Unwaxed floss filaments are not impregnated with wax and tend to fan out over the tooth and break up the microcosms as they cut through and dislodge the plaque deposits.

2. Some dental professionals believe that unwaxed floss helps carry away the plaque and debris from the teeth and sulcus.

3. Waxed floss is advantageous for tight contacts and roughened surfaces; unwaxed floss might fray in these areas.

B. Extra fine, flat tape, or tufted

C. White versus colored

D. Plain versus flavored

V. Recommendation of a particular floss product should be based on the patient's dentition, age, and manual skills.

VI. The technique for flossing is as follows:

A. Begin with a 12- to 18-inch piece of dental floss.

B. Wrap the floss around the middle fingers of both hands, leaving a short span (1 to 2 inches) between the hands, with no slack.

C. The ends of the floss are kept wound on the fingers or held in the palm of the hand.

D. The thumb and forefingers guide the floss into the interdental space.

E. A gentle sawing motion of the floss inserts it between the teeth and into the sulcus. Caution must be taken to avoid snapping the floss into the interproximal area.

F. The floss is wrapped around the tooth in a C shape so that it can slide up and down the proximal surface of the tooth to remove the plaque.

G. The floss is advanced on the fingers to a new area after each tooth is cleaned.

H. The mesial and distal surfaces of all teeth are flossed.

I. The patient is instructed not to neglect areas without adjacent teeth, such as third molars.

AUXILIARY ORAL HYGIENE AIDS

I. Dentifrices

A. A **dentifrice** is a compound used in conjunction with a toothbrush to clean the teeth.

B. Most dentifrices contain a mild abrasive, a detergent, a flavoring agent, coloring, optimal deodorants, and/or various medicaments (such as fluoride) that are designed to prevent dental caries.

C. Some dentifrices are designed to prevent tartar accumulation or desensitize teeth.

D. When toothpaste or any other product is suggested to the patient, make certain that it has earned American Dental Association (ADA) approval. This ensures that the product has been tested extensively and is proven to do what the manufacturer claims.

E. Most ADA-approved fluoride toothpastes contain 1000 to 1100 ppm of fluoride in one average application of paste.

II. A **disclosing agent** is a colored substance that is applied to the teeth on which bacterial plaque is not ordinarily visible to the patient.

A. Liquid disclosing agents can be used in the office; a tablet form is available for home use.

B. The main ingredient of this agent is a harmless dye, usually red; it stains any plaque or debris that remains on the teeth and helps illustrate for the patient that plaque is present on the teeth even though it wasn't visible before.

C. The disclosing agent shows where the patient needs to brush and floss better.

D. A disclosing agent can be used in conjunction with a plaque control chart (Fig. 18-1) as a visual aid that shows the patient the areas in the mouth where debris remains after flossing and brushing.

E. When marked on the plaque control chart, an **oral hygiene score** indicates the percentage of teeth on which plaque is present.

F. This percentage can be determined with the following simple formula: total number of disclosed tooth surfaces ÷ total number of tooth surfaces × 100% = oral hygiene score %; or it can be determined with the following formula: x/t100 = % index.

G. Obtain the oral hygiene score as follows:

1. Instruct the patient to brush thoroughly.

2. Apply lubricant to the patient's lips to avoid staining.

3. Using a cotton-tipped applicator, paint the solution onto the teeth. If the tablet form is used, instruct the patient to chew one tablet thoroughly and swish the dye around the mouth completely.

4. Rinse the area thoroughly.

5. Use a mouth and hand mirror to illustrate the areas that are disclosed.

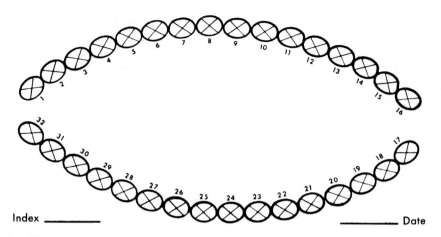

Fig. 18-1 Plaque control chart. (From Woodall IR: *Comprehensive dental hygiene care*, ed 3, St. Louis, 1993, Mosby.)

INTERDENTAL AIDS

I. **Interdental aids** are devices that stimulate the tissue between the proximal surfaces of adjacent teeth or aid in cleaning the interproximal surface of the teeth.

II. Interdental aids include the following:
   A. Floss holder—a Y-shaped plastic device that holds the floss in a short, taut span to aid in flossing
   B. Rubber stimulator—small, cone-shaped rubber device on the end of the toothbrush handle or on a separate handle
      1. This is used when a large interproximal space exists and/or loss of papillae occurs.
      2. Place the rubber tip in the interdental space, angle it toward the occlusal surfaces, and use a gentle rotary motion.
      3. The gingiva is massaged and stimulated, and some plaque is removed.

III. Wood stimulator—interdental aid made of soft wood, usually balsam, in an elongated wedge shape.
   A. This is used when loss of papillae occurs or a large interdental space is present.
   B. Before the wood stimulator is used, it is softened with water or saliva and placed between the teeth, angled toward the occlusal.
   C. Use an in-and-out motion, rubbing the wood against the tooth surface.

IV. Interproximal brush—a brush with soft nylon bristles, usually cone shaped, on a plastic or twisted wire handle
   A. This is recommended for the following:
      1. Cleaning in and around orthodontic wires and brackets

      2. Cleaning an open bifurcation or trifurcation
      3. Stimulating and cleaning an open contact area or site where there is a loss of papillae
   B. For proper use, place the brush in the desired area, apply light pressure, and use a rotary motion.

V. Water irrigation device—device with a steady or pulsating stream of water that helps remove nonadherent debris and food
   A. This is especially useful for patients with fixed bridges or orthodontic appliances.
   B. It is not a substitute for proper brushing and flossing because it does not eliminate adherent plaque.
   C. Point the water stream in a horizontal direction perpendicular to the tooth and gingiva; never direct the water into the gingival sulcus because this could cause damage to the gingiva and periodontium by forcing debris further into the sulcus.
   D. It is not recommended for patients who have subacute bacterial endocarditis (SBE).

VI. Floss threader—a stiff, plastic device, available in numerous sizes and shapes; designed like a small needle with an eye through which the floss is threaded
   A. This helps remove plaque and debris from under fixed bridges and retainers and between orthodontic wires.
   B. Instruct the patient to thread the floss or tape (or a piece of synthetic yarn if the opening is large) through the eye of the device.
   C. The patient can direct the stiff end of the threader with the floss under or through the

contact and then remove the threader, leaving the floss.

D. The floss is now in position in the hard-to-reach area, and effective cleaning can take place.

VII. Oral Rinses

A. The ADA has approved oral rinses that contain fluoride and help reduce dental decay, supragingival plaque, and gingivitis.

B. The dental professional should advise the patient that the rinse may contain substances that could cause harm if ingested.

C. They are intended (as the label states) to be placed in the mouth, swished about, and expelled from the oral cavity.

D. They are not recommended for use by young children or persons who are unable to effectively expectorate.

CARE OF PROSTHETIC DEVICES

I. Fixed bridge

A. Extra care is required to maintain optimal oral health.

B. Cleaning under the pontic of the fixed bridge is essential; one of the auxiliary aids can be used for this purpose.

II. Orthodontic bands and appliances

A. For the orthodontic patient with fixed appliances, a special orthodontic toothbrush can be suggested.

B. The orthodontic toothbrush has a center row of shorter bristles to fit over the orthodontic brackets and aid in cleaning.

C. Instruct the patient to use short vibrating strokes with the toothbrush to clean and stimulate the gingiva.

D. Caution the patient that if proper care is not taken during active orthodontic treatment, carious lesions can occur around and under the brackets and bands.

E. Regular fluoride treatments are often prescribed for the patient during the course of orthodontic treatment to reduce the risk of carious activity.

III. Removable prostheses

A. Removable dentures and appliances should be taken out of the mouth and cleaned at least once a day.

B. They should be rinsed after a meal.

C. Cleaning can be accomplished by the following methods:

1. Rinse under water only when other methods are not available.

2. Brush with a denture brush and a mild soap or toothpaste. Avoid coarse abrasives—they may be damaging to the appliance or soft tissue.

3. Immerse in a commercial chemical soaking solution or a solution that is made at home with the following ingredients: 1 tsp bleach, 2 tsp anticorrosive agent (Calgon), 1 cup warm water.

D. If calculus is observed, the appliance can be soaked in a dilute vinegar solution that contains 1 to 2 tsp white vinegar and 1 cup warm water.

E. Such solutions should be used only occasionally and not on a daily basis.

F. At least once a day the tissue should be cleansed with a soft-bristle brush to maintain circulation and help fight tissue trauma.

ORAL HYGIENE FOR PATIENTS WITH SPECIAL NEEDS

I. Oral hygiene instructions must be customized for patients with special needs, including disabled individuals, those with cancer, older adults, and pregnant patients.

A. Physically challenged patients

1. Instruction and home care depend on the type and severity of the disability.

2. A patient with a mild physical or mental disability can be taught a simple brushing method, such as the Fones or the press-roll method.

3. Supervision by the parent or caregiver may be required at one of the daily brushings, preferably the evening one.

4. A more seriously disabled patient may be taught to use an electric toothbrush.

5. The patient should be encouraged to brush the teeth by himself or herself during the day for two reasons:

a. To reinforce the concept that the teeth should be cleaned at least twice daily

b. To give the patient a sense of responsibility for his or her own care

6. Toothbrushes can be personalized according to the patient's needs.

7. Severely physically challenged patients and some bedridden patients may require that the caregiver provide all oral hygiene care.

8. An *aspirating toothbrush* might be considered for some patients. It consists of a flexible tube that is connected at one end to a suction device; the opposite end is con-

nected to the back of the head of a manual toothbrush. This system allows for simultaneous brushing and removal of oral fluids and debris, providing a clear working field.

B. Cancer patients
1. Rampant or root caries may be present.
2. Xerostomia may be a problem for the patient.
3. Gingival bleeding may occur.
4. The patient may have loss of facial and masticatory muscle function.
5. The patient's immune system may be impaired.

C. Older adult patients
1. Older adults may have limitations or problems.
   a. Gingival fragility
   b. Recession
   c. Cervical abrasion
2. Recommend a soft toothbrush to avoid aggravating existing conditions.
3. Recommend a brushing method that concentrates on the cervical area.
4. Home fluoride therapy may be necessary to deter root surface caries and lessen tooth sensitivity.
5. Patients with arthritis or reduced motor function caused by a stroke may need a modified toothbrush handle or an automatic toothbrush.
6. Dental flossing needs to be encouraged but may be difficult for these patients.

D. Pregnant patients
1. Pregnancy gingivitis is common.
2. Inform the patient why this gingivitis is occurring.
3. Thorough daily brushing and flossing are essential to avoid serious gingival problems that are complicated by hormonal changes.
4. Toothpaste odors and flavorings may be difficult to tolerate and may cause nausea.
5. Morning sickness or vomiting creates an acidic environment in the mouth; this may cause tooth erosion or increased dental caries.
6. Encourage the patient to brush or rinse frequently to lessen the chance of this happening.
7. Offer suggestions about the new baby's teeth and their care.
   a. Explain to the patient that she must brush the baby's teeth or wipe them with a moist gauze daily as soon as they erupt.
   b. Caution her to eliminate the possibility of *nursing bottle decay* by never putting the baby to bed with a bottle filled with anything but water.
   c. Provide educational materials.

ORAL PROPHYLAXIS

I. **Oral prophylaxis** refers to the prevention of dental disease; consequently, it is more than just having the teeth cleaned.

II. It is the removal of calculus (subgingival and supragingival, from all surfaces of the teeth), removal of stains, polishing of the teeth, thorough examination of all intraoral soft and hard tissues, and examination of the extraoral tissue.

III. It is a procedure intended to prevent periodontal disease and to examine oral tissue for early signs of oral disease, lesions, and other anomalies.

IV. A professional oral prophylaxis should be done on a regular basis depending on the patient's needs.

V. The basic steps in an oral prophylaxis procedure include the following:
A. Initial oral examination
B. Disclosing procedure
C. Patient education
D. Scaling
E. Polishing
F. Flossing
G. Final examination and charting of oral conditions

VI. Basic prophylaxis instruments include the following:
A. The *periodontal probe* is the primary instrument used in periodontal examination; used to examine the gingiva for bleeding and determine the depth of the gingival sulcus.
B. The manual **scaler**—to remove supragingival and subgingival calculus from the tooth; most common shapes are the curet and sickle; chisel and hoe scalers also available for use in specific areas.
   1. The *curet scaler* is the most effective instrument for removal of calculus and for smoothing root surfaces; supplied as single-ended or double-ended instruments. Two types of curets are available: universal and area specific (Gracey).
   2. The *sickle Scaler* is designed for removal of supragingival calculus or removal of deposits that extend only slightly below the free gingival margin; two basic types of

sickle scalers are the *straight* (anterior) and the *modified* (contra-angle or universal). The difference in these two types of sickle scalers is the angle of the blade—the blade of the modified scaler sits at a right angle to its shank.

3. The *hoe scaler* is designed for removing or dislodging heavy supragingival and subgingival calculus in easily accessible areas. It is not a routine instrument for a prophylaxis tray setup; it is designed with a single straight cutting edge and is used primarily for the removal of heavy supragingival calculus in anterior areas.

C. The *mechanical* or *ultrasonic scaler* can be useful in gross calculus removal in specific situations. It removes calculus with a high-frequency vibrating, scaler-shaped tip; generates heat; and is supplied with a built-in water coolant. It is effective for the following uses:
   1. Removal of heavy, tenacious supragingival calculus
   2. Removal of heavy staining, which is difficult to remove with conventional hand instruments
   3. Treatment of acute necrotizing ulcerative gingivitis (ANUG). Manual scaling may cause discomfort to the inflamed tissues.

D. Polishing devices are used as follows:
   1. Polishing is achieved with the use of manual or power-driven polishing devices and dental floss.
   2. Polishing the teeth during oral prophylaxis is done to accomplish the following:
      a. Remove extrinsic stains for improved esthetics
      b. Create a smooth finish on existing restorations to enhance their longevity
      c. Remove plaque from the tooth surface to create a less adherent surface and a fresh, clean mouth
   3. The porte-polisher is still available but is rarely used today
   4. Prophylaxis angles or contra-angles are supplied in a sterilizable metal or a disposable style and hold either a rubber cup or a polishing brush.

E. Polishing paste is used as follows:
   1. Polishing paste is basically flour of pumice with flavoring, coloring, and glycerine matrix to hold it together; it may or may not contain fluoride.
   2. It is supplied in bulk and placed in a regular or disposable dappen dish with paste that can be placed into a small finger ring.
   3. Avoid using fluoridated pastes when sealants are to be placed during the same appointment.
   4. Coarse, abrasive polishing pastes may be contraindicated when used in areas of a fixed prosthesis, such as porcelain surfaces.
   5. Automatic polishing devices, such as prophy-jets, which can be less abrasive to the enamel in the removal of debris, provide a jet of water simultaneously to rinse the area.

F. Dental floss may be used for polishing the interproximal surfaces of the teeth before a final rinsing of the patient's mouth is completed.

VII. Oral prophylaxis procedure is described in the box on page 300.

CORONAL POLISHING

I. The dental assistant may assist the operator or perform the task if legally delegated.

II. The responsibilities of the assistant include the following:
   A. Prepare the armamentarium
   B. Maintain access and visibility to the treatment site
   C. Provide patient comfort
   D. Floss interproximal surfaces with the polishing abrasive after the polishing procedure

III. Coronal polishing involves the following:
   A. It is done to remove extrinsic stains on the coronal surfaces (including the free gingival space) after scaling or root planing.
   B. It may include polishing all the teeth and their surfaces or selective polishing of specific teeth.
   C. Selective polishing includes only teeth with stains.
      1. This minimizes polishing away the fluoride-rich enamel layer.
      2. It diminishes the potential for changes in tooth morphology.
      3. It allows the patient to realize the importance of maintaining oral hygiene.
   D. It is done before application of acid etch solution for placement of sealant or other material.
   E. It is done before placement of temporary or permanent coverage restorations.
   F. It is done during bonding of orthodontic bands or brackets.

ORAL PROPHYLAXIS PROCEDURE

- Are all universal barrier techniques being used?
- Is all of the armamentarium available and prepared for use?
- Are the instruments arranged in sequence of use?
- Are you prepared for alternative treatment plans?
- Is the necessary equipment turned on and ready to operate?

Responsibilities of the dental assistant during manual scaling and polishing include the following:

1. Seat and drape the patient with a patient napkin or apron, and offer safety glasses.
2. The mirror and explorer are used for the initial oral examination.
3. Tissues are probed with the periodontal probe; then lubricant is placed on the lips before the disclosing solution is applied.
4. Rinse the patient's mouth.
5. Give the hand mirror to the patient so that the operator may show the disclosed area to the patient.
6. Pass the scalers in sequence of operator's choice.
7. Keep the mirror clean of debris and evacuate the mouth as necessary.
8. Be prepared to rinse the site as bleeding occurs.
9. Keep instruments free of debris.
10. Rinse and evacuate as necessary; constantly observe the patient's mouth as bleeding occurs or saliva accumulates in the mouth.
11. When scaling is completed, pass the handpiece with the prophylaxis angle and cup attached; position the handpiece for the appropriate arch.
12. Hold the polishing paste in the transfer zone so that it is always available for operator use.
13. Evacuate saliva and polishing paste.
14. Change from the polishing cup to a brush as needed.
15. Pass the dental floss.
16. Perform a complete mouth rinse.
17. Pass the mirror and explorer for the final oral examination.
18. Pass a 2 × 2 gauze for soft-tissue examination of the tongue and the floor of the mouth.
19. Chart oral conditions as dictated; this may be done before scaling and at the option of the operator.
20. Offer the patient a cup of water for rinsing.
21. Check the patient's face for debris and wipe with a damp tissue.
22. Reposition and release the patient.
23. Follow the suggested disinfection and sterilization procedures.

- Have the appropriate universal barrier techniques been removed?
- Have all the appropriate surfaces been cleaned and disinfected?
- Has all of the armamentarium been removed?
- Has all equipment been repositioned?
- Has all equipment been disinfected/sterilized according to OSHA guidelines?

G. It is optional before rubber dam isolation placement.

IV. Contraindications for coronal polishing include the following:
 A. Patient with active tuberculosis not controlled by an antibiotic regimen
 B. Weakened tooth surfaces from decalcification or abrasion
 C. Patient with a condition (such as a prolapsed valve/joint replacement) who has not taken required premedication

V. Objectives of coronal polishing include the following:
 A. Remove surface discolorations
 B. Provide minimal removal or abrasion of tooth structure
 C. Minimize trauma to the gingiva
 D. Minimize heat production to the tooth surface
 E. Prevent damage to restorations

VI. Manual polishing can be performed using the porte-polisher
 A. Hand instrument with a thick handle and an adjustable working end that holds a wood point at a contra-angle
 B. Technique

1. Use a modified pen grasp for all surfaces except the maxillary anterior.
2. Use a palm grasp for maxillary anterior, using the thumb as the fulcrum finger.

C. Manipulation or stroke used
   1. Strokes in round or small circles about 1/8 inch in diameter are applied to the cervical third.
   2. Vertical, oblique, and horizontal strokes may be used on all other surfaces except near the gingival margins, depending on access.
   3. Use arm and wrist motion with firm pressure and slow, controlled strokes.

D. Applications
   1. Homebound patient
   2. Application of desensitizing agents
   3. Patient with active communicable disease; manual polishing to prevent aerosols
   4. Tooth surfaces that may be inaccessible for prophylaxis angles; distal surfaces of maxillary molars; lingual surfaces of lingually inclined mandibular posterior teeth; long proximal surfaces that may be exposed by gingival or periodontal surgery
   5. For use on patients with a titanium implant

VII. An air-power/airbrasive device uses air and water pressure to deliver a controlled stream of sodium bicarbonate in a slurry to the tooth surface.
   A. The operation should be precise and well controlled to prevent potential damage.
   B. Applications include the following:
      1. It protects the patient with full drape, hair cover, eye protection, and lip lubrication.
      2. It protects the operator and assistant using personal protective devices
      3. It directs the spray in constant motion for only 3 to 5 seconds at any area on the enamel, directing the device away from the gingival margin.
      4. It uses high-velocity evacuation.
   C. Take precautions.
      1. This type of polishing is contraindicated for patients with a communicable disease.
      2. Avoid using it for patients who have a respiratory disease, a condition that limits swallowing, or a restricted sodium diet.
      3. Avoid contact with exposed cementum or dentin, soft spongy gingival tissues, all nonmetallic restorative materials, and all gold restorations.

VIII. Automatic polishing can be performed using power driven devices
   A. Armamentarium

1. Low-speed handpiece with variable speed
2. Prophylaxis angle—sterilizable or disposable prophylaxis angle or contra-angle
3. Rubber cups—variable stiffness, webbed or nonwebbed; various shank styles
4. Bristle brushes—attached to mandrel or threaded stem
5. Polishing paste—pumice mixed with water to slurry consistency; premixed in disposable cups or in tubs; with or without fluoride; flavored or unflavored
6. Disclosing agent
7. Dental floss or tape or a hybrid floss; floss threader optional
8. Gauze sponges for debris removal

B. Technique for using rubber cup
   1. Use a pen or modified pen grasp; position the middle finger pad to provide support; rest the hand piece in the V between thumb and index finger.
   2. Fulcrum or finger rest—establish intraoral rest on firm teeth; avoid mobile teeth or pontics.
   3. Dip the rubber cup into the polishing paste.
   4. Apply the paste-filled cup to individual teeth.
   5. Activate the rubber cup; bring it almost in contact with the tooth surface before turning on the power.
   6. Use a polishing stroke from the gingival one third to the incisal one third of the tooth.
   7. Use the lowest possible speed.
   8. Apply the cup to the tooth with light, intermittent pressure; the edges of the cup should barely flare.
   9. Use continuous motion; avoid holding the cup in a single spot for a long time to prevent frictional heat.
   10. Progress from the posterior distal aspect to the mesial aspect and from the cervical aspect to the occlusal aspect.
   11. Apply only where needed to remove stain.

C. Bristle brush
   1. Use this only when the rubber cup cannot accomplish stain removal; use it for occlusal and smooth surface pits.
   2. Avoid using it near the gingival margin.
   3. Avoid using it on cementum.
   4. Soak the brush in water to soften it before use.
   5. Grasp, fulcrum, and other techniques are

similar to those for the rubber cup procedure.

IX. Explain the procedure to the patient.

A. Explain the reason for the polishing procedure.

B. Point out areas in which stain has occurred and give possible explanation for the stain.

C. If the patient is a child, allow him or her to see the handpiece and possibly feel the rubber cup rotating on the finger.

X. Chair and patient positions for each quadrant for a right-handed operator are as follows.

A. Using direct and indirect vision

B. Positioning for the maxillary right quadrant
   1. Operator position—8 to 9 o'clock position
   2. Patient position—head turned away and slightly up for buccal surfaces; head turned toward operator and up for lingual surfaces

C. Positioning for the maxillary anterior area
   1. Operator position—8 to 9 o'clock position; use mouth mirror for lingual, may need 11 to 12 o'clock position
   2. Patient position—head tipped up slightly for facial surfaces

D. Positioning for the maxillary left quadrant
   1. Operator position—8 to 9 o'clock position
   2. Patient position—head turned toward operator and slightly up for buccal surfaces; head turned away from operator for lingual surfaces

E. Positioning for the mandibular left quadrant
   1. Operator position—8 to 9 o'clock position
   2. Patient position—head turned toward operator for buccal surfaces; head turned away from operator for lingual surfaces

F. Positioning for the mandibular anterior area
   1. Operator position—8 to 9 or 11 to 12 o'clock position
   2. Patient position—head in various positions for operator to gain access

G. Positioning for the mandibular right quadrant
   1. Operator position—8 to 9 o'clock position
   2. Patient position—head turned slightly away for the buccal surfaces; head turned toward operator for the lingual surfaces

H. Positioning for a left-handed operator
   1. approximately the 3 to 4 o'clock position.

XI. After coronal polishing is completed, the interproximal surfaces may be polished with the abrasive still in the mouth with dental floss or tape.

A. Dental floss or tape is worked into each interproximal area using a back-and-forth action.

B. The floss should be worked against both the mesial and the distal surfaces of the teeth to remove stain.

C. The floss is moved along the fingers, using a new area often avoiding tearing and shredding the floss.

D. If necessary, a floss threader may be used under fixed prosthetic devices.

E. After flossing is completed, the patient is given a complete mouth rinse to thoroughly remove all debris.

XII. General suggestions and precautions include the following:

A. Follow a consistent sequence for the polishing procedure to ensure polishing all surfaces.

B. Prevent contaminated aerosols; have patient rinse with antibacterial mouth rinse.

XIII. After completion of the procedure, the following should be apparent:

A. The patient should be free of debris inside and outside of the mouth.

B. The tooth surfaces should be without evidence of disclosing solution, clean and smooth.

C. Tissue trauma should not exist as a result of the coronal polishing procedure.

FLUORIDE

I. Application of **fluoride** is described (boxes).

II. Application of **pit and fissure sealant** is described (box on page 303).

APPLYING ACIDULATED PHOSPHATE FLUORIDE (4-MINUTE FORM)

1. Seat the patient in an upright position.
2. Try in the trays for proper fit.
3. Fill trays one third full with the acidulated phosphate fluoride gel.
4. Place cotton rolls in vestibule areas if necessary.
5. Dry the teeth thoroughly with compressed air.
6. Insert foam trays (one at a time or as a set) in the patient's mouth.
7. Insert a saliva ejector and cotton rolls at the corner of the patient's mouth and instruct the patient to gently chew for 1 minute.
8. Four minutes after the saliva ejector has been inserted, remove it and discard the cotton rolls; remove the foam trays.
9. Remove excess fluoride from the patient's mouth with the saliva ejector; direct the patient to empty excess gel from the mouth before swallowing.
10. A piece of dry gauze may be used to further wipe off the teeth and tongue if necessary.
11. Instruct the patient not to eat, chew, drink, smoke, or rinse for 30 minutes after this treatment.

APPLYING STANNOUS FLUORIDE

1. Isolate one quadrant or one half of the mouth with cotton rolls and holders.
2. Dry the teeth thoroughly with compressed air.
3. Place saliva ejector in the mouth.
4. Apply stannous fluoride solution with cotton-tipped applicators repeatedly to keep the teeth moist for 4 minutes.
5. After 4 minutes, remove excess fluoride and cotton rolls.
6. Repeat the procedure for the remaining quadrants.
7. The patient should be instructed not to eat, chew, drink, smoke, or rinse for 30 minutes after this treatment.

APPLYING SODIUM FLUORIDE

1. One arch at a time is treated.
2. Isolate the arch to be treated with cotton rolls and holders.
3. Place the saliva ejector into the mouth.
4. Dry the teeth thoroughly.
5. Apply sodium fluoride solution with cotton-tipped applicator to wet all of the isolated teeth.
6. Allow the fluoride solution to dry on the teeth for 3 minutes.
7. Remove cotton rolls and any excess fluoride after 3 minutes.
8. Repeat the procedure for the remaining arch.
9. Instruct the patient not to eat, chew, drink, smoke, or rinse for 30 minutes after this treatment.

APPLYING PIT AND FISSURE SEALANT

1. Prepare armamentarium.
2. Update medical history.
3. Examine and determine absence of caries in teeth that will receive pit and fissure sealants.
4. Pumice tooth with nonfluoridated pumice.
5. Rinse and evacuate.
6. Check occlusal relationship.
7. Isolate.
8. Dispense and place acid etchant.
9. Rinse thoroughly, evacuate, and dry the teeth.
10. Isolate again with dry cotton rolls.
11. Dispense and apply pit and fissure sealant.
12. Check occlusal relationship and correct if necessary.

MOUTH GUARDS

I. Mouth guards are protective devices used in contact sports or other physical activities.
II. Fig. 18-2 illustrates the potential areas of trauma that can be prevented or reduced by the use of a mouth guard.

Questions

Preventive Dentistry

1 Which of the following preventive regimens is most likely to control dental caries?
  a. Topical fluoride application
  b. Use of dental floss
  c. Pit and fissure sealants
  d. Dietary control of sucrose
  e. Combination of all of the above

2 An undesirable result of using waxed dental tape or floss before topical application of fluoride is
  a. Shredding
  b. Coating on the proximal surfaces
  c. Excessive absorption of moisture
  d. Sliding of material through contacts

3 A patient has had extensive periodontal involvement and surgery. Some teeth have furcation involvement. The dentist has asked you to instruct this patient in the proper method of keeping the furcation plaque free. Which of the following auxiliary aids would you demonstrate?
  a. Bridge cleaner with floss
  b. Interproximal brush
  c. Pipe cleaner
  d. All of the above

4 The clinical appearance of dental fluorosis or mottled enamel might include which of the following?
  a. White, opaque areas
  b. Pitting of the tooth surface
  c. Brown staining
  d. All of the above

5 After fluoride application the patient should be instructed to not eat, drink, smoke, rinse or brush the teeth for *at least* _____ minutes.
  a. 10
  b. 20
  c. 30
  d. 40
  e. 60

6 Nursing bottle decay is caused by
  a. Breastfeeding a newborn child
  b. Putting a baby to bed with a bottle of sugared liquids
  c. Sucking a pacifier past 1 year of age
  d. Excessive consumption of sticky sweets

7 Fluoride content in acidulated phosphate fluoride is approximately _____ percent.
  a. 2.31%
  b. 1.23%

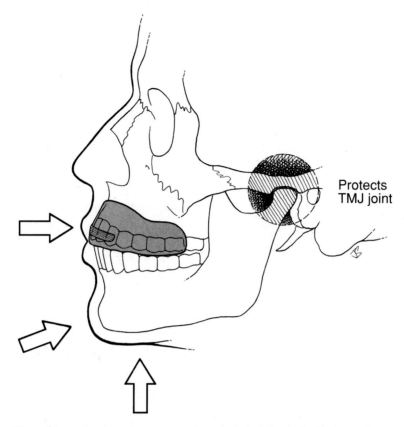

Fig. 18-2 Sites of impact where trauma can be prevented through the use of a mouth guard. Arrows represent points of impact. A mouth guard may prevent oral lacerations, tooth injury, jaw fractures, TMJ trauma.

c. 1.32%
d. 3.12%

8 Compared with acidulated phosphate fluoride, sodium fluoride
   a. Has an unpleasant taste
   b. Is not a stable solution
   c. Stains anterior composite restorations
   d. Requires a series of four applications

9 What is the rationale for the topical application of fluorides in dental caries prevention?
   a. Fluorides penetrate the enamel through the lamellae.
   b. Primary cuticle, being less calcified, absorbs the fluorides.
   c. Acid solubility of the surface enamel is reduced by fluorides.
   d. Keratin content of the enamel is made more resistant to solubility.

10 Plaque consists of
   a. Calculus
   b. Debris that adheres to the acquired pellicle
   c. Calcium bacteria
   d. Calcium and phosphate salts

11 The recommended fluoride concentration in a water supply is
   a. 0.1 ppm
   b. 1 ppm

c. 2 ppm
d. 100 ppm

In items 12-18, match the term in column A with the correct definition in column B.

Column A	*Column B*
_____ **12** Sealant	a. Is absorbed by all teeth
_____ **13** Fluoride	b. Identifies presence of plaque
_____ **14** Disclosing	c. Removes calculus from all surfaces of teeth
	d. Protects deep grooves in premolars and molars

Column A	*Column B*
_____ **15** Modified sickle scaler	a. Removes calculus from all surfaces of teeth
_____ **16** Periodontal probe	b. Marks pocket depth
_____ **17** Rubber cup	c. Used for coronal polishing
_____ **18** Curet scaler	d. Removing calculus from subgingival areas of teeth
	e. Removes deposits from posterior interproximal areas

19 Selective coronal polishing is performed because
   a. The patient may not want all the teeth polished.
   b. It minimizes wearing away the enamel surface.
   c. Insurance companies will only reimburse for this procedure.

20 Which of the following is *not* a technique for coronal polishing?
   a. Porte-polisher
   b. Rubber point polishing
   c. Rubber cup polishing
   d. Air powder polisher
   e. All of the above

Arrange the steps for the coronal polishing in order of sequence. Place the first step in item 21 and continue to the last step in item 25.
   a. Floss with paste in place.
   b. Maintain fulcrum.
   c. Position your hand on hand piece as you would for holding a pen.
   d. Move the rubber cup with polishing paste from the gingival one third to the incisal one third of the tooth.
   e. Rotate the cup prior to placement on the tooth surface.

   _____ **21**
   _____ **22**
   _____ **23**
   _____ **24**
   _____ **25**

Rationales

Preventive Dentistry

1 E No one technique can control dental caries; this type of prevention requires the combination of a variety of techniques.

   Topical fluoride helps reduce dental caries by combining with the hydroxyapatite of the hard tooth structure to form fluoroapatite, which is more resistant to carious breakdown.

   The use of dental floss helps to break down the bacterial colonies at the interproximal surfaces, where the patient is unable to brush during routine home care.

   Pit and fissure sealants are applied to susceptible occlusal surfaces of posterior teeth to seal the surface irregularities and prevent ingress of oral fluids, food, and debris.

   Dietary control of sucrose can decrease the amount of sugar that can react with bacteria to create an acid in the mouth that reacts with the tooth surface to create a carious lesion.

2 B Waxed dental tape or floss may leave a film of wax on the tooth surface. Done prior to application of fluoride, it would be a contraindication to the success of a fluoride application.

3 B Because the patient has no fixed prosthesis or missing teeth in the area of treatment, an interproximal brush would benefit the patient during home care in this area.

4 D When an excess of fluoride is ingested, it can result in fluorosis. This condition results in defective calcification of teeth, giving a white chalky appearance that gradually undergoes brown discoloration.

5 C Because the effect of the application of topical fluoride is not effective immediately, it is suggested that the patient not eat, drink, smoke, rinse or brush the teeth for at least 30 minutes.

6 B Putting a baby to bed at night with a bottle of sugared liquid allows the sugar to react with bacteria in the mouth to create nursing bottle decay. To prevent this condition, the caregiver should be advised to put the baby to bed with clear water rather than a sugared substance.

7 B Acidulated phosphate fluoride is available in a 1.23% gel in both 1- and 4-minute formulas. A 4-minute single professional application of this gel twice a year gives valuable caries protection.

8 D For maximum effectiveness it is necessary to apply sodium fluoride in four 3-minute applications, 2 to 7 days apart.

9 C Topical fluoride helps reduce dental caries by combining with the hydroxyapatite of the hard tooth structure to form fluoroapatite, which is more resistant to carious breakdown.

10 B Plaque is a structured yellow-gray, transparent, or near transparent mass of colonizing bacteria that adheres to the acquired pellicle and supporting tissues. This layer of plaque is not visible to the patient.

11 B One ppm of fluoride in a water supply is the recommended concentration. Studies indicate that significantly less than this amount provides no noticeable effect in carious reduction. Excessive amounts of ingested fluoride should be avoided because this could cause dental fluorosis or mottled enamel.

12 D Sealants as a preventive agent are most effective when used in the deep pit and fissure grooves of premolars and molars.

13 A Fluoride as a topical application can be absorbed by all teeth.

14 B Disclosing solution or tablets are used to identify the presence of plaque.

15 E A modified sickle scaler has a blade at a right angle to the blade. It allows for removal of deposits from posterior interproximal surfaces of the teeth.

16 B A calibrated instrument, the periodontal probe is used to measure the depth of periodontal pockets.

17 C A rubber cup can be used on a rotary hand piece to polish coronal surfaces of the teeth. It is most effective on the smooth surfaces of the teeth.

18 A The curet scaler is a universal scaler and can be used to remove calculus from all surfaces of the teeth.

19 B Selective coronal polishing is done to ensure that unnecessary polishing does not occur that might wear away enamel.

20 B A porte-polisher is a manual polishing device. Rubber cups and air powder polishers are rotary devices that allow for coronal polishing. There is no rubber point used for coronal polishing.

21 C See No. 25.

22 B See No. 25.

23 E See No. 25.

24 D See No. 25
25 A The operator grasps the handpiece with the rubber cup in place and holds it in a pen grasp. A fulcrum is then established to stabilize the hand. The cup should be rotated prior to placement on the tooth surface. The cup is placed on the tooth, moving the cup with the polishing paste from the gingival one third of the tooth to the occlusal/incisal one third. When the rotary polishing is complete, the interproximal surfaces are polished with floss while the abrasive paste is still in place.

To enhance your understanding of the material in this chapter refer to the illustrations in Chapter 26 of Finkbeiner/Johnson: *Mosby's Comprehensive Dental Assisting: A Clinical Approach.*

CHAPTER 19

Common Restorative Procedures

OUTLINE

Dental Amalgam
  Cavity Forms
  Common Armamentarium for an
    Amalgam Restoration
  Amalgam Procedure

Pin-Retained Amalgam
    Restoration
Composite Restorations
  Cavity Preparation for Composite
    Procedure

Armamentarium for Composite
    Procedure
Composite Procedure

KEY TERMS

Bonding

Caries removal

Convenience form

Extension for prevention

Outline form

Polymerized

Resistance form

Retention form

Shade selection

Smooth surface carvers

A restorative procedure is one in which tooth structure is restored with a manufactured substance. The substance is used to re-create anatomy that no longer exists on a tooth. Two common restorative materials are used routinely: *amalgam* and *composite*. The placement of either of these materials as a tooth restoration involves a single appointment. With minor differences, the procedure for each of these is similar as shown (box on page 308).

Both amalgam and composite restorations can be placed on teeth to restore surfaces that have been lost to trauma, defects, or carious lesions. Amalgam restorations are placed in cavity preparations that are predominantly on posterior tooth surfaces of the primary and permanent dentition, including carious lesions of Classes I, II, V, and VI. Amalgam is not a particularly esthetic material, and its use in the anterior segment of a patient's mouth would be prohibitive. An exception could be the use of amalgam in a Class III preparation on the distolingual surface of a cuspid or a Class I pit on the lingual of an anterior tooth. Amalgam does not possess adequate compressive strength to be used when the crown of a posterior tooth needs to be completely restored. However, amalgam may be used as a core material to rebuild tooth structure that has been extensively lost due to fracture or decay. The core of amalgam placed on the tooth usually serves as a base for a cast metal restoration.

Today, it is estimated that the average dental practitioner spends 10% to 15% of treatment time on procedures that are related to a patient's appearance. It is projected that by the end of this decade the per-

RESTORATIVE PROCEDURES	
AMALGAM	COMPOSITE
History update	History update
Examination of the treatment site	Examination of the treatment site
Anesthesia	Anesthesia
Isolation	Isolation
Preparation of the area	Preparation of the area
Medication of the prepared tooth	Medication of the prepared tooth
Placement/condensation of the amalgam	Acid etching of the prepared tooth
Finishing of the amalgam material	Placement of the composite
Postoperative instructions	Finishing of the composite
	Postoperative instructions

centage of time allocated to esthetic dentistry will triple.

Esthetic filling materials usually are placed in areas of the oral cavity that are readily visible during smiling or talking. Obtaining the best esthetic restorative material has been a goal of the dental profession. Materials used include veneers, glass ionomers, and chemically and light-cured composite resins. Microfilled composite restorative material provides the best esthetic restoration in a single-appointment procedure. Placement of the composite materials in anterior teeth is as common as placement of amalgam in the posterior teeth. A positive aspect of the material is its ability to obtain the correct color and translucency match. The microfilled composites are among the most commonly used composite materials because the surfaces can be finished to an extreme level of smoothness. Macrofilled and minifilled composite materials are also available.

Microfilled composite resin materials are usually bonded in place on a tooth. **Bonding** is a common procedure used to attach the restorative material to the tooth surface. Before the development of the bonding technique, restorative materials were held in place through a system of mechanical lock. The bonding technique involves the placement of an acid etchant on the enamel surface of the tooth. The etched enamel provides a slightly porous surface to which the bonding material will adhere. The composite resin material then adheres to the bonded resin. With the use of a bonding material, less tooth surface has to be removed to retain a restorative material. In some circumstances burs are not even used to create a preparation before the placement of the restorative material; the surface is simply acid etched and bonded.

The common classifications of cavities usually restored with composite material include Classes I, III, IV,

and V. Composite filling material is also used on a regular basis as a core material to reconstruct major tooth structures before crown preparation. Failure of a composite resin restoration is usually attributed to color change and excess washing or to wear in the contour of the material.

DENTAL AMALGAM

I. Cavity Forms
   A. Cavity form is the actual shaping of the cavity walls and floors as the tooth is prepared to receive various types of restorative materials.
   B. Cavity form phases require different designs and various instruments depending on the type of restorative material that is to be placed.
   C. The cavity forms that provide guidelines for a cavity preparation lead to a successfully retained restoration (box on page 309).
   D. **Extension for prevention** allows for the extension of margins of cavity preparations to a point that the patient can easily reach with a toothbrush.

II. Common Armamentarium for an Amalgam Restoration
   A. The armamentarium for an amalgam procedure is grouped into phases according to the fundamental steps listed (box on page 309).
   B. Categories of instruments needed during an amalgam procedure include the following:
      1. Examination
         a. Explorer
         b. Mirror
         c. Cotton pliers
      2. Preparation and placement
         a. Spoon excavator

CAVITY FORMS
OUTLINE FORM
The form of the cavity preparation is performed after the opening phase as it meets the tooth surface when it has been expanded to include all carious areas
RESISTANCE FORM
A shape that is given to a cavity that enables a restoration to withstand the stress that occurs during mastication
RETENTION FORM
Shaping the cavity preparation to prevent the restoration from being displaced (a large part of this is provided by the resistance form; in most cavities the retention form is made by shaping certain opposing walls so that they will be parallel or slightly undercut)
CONVENIENCE FORM
The changes that are made in the basic outline form to facilitate visibility and placement of the restorative material
REMOVAL OF CARIES
The actual removal of carious or decalcified tissue from the tooth
FINISHING ENAMEL WALLS AND MARGINS
The placement of angles and bevels in the cavity preparation and the final smoothing of the cavity walls
EXTENSION FOR PREVENTION
The extension of the original cavity preparation that includes pits and fissures that could become carious at a later time

STEPS OF AMALGAM RESTORATION
1. Prepare armamentarium.
2. Update medical history.
3. Examine treatment site.
4. Determine occlusal relationship.
5. Administer anesthetic.
6. Isolate with rubber dam.
7. Open cavity preparation.
8. Outline/resistance form.
9. Remove caries.
10. Place retention form.
11. Isolate with cotton rolls (alternative isolation).
12. Place cavity medication.
13. Place matrix band, retainer, and wedge(s).
14. Insert and condense amalgam.
15. Perform initial carving.
16. Remove matrix retainer, wedge, and band.
17. Perform interproximal carving.
18. Complete final carving.
19. Remove isolation.
20. Check articulation.
21. Burnish margins.
22. Give postoperative instructions.
23. Finish and polish (optional).

      b. Enamel hatchet

      c. Mesial and distal gingival margin trimmers

      d. Burs

      e. Amalgam carrier/syringe/gun

      f. Matrix retainers, bands, and wedges

      g. Anatomic carvers

      h. **Smooth surface carvers**

      i. Ball burnishers

      j. Anatomic burnishers

      k. T-ball/beaver-tail burnisher

      l. Dappen dish/amalgam well

     m. Articulating paper

      n. Cotton rolls

      o. Cotton pellets

      p. Cotton gauze

      q. Articulating paper holder

      r. Rubber dam armamentarium

      s. Anesthesia armamentarium

      t. Finishing and polishing armamentarium

      u. Dental materials armamentarium

  C. Prepare the matrix band and retainer.

     1. A circumferential matrix band and retainer, such as the Tofflemire band and retainer, are commonly used in Class II and Class VI amalgam procedures (box on page 310).

     2. Assembly of the Tofflemire retainer and band is shown (box on page 310).

     3. Assembly of the universal matrix band in the retainer is shown (box on page 311).

III. Amalgam Procedure

  A. Prepare the armamentarium.

  B. The procedural steps are described (box on pages 311-313).

  C. The team approach for four-handed dentistry is shown (box on pages 314-315).

PARTS OF THE TOFFLEMIRE RETAINER

Outer knob—A knob used to adjust the tightness of the spindle on the band inside of the vise

Inner knob—A knob used to move the vise to increase or decrease the size of the band to accommodate the size of the tooth

Frame—The part of the retainer that connects the outer and inner knobs, vise, and spindle

Spindle—A threaded rod that holds the end of the matrix band in the vise

Vise—The device that clamps tight to hold the ends of the matrix band in the retainer

Guide slots—Slots at the end of the retainer and in the area of the vise that allow the band to be directed to certain areas as selected

PREPARATION OF THE TOFFLEMIRE RETAINER

When the retainer is assembled, two orientations of it should be considered: the gingival aspect and the occlusal aspect.

Gingival aspect—from the side of the retainer that will be placed near the gingival openings, the guide slots and diagonal slots are visible.

Occlusal aspect—from the side of the retainer that will be placed near the occlusal surface, openings of the guide slots and diagonal slots are not visible.

It is necessary to understand these orientations when the assembly and placement of the matrix band into the retainer are discussed.

The retainer should be prepared first in the following stages of assembly:

- Hold the retainer with the gingival aspect facing upward.
- Adjust the outer knob by turning it clockwise; stop turning the knob before the spindle enters the vise slot.
- If the knob is turned too far, entry to the diagonal vise slot is blocked, and the matrix band will not slide into place.
- Turn the inner knob clockwise to move the vise inch from the end of the retainer.
- If the outer knob needs to be adjusted, move the spindle to the end of the diagonal vise slots.

PLACING THE UNIVERSAL MATRIX BAND IN THE RETAINER

The universal matrix band, like the contoured and ivory band, have a gingival and an occlusal edge. (Because the T-band has equal surface area on both sides, it can be placed toward the gingiva or the occlusal surface.)

The following steps are provided as guidelines for the assembly of the matrix band and retainer:

- Hold the band with the gingival aspect above the occlusal aspect. (The band position simulates a smile toward the operator)
- Pull the two ends of the band toward you.
- The larger part of the circle (the occlusal edge) is down; the smaller part of the circle (the gingival edge) is up. (Note: This size correlates with the shape of the tooth; it is narrow at the gingiva and wide at the occlusal.)
- Place the occlusal edge of the band into the diagonal slot first, with the loop extending toward the end of the retainer.
- With the gingival aspect of the retainer and the band facing up, place the thumb over the slots to stabilize the band. The opening of the loop should be as close as possible to the size of the tooth on which it is to be placed. For instance, if a premolar is being prepared, the loop, when it is first placed into the retainer, should be smaller than it is for a molar.
- Force the loop of the band up, lifting it through the right side opening of the retainer and sliding it firmly into place.
- Tighten the outer knob into the ends of the band by turning it clockwise; this secures the band and ensures that it will not fall out when placed in the patient's mouth.
- Increase or decrease the size of the band to accommodate the tooth being treated. (For a molar, use a large opening; for a premolar, use a moderate or smaller opening.) Do this by moving the inner knob clockwise or counterclockwise. A band that is not correctly sized or shaped to the contour of the prepared tooth causes loss of time and motion for the operating team at chairside.
- The loop of the band may become crimped during preparation; this can be smoothed by taking the end of a mirror handle and running it around the inside the loop, while it is tightly held by the retainer. The thumb is used to create a controlled pressure on the mirror handle against the band. This establishes again the round shape of the band needed to obtain a good contour around the tooth. Because bands are sterilizable, they can be distorted through repeated use.
- The band and retainer are now prepared for the maxillary right or the mandibular left quadrant.

MATRIX BAND AND RETAINER PREPARATION

1. Adjust the outer knob so that the spindle is short of entering the vise slot.
2. Turn the inner knob clockwise so that the vise is ³⁄₁₆ inch from the end of the retainer.
3. Hold the matrix band with the gingival aspect above the occlusal aspect. (The band position simulates a smile.)
4. Pull the free ends of the band toward you, with the occlusal aspect below the gingival aspect.
5. Place the occlusal, larger part of the circle into the slots of the retainer first. (The size of the circle that extends from the retainer should correlate with the size of the tooth on which it will be placed.)
6. Look at the gingival aspect of the retainer and band and place the loop out the right side of the retainer for the mandibular left quadrant or the maxillary right quadrant. If the loop is out the left side of the retainer, assemble it for the mandibular right and maxillary left quadrants.
7. Tighten the outer knob, securing the spindle against the band.
8. Smooth the loop of the band with a mirror handle if it is crimped.

AMALGAM PROCEDURE

- Are all universal barrier techniques being used?
- Is all of the armamentarium available and prepared for use?
- Are the instruments arranged in sequence to use?
- Are you prepared for alternative treatment plans?
- Is the necessary equipment turned on and ready to operate?

The Class II amalgam restoration is a common procedure. Because this particular type of cavity classification encompasses most of the basic concepts of an amalgam procedure, the procedure for placing a Class II amalgam restoration on a posterior tooth is described.

MEDICAL HISTORY UPDATE

A current health history is obtained from the patient being seen for restorative treatment.

EXAMINATION OF TREATMENT SITE

The treatment site is examined by the operator as the assistant passes the explorer and mirror. The operator confirms the area and the extent of treatment to be rendered.

DETERMINATION OF OCCLUSAL RELATIONSHIP

The first step completed before any restorative procedure is begun determines the occlusal relationship and any interference. The surfaces of the teeth are dried with a 2 × 2 gauze sponge, and articulating paper is held between the arches with articulating paper forceps or cotton pliers; the patient is directed to bite firmly and side to side.

ANESTHESIA ADMINISTRATION

After the occlusion has been established, the anesthetic is administered. The operator palpates the site of the injection. Pass the 2 × 2 gauze sponge to dry the site. Exchange the gauze with a cotton-tipped applicator with topical anesthesia. Retrieve the applicator and slightly raise the operating light. Pass the syringe using the hidden syringe technique. Retrieve the syringe and recap using OSHA accepted techniques, and pass a 2 × 2 gauze to dry the site.

RUBBER DAM ISOLATION

During the few minutes it takes for complete anesthesia to occur, the rubber dam isolation procedure may begin. Holes are punched for four teeth: one posterior to the tooth to be prepared, the tooth that is to be treated, and the two teeth anterior to the tooth that is being prepared. The assistant flosses the interproximal spaces of the teeth to determine that the contacts are not too tight.

The rubber dam assembly is passed to the operator, and the clamp is placed on the second molar. The operator positions the holes over the first molar, second premolar, and the first premolar as the assistant flosses the dam down in the interproximal spaces. An anterior ligature is placed in the mesial contact of the first premolar, stabilizing the rubber dam assembly.

The rubber dam napkin or gauze is placed under the assembly. The spoon excavator, beaver-tail burnisher, or plastic instrument is used to invert the dam into the gingival sulcus.

Continued

AMALGAM PROCEDURE—cont'd

CAVITY PREPARATION

Opening phase

Throughout the rest of the procedure the assistant maintains a clear field through the use of the HVE and the A/W syringe. The operator uses a high-speed handpiece with either a #34 FG inverted cone or a #1 or #2 FG round bur to open the enamel on the occlusal surface.

OUTLINE OR RESISTANCE FORM PHASE

The operator continues the opening, and, when that is completed, begins the outline phase, which is an extension of the preparation that includes shaping and designing the wall and floor of the preparation. This may be accomplished with a #55, #56, or #57 FG straight fissure on the high-speed handpiece. The process of the outline phase could also result in development of the resistance form.

When the opening of the preparation is adequately expanded from the occlusal surface across to the distal proximal wall, the operator may use hand-cutting instruments to continue the preparation procedure. When all unsupported enamel has been removed by the planing and cleaving process with the enamel hatchet, the operator uses the distal gingival margin trimmer to place bevels on the line angles of the cervical and pulpal floors.

CARIES REMOVAL

Caries removal involves the removal of any carious tissues through mechanical or manual means. By manual means, a spoon excavator is used to remove carious tissue. Mechanically, caries are removed through the use of the slow-speed handpiece with a round bur.

The low-speed handpiece with a #2, #4, or #6 FG or RA bur is used for caries removal.

RETENTION PHASE

The retention form assists with the retention of the restoration in the preparation. Usually the retention phase involves the placement of small grooves on the pulpal and cervical floors of the preparation to assist in mechanically locking the amalgam in place.

Retentive grooves are usually placed with a #¼ or #½ FG or RA round bur on a low-speed handpiece.

COTTON ROLL ISOLATION

If cotton roll isolation is used instead of rubber dam isolation, the cotton rolls are placed at this point.

CAVITY MEDICATION PLACEMENT

The cavity medication phase may proceed as indicated by the depth of the prepared tooth and the closeness of the pulpal tissues. Cavity depth determines the type of medication needed to seal the dentinal tubules, provide insulation, act as an obtundent, stimulate the pulp, and create an ideal depth in the preparation. Table 19-1 lists various cavity depths and medications needed to provide patient comfort.

MATRIX BAND, RETAINER, AND WEDGE PLACEMENT

The next step in the procedure is the placement of the prepared matrix band and retainer. It may be necessary to place a wedge first for a few minutes to force the teeth apart and allow easier placement and adaptability of the matrix band and retainer. If this step is not needed, the band and retainer are placed on the first molar. Once the band is adapted to the cervical and completely surrounds the tooth, the retainer is tightened and the band circumference reduced to a snug fit.

The wedge is placed against the base of the interdental space or the cervical, directed from the lingual into the proximal space.

AMALGAM INSERTION

After the matrix band, retainer, and wedge are placed, the insertion phase begins. The activated amalgam capsule is placed in the amalgamator and mixed for the proper length of time. The amalgam is placed in the amalgam carrier, and the operator places the first increment in the least accessible area. The #1 amalgam condenser is used to condense the increments into the cavity preparation. As the preparation becomes full, a larger condenser may be used.

AMALGAM PROCEDURE—cont'd

INITIAL CARVING

When the preparation is sufficiently overfilled, the initial carving phase begins. The instrument of choice (a #7 cleoid-discoid carver, a #26 spoon, or even a #21B anatomic burnisher) is used to remove the gross amount of amalgam and surface mercury. The carver should be placed on the cavosurface margin. This position functions as a fulcrum, to counteract the tendency to overcarve the amalgam and create an underfilled area at the cavosurface margins.

Next, the #7 carver is exchanged for the explorer or Ward's C carver to remove amalgam from the contact at the marginal ridge and the band. Care must be taken during this step to avoid any fractures of the amalgam. Additional amalgam that was forced down around the band in other areas (such as the buccal or lingual) is removed by slightly rotating the instrument through these areas.

MATRIX RETAINER, WEDGE, AND BAND REMOVAL

The wedge is removed with the cotton pliers; then the retainer is loosened and removed. The operator removes the matrix band.

INTERPROXIMAL CARVING

The assistant receives the band by exchanging the Ward's C carver or the explorer for the interproximal carving to contour the least accessible area.

The blade of the carver is positioned interproximally and raised toward the occlusal until resistance is met. The operator uses the explorer to check the area carved with the Ward's C carver.

FINAL CARVING

The operator exchanges the explorer for the #5 C carver for the final carving of the occlusal surface. The original tooth anatomy is reestablished in the amalgam with a #5 C carver, deepening and accentuating the grooves and fissures that were placed with the #7 C carver. The operator often uses the explorer to check the margins after carving with the #5 C carver.

ISOLATION REMOVAL

The rubber dam is removed and the assistant completes a full mouth rinse.

CHECKING THE ARTICULATION

The articulating paper is used to check the occlusion of the newly restored surfaces. If the paper marks the amalgam surface, the assistant passes the #5 C carver to the operator to remove the excess amalgam where the occlusion is too heavy. The articulation may be checked and the occlusal surface may be carved several times before the occlusal contact is correct and comfortable for the patient.

BURNISHING

The operator receives the ball burnisher (or burnisher of choice) and smooths the cavosurface margins and all other areas. Occasionally, the operator needs to exchange the burnisher for the explorer to remove any flash of amalgam.

FINISHING AND POLISHING

With certain types of amalgam, finishing and polishing can be accomplished at this appointment. With the use of other types of amalgam a longer setting time may be required, necessitating another appointment. The assistant receives the handpiece and provides the patient with a complete mouth rinse.

POSTOPERATIVE INSTRUCTIONS

The patient is given postoperative instructions by the assistant or the operator regarding the length of time that the anesthetic may remain in effect.
- Have the appropriate universal barrier techniques been removed?
- Have all appropriate surfaces been cleaned and disinfected?
- Has all of the armamentarium been removed?
- Has all equipment been repositioned?
- Has all equipment been disinfected/sterilized according to OSHA guidelines?

AMALGAM PROCEDURE: TEAM APPROACH	
OPERATOR	**ASSISTANT**
	Select and prepare all armamentaria.
	Prepare the treatment room and escort the patient in to be seated.
	Assist in administration of anesthetic and placement of isolation.
	Pass mirror and explorer.
Examine treatment site.	Exchange instruments for opening bur in high-speed handpiece.
Open the preparation.	Place HVE and A/W syringe to maintain clear field of operation.
	Prepare explorer to pass.
	Exchange explorer for handpiece.
Examine site with explorer.	Insert outline and resistance form bur in handpiece and exchange handpiece for explorer.
Create outline resistance form.	Maintain clear field of operation.
	Exchange hand-cutting instruments for handpiece.
Receive and use hand-cutting instruments to place bevels and remove unsupported tooth structure.	Exchange slow-speed handpiece with caries removal bur for hand-cutting instruments.
Remove caries.	Maintain clear field of operation.
	Exchange explorer for handpiece.
Check preparation for complete caries removal of explorer.	Exchange retentive bur in handpiece for explorer.
Place retentive grooves.	Maintain clear field of operation.
	Exchange explorer for handpiece.
Place cavity medication.	Prepare cavity medication and exchange placement instrument for explorer.
	Keep 2 × 2 gauze and medication in transfer zone for easy operator access.
	Exchange instrument for explorer.
Use the explorer to remove excess cement.	Maintain clear field of operation.
	Exchange prepared matrix retainer and band for explorer.
Place matrix retainer and band.	Pass cotton pliers and wedge.
Place wedge interproximally.	Exchange explorer for cotton pliers.
Evaluate placement of retainer, band, and wedge.	Mix amalgam and receive explorer.
	Fill amalgam carrier and pass.
Place amalgam preparation.	Exchange carrier for condenser and fill carrier.
	Continue exchange of the amalgam carrier and condenser until the preparation is overfilled with the HVE in the area to remove excess pieces of amalgam.
	Exchange anatomic carver for condenser.
Initially carve restoration removing gross amounts of excess.	Maintain clear field of operation.
	Exchange carver for explorer.
Remove excess from marginal ridge area.	Exchange explorer for cotton pliers.
Remove wedge.	Receive wedge.
Remove retainer.	Receive retainer.
Remove band.	Exchange smooth surface carver for band and cotton pliers.
Carve smooth surface.	Exchange carver for explorer.
Check smooth surfaces with explorer.	Prepare anatomic carver.
	Exchange explorer for anatomic carver.

AMALGAM PROCEDURE: TEAM APPROACH—cont'd	
OPERATOR	ASSISTANT
Refine anatomic carving.	Maintain clear field of operation.
	Exchange carver for burnisher.
Burnish the restored surfaces.	Exchange burnisher for explorer.
Remove flash.	Remove carved flash with HVE.
Remove isolation.	Assist in removal of isolation.
	Exchange articulating paper and paper holder for explorer.
Check articulation.	Exchange holder for carver.
Remove excess with carver.	Exchange carver for articulating paper.
Check articulation.	Exchange articulating paper for carver or burnisher.
Carve or burnish as needed.	Receive instruments.
	Remove debris and provide full mouth rinse.
	Provide postoperative instructions and dismiss patient.
	Record treatment on the patient's chart.
	Follow OSHA guidelines for cleanup.

D. Modifications of the procedure will be required as changes take place in the cavity preparation.
1. Cavity depth may range from ideal to a pulp exposure and would be treated with medications according to the specific depth.
2. Different cavity classifications may require different burs to establish the outline form.
3. **Caries removal** could be performed with different size burs according to the size of the lesion.
4. A single spill of amalgam would likely be used on Class I, Class V, and small Class II lesions and a double spill on a large Class II and Class VI lesions.
5. Both gingival margin trimmers will be used on Class VI and either the mesial or distal on a Class II lesion, depending on the missing wall.
6. Matrix bands, retainers, wedges, occlusal anatomic carvers, anatomic burnishers, and smooth surface carvers will vary according to the surfaces involved.
7. See Table 19-1 for instruments used in various situations.

IV. Pin-Retained Amalgam Restoration
A. If a tooth is not structurally capable of retaining the restorative material—whether it is amalgam or composite—a pin technique is used to aid retention with amalgam or composite restorative procedures.
B. The procedure is as follows:

1. The operator makes a starter hole with a round bur and then expands the hole with a spirec drill on the slow-speed handpiece.
2. Each type of pin system provides or recommends the use of a particular spirec drill for the pin technique.
3. The pin is placed in the hole with a pin wrench or an autoclutch (a mechanical means of pin placement).
4. If an autoclutch is used, it is placed on the slow-speed handpiece with a plastic latch-type, shanked pin, allowing the pin to be twisted in automatically.
5. Because the pin is a self-shearing device, it will shear off as the pin reaches the correct pinhole depth.
6. Placing more than one pin requires a multipin threading system; two pins attached to a plastic latch-type shank device (piggy back pins) allow placement of the pins without removing the device from the autoclutch.
7. After all the pins are placed in the preparation, the procedure continues as would any other Class II or Class VI procedure.

COMPOSITE RESTORATIONS ■

I. The composite procedure is similar to the amalgam procedure (i.e., retention form, caries removal) but is generally less extensive.
II. The common armamentarium used in a composite procedure involves the following:

Table 19-1 Amalgam tray usage

	2^B	12°	14^6	19MO	21DO	30^MOD	32^L
Anesthesia							
Long	—	—	—	X	X	X	X
Short	X	X	X	—	—	—	—
Rubber dam							
Teeth isolated	1, 2, 3, 4*	10, 11, 12, 13	12, 13, 14, 15	18, 19, 20, 21	20, 21, 22, 23	28, 29, 30, 31	30, 31, 32
Clamp on	1	13	15	18	20	31	32
Explorer	X	X	X	X	X	X	X
Mirror	X	X	X	X	X	X	X
Cotton pliers	X	X	X	X	X	X	X
Spoon excavator	X	X	X	X	X	X	X
Hatchet/chisel	X	X	X	X	X	X	X
Mesial margin trimmer	—	—	—	X	—	X	—
Distal margin trimmer	—	—	—	—	X	X	—
Amalgam carrier	X	X	X	X	X	X	X
#1 condensor	X	X	X	X	X	X	X
#2 condensor	X	X	X	X	X	X	X
Ward's C carver	X	—	—	X	X	X	X
7C	—	X	X	X	X	X	—
5C	—	X	X	X	X	X	—
Ball burnisher	X	X	X	X	X	X	X
Anatomic burnisher	—	X	X	X	X	X	—
Matrix band	—	—	—	X	X	X	—
Matrix retainer	—	—	—	X	X	X	—
Wedges							
1.	—	—	—	X	X	—	—
2.	—	—	—	—	—	X	—
Dappen dish/amalgam well	X	X	X	X	X	X	X
Cotton pellets	X	X	X	X	X	X	X
Articulating paper	—	X	X	X	X	X	—

*Rubber dam optional; additional teeth may be isolated at operator's preference.

A. The armamentarium is grouped into phases according to the fundamental steps outlined (box on page 317).
B. Categories of instruments needed for a composite restorative procedure include the following:
   1. Examination instruments
      a. Explorer
      b. Mirror
      c. Cotton pliers
   2. Preparation and insertion
      a. Shade guides
      b. Rubber cup and pumice
      c. Spoon excavator
      d. Wedelstaedt chisel
      e. Triple-angle chisel
      f. Burs
      g. Acid etch
      h. Bonding agent
      i. Light-activating device

j. Teflon/plastic instrument
k. Composite (centrix) syringe, tip (compules), and plunger
l. Mylar/celluloid matrix strip
m. Wedge(s)
n. Matrix strip holder
o. Skubes/disposable brushes/cotton pledgets
p. 12B scalpel blade and handle
q. Finishing strip
r. Articulating paper
s. Articulating paper holder
t. Assorted stones
u. Mandrel
v. Composite finishing points
w. Composite finishing disks
x. #7900 finishing burs
y. Rubber dam armamentarium or cotton rolls (used for isolation)
z. Cotton pellets

STEPS OF COMPOSITE RESTORATION

1. Update medical history.
2. Examine treatment site.
3. Determine occlusal relationship.
4. Administer anesthetic.
5. Polish tooth with pumice.
6. Select shade.
7. Isolate with rubber dam/cotton roll(s).
8. Open cavity preparation.
9. Place outline and resistance form.
10. Remove caries.
11. Place retention.
12. Place cavity medications (base).
13. Place matrix strip and wedge(s).
14. Acid etch (reisolate if necessary).
15. Apply bonding material.
16. Insert filling material.
17. Remove matrix and wedge.
18. Finish and polish.
19. Remove rubber dam/cotton roll(s).
20. Check articulation.
21. Give postoperative instructions.

aa. Cotton gauze
bb. Anesthesia armamentarium
cc. Composite resin armamentarium
III. The composite procedure is as follows:
  A. Prepare armamentarium.
  B. The procedure is described (box below and on pages 318-319).
  C. The team approach for four-handed dentistry is shown (box on page 320).
  D. Modifications of the procedure will be required as changes take place in the cavity preparation.
    1. In some locations **shade selection** may not be as critical.
    2. Determination of the occlusal contact is not as necessary when there are no contact areas with an opposing tooth.
    3. The type and use of a matrix strip may vary according to the surfaces involved.
    4. Sometimes finishing and polishing may not be completed with disks if a surface is difficult to reach, but stones and points are possible alternative choices.
    5. A matrix strip or a preformed celluloid

CLASS III COMPOSITE PROCEDURE

One of many forms of composite procedures performed daily in a general dentistry practice is a Class III restoration. Following is a description of the procedure for placing an acid-etched and bonded composite resin using light-cured composite resin.
- Are all universal barrier techniques being used?
- Is all of the armamentarium available and prepared for use?
- Are the instruments arranged in sequence of use?
- Are you prepared for alternative treatment plans?
- Is the necessary equipment turned on and ready to operate?

MEDICAL HISTORY UPDATE

A current health history is obtained from the patient being seen for treatment on the distal surface of an anterior tooth.

EXAMINATION OF TREATMENT SITE

The treatment site is examined by the operator with the explorer and the mirror.

DETERMINATION OF OCCLUSAL RELATIONSHIP

The occlusal relationship is examined to identify any interferences that may exist between the arches.

ANESTHESIA ADMINISTRATION

After the occlusion has been established, the anesthetic is administered. The assistant then provides a full mouth rinse.

POLISHING THE TOOTH WITH PUMICE

For a routine preparation this step may not be performed. If bonding is being done, the tooth to be restored must be cleansed of all debris and any fluoride remnants before the acid etched composite procedure is performed.

Continued

CLASS III COMPOSITE PROCEDURE—cont'd
SHADE SELECTION
After the tooth has been polished, the shade selection, which determines tooth color, is easier to match with the resin. It is important to ensure that the correct shade is selected under natural conditions. The shade is selected without the rubber dam in place, with saliva moistening the shade button, and in natural light. The assistant retrieves the material that corresponds to the selected shade of restorative material from the available selections with either overgloves or noncontaminated thumb forceps.
ISOLATION WITH RUBBER DAM
A composite restorative procedure is an excellent example of the ideal use of rubber dam isolation because total isolation must be maintained during various phases of the procedure.
CAVITY PREPARATION
Cavity preparation in a composite restorative procedure may not be necessary in some circumstances. If the patient has a fractured incisal edge, the extent of treatment may be pumicing, etching, bonding and placement, curing, and finishing of the restorative material. Other situations warrant the removal of tooth structure, as in this example.
OPENING PHASE
Throughout the rest of the procedure the assistant maintains a clear field through the use of the HVE and the A/W syringe. In this treatment situation the decay has begun on the facial surface and penetrated to the lingual, forcing the removal of the proximal area completely. The preparation is started with the penetration of a #½ or #1 round FG bur on the high-speed handpiece through the lingual surface on the tooth.
OUTLINE AND RESISTANCE PHASE
The operator uses the high-speed handpiece, with the #55 straight fissure FG bur, to extend the preparation in the outline form. The handpiece is exchanged for a Wedelstaedt, binangle, or triple-angle chisel, or even an enamel hatchet, to cleave the unsupported enamel and to finish the walls. The operator may use #7901 finishing bur or diamond bur on the high-speed handpiece on the cavosurface margins to place bevels on the enamel surface.
CARIES REMOVAL
If all the carious tissue was not removed, the low-speed handpiece with a #1 or #2 RA round bur is commonly used to preserve as much tooth structure as possible. An optional instrument for caries removal is a spoon excavator.
PLACEMENT OF RETENTIVE GROOVES
The #¼ or #½ RA round bur in the conventional-speed handpiece is used to place retentive grooves in the dentin along all existing walls.
PLACEMENT OF CAVITY MEDICATION
The selection of cavity medication is predicated on several factors, including the thickness of the remaining dentin, the pulpal protection, and the type of restorative material that is to be placed.
PLACEMENT OF MATRIX STRIP AND WEDGE
A curved or straight celluloid matrix strip is placed interproximally and contoured properly to the tooth surface. The wedge is placed from the lingual or facial aspect to secure the position of the matrix strip during the insertion of the restorative material.

CLASS III COMPOSITE PROCEDURE—cont'd

ACID ETCHING

The acid etching procedure is performed to obtain an ideal bond of the surfaces when composite resin materials are used. The applicator is passed, and the acid is held in the transfer zone for the operator to dip the instrument into the etchant and apply it to the thoroughly dried tooth surface. The application technique varies, depending on the type of etchant. If the etchant is in liquid form, it should be applied to the surface and then reapplied every 20 seconds for 1 minute. If the etchant is in gel form, a single application left on the surface for 1 minute is adequate. After 1 minute the tooth is thoroughly rinsed from the etched enamel surface for at least 30 seconds and then dried. If rubber dam is not used for isolation, cotton rolls are removed and replaced at this time.

PLACEMENT OF BONDING MATERIAL

The operator maintains complete isolation while the material is placed on the etched surfaces. The material may be self-cured, chemically cured, or light cured.

INSERTION OF FILLING MATERIAL

Composite filling materials are available as chemically cured two-paste systems or as light-cured single-paste systems. The preselected light-cured filling material is dispensed. The incremental amounts placed in the preparation normally should not exceed 2.0 mm in thickness before the material is cured or **polymerized.** The curing wand is placed approximately 1 mm from the restorative material, and the time is set for 20 to 30 seconds.

REMOVING MATRIX STRIP AND WEDGE

After curing is completed, the wedge, matrix holder (if used), and matrix strip are removed.

FINISHING AND POLISHING

The finishing and polishing procedure is extremely important. Finishing begins with the removal of excess material; this can be accomplished by hand or mechanically. The #12B Bard-Parker scalpel is used to remove flash from the tooth surfaces.

Other devices may be used for gross removal of excess restorative material. Coarse disks placed on mandrels in the low-speed handpiece remove excess amounts of material more quickly than do finer disks. The stones have shapes that match the areas to be contoured, such as round, carrot, or biscuit.

Other rotary devices that may be used are the #7901 finishing bur series or diamonds. These devices provide a smooth surface when used with the high-speed handpiece.

Various composite finishing and polishing points, disks, and tones are available in kits that are specific to certain resins. These kits provide various rotary devices that perform well during the finishing and polishing procedure.

REMOVAL OF RUBBER DAM

The rubber dam or cotton rolls are removed. If a rubber dam has been used for isolation, dehydration of the tooth can occur, resulting in a temporary change in color of the tooth surface.

CHECKING ARTICULATION

After the rubber dam is removed, the patient should receive a complete mouth rinse. The site is thoroughly dried and the articulation is checked. If the restored surface is excessively marked, the operator will want to smooth the surface. The tongue is extremely sensitive to that which the eye cannot see. If any roughness is indicated, the operative team continues to make adjustments.

POSTOPERATIVE INSTRUCTIONS

The tissue in the area may still be anesthetized, and the patient should be informed of the expected duration of the anesthetic.
- Have the appropriate universal barrier techniques been removed?
- Have all the appropriate surfaces been cleaned and disinfected?
- Has all of the armamentarium been removed?
- Has all equipment been repositioned?
- Has all equipment been disinfected/sterilized according to OSHA guidelines?

| COMPOSITE PROCEDURE: TEAM APPROACH ||
OPERATOR	ASSISTANT
	Select and prepare all armamentaria.
	Prepare the treatment room and escort the patient in to be seated.
	Assist in administration of anesthetic.
Examine treatment site.	Pass mirror and explorer.
Select composite shade.	Receive instruments and pass shade guide.
	Assist in shade selection.
Place isolation.	Pass isolation setup and assist in placement.
	Pass opening bur in high-speed handpiece and mirror.
	Place HVE and A/W syringe to maintain clear field of operation.
Open the preparation.	Evacuate and dry the site.
	Exchange explorer for handpiece.
Examine site with explorer.	Insert outline/resistance form bur in handpiece and exchange for explorer.
Create outline/resistance form.	Maintain clear field of operation.
	Exchange hand-cutting instrument for handpiece.
Place bevels and remove unsupported tooth structure.	Exchange low-speed handpiece with caries removal bur for hand-cutting instrument.
Remove caries.	Maintain clear field of operation.
	Exchange explorer for handpiece.
Check preparation for complete caries removal with explorer.	Exchange retentive bur in handpiece for explorer.
Place retentive grooves.	Maintain clear field of operation.
	Exchange finishing bur in high-speed handpiece for explorer.
Feather preparation cavosurface margin.	Maintain clear field of operation.
	Pass matrix strip.
Place matrix strip.	Prepare and pass etching agent.
Etch tooth structure.	Thoroughly rinse, dry, and evacuate field.
Remove matrix strip.	Exchange used matrix strip for new strip.
	Prepare and pass bonding agent.
Place bonding agent.	Maintain clear field of operation.
	Pass composite resin material and placement instrument.
Place composite material.	Exchange curing device for placement instrument.
Cure the composite material.	Exchange explorer for curing device.
Check for set of composite.	

crown form can be used to provide a mould for the lost tooth structure in a Class IV lesion; a hole is usually placed in the mesial or distal-incisal corner to allow excess material to extrude from the form; incisal and mesial or distal surfaces of the crown form may be cut away from the rest of the form and used as a matrix to hold the material on the tooth during the placement and curing.

6. A threaded pin can be placed to provide support for the restorative material in an extensive lesion.

Questions

Common Restorative Procedures

1 What instrument is *not* used in the placement of a Class I amalgam restoration?
   a. Amalgam carrier
   b. Condenser
   c. Spoon excavator
   d. Matrix band retainer
2 A wooden wedge is used to
   a. Prevent gingival amalgam overhang

b. Condense amalgam into small preparations

c. Aid in surgical removal of root tips

d. Splint loose teeth

3 In a mesioocclusal cavity preparation, where is the amalgam placed first?

a. On the occlusal surface

b. In the proximal box

c. In the distal portion of the preparation

d. It does not matter which part of the cavity preparation is filled first

4 Place the following stages of restorative dentistry in proper sequence:

1. Administration of local anesthetic

2. Contouring and placement of matrix

3. Seating the patient

4. Entering the treatment data

5. Completion of the cavity preparation

6. Application of the rubber dam

7. Placement and condensation of restorative material

8. Placement of cavity medications

9. Carving and contouring of the restorative material

a. 3, 1, 5, 2, 6, 7, 8, 9, 4

b. 3, 4, 1, 5, 6, 2, 7, 8, 9

c. 3, 1, 6, 5, 8, 2, 7, 9, 4

d. 1, 3, 6, 5, 8, 2, 7, 9, 4

5 Which of the following cavity classifications would be candidates for an amalgam restoration?

1. Class I

2. Class II

3. Class III

4. Class IV

5. Class V

a. 1 and 2

b. 2 and 3

c. 3 and 4

d. 1, 2, and 4

e. 1, 2, and 5

6 Which of the following instruments and materials are not necessary for a Class III composite restoration with ideal cavity depth?

1. Cavity varnish

2. Articulation paper

3. Plastic instrument

4. Cleoid-discoid carver

5. Finishing strip

6. Finishing disks and mandrel

7. Cavitec

8. White stones

9. Rubber wheel

10. Carbide burs

a. 1, 4, and 7

b. 1, 4, and 9

c. 2, 7, and 9

d. 4, 7, and 9

7 Which of the following hand instruments might be used to plane the walls and floors of the cavity preparation for a composite restoration?

1. Binangle chisel

2. Cleoid-discoid carver

3. Hoe

4. Gingival marginal trimmer

5. Wedelstaedt chisel

a. 1 and 3

b. 2 and 4

c. 1, 3, and 5

d. 1, 2, 3, and 4

8 When necessary, the preferred lining agent before insertion of a composite restoration is

a. Calcium hydroxide

b. Zinc oxide-eugenol

c. Cavity varnish

d. Zinc phosphate

9 After inserting, when can the final polish of light-cured composite be accomplished?

a. Within 10 minutes

b. Within 20 to 30 minutes

c. After 8 hours

d. As soon as polymerized

10 Which of the following statements are true regarding acid etching of enamel for a composite restoration?

1. The acid-etching agent forms a mechanical bond with the enamel.

2. The acid etching is flooded onto the surface and rubbed vigorously.

3. The material is applied with cotton pellets or small sponges that are supplied with the kit.

4. The composite resin is placed before acid etching of enamel.

5. Acid etching is rinsed from the tooth after the recommended time, to stop the etching process.

a. 1 and 3

b. 2 and 4

c. 1, 3, and 5

d. 1, 2, 3, 4, and 5

11 When a composite restoration is being placed on the buccal one third of tooth #30, which of the following is the matrix of choice?

a. Universal circumferential Tofflemire

b. Ivory noncircumferential

c. Class V composite

d. Celluloid strip

Use the tray-setup diagram (on page 322) to answer items 12-17.

12 Instrument 7 would be used to

a. Remove caries

b. Condense amalgam

c. Place bevels

d. Remove unsupported enamel

13 Instrument 12 would be used to

a. Condense amalgam

b. Carve smooth surface amalgam

c. Remove unsupported enamel

d. Carve grooves and fissures in the amalgam

14 Instrument 19 is a/an

a. Ball burnisher

b. Anatomic burnisher

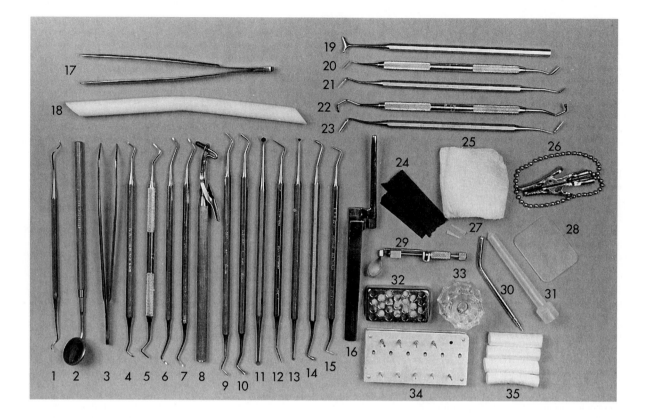

c. Contoured condenser

d. Beaver-tail burnisher

15 Instrument 11 is a

a. Spoon excavator

b. Larger ball burnisher

c. #5 cleoid-discoid carver

d. #7 cleoid-discoid carver

16 Instrument 29 is used to

a. Replace occlusal walls

b. Circumferentially surround tooth

c. Provide a single wall to restore against

17 Which instrument is commonly used for forming retention in the preparation?

a. ½

b. 2

c. 34

d. Spoon excavator

In items 18-21, match the term in column A with the appropriate definition in column B.

Column A	Column B
_____ **18** Double spill	a. Amalgam for a Class I
_____ **19** Explorer	b. Amalgam for a Class II
_____ **20** Hollenback carver	c. Check for caries
_____ **21** #7C carver	d. Initial carving
	e. Smooth surface

Place an A for *True* or a B for *False* as it refers to each of the following statements:

_____ **22** Only light-cured composite restorative material may be placed in layers.

_____ **23** Composite restorative material may be placed in the anterior and posterior preparations.

_____ **24** When a celluloid crown form is being used during a composite procedure, a hole should be made in the incisal edge of the form.

_____ **25** Composite restorative materials may be placed with an FP1 instrument.

Rationales

Common Restorative Procedures

1 D A Class I amalgam restoration is placed in pit and fissure cavity preparations. It does not involve a proximal wall. Therefore, the matrix band retainer would not be used.

2 A A wooden wedge is placed at the interproximal gingival area to adapt the matrix band to the contour of the tooth. When the band is tightly adapted to the tooth, the potential for cervical overhangs is eliminated.

3 B It is common to place the first increment of amalgam in the least accessible area. Therefore, in a mesioocclusal cavity preparation, the most difficult access is in the proximal box. Therefore, this area is filled first, before the pulpal floor.

4 C The common steps of an amalgam restoration include the following:

Updating the medical history

Preparing the armamentarium

Examining the site

Determining occlusal relationship

Administering anesthetic

Isolation of the site

Opening the cavity preparation

Outlining the cavity preparation

Removing caries

Placing retention form

Isolating with cotton rolls (alternative isolation)

Placing cavity medication

Placing the matrix retainer, band and wedge (if needed)

Inserting and condensing the amalgam

Initial carving of the amalgam

Removing the matrix assembly (if used)

Interproximal carving

Completing final carving

Removing isolation

Checking the articulation

Burnishing the margins

Giving postoperative instructions

Finishing and polishing (optional)

5 E Amalgam is not considered an esthetic restoration. Classes III and IV are cavity preparations on anterior teeth. The remainder of the classifications are on posterior teeth.

6 A 1 and 7 are cavity medications that are contraindicated with a composite restoration. Their use can affect the properties of the material. The cleoid-discoid carver is an anatomic carver used only with amalgam restorations. All of the other instruments can be used in the placement and finishing of the composite restoration.

7 C Chisels are widely used in the preparation of a tooth for a composite restoration. The hoe, though, is actually a chisel that has a blade at a right angle to the shank of the instrument but is used in the same manner as other chisels. A cleoid-discoid carver is used in an amalgam restoration, and the gingival marginal trimmer places bevels at the cervical margins of an amalgam cavity preparation.

8 A Calcium hydroxide has no adverse effects on the setting of a composite restoration. Refer to item 6 for the adverse effect of zinc oxide-eugenol and cavity varnish. Zinc phosphate is not a cavity liner.

9 D Once the light-cured composite has been polymerized, hand and rotary instruments can be used to finish the restoration without fear of damage.

10 C The effect of the acid etching of the enamel is to leave a cleansed surface of enamel microporosities that provide a source of mechanical retention for the restorative material. Prior to placement of the restorative material the acid etchant is applied with small sponges or cotton pellets and then rinsed thoroughly for a recommended time to stop the etching process.

11 C A small Class V composite matrix is available to adapt the material to this cavity preparation. Metal bands used with amalgam are contraindicated, and the standard celluloid strip will not provide the contour needed in this area.

12 C This is a gingival marginal trimmer; it is used during cavity preparation to place bevels at the cervical margin and at the pulpoaxial line angle.

13 B This is a Ward's carver designed primarily to carve excess amalgam from the buccal, lingual, and proximal surfaces.

14 D The beaver-tail burnisher has a Y-shaped configuration that can be used to burnish occlusal surfaces.

15 D The larger of the anatomic carvers is the #7 cleoid-discoid carver.

16 B This circumferential matrix band can be used to completely circumscribe the tooth. It can be used in cavity preparations with either one or two proximal surfaces involved.

17 A A small round bur is used to place a retentive groove around the floor of the cavity preparation.

18 B A Class II or VI restoration will warrant mixing a double-spill amalgam capsule. This allows for the extra material that probably will be needed in the proximal box.

19 C This sharp, pointed instrument can be used to detect anomalies in the tooth.

20 E A Hollenback carver is a sharp, flat-bladed instrument that allows for contouring smooth surfaces of the tooth during an amalgam procedure.

21 D This larger cleoid-discoid carver can be used in the initial carving phase, when excess amalgam is removed from the occlusal surface.

22 A When a preparation warrants a large amount of composite material, it can be placed in layers with light-cured material. Such a bond is effective with this material but not possible with chemically cured composite.

23 A The physical and esthetic properties of this material make it an acceptable restoration in anterior and posterior areas of the mouth.

24 A Class IV cavity preparations warrant the re-creation of the incisal angle. A matrix that would aid in this placement would be a celluloid crown that is anatomically correct for the tooth being treated. To allow trapped air to escape, a small hole can be placed near the incisal edge of the form.

25 B A metal instrument such as an FP1 is contraindicated with the use of composite material. Most manufacturers recommend a plastic or Teflon instrument to prevent discoloration of the material.

To enhance your understanding of the material presented in this chapter refer to the illustrations in Chapter 27 of Finkbeiner/Johnson: Mosby's Comprehensive Dental Assisting: A Clinical Approach.

CHAPTER 20

Prosthodontics

OUTLINE

Objectives of Prosthodontics
Definition of Prosthodontics
Types of Prosthodontics
Factors to Consider When Selecting
  a Prosthesis
Preliminary Treatment
Model Surveying
Case Presentation
Mouth Preparation
Fixed Prosthodontics

Principles of Tooth Preparation
Procedure for Fixed Prosthesis
Removable Prosthodontics
Types of Removable Prosthodontic
  Restorations
Components of a Partial Denture
Two Basic Components of a Den-
  ture
Typical Appointment Schedules for
  Removable Prostheses

Preliminary/Final Impressions
Interim Laboratory Procedures
Jaw Relationships
Denture Try-In
Final Laboratory Procedures
Prosthesis Insertion
Home Care Instructions
Initial Adjustment
Relining and Rebasing

KEY TERMS

Abutment
Adjustment
Alveolar ridge
Bar
Base
Baseplate
Bilateral
Biologic principle
Bite registration
Border molding
Bridge
Burnishing
Cantilever
Cast
Cementation
Centric relationship
Clasp
Complete denture
Connector

Conventional denture
Coping
Cosmetic imaging
Crucible former
Denture
Denture base
Diatoric hole
Draw
Duplicate denture
Edentulous
Endosteal
Esthetic principle
Face-bow
Facing
Film thickness
Fixed partial denture
Fixed prosthodontics
Flask

Framework
Freeway space
Full-coverage crown
Immediate denture
Implant
Inlay
Investing
Ischemia
Laboratory prescription/requisition
Laminate
Luxate
Maryland bridge
Margin design
Mechanical principle
Mortise
Mould
Muscle trimming
Obturator
Occlusal clearance

Occlusal rim	Rebasing	Sprue
Onlay	Relining	Stippling
Opposing model	Removable prosthodontics	Subperiosteal
Osseointegration	Resistance form	Surfactant
Overdenture	Rest	Surveying
Partial denture	Retainer	Tenon
Pontic	Retention form	Three-quarter crown
Porcelain crown	Retentive area	Tissue conditioning
Post and core	Ridge	Tissue retraction
Precision attachment	Saddle	Undercut
Prosthesis	Shade	Unilateral
Prosthodontics	Shimstock	Vertical dimension

As noted in the previous chapters on restorative dentistry, a dental material such as amalgam or composite is used to restore a diseased or injured tooth to its normal function. This is accomplished by placing the material directly into a cavity preparation that is designed to retain the material as an intracoronal restoration. When the intracoronal restoration is inserted, the dental material is in a malleable or moldable state, which allows the material to be placed into the tooth. As the restorative material hardens, it is carved or trimmed to normal anatomic structure.

This chapter describes the dental **prosthesis**—the device used to replace missing teeth and tissues. Prostheses are constructed outside the oral cavity after a series of appointments. They require various methods of insertion, depending on the type of prosthesis used. The materials used in dental prosthetics include various precious and nonprecious metals, plastic, and porcelain.

This chapter presents an overview of **prosthodontics,** both **fixed** (cannot be removed from the oral cavity) and **removable** (can be removed from the mouth by the patient). Through a series of descriptions and illustrations, the dental assistant should understand the reasons a dentist prescribes a specific type of prosthesis for a patient with certain oral conditions.

OBJECTIVES OF PROSTHODONTICS

I.   Definition of Prosthodontics: the Art and Science of Designing and Fitting Artificial Substitutes to Replace Lost or Missing Tissues

     A. When properly designed, a fixed or removable prosthesis can meet the objectives of prosthodontic service listed (box).

B. When a patient loses a significant number of teeth, it can be difficult to carry on normal oral functions of teeth, which include the following:

    1. Aid the tongue and lips to form sound in speech

    2. Give support to the facial musculature, which aids the lips and cheeks in performing the function of manipulating food and expressing emotion

    3. Divide food finely into a larger surface area for the natural action of digestive juices

C. The loss of a single tooth can initiate the collapse of a dental arch.

D. When a patient loses all the teeth, becoming **edentulous,** the following problems arise:

OBJECTIVES OF PROSTHODONTIC SERVICE

Replace lost tissues with like tissues

Replace missing teeth and tissues with biologically acceptable restorations

Improve phonetics and aesthetics

Provide restorations that are comfortable to the patient

Improve masticatory function

Preserve teeth and tissues that will enhance either a fixed or removable prosthesis design

Prevent future dental disease or loss of oral structures

Promote good oral health

Improve the general health and well-being of the patient

1. Limitations in the daily diet—hard and fibrous foods must be finely chopped or potential digestive problems can occur.
2. Difficulty with speech—the tongue cannot come to proper rests on the teeth to form certain consonant sounds.
3. The appearance of premature aging—musculature support is lost, causing the cheeks and lips to sag, the soft tissues to bunch up around the mouth, and the chin and nose to become abnormally close.

E. A fixed or removable partial or full **denture** prosthesis for a patient can literally add years of life by performing the following functions:
1. Improving dietary consumption
2. Providing mastication
3. Assisting in normal speech
4. Preserving the health of the soft oral tissues
5. Eliminating the potential for future dental disease
6. Improving esthetics, which not only creates an improved appearance but can result in improved self-image

---

ADVANTAGES AND DISADVANTAGES OF A FIXED PROSTHESIS

ADVANTAGES

- Greater retention can be achieved with full versus conservative coverage.
- Most fixed prostheses provide increased strength for the tooth.
- Access to the furcation can be achieved in certain restoration designs, particularly with single-unit coverage compared with multiple-unit coverage.
- Close match of color can be obtained for natural esthetic appearance by using ceramic or ceramic that is fused to metal materials.
- Shade, contour, and staining can be customized.

DISADVANTAGES

- Extensive removal of tooth structure may be necessary, depending on the type of restoration that is placed.
- Gingival irritation can be created at the cervical margin by the introduction of an unnatural material.
- With certain restorations the ability to perform electric vitality tests is eliminated.
- Galvanism can be created under some conditions.
- If ceramic material is used in certain areas of the mouth, the prosthesis may be susceptible to fracture from force.

F. A fixed prosthesis might be preferred over a removable prosthesis but may not be feasible because of the anatomic structure of a patient's mouth or ability to maintain good oral hygiene, or because the cost may be prohibitive.

II. Types of Prosthodontics
A. **Fixed prosthodontics** involves creating an artificial replacement for missing teeth and associated structures that is secured to the supporting teeth in the mouth.
1. This type of restoration cannot be removed to clean or inspect.
2. Fixed prostheses include a variety of extracoronal restorations, such as **bridges, implants,** and **fixed partial dentures.**
3. Extracoronal restorations, referred to as *fixed restorations,* are designed to replace missing tooth structures and may provide partial or complete coverage of a tooth. They include **inlays, onlays, three-quarter** and **full-coverage crowns, bridges, laminates, implants,** and **post and cores.**
4. An extracoronal restoration may be fabricated from several materials, including precious and nonprecious metals, plastic, and porcelain.
5. Advantages and disadvantages of fixed prostheses are listed (box in left column).

B. Removable prosthodontics involves creating an artificial substitute for missing teeth and supporting tissues that can be removed by the patient for cleaning and inspection.
1. Removable prosthodontics can be classified as complete, partial, overdenture, fixed removable, or interim denture.
2. The advantages and disadvantages of removable prostheses are listed (box on page 327).

C. Maxillofacial prosthodontics involves replacing missing parts of the stomatognathic system.
1. This includes structures responsible for speech, mastication, and deglutition of food.
2. It is not uncommon in this phase of prosthodontics to see patients who have cleft palate, who have lost portions of head and neck tissue because of cancer or other disease, or who are trauma victims.
3. Specialized prostheses, including **obturators** and other devices, are designed to replace missing tissues in the maxillofacial region.

III. Factors to Consider When Selecting a Prosthesis
A. Esthetics
B. Oral hygiene practices

ADVANTAGES AND DISADVANTAGES OF A REMOVABLE PROSTHESIS
ADVANTAGES
• Improves mastication. • Eliminates aging appearance. • Prevents drifting. • Improves speech. • Improves self-image.
DISADVANTAGES
• Clasp-type attachments of partial dentures can cause trauma to abutment teeth. • It can create gingivostomatitis. • The use of clasps can create poor aesthetics. • If not cleaned regularly, the prosthesis can create tissue trauma or decay to the abutment teeth. • If not worn routinely, drifting and hypereruption can occur. • It could be lost or damaged if left out of the mouth.

    C. Level of function needed to correct the condition that requires the prosthesis

    D. Patient's attitude toward oral health

    E. Patient's financial ability to make the investment

    F. Skill of the dentist

    G. Technical laboratory support services

IV. Preliminary Treatment

    A. Several preliminary steps must be completed before a thorough diagnosis can be made or any form of prosthodontic treatment can begin, including the following:

      1. Complete medical and dental history

      2. Intraoral and extraoral examination

      3. Radiographic examination

      4. Diagnostic models

      5. Case presentation

      6. Oral cavity preparation, including periodontal, endodontic, orthodontic, occlusal equilibration, or surgical treatment

    B. Combined with clinical information, the dentist must determine answers to many of the following questions from diagnostic models:

      1. Are the proposed **abutment** teeth favorable for clasping or for use as abutment teeth?

      2. Are there any interferences, such as undercuts, tori, or malposed teeth?

      3. Will restorative treatment be necessary to achieve the required retention or articulation?

      4. What are the best types of connectors or retainers to use?

      5. Is clearance adequate for the proposed prosthesis? Will the vertical dimensions have to be opened or the teeth reduced?

      6. Will the ridge, as it exists, provide stability for the prosthesis?

      7. Is the occlusion adequate, or will it have to be adjusted?

V. Model Surveying

    A. **Surveying** is the process of studying the parallelism or lack of parallelism of the teeth and associated structures to select a path for placement of the components of the prosthesis.

    B. Models should be poured in stone rather than plaster to provide a more rigid surface for surveying.

    C. This process ensures that the **clasps, rests, retainers,** and **connectors** are placed in positions that will provide adequate and balanced retention without causing stress or interference to the teeth and soft tissues and yet will provide a prosthesis that is esthetically acceptable.

VI. Case Presentation

    A. The patient must understand what the treatment involves and what his or her responsibility is to maintain the prosthesis and oral tissues.

    B. The patient must have a positive attitude about the prosthesis that is to be constructed and a willingness to maintain this device.

    C. A dissatisfied patient is often one who did not thoroughly understand the process or did not accept the treatment plan in the beginning.

    D. The patient must be involved in the treatment selection and have a thorough understanding of the processes, advantages, and disadvantages of proposed treatment; the consequences of neglect; and the alternative options that are available.

    E. Effective treatment planning and case presentation requires the use of visual aids, including the following:

      1. The patient's diagnostic models

      2. Comparative models

      3. Radiographs

      4. **Dental** or **cosmetic imaging** (an esthetic reproduction system)

      5. Examples of various types of dental prostheses

      6. Photos of completed cases

      7. Pamphlets or video materials

VII. Mouth Preparation

    A. Two goals of mouth preparation in planning

for prosthodontic treatment are the following:

1. To obtain optimal health of the foundation tissues
2. To provide adequate mouth preparation for the insertion of a fixed prosthesis or a full or partial denture

B. Depending on the type of prosthesis, any of the following treatments may be necessary in mouth preparation.

1. Preparatory surgery
   a. Provide the patient with relief from pain.
   b. Remove teeth that cannot be retained because they are nonusable and nonvital, severely malpositioned, unerupted, or nonrestorable because of extreme caries or periodontal disease.
   b. Remove root remnants, cysts, or tumors.
   c. Perform electrosurgery around abutment teeth to remove excess soft tissue that may impinge on cervical marginal areas.
   d. Recontour hard tissues, including knife-edged ridges, tori, bone nodules, undercuts, and prominent tuberosities; soft tissues, such as prominent frena or hyperplasia from previous dentures; or flabby, fibrous ridges.
2. Oral prophylaxis and periodontal treatment
   a. For the patient who is retaining teeth in the oral cavity and will receive a fixed bridge or partial denture, a thorough oral prophylaxis must be performed.
   b. The prophylaxis and any necessary periodontal treatment should be completed as soon as possible.
3. Endodontic treatment
   a. This procedure should be completed before prosthetic treatment.
4. Restorative procedures
   a. Restorative treatment of all nonabutment teeth should be done before beginning the prosthodontic procedures.
   b. When a partial denture is placed in conjunction with fixed bridgework, the fixed prosthesis is completed before the removable prosthesis.
5. Orthodontic treatment
   a. Unless orthodontic factors such as malocclusion, oral habits, or jaw formation are considered, the prosthetic restoration may result in additional problems.
6. Occlusal equilibration

a. The elimination of occlusal interference through occlusal equilibration techniques or the use of an intraoral occlusal appliance may be suggested before additional care is offered.

7. Tissue conditioning
   a. **Tissue conditioning** is the process of removing irritants and treating the soft tissues so that they can return to a healthy state.
   b. The three approaches to tissue conditioning are as follows:
      (1) Complete tissue rest
      (2) Surgical intervention
      (3) Use of a tissue treatment agent

FIXED PROSTHODONTICS

Fixed prosthodontics involves the preparation or shaping of a tooth or teeth for a prosthesis that will be cemented into the mouth as a permanent restoration. This type of restoration may be an *intracoronal* or *extracoronal* restoration and usually requires a minimum of two appointments: one for tooth preparation and another for **cementation** or final insertion of the restoration. In some instances interim appointments are necessary to try in the restorations or components of the prosthesis.

I. Principles of Tooth Preparation
   A. Preparing a tooth to receive a fixed restoration involves the following steps:
      1. Reduce the tooth shape to remove a portion of the occlusal surface from contact with the opposing tooth.
      2. Decrease the circumference of the tooth.
      3. Create a margin that allows for smooth transition from the tooth to the restoration.
      4. Remove any carious lesion and rebuild with core material if necessary.
   B. Several design factors or principles must be considered when a fixed prosthesis is constructed, including the following:
      1. **Biologic principle** of tooth preparation refers to creating a balance between tooth conservation and retention of the restoration.
      2. **Mechanical principle** refers to the components in the preparation design that aid in retention of the restoration.
      3. **Esthetic principle** refers to the theory of beauty and fine arts and requires concern for the creation of a pleasant smile and appearance while maintaining a functional dentition.
   C. Each design principle interrelates with the other two and may affect the integrity of the

restoration, which can result in success or failure.

D. Design factors are applied to the fixed restorative procedure as follows:
1. **Retention** and **resistance form**—in fixed prosthodontics it differs from an amalgam and composite preparation because it includes the use of grooves and pinholes instead of undercuts to ensure retention.
2. **Draw**—a taper or divergence of the intracoronal or extracoronal walls of a preparation must be present to allow for the insertion of the cemented restoration.
3. Pins—when used as part of a **cast** restoration, pins must be parallel to each other for placement and removal of the casting.
4. Occlusal forces—concern for natural occlusal forces must be noted; otherwise the new restoration may interfere with the patient's normal chewing patterns and could result in damage to the teeth and associated structures.
5. **Occlusal clearance**—the amount of space between the prepared and opposing tooth/teeth must be adequate.
6. **Margin design**—ideally, the margin of a preparation is placed supragingivally because periodontal disease has been related to subgingival margin placement; this provides easier access for the operator during the preparation and seating appointment and makes it easier for the patient to maintain good oral hygiene.
7. Dental material—the appropriate dental material must be chosen to withstand the patient's occlusal forces.
8. Internal surface roughness—surface roughness on the inside of the cast restoration is necessary to achieve an interface with the luting cement.
9. Dental cement—the type of cement used and its luting consistency is important to retention; a thin layer of cement, referred to as **film thickness,** is placed on the inner surface of the restoration.

II. Procedure for Fixed Prosthesis
A. The procedure for creating a fixed prosthesis includes three major phases:
1. *Preparation* includes reducing the tooth structure, creating retention, taking the **bite registration,** taking the impression and opposing impression, and temporization.
2. *Laboratory processing* includes creating casts and dies; fabricating the wax pattern;

investing the pattern; and creating, finishing, and polishing the casting.
3. *Cementation* includes removal of the temporary restoration, trying in the cast restoration, checking margins and occlusion, and cementing the cast.

B. A fixed prosthodontic procedure is performed in multiple appointments.
1. Preparation is done at the first appointment, and the patient is dismissed with some form of temporary restoration on the prepared tooth.
2. During the interim, the restoration is created at the laboratory.
3. Sometimes additional appointments are necessary for trying in the castings before soldering the units together to determine appropriate fit or before porcelain is fired to the casting to create a **porcelain crown.**
4. The final appointment is for cementation or seating, when the temporary restoration is removed and the fixed prosthesis is tried in and cemented in place.

C. The procedures for completing each phase of fixed prosthodontics for a full-cast restoration are listed (box on page 330).

D. The responsibilities of the dental assistant in this procedure include the following:
1. Preparing the armamentarium for each phase of the preparation and cementation
2. Performing basic laboratory procedures
3. Communicating with laboratory staff
4. Scheduling appointments
5. Providing patient education
6. (In some states) taking opposing impressions; placing tissue pack for gingival **tissue retraction;** fabricating, placing, and removing temporary restorations

E. Procedural modifications for various fixed prostheses are shown in Table 20-1.

F. The armamentarium is prepared.
1. The armamentarium for the preparation appointment is provided (box on page 330).
2. The armamentarium for the laboratory procedures is provided (box on page 331).
3. The armamentarium for the cementation procedure is provided (box on page 331).

G. The procedure for a preparation for a full-cast crown is described (box on pages 332-334).

H. The procedure for seating the cast restoration is provided (box on pages 334-335).

I. A **laboratory prescription/requisition** is required as follows:
1. A laboratory prescription (specific direc-

PROCEDURES FOR FIXED PROSTHODONTICS

PREPARATION

1. Prepare armamentarium.
2. Update patient's medical history.
3. Examine treatment site.
4. Determine occlusal relationship.
5. Administer anesthetic.
6. Prepare tooth.
   a. Remove caries and place core material to build up tooth as necessary.
   b. Reduce occlusal surface.
   c. Place occlusal grooves.
   d. Check occlusal clearance.
   e. Reduce axial walls.
   f. Place axial grooves.
   g. Remove caries as necessary.
   h. Refine and finish margins.
7. Dry and isolate site.
8. Place cavity medication if needed.
9. Retract gingiva.
10. Obtain final and opposing impressions.
11. Obtain bite registration.
12. Fabricate and place temporary restoration.
13. Provide postoperative instructions.
14. Prepare case (according to OSHA guidelines) and prescription for laboratory.

LABORATORY

1. Disinfect impression according to OSHA guidelines.
2. Produce die and cast from impression.
3. Articulate casts.
4. Fabricate wax pattern on die.
5. Invest wax pattern.
6. Eliminate wax.
7. Cast alloy.
8. Recover cast.
9. Remove **sprue.**
10. Remove imperfections.
11. Finish cast restoration.

CEMENTATION

1. Disinfect cast and restoration.
2. Administer anesthetic if necessary.
3. Remove temporary restoration and excess cement.
4. Try in cast restoration.
   a. Assess stability.
   b. Check contacts.
   c. Check occlusion.
   d. Determine margin integrity.
   e. Make necessary adjustments.
5. Finish margins.
6. Complete final laboratory finish and polish.
7. Disinfect cast restoration.
8. Isolate tooth.
9. Prepare final cement.
10. Place thin film of cement on inner surface of casting.
11. Cement cast restoration on tooth.
12. Remove excess cement.
13. Reevaluate occlusal contact and margins.
14. Make final adjustments as needed.
15. Provide postoperative instructions.

ARMAMENTARIUM FOR PREPARATION APPOINTMENT

Explorer
Mirror
Cotton pliers
Cotton rolls
2 × 2 gauze
Anesthetic setup
Spoon excavator
Gingival retraction packing instrument (Geyer 7, FPI)
Retraction cord
Astringent agent
Scissors
Rotary instruments for high- and low-speed use
   Diamond burs or stones
   Fissure burs (tapered and straight)
   Diamond disks
   Mandrels and assorted finishing disks

28-gauge casting wax
Maxillary and mandibular impression trays (quadrant or full arch as needed)
Impression material for **opposing model** and final impression
Mixing pads/bowls, spatulas, and syringes for impressesions
Bite registration material and armamentarium
Means of temporization (acrylic, preformed aluminum crown, coping)
Temporary cement
Floss
Articulating paper
Articulating paper forceps
Thumb forceps
Cement placement instrument

Table 20-1 Procedural modifications for various fixed prostheses compared with full-cast crown

Type of restoration	Preparation	Laboratory	Cementation
Inlay/onlay	More conservative	Same as cast crown; no lab work needed if CAD/CAM design	Same
Three-quarter crown	Less tooth preparation	Same	Same
Porcelain jacket	Modified margin design; shade selection	Not a cast procedure; porcelain is baked	Same; dependent on type of cement
Porcelain veneer	Modified margin design; shade selection	May need an opaque liner	Same
Fixed bridge	Multiple tooth preparation; possible shade selection	Possible try-in appointment; opaque liner when needed	Same
Cantilever bridge	Conservative preparation	Same	Same
Resin-retained bridge	Minimal tooth reduction	Wax and cast framework and create and bake porcelain pontic	Rubber dam preferred; use of resin cement
Post and core	Canal preparation at first appointment, impression of cemented post and core at second appointment	Create two working casts and dies; possible opaque liner	Cement post with core; cement crown over post and core

ARMAMENTARIUM FOR LABORATORY PROCEDURE

The following list includes instruments and materials used to fabricate a full-cast crown. The armamentarium is divided into four phases.

Phase 1—creating casts and dies
Impression of prepared areas of the mouth
Opposing impression or model
Die material
High-strength stone
Mixing bowls and spatulas
Dowel pin
Separating agent
Die space
Articulator
Sticking wax and sticks
Bite registration
Phase 2—fabricating the wax pattern
Casting wax for patterns
Waxing instruments, including #7 spatula
Bunsen burner

Phase 3—investing the wax pattern
Crucible former
Sprue material
Ring liner
Casting ring
Surfactant
Sable brush
Investment material and armamentarium
Phase 4—making the casting
Furnace
Centrifuge and crucible
Air/gas torch
Flux
Alloy
Tongs
Pickling solution
Finishing and polishing devices

ARMAMENTARIUM FOR CEMENTATION PROCEDURE

Cast restoration and working cast
Explorer
Mirror
Cotton pliers
Cotton rolls and gauze
Rubber dam setup (optional procedure)
Spoon excavator
Instruments required for removing the temporary restoration and the final restoration before cementation (modified sickle scaler, curet scaler, large spoon excavator, crown remover)

Finishing and polishing devices (such as rubber wheels, finishing burs and stones, mandrels, and disks)
Articulating paper and holder
Shimstock
Floss
Burnishers (ball/2 to 3S)
Tripoli and rag wheel
Cement and necessary armamentarium
Cooley peg
Orangewood stick
Lubricant

PROCEDURE FOR A FULL-CAST CROWN

- Are all universal barrier techniques being used?
- Is all of the armamentarium available and prepared for use?
- Are the instruments arranged in sequence to use?
- Are you prepared for alternative treatment plans?
- Is the necessary equipment turned on and ready to operate?

PREPARATION PROCEDURES

The following discussion presents a step-by-step procedure for the preparation appointment.

EXAMINATION OF THE TREATMENT SITE

Before treatment begins, the updated medical and dental history is reviewed to alert the dental team to any health contraindications. The operator examines the tooth and determines the expected level of margin placement, furcation involvement, relation of opposing and hypererupted teeth, and any other factors to be considered in the preparation design.

DETERMINATION OF OCCLUSAL RELATIONSHIP

The occlusal relationship of the arches before the preparation is an important factor for the operator to consider. To determine the occlusal relationship, articulating paper is placed in the mouth to mark the occlusal contacts.

ADMINISTRATION OF ANESTHETIC

Anesthetic is administered to achieve patient comfort for the dental procedure.

PLACEMENT OF OCCLUSAL GROOVES AND SURFACE REDUCTION

The reduction of the tooth is performed with various rotary instruments. Most commonly, a wheel-shaped diamond is used to reduce the occlusal cusps, and tapered diamonds and carbide burs are used to form walls of the preparation. The functional cusp depth must be reduced to 1.5 mm; nonfunctional cusp depth to 1 mm.

The occlusal reduction can be completed in two steps. The tooth structure is removed on either the mesial or the distal half of the tooth; the other half remains intact, providing the operator with a reference point because one half of the tooth is maintained intact with original tooth structure and the other half is reduced for occlusal clearance. The other half of the occlusal reduction is completed in the same manner as the first half. During the procedure the dental assistant performs constant oral evacuation and retraction of the soft tissues. Once the handpiece is removed, the site is rinsed and dried so that the operator can examine the progress of the preparation. This step is repeated throughout the procedure.

CHECK OCCLUSAL CLEARANCE

Occlusal clearance may be determined using a piece of 28-gauge casting wax that is folded into three thicknesses (slightly larger than the occlusal surface of the tooth). The wax is placed on the reduced occlusal surface, and the patient is directed to close the arches firmly. The wax is removed from the mouth and evaluated for thin areas in which the teeth are occluded.

PLACEMENT OF AXIAL GROOVES AND REDUCTION

The axial reduction is done with the removal of tooth surface and placement of at least a minimum 5 degrees of taper on the axial walls from the occlusal to the cervical.

REFINE MARGIN AND FINISH

Placement of the cervical margin is often completed as the operator performs the axial reduction. Regardless of the design of the cervical margin, the width of the margin should be uniform throughout the tooth and should be a smooth, continuous line completely around the tooth. If additional retentive features are desired, they can be placed at this time.

DETERMINE DRAW AND ACCURACY

At this point, the preparation can be evaluated for accuracy through the use of a snap impression technique. After it has hardened, the impression compound is removed from the preparation and inspected for taper or draw, margin definition, and fracturing.

PROCEDURE FOR A FULL-CAST CROWN—cont'd

BITE REGISTRATION

Re-creating the correct occlusion of the patient on the models being obtained requires a bite registration. The bite registration material is placed in the mouth, and the patient is directed to close the arches and hold them together. After the material hardens to a rubberized state, it can be removed and disinfected as directed.

TISSUE MANAGEMENT AND RETRACTION

A cast (the replica of the prepared structures) is fabricated from the impression, and the fixed prosthesis is made from the case and die. Thus, an impression or a negative production of the area must be obtained. The die is a replica of a single tooth or several teeth. A wax pattern of the actual shape of the future restoration is fabricated indirectly on a die outside the patient's mouth. A wax pattern is constructed on the replica of the teeth that becomes the pattern for the cast restoration. To arrive at an acceptable finished restoration, an accurate impression must replicate the prepared tooth or teeth; adjacent tissues surrounding the preparation must be free of voids. Before an accurate impression can be obtained, three factors must be considered: tissue health, isolation of the site, and gingival retraction.

TISSUE HEALTH

Before the impression is taken, the health of the soft tissue surrounding the prepared tooth is accessed. Implementing measures to remove the excess tissue or reduce the inflammation before taking the impression can minimize time and motion later. The dentist may opt to perform an electrosurgery procedure.

MOISTURE CONTROL

To maintain the patient's comfort and ensure an accurate impression, a dry field must be maintained in the preparation during the impression procedure. The most common method for doing this involves the use of cotton rolls. A svedopter with a tongue flange can be used in the mandibular arch to retract the tongue and to aid in removing saliva.

TISSUE RETRACTION

To obtain an accurate impression of the prepared area, the soft tissue surrounding the gingival margins must be displaced. Not only is access to the margins increased, but the space for placement of the impression material is also increased to ensure adequate thickness of the impression material.

Tissue retraction or displacement of the gingival tissue is accomplished with the placement of retraction cord in the sulcus.

Placement of retraction cord involves cutting a piece of cord long enough to encircle the prepared tooth. The operator gently forces the cord into the sulcus area with an instrument such as a Geyer 7 or a FP1 plastic instrument.

FINAL IMPRESSION OPPOSING IMPRESSION

The final impression is necessary to obtain an accurate recording of the tissues. The impression is usually obtained using the syringe-tray technique or the putty/wash system.

Using a custom acrylic tray ensures that the tray will fit the configuration of the patient's mouth, reducing the amount of impression material needed.

As the operator injects the syringe material, the assistant mixes and places the tray material in the impression tray. The operator places the tray in position over the prepared area.

Once the impression reaches the final set, it is removed from the mouth, rinsed thoroughly under water, dried, and evaluated for accuracy. If voids or tears are present or definition of the margins is inadequate, it may be necessary to repeat the previous steps and to retake the impression.

An impression of the opposing arch may need to be taken at this time if this was not done at a previous appointment, or if treatment was provided after the diagnostic models were constructed. When all of the impressions have been taken and are acceptable, they are disinfected according to OSHA guidelines.

TEMPORIZATION

Temporary coverage of the prepared tooth or teeth is made to (1) protect the pulp, (2) maintain periodontal health, (3) prevent the drifting of teeth, (4) prevent fracture of the preparation, and (5) maintain the occlusal relationship. The temporary restoration also restores masticatory and phonetic function of the tooth and provides an esthetic appearance. The choice of a temporary restoration is determined by the operator's preference, the period of time the temporary restoration must remain in the mouth, and the location of the preparation.

Continued

PROCEDURE FOR A FULL-CAST CROWN—cont'd

POSTOPERATIVE INSTRUCTIONS

At the end of the treatment, the anesthetic may still be effective, creating a false sense of comfort. It is important for the patient to understand the conditions in the mouth before leaving the treatment room.

The temporary restoration may also be more sensitive than tooth tissue to temperature changes. The patient must be informed of the importance of maintaining the temporary restoration in the mouth. The patient should also be told to avoid eating or chewing sticky or extremely hard foods in the area of the temporary restoration because each may contribute to displacement of the restoration.

- Have the appropriate universal barrier techniques been removed?
- Have all appropriate surfaces been cleaned and disinfected?
- Has all of the armamentarium been removed?
- Has all equipment been repositioned?
- Has all equipment been disinfected/sterilized according to OSHA guidelines?

PROCEDURE FOR SEATING THE CAST RESTORATION

REMOVING THE TEMPORARY RESTORATION

The temporary restoration and any remaining cement are removed from the prepared tooth. Excess cement left in place interferes with the try-in of the cast restoration. The tooth may be lightly polished with a polishing paste and cup to remove any residual cement. If the preparation is an intracoronal restoration, the procedure is not significantly different. A scaler may be used to loosen the cement, followed by removal of any remaining cement.

TRYING IN THE CAST RESTORATION

The initial try-in involves checking the contact relationship, checking the occlusion, and determining the margin integrity.

CHECKING THE CONTACT

If the crown does not go into place, the first area of adjustment is usually the proximal contact. The contact may be heavy, which results in the incomplete seating of the casting, inability to pass floss through the contact, and pressure at the contact points. If the contact is light, the restoration will fall into place without any resistance. An ideal contact allows for a snapping action of the floss as it is passed through the contact.

If the contact is too light, solder must be added to establish a contact. An improper contact can result in damage to the tissues later. If a contact is left open or is light, food can be trapped, causing trauma to the interdental papilla. If it is too tight, the patient will be unable to pass floss through the contact area to maintain healthy oral tissues.

CHECKING MARGIN INTEGRITY

Once the proximal contact is established and the restoration is seated on the tooth, the margin integrity is assessed. If the casting has inadequate margins, a new impression must be obtained and the laboratory procedure repeated to create a new casting.

CHECKING OCCLUSION

The occlusal contact of the maxillary and mandibular teeth is evaluated to ensure that distribution of contact exists throughout the mouth; the operator can determine this by having the patient close on the restoration and by visually assessing the areas. **Shimstock** (a narrow strip of silver Mylar) is placed throughout the mouth at contact areas. If resistance is met when an attempt is made to pull the Mylar strip from the closed mouth, contact is confirmed in this area.

Articulating paper is used to mark any interference in the relationship of the arches. Occlusal contacts can be evaluated with a technique that is similar to that used for the proximal contact: a matte finish is placed on the surface with rotary instruments or a sandblast unit. The patient is directed to occlude; heavy contact areas will appear scratched, giving the operator guidance for relief of the area. Occlusal indicator pastes and other such systems can also be used.

When all the adjustments for seating have been made, the final finish and polish of the restoration is complete. The restoration is brought to a high polish to reduce the possibility of food and plaque adhering to the surface. The cast restoration is disinfected after polishing to remove any contaminants before cementation.

PROCEDURE FOR SEATING THE CAST RESTORATION—cont'd

CEMENTING THE CAST RESTORATION

The permanent cementation of the restoration involves the selection of a luting agent that has a relatively long working time, adheres well to the tooth and the restoration, establishes a good seal, has compressive strength, is nonirritating to the pulp, and has low viscosity and solubility characteristics. Currently, no cement has all of these characteristics, but many cements provide most of them, including the most commonly used luting agents (such as zinc phosphate, glass ionomer, and zinc polycarboxylate cements).

CEMENTATION

The restoration and the tooth are inspected for any debris or contaminants. The field must be isolated; the tooth is dried, and the patient is directed to keep the mouth open. A thin coat of cement is placed to cover completely all internal surfaces of the restoration. The tooth is dried again. The restoration is seated on the tooth, and the patient is directed to bite on an orangewood stick that is rocked back and forth across the occlusal surface of the restoration. The margins are checked with an explorer to ensure that the crown is seated completely.

At this time, the operator may opt to use a hand **burnisher** (such as a ball burnisher or 2 to 35 burnisher) to burnish the margin. A burnisher that is mounted on a slow-speed handpiece can also be used. The burnishing activity spins the gold to create a desirable surface to the alloy. As the cement becomes elastic, its removal can begin. Dental floss is forced through the proximal contact and pulled to the side.

An explorer, curet, spoon excavator, or other instrument of choice is used to remove cement from the exterior of the crown; all cement must be removed, especially from the gingival sulcus. The restoration is checked again for proper occlusal contact. Once the crown is cemented and cleaned of cement, the patient is given postoperative instructions.

---

tions from the dentist to the laboratory technician) must be sent to a commercial laboratory with each case.

2. The impression, casts, bite registration, and other materials (such as a shade button) are sent with the prescription.
3. The following information must be included in the prescription:
   a. Description of the type of prosthesis to be constructed
   b. Type of alloy or other dental material to be used
   c. Shade selection
   d. Diagram of the device
   e. Dentist's name, address, and phone number
   f. Patient's name and case number
   g. Appointment dates

REMOVABLE PROSTHODONTICS ■■■■

When properly designed, a removable prosthesis can meet the objectives of prosthodontic service by replacing lost tissues with prostheses that simulate missing tissues, by improving phonetics and esthetics, and by providing restorations that are comfortable for the patient. The purpose of these prostheses is to improve masticatory function, preserve teeth and tissues (which will enhance and promote oral health), and improve the health and general well-being of the patient. Although a patient may prefer to have a fixed prosthesis, it may not be feasible because of the anatomic structure of the mouth, the patient's ability to maintain good oral hygiene, or prohibitive cost. Consequently, some form of removable prosthesis offers an alternative that provides function and aesthetics.

I. Types of Removable Prosthodontic Restorations
   A. **Complete denture**—This denture replaces all of the natural teeth and associated structures of the maxillae and mandible; it can be prepared for insertion by two different methods:
      1. **Immediate**—the denture is delivered at the time the natural teeth are extracted
         a. It is common to remove some of the posterior teeth before taking impressions for this type of denture.
         b. This process generally involves removing the posterior teeth, allowing these tissues to heal, taking impressions, and designing the denture.
         c. A try-in of the denture setup is done with the anterior teeth still intact.
         d. On the day the denture is delivered, the remaining teeth are extracted and the denture is inserted immediately.
         e. The patient is encouraged to leave the denture in place for the next 24 hours to restrict edema, promote healing, and aid the patient in maintaining aesthetics during this time.

2. **Conventional**—all of the natural teeth are removed before denture construction.
   a. Tissues are allowed to heal for 6 to 8 weeks; then the patient returns for the denture construction process.
   b. This is an option for the patient who has a severely diseased mouth and is not gravely concerned about aesthetics for a few weeks or for the patient who has had a previous denture.
   c. If the patient has a denture that is not injurious to the tissues, it can be worn during the construction of the new denture.
B. **Duplicate denture**—A second denture is constructed to be a copy of the first denture. It acts as a spare or backup denture.
C. **Overdenture** (sometimes referred to as a *fixed removable partial denture*)—This complete or partial denture is supported by retained roots that provide improved support, stability, and tactile sensation and reduce **alveolar ridge** resorption.

D. An interim partial or full denture is a denture that is used for only a short period of time, sometimes called a "flipper".
E. **Partial denture**—This replaces one or more missing teeth; it can be prepared in many styles.
   1. The most typical style is the extracoronal clasp retainer style.
   2. The intracoronal semiprecision attachment or the **precision attachment** partial (which has no visible external components) provides a more esthetic approach but involves a greater initial investment for the patient.
F. Edentulous conditions in a patient's mouth can be classified according to the Kennedy classification system as illustrated in Table 20-2 and Fig. 20-1.

II. Components of a Partial Denture
A. The components of a typical clasp partial denture are described (box on page 337).
B. Components of an intracoronal partial denture include the following:

Table 20-2 Kennedy classification system for partially edentulous conditions in the oral cavity

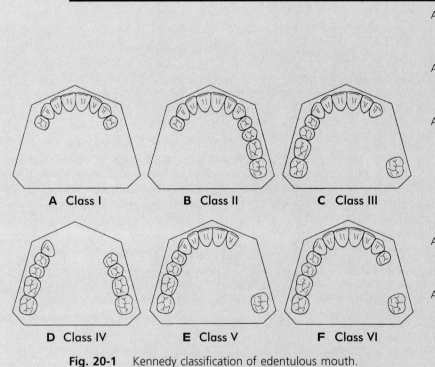

A Class I   **B** Class II   **C** Class III

D Class IV   **E** Class V   **F** Class VI

Fig. 20-1 Kennedy classification of edentulous mouth.

An edentulous situation in which all remaining teeth are anterior to the **bilateral** edentulous areas (Fig. 20-1, *A*).

An edentulous situation in which the remaining teeth of either the right or the left side are anterior to the **unilateral** edentulous area (Fig. 20-1, *B*).

An edentulous situation in which the edentulous area is bounded by teeth that are *unable* to assume total support of the prosthesis. These abutments require the aid of teeth that are remotely located, so that the principles of cross-arch splinting and counter leverage can be used to resist lateral tilting forces (Fig. 20-1, *C*).

An edentulous situation in which the remaining teeth bound the edentulous area posteriorly on both sides of the median line (Fig. 20-1, *D*).

An edentulous situation in which teeth bound the edentulous area anteriorly and posteriorly but where the anterior abutment tooth is *not* suitable for normal abutment service (Fig. 20-1, *E*).

An edentulous situation in which the boundary teeth are capable of total support of the required prothesis (Fig. 20-1, *F*).

1. Intracoronal components of a partial denture provide retention by internal frictional resistance.
2. The terms *precision, semiprecision,* and *spring lock attachment* refer to some type of prefabricated interlocking mechanism with two matched parts.
3. Typically, a crown covers the abutment tooth, into which is imbedded one part (the **mortise** [female] portion) of the attachment.
4. The removable partial denture houses the **tenon** (male) portion of the attachment instead of a clasp.

COMPONENTS OF A CLASP PARTIAL DENTURE

1. Direct retainer—a clasp or an attachment on the removable prosthesis that is applied to an abutment tooth to provide retention to the removable prosthesis. Clasps can be categorized as follows:
   a. The *circumferential clasp* encircles more than 180 degrees of the tooth; one terminal end is placed in the infrabulge area or in the **undercut** of the crown of the tooth.
   b. The bar clasp originates from the denture base or from a major connector and approaches the undercut from a cervical direction.
2. Major connector—part of the device that is generally a plate, strap, or **bar** that connects the sides or bases of a partial denture.
3. Minor connector—connecting link between the major connector or base and the other parts of the prosthesis, such as the clasps and rests.
4. Rest—a rigid extension of the partial denture that contacts a tooth to dissipate vertical and horizontal forces; incisal, occlusal, cingulum, or ball rest may be placed.
5. Indirect retainer—part of the partial denture that functions as a lever to prevent displacement of the partial denture.
6. Plastic retention area—loop or mesh-like area designed to retain the acrylic base material.
7. Base—part of the partial denture that rests on the oral mucosa to which teeth are attached; the term **saddle** is often used to describe this portion of the appliance.
8. Teeth—may be made of resin, porcelain, or even metal; may be denture teeth, tube teeth, facings, or metal teeth.

---

5. Advantages of the precision attachments include the following:
   a. Improved aesthetics
   b. Reduction of food impaction, plaque, and caries
   c. Resistance to rotational forces to displace the partial denture
   d. Improved patient comfort
   e. Improved support of the forces of mastication
6. The precision attachment requires more clinical and laboratory time, more abutment tooth considerations, and a greater investment on the part of the patient.

III. Two Basic Components of a Denture
   A. **Base**
      1. The base is the part of the denture that simulates the gingival mucosa, alveolar mucosa, and hard palate; it is available in a variety of tissue colors that reflect the patient's complexion and can be characterized to create a natural appearance.
      2. Placing special characteristics in the denture base can be as important in personalizing the denture as it is in selecting the correct type of teeth to create a natural appearance.
      3. The patient's complexion dictates the type of base material to use.
      4. Various shades of acrylic are available to match the patient's tissue tone.
      5. **Stippling**—the orange-peel, pebblelike appearance of the natural attached gingiva—can be re-created in the denture base by contouring the finished denture.
      6. Small colored fiberglass fibers are added to some acrylic bases to simulate capillaries.
      7. Acrylic resin is most often used as a denture base, but metal may be chosen as an alternative.
   B. Teeth
      1. The teeth provide the functional portion of the denture; they are available in various shades or colors, shapes or moulds, sizes, and arrangements that enable the operator to re-create the patient's natural look.
      2. The types of teeth used in removable prosthetics include the following:
         a. **Facings**—most commonly used for anterior teeth in partial dentures; attach to a metal slot on a metal-backed prosthesis; often used for a single tooth re-

placement or where minimal space is available; poor aesthetics because of their opacity when backed with metal.

    b. Tube teeth—designed by altering a resin or porcelain denture tooth to fit onto a metal partial base; a hole is ground in the denture tooth that fits over a projection in the cast partial **framework;** can be attached to the partial denture with autopolymerizing resin or traditional crown and bridge cement.

    c. Denture teeth—carded in full sets of maxillary or mandibular anteriors (1 × 6s) and maxillary and mandibular posteriors (1 × 8s); arch can be distinguished on the card because the teeth are set in the same position as in the mouth.

3. Four different sets of teeth must be ordered for a complete set of dentures: one maxillary 1 × 6, one mandibular 1 × 6, one maxillary 1 × 8, and one mandibular 1 × 8.

4. Teeth are made of porcelain, plastic, or metal.

5. The differences between plastic and porcelain teeth are listed (box).

6. Metal occlusals
    a. Metal occlusals are waxed and cast in the same manner as any other metal casting, but all occlusal surfaces are attached together as one unit.
    b. Metal occlusals provide strength and can be designed to occlude with the patient's existing teeth.
    c. Metal occlusals are often indicated when the occlusion in the removable prosthesis opposes cast gold restorations.

7. Shade selection
    a. A variety of selection systems can be used to determine tooth **shade** (color).
    b. A shade guide is provided to aid in determining the color of the teeth.
    c. The shade guide provides a complete range of natural tooth colors to aid in selecting the tooth shade that will harmonize with the patient's hair, eyes, and complexion.
    d. The shade is selected under the same conditions as shades for any other aesthetic restorations.

PLASTIC VERSUS PORCELAIN TEETH

PLASTIC

Easily adjusted

Will not wear opposing natural tooth structure or gold

More commonly used in a removable prosthesis

Can withstand considerable grinding and adjusting

Greater resistance to breakage

Less noisy during occlusion

Easily polished to smooth finish

Anterior denture held in the base by a chemical bond with the plastic base

PORCELAIN

Difficult to grind and adjust; grinding leaves unglazed surface on the porcelain.

Do not readily wear but cause wear to natural tooth structure, including gold and resin teeth in opposing arch

More translucent

Anterior porcelain denture teeth are distinguished from plastic anterior teeth by small pins that project from the lingual surface.

Porcelain posterior denture teeth have no pins, but rather a **diatoric hole** that is molded into the center back of the tooth.

Small vent holes provided in porcelain teeth allow air to escape as the denture base material flows into the diatoric hole.

---

8. Mold selection
    a. **Mould** is the shape of the teeth. Four basic face forms—square, square tapering, tapering, and ovoid—are described in Table 20-3.
    b. A mold number is placed on each tooth and on the carded set of teeth; the manufacturer will correlate the anterior moulds to the opposite arch and to the appropriate shape of the posterior teeth.

9. Tooth arrangement
    a. Teeth are not naturally arranged perfectly.
    b. Individualized anterior arrangements for teeth are available.

10. Anatomic versus nonanatomic posterior teeth
    a. Posterior teeth are manufactured with anatomic, semianatomic, and nonanatomic characteristics.

Table 20-3 Face form used
in selecting natural anterior tooth arrangement

Facial descriptions	
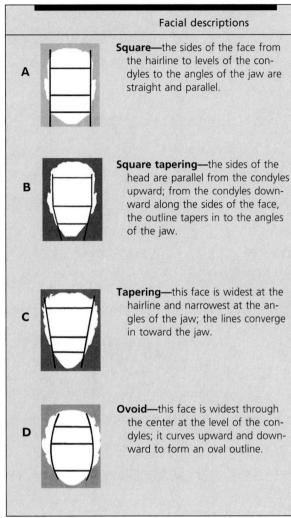 A	**Square**—the sides of the face from the hairline to levels of the condyles to the angles of the jaw are straight and parallel.
B	**Square tapering**—the sides of the head are parallel from the condyles upward; from the condyles downward along the sides of the face, the outline tapers in to the angles of the jaw.
C	**Tapering**—this face is widest at the hairline and narrowest at the angles of the jaw; the lines converge in toward the jaw.
D	**Ovoid**—this face is widest through the center at the level of the condyles; it curves upward and downward to form an oval outline.

USES OF ANATOMIC VERSUS NONANATOMIC DENTURE TEETH

1. Anatomic posterior teeth are used for younger denture patients whose natural teeth are still fully formed, for single dentures that oppose fully formed natural teeth, and for partial dentures.
2. Semianatomic posterior teeth are more often used for middle-aged patients whose natural teeth are partially worn down or whose supporting structures will not accommodate anatomic posteriors.
3. Nonanatomic teeth are used for older patients whose natural teeth have worn down or are nearly flat.

ESTHETIC FACTORS TO CONSIDER IN DENTURE CONSTRUCTION

1. Basic coloring, including complexion, eyes, and hair
2. Size and shape of the face
3. Variations in symmetry from right and left sides
4. Prior dental records indicating dental anomalies or restorations
5. Age of the patient
6. Alterations in shade of various teeth (the cuspid, for instance, may be much darker than the other anterior teeth, or there may be a darkness at the cervical area of the teeth)

APPOINTMENT SCHEDULE FOR A PARTIAL DENTURE

The following appointments are scheduled after the complete oral examination, surveying of the models, consultation, and acceptance of the treatment plan:
- Mouth preparation, including surgical, endodontic, periodontal, and restorative procedures
- Tooth preparation for partial denture retention
- Preliminary impressions
- Final impressions of prepared teeth, remaining teeth, and edentulous ridges
- Trying in framework and adjusting as necessary
- Final impression of edentulous ridge (if required)
- Bite relationships
- Shade and mould selection as needed
- Insert partial denture
- Adjustment appointments as necessary

b. The uses of anatomic versus nonanatomic denture teeth are listed (box).
 11. Esthetic factors to consider in denture construction (box).
IV. Typical Appointment Schedules for Removable Prostheses
 A. Partial denture (box)
 B. Conventional denture (box on page 340)
 C. Immediate denture (box on page 340)
V. Preliminary/Final Impressions
 A. Before any treatment begins, preliminary impressions must be taken.
 B. Custom trays are constructed for final impressions and must fit each arch accurately.
 C. Final impressions are taken from which a master cast is made to begin prosthesis construc-

---

APPOINTMENT SCHEDULE FOR A CONVENTIONAL DENTURE

The following appointments are scheduled after the complete oral examination, consultation, and acceptance of the treatment plan:
- Tissue conditioning as needed
- Initial impressions of arches and edentulous ridges
- Final impressions of arches and edentulous ridges
- Jaw relationships, shade and mould selection
- Try-in and setup approval
- Denture insertion
- Adjustment appointments as necessary

APPOINTMENT SCHEDULE FOR AN IMMEDIATE DENTURE

The following appointments are scheduled after the complete oral examination, consultation, and acceptance of the treatment plan:
- Extraction of posterior teeth on one side of the mouth
- Extraction of posterior teeth on opposite side of the mouth
- Taking initial impressions of arches with remaining teeth and edentulous ridges (4 to 6 weeks later)
- Jaw relationships, shade and mould selection
- Try-in and setup approval
- Extraction of remaining teeth and insertion of dentures, surgery by maxillofacial oral surgeon if necessary
- Follow-up visit to examine denture and tissues (day after surgery)
- Adjustment appointments as necessary
- Recall visit to examine denture fit and need for reline (6 to 8 months later)

ARMAMENTARIUM FOR BORDER MOLDING AND FINAL IMPRESSIONS

Prepared custom-made trays
Low-fusing compound
Heating bath
Laboratory knife
#7 wax spatula
Bunsen burner
Matches
Cold cream or petroleum jelly

Impression materials: zinc oxide-eugenol impression paste or elastomer-type impression material (such as polyvinylsiloxane, polysulfide rubber base, or polyether materials)
Mixing pads and spatulas

CRITERIA FOR ACCURATE FINAL IMPRESSIONS IN DENTURE CONSTRUCTION

- Close contact with the surface of the mucous membrane on which the denture will rest
- Complete registration of the mucolabial fold
- Extension of the impression distally to include all tissues that will be involved in the design of the denture to obtain an adequate seal
- Detailed reproduction of all soft and hard tissues
- Absence of voids

INTERIM LABORATORY ACTIVITIES

- Survey of casts
- Custom tray construction
- Master cast construction
- Casting framework (for partial denture)
- Construction of baseplates and occlusal rims
- Setup for trial, full, or partial denture
- Processing final, full, or partial denture
- Processing reline for full or partial denture

---

tion. The final impressions appointment includes two phases:
1. *Border molding* of the periphery of the tray (box on page 341)
2. *Final impressions* of the soft and hard tissues of the arch
D. The armamentarium for the border molding and final impressions appointment is listed (box).
E. Criteria for accurate final impressions are listed (box).
VI. Interim Laboratory Procedures
A. Laboratory activities (box)
B. Boxing the impression

1. The impression is thoroughly dried.
2. The mandibular impression tongue area is blocked out with wax and sealed to the lingual border of the impression.
3. A wax rope, approximately 4 mm wide, is adapted around the periphery of the impression approximately 3 to 4 mm beneath the border of the impression.
4. The wax is carefully sealed with a warmed spatula.

BORDER MOLDING

- Are all universal barrier techniques being used?
- Is all of the armamentarium available and prepared for use?
- Are the instruments arranged in order of use?
- Are you prepared for alternative treatment plans?
- Is the necessary equipment turned on and ready to operate?

  Border molding, or **muscle trimming,** is a common procedure for complete dentures. It is also performed on the tissue areas of partial dentures, such as the saddle or tuberosity areas. The primary objective of border molding is to obtain an impression that replicates the border of the denture, while the tissues are being manipulated or are actively moving. The patient must activate the tongue in many different positions to create action that might cause denture movement.

To achieve border molding the dentist performs the following steps:
1. Coat the periphery of the custom-made tray with warmed dental compound.
2. Place the tray into the patient's mouth.
3. Manipulate the soft tissues.
4. Ask the patient to move the lips, cheeks, or tongue in various directions.

The custom-made tray relieves peripheral borders used during the border molding. The tray is trimmed about 2 to 3 mm short of the planned denture border to allow for the extension of the borders in dental compound.

STEPS IN THE BORDER-MOLDING PROCEDURE

1. Warm the compound in a flame from a Bunsen burner until it is softened.
2. Fill the relieved areas on the peripheral border of the tray with dental compound.
3. Use a flame from an alcohol torch to soften the compound on the tray.
4. Dip the tray into a water bath at the working temperature of the dental compound to temper and soften the material so that it will be comfortable when placed in the patient's mouth.
5. Place the tray slowly into the patient's mouth and seat it firmly in place. This will allow the compound to flow.
6. Remove the tray from the mouth and chill in cold water to harden the compound.
7. Remove the excess compound from the peripheral border with a laboratory knife or wax spatula.
8. Rewarm the compound in the water bath and reinsert the tray in the patient's mouth.
9. Instruct the patient to activate various muscle groups by extending the tongue, opening the mouth wide, swallowing, everting the lips, or biting down.
10. In addition, the dentist will massage various groups of muscles and feel and observe the cheeks, frena, and various flange areas to ensure that no overextensions of the tray will create poor denture design.
11. This process is continued until the dentist has ensured that all border extensions are adequate to provide the necessary support and retention in the denture.
12. Once the border molding is completed, a wash-type impression of zinc oxide eugenol, rubber base, or silicone is taken of the ridges and supporting structures.
13. The impression is disinfected (according to OSHA guidelines) before being sent to the laboratory for the master cast to be poured.
- Have the appropriate universal barrier techniques been removed?
- Have all appropriate surfaces been cleaned and disinfected?
- Has all of the armamentarium been removed?
- Has all equipment been repositioned?
- Has all equipment been disinfected/sterilized according to OSHA guidelines? Note: Be certain to follow the laboratory guidelines as well as the clinical OSHA guidelines when working with prosthetics.

5. A strip of boxing wax is warmed and adapted around the wax rope to form the base of the cast.
6. The boxing wax strip is sealed with a hot spatula, and the finished boxed impression is ready to be poured with a high-strength stone.
7. When the models are separated, they are prepared by the laboratory technician and mounted on an articulator.
8. From these models a baseplate is constructed for each arch.
C. Constructing baseplates and occlusal rims
   1. A record base or **baseplate** is an acrylic

resin or shellac substance used as the denture base in making maxillomandibular jaw relationship records.

2. An **occlusal rim** or bite rim, built from wax, is secured on the baseplate and used to determine the maxillomandibular jaw relationships that will later be used as a base into which the teeth will be set for the prosthesis.

3. The baseplate must be adapted closely to the master cast to ensure proper retention.

4. Typically, the laboratory technician performs the following steps:
   a. Block out all undercuts on the model with wax.
   b. Place aluminum foil over the master cast.
   c. Place a thin layer of zinc oxide-eugenol impression paste into the tissue side of the baseplate.
   d. Seat the tray on the foil-covered model.
   e. When set, remove the baseplate.
   f. Peel off the aluminum foil.
   g. Remove all excess material from the peripheral borders.
   h. Store the baseplate back on the master cast.
   i. Return the case to the dental office.

VII. Jaw Relationships
   A. The armamentarium for jaw relationships is provided (box).
   B. The procedure for this appointment is provided (box below and page 343).

ARMAMENTARIUM FOR JAW RELATIONSHIPS

Articulated setup with the baseplates and occlusal rims	Baseplate wax
	Millimeter ruler
Sharp laboratory knife	Caliper or Boley gauge
Hanau torch	Bite wax (such as Alu-wax)
Wax spatula	Tongue blade
Face-bow assembly	

PROCEDURE FOR JAW RELATIONSHIPS

CHECKING THE FIT OF THE BASEPLATES

The dentist places the baseplates in the patient's mouth to ensure that they are stable and comfortable. If the bases are not stable to finger pressure, it may be necessary to correct the baseplate or even begin with a new final impression. To determine tissue comfort, some pressure indicator paste is placed on the inner surface of the baseplate with a small brush. Any pressure areas should be relieved before continuing with jaw relationships.

ATTACHING THE OCCLUSAL RIMS

Once the baseplates have been deemed stable, the dentist attaches the occlusal rims by using either a sheet of baseplate wax, which has been rolled into a tight rope, or a preshaped wax occlusal rim. The occlusal rim is attached to the ridge of the baseplate.

MAKING A FACE-BOW RECORD

A **face-bow** is a caliperlike, adjustable device used to establish the relationship between the mandibular condyle of the temporomandibular joint and the maxillary dental arch. This dimensional relationship is transferred to the articulator to simulate jaw movement during the construction of the dental prosthesis. Making the face-bow record includes the following steps:

1. Place the ear rod of the face-bow into the external auditory meatus.
2. Place the maxillary baseplate, to which the bite fork has been attached, in the patient's mouth.
3. Position the face-bow apparatus to fit into the bite fork arm, and adjust the side axis arms so that they are an equal distance from the axis points that have been marked on the face. The arms should just touch the marked points.
4. Readjust the arms until they lightly touch the face, and take a reading on the numbered index scale. This number is recorded on the patient record.
5. Remove the face-bow and baseplate from the patient's mouth and attach it to the articular condyle rods of the articulator.

C. The case is disinfected (according to OSHA guidelines) and transferred to the dental laboratory with the appropriate instructions on the laboratory requisition.

D. The laboratory technician arranges and articulates artificial teeth on the occlusal rims according to data provided by the dentist.

E. The trial denture is contoured in wax on the gingival mucosa areas to reproduce the contours of the original tissues in the dentulous mouth.

F. When the trial denture has been completed, it is returned to the dental office for a try-in appointment.

VIII. Denture Try-In Appointment

A. At this appointment the dentist checks the tooth arrangement to ensure that the denture provides for adequate speech and mastication and that a pleasing appearance has been achieved.

B. This is the final appointment before the completion of the denture; any necessary changes must be made at this appointment.

C. The denture is evaluated to confirm the following:
   1. Adequate tongue space for proper speech
   2. Correct fullness in the cheek and lip areas

PROCEDURE FOR JAW RELATIONSHIPS—cont'd

6. Adjust the anterior height of the maxillary occlusal rim by moving the face-bow up and down so that the incisal edge of the maxillary occlusal rim is level with the line on the incisal guide pin.
7. Mount the ring of the articulator to the prepared maxillary cast with stone.
8. Remove the bite fork from the setup by warming the handle of the fork in a direct flame. The heat is transferred to the bite portion of the fork and allows for easy removal. A wax spatula can aid in smoothing any voids in the occlusal rim.

   The next step in the procedure is to obtain vertical-dimension relationships. **Vertical dimension** refers to the distance between two arbitrary fixed points—one on the maxilla and one on the mandible when the jaws are at rest. This measurement is used to establish the height of the occlusal tables and the freeway space in denture construction. The **freeway space** is the amount of space between the maxillary and mandibular teeth when the jaws are at rest. The *vertical dimension of occlusion* refers to the face height that exists when the teeth are in occlusion. The *vertical dimension of rest* is defined as the habitual postural position of the mandible when the patient is resting comfortably in an upright position and the condyles are in a neutral unstrained position. To obtain vertical dimension the dentist performs the following steps:

1. Select two points to determine facial height—one on the mandible and the other on the maxilla.
2. Take a measurement of the patient's vertical dimension while at rest and in occlusion, using a millimeter ruler and tongue blade.
3. Record the measurements.

   Once the vertical dimension has been obtained, the dentist obtains a **centric relationship.** Two factors are considered in this relationship: centric occlusion and centric jaw relation. *Centric occlusion* is the relationship of opposing occlusal surfaces that provides the maximum contact or intercuspation. The *centric jaw relationship* is more complex and includes the relationship of the mandible to the maxilla when the condyles are in their most posterosuperior, unstrained positions in the glenoid fossae, from which lateral movements can be made at the occluding vertical relationship that is normal for the patient. The centric relationship exists at any degree of jaw separation.

   To determine the centric relationship the dentist performs the following steps:

1. Make a V-shaped notch approximately 1 to 3 mm in the mandibular occlusal rim.
2. Rub the surface with petroleum jelly and insert the mandibular occlusal rim into the patient's mouth.
3. Prepare the maxillary occlusal rim by relieving the wax occlusal rim vertically, approximately 4 mm in the posterior area that opposes the mandibular occlusal rim.
4. Add a warmed, softened bite wax to the relieved area on the maxillary rim and instruct the patient to bite the wax. Ask the patient to remain in this position until the wax is hardened.
5. Remove the occlusal rims and cool to set the wax.

   The dentist returns the baseplates and bite rims to the articulator frequently, until all vertical, centric, excursive, and protrusive recordings have been completed. Each time a relationship is recorded on the articulator, the dentist adjusts various settings on the condylar element to simulate the patient's various jaw relationships.

   In addition, at this appointment appropriate shade guides must be made available for shade and mould selection. A Trubyte Tooth Indicator is optional.

3. Proper vertical and centric dimension
4. Correct shade and mould
5. Adequate buccal and labial tooth position to avoid biting the cheeks and lips

D. The armamentarium for the denture try-in appointment is listed (box).

E. The procedure for the denture try-in is described (box).

ARMAMENTARIUM FOR THE DENTURE TRY-IN APPOINTMENT

Waxed dentures on the articulator
Millimeter ruler
Bunsen burner
Wax spatula
Wax knife

Baseplate wax
Bowl of cold water
Boley gauge
Hand mirror (or access to wall mirror)

PROCEDURE FOR DENTURE TRY-IN

The denture is disinfected before it is tried in the patient's mouth. The denture is then passed to the dentist for insertion. The following points are checked:

1. Occlusal vertical dimension, using the caliper and millimeter ruler. The patient is asked to perform the same type of verbal activities as done during the initial appointment.
2. Centric occlusion.
3. Tooth position. Ask the patient to speak to verify that the lingual position is adequate.
4. Appearance. Observe the lip and cheek fullness to ensure that adequate bulk is present. If the cheeks are too full, the teeth may need to be repositioned or some of the wax removed. If the cheeks are too shallow or a sunken appearance is evident, the teeth may need to be repositioned or new teeth added.
5. Orientation of the occlusal plane to ensure that it is even with the lip line and that an adequate amount of tooth length is showing.
6. Shade and mould of the teeth for a blend with the patient's complexion and face shape.
7. Arrangement of the teeth to verify that they provide a pleasing appearance.

If any of these check points are not satisfactory, it may be necessary to heat a wax spatula or knife, remove or reset the teeth, or recontour the mucosa wax. When the trial denture is accepted by the dentist and the patient, it is disinfected and returned to the laboratory for final processing. A laboratory requisition accompanies the case with details regarding the final insertion.

IX. Final Laboratory Procedures

A. Denture processing involves converting the wax pattern of a denture or trial denture into a denture with a base that is made of another material, such as acrylic resin.

B. The denture goes through a flasking process in which the cast and wax dentures are placed into a **flask** to prepare for molding the denture base material into the form of the denture.

X. Prosthesis Insertion

A. Complete immediate dentures are delivered to the maxillofacial oral surgeon, who performs the surgery and inserts the dentures initially.

B. Nonimmediate dentures or partial dentures are sent directly to the dentist who has been preparing the prosthesis for insertion.

C. The procedural description for inserting full nonimmediate dentures is described (box below).

D. The armamentarium for prosthesis insertion is shown (box on page 345).

PROSTHESIS INSERTION

The denture is disinfected before insertion. The following steps are performed during insertion:

1. The denture is examined to ensure that no nodules or sharp edges are present that could injure the soft tissues.
2. The maxillary denture is inserted with a firm upward and backward motion. With a finger in the palatal area, the dentist seats the denture firmly.
3. The denture is removed to verify retention by grasping the buccal surfaces of the denture with thumb and forefinger; pressure is applied in a downward pulling motion.
4. The maxillary denture is reinserted; the mandibular denture is then inserted.
5. The retention of the lower denture is tested by applying force in an upward direction.
6. Internal tissues are checked by brushing pressure-indicator paste inside the denture. Where evidence of extreme pressure is apparent, the acrylic is removed with a small bur or stone.
7. The occlusion is checked with the use of articulating paper. High contact points are adjusted with stones or burs.
8. The markings are removed with a tissue or 2 × 2 gauze. If the marks cannot be removed manually, it may be necessary to transfer the denture to the polishing wheel in the office laboratory.

The patient is shown a mirror and is allowed to practice putting the dentures in and taking them out to ensure proper placement and comfort.

ARMAMENTARIUM FOR PROSTHESIS INSERTION

Completed dentures
Burs and stones
Slow-speed handpiece
Millimeter ruler

Articulating paper and
forceps
Pressure indicating paste
setup

RECOMMENDATIONS FOR PROSTHESIS HOME CARE

- Use a soft brush.
- Clean over a water-filled bowl to avoid breakage.
- Use a recommended cleaning agent to dissolve calculus.
- Avoid wearing the prosthesis at night.
- Store the prosthesis in water when it is not being worn.

XI. Home Care Instructions
  A. Soreness and discomfort
    1. The patient needs to know that the soft tissues may be sore for a few days after insertion of the prosthesis.
    2. If the prosthesis is a partial denture, discomfort may occur in some of the natural teeth.
    3. Discomfort that occurs after several weeks or months may be due to tissue changes, and the dentist must see the patient to determine what changes have occurred.
    4. The patient should be instructed not to use home remedies to avoid an office visit.
  B. Potential damage from denture neglect
    1. Encourage the patient to observe changes taking place in the mouth; neglecting symptoms may cause damage to the surrounding tissues and existing teeth and gingiva.
    2. Acute conditions are often evidenced by pain, redness of tissues, and ulcerated tissue and may be the result of discrepancies in the fit of the prosthesis.
    3. Chronic conditions are generally the result of a lack of attention to home care and may cause chronic damage to the oral tissues.
    4. A recall system for denture patients is encouraged and can become part of the education program.
  C. Coping with the prosthesis
    1. The new prosthesis wearer must learn coping techniques for specific areas, including speaking distinctly, eating, and managing an increased salivary flow and excessive bulk in the mouth.
    2. Sensory receptors in the tongue are stimulated, causing the patient to be aware of the new prosthesis, and for a short time these receptors may also induce increased salivary flow.
    3. The patient must understand that these reactions are normal and will subside after the prosthesis has been worn for a time.

ARMAMENTARIUM FOR INITIAL ADJUSTMENT

Mouth mirror
Mouthwash
Pressure-indicating paste
Articulating paper

Articulating paper forceps
Assorted burs and stones
Slow-speed handpiece

---

    4. The patient needs instruction in maintaining the oral tissues beneath the prosthesis and in caring for the prosthesis.
    5. The patient with a partial denture must learn how to care for the natural teeth as well.
    6. To promote healthy capillary action, the tissues need to be exposed for several hours at a time.
    7. The easiest and most convenient tool for cleaning and massaging the soft tissues is a soft tooth brush; a moist washcloth may also be used.
    8. Recommendations for prosthesis home care are listed (box above).
XII. Initial Adjustment
  A. A denture **adjustment** involves removing excess denture base to relieve an area of soft-tissue irritation or to alter the occlusion.
  B. The follow-up appointment is generally scheduled within 24 to 48 hours after insertion of the prosthesis.
  C. The armamentarium for the initial adjustment is provided (box above).
  D. The procedure for the initial adjustment is provided (box on page 346).
XIII. Relining and Rebasing
  A. **Relining** is the process of adding denture base material to the tissue side of the removable prosthesis to improve its adaptation to the tissues. A complete denture is relined to improve retention and stability.

PROCEDURE FOR INITIAL ADJUSTMENT

1. The denture is gently removed.
2. The patient is allowed to rinse the mouth gently, without forcefully swishing the mouthwash about, to avoid dislocation of any blood clots. The mouthwash is removed gently with the HVE tip, avoiding contact with the soft tissues.
3. The assistant rinses the denture.
4. The dentist examines the oral tissues to identify any areas that may be irritated by the denture.
5. The denture can be dried and pressure-indicating paste inserted in the tissue portion of the denture. The denture is reinserted and removed to identify pressure points. These pressure points can be relieved with a bur or stone.
6. The denture is reinserted and the occlusion adjusted. Minor adjustments may be made at this appointment because discomfort from the surgery or other sore spots may impede a realistic occlusal registration.
7. The patient is shown how to put the denture in and take it out of the mouth and is allowed to practice this procedure.
8. The home care procedure and the need to observe changes in oral tissues is reviewed for the patient.
9. The patient is informed of the need for future follow-up appointments and is encouraged to contact the office if discomfort occurs.

ARMAMENTARIUM FOR RELINING AND REBASING

Prosthesis to be relined
Acrylic bur or flange
Petroleum jelly or cold cream
2 × 2 gauze sponges
Impression material—zinc oxide-eugenol, polyvinyl siloxane, or polysulfide

PROCEDURE FOR RELINING AND REBASING

1. Clean the tissue surface of the denture manually or in the ultrasonic cleaner.
2. Remove all undercuts from the denture to ensure that the denture can be removed from the stone casts after the reline has been cast.
3. Remove flanges of the denture with an acrylic bur or stone to avoid overextension.
4. Correct minor defects or base extension with low-heat stick compound.
5. Take an impression by placing the impression material in the tissue side of the denture and inserting it into the patient's mouth. If a zinc oxide-eugenol paste is used, lubricate the patient's extraoral tissues before insertion.
6. Remove the denture from the patient's mouth.
7. Disinfect the denture and transfer it to the laboratory with instructions for the reline and delivery time.

B. **Rebasing** is replacing all the acrylic resin base material without changing the occlusal relationships.
C. Indications for relining or rebasing include the following:
  1. Noticeable movement in a partial denture, causing the retainer rests to be raised or even unseated
  2. Instability in a denture, over which a patient has no control
  3. Irritation of the soft tissues, caused by the unstable denture
D. The patient needs to be informed of the length of time it will take to complete this process. A patient may come to the office early in the day and have the prosthesis returned later in the day.
E. The armamentarium for this procedure is provided (box).
F. The procedure for relining and rebasing is provided (box).
XIV. Osseointegration
  A. **Osseointegration,** the growth of the alveolar process around the mortise of a dental implant, is an integral aspect of prosthetic dentistry.
  B. Implanting single tooth restorations or multiple teeth in combination with bridges or a partial or full denture is an alternative for some patients.
  C. Certain oral conditions must exist for successful implants, including the following:
    1. An alveolar process that is of adequate height, width, and density
    2. Healthy gingival tissues
  D. Two common dental implants are the **endosteal** and **subperiosteal** implants.
    1. The endosteal implant involves the use of screws, cylinders, or blades that are im-

planted in the alveolar process. Each implant is capable of holding a single restoration or a combination of prosthetic teeth.

2. The subperiosteal implant is positioned over the alveolar process, and a framework of metal posts extends from the gingival tissue after implantation to assist in retaining a prosthesis.

E. The implant process requires the following appointments:
1. Anchor placement
2. Postsurgical care: first appointment
3. Abutment connection
4. Postsurgical care: second appointment
5. Restorative procedure

Questions

Prosthodontics

1 Which of the following restorations can be used to retain a fixed bridge?
1. Porcelain crowns
2. Three-quarter crowns
3. Inlays
4. Full crowns
5. Amalgam restorations
a. 1, 2, and 3
b. 2, 3, and 4
c. 2, 3, and 5
d. 3, 4, and 5

2 The following is true of an immediate denture: It is
a. Constructed in one visit
b. Made of shellac
c. Used to replace only the anterior teeth
d. Inserted during the same appointment in which the remaining teeth are extracted

Place the following steps for a preparation appointment for a cast metal restoration in the correct order. Place the first step in item 3 and continue to the last step in item 7.
a. Administer anesthetic.
b. Retract gingiva.
c. Fabricate and place temporary restoration.
d. Prepare tooth.
e. Obtain impressions.
_____ **3**
_____ **4**
_____ **5**
_____ **6**
_____ **7**

Place the following steps for a cementation procedure for a cast metal restoration in the correct order. Place the first step in item 8 and continue to the last step in item 12.
a. Cement restoration

b. Try in restoration
c. Finish margins
d. Disinfect cast and restoration
e. Place thin film of cement on inner surface
_____ **8**
_____ **9**
_____ **10**
_____ **11**
_____ **12**

13 When a crown preparation is being performed on a patient who has mitral valve dysfunction and a sensitivity to epinephrine, which of the following would most likely be used?
1. Premedication
2. Gingival retraction cord with clotting ability
3. Anesthetic with a vasoconstrictor
4. Anesthetic without a vasoconstrictor
5. Nitrous oxide
a. 1 and 3
b. 1 and 4
c. 1, 2, and 4
d. 2, 4, and 5
e. 5 only

14 After the patient has been anesthetized and the tooth to be treated has been isolated and prepared, the next steps usually are which of the following?
a. Check occlusal clearance, determine draw, take bite registration, place gingival retraction cord, take final impression, and temporize.
b. Determine draw, check occlusal clearance, place gingival retraction cord, make temporary restoration, and take final impression.
c. Check occlusal clearance, determine draw, place gingival retraction cord, take diagnostic impressions, and temporize.
d. Check occlusal clearance, determine draw, place gingival retraction cord, take final impression, and temporize.

Place an A for *True* or a B for *False* in the space provided as it relates to each statement.
_____ **15** When teeth for a removable prosthesis are selected, the shape of a patient's face contributes to the selection of a mould.
_____ **16** A person's complexion relates to selection of shade of teeth for a prosthesis.
_____ **17** The objective of border molding is to replicate the border of the denture while tissues are being manipulated or are actively moving.
_____ **18** Gutta-percha is placed on the peripheral border of a tray during border molding.
_____ **19** *Clasp* and *rest* are synonymous terms.
_____ **20** *Immediate* and *conventional* (dentures) are synonymous terms.
_____ **21** The loss of a single tooth in an arch can be the initial stage in becoming a dental cripple.
_____ **22** The lingual bar on a maxillary denture is a major connector.

_____ **23** The palatal bar on a maxillary denture is a minor connector.

_____ **24** An extension from the lingual bar to a clasp or rest would be a minor connector.

_____ **25** Stippling is done on the internal portion of a denture.

Rationales

Prosthodontics

1 B Inlays, three-quarter crowns, and full cast or porcelain fused to metal crowns are the most effective retainers for a fixed bridge. Porcelain crowns are more susceptible to fracture, whereas amalgam restorations cannot be cast.

2 D Two types of dentures are available for insertion: conventional and immediate. The immediate denture is inserted immediately after the removal of the teeth. Generally, posterior teeth are extracted about 6 to 8 weeks prior to final impressions. Healing takes place while the anterior teeth are retained. After preparatory procedures in denture construction are completed, the teeth are removed in the anterior and the denture is inserted.

A conventional denture may be a replacement or new denture. If it is a new denture, all the patient's teeth are removed, healing takes place, and the preparatory construction begins for the denture. During this procedure the patient remains completely edentulous.

3 A

4 D

5 B

6 E

7 C The procedural steps for preparation of a tooth for a cast restoration include the following:
Prepare the armamentarium
Update patient's medical history
Examine treatment site
Determine occlusal relationship
Administer anesthetic
Prepare tooth
Remove caries and place core material to build up tooth as necessary
Reduce occlusal grooves
Check occlusal clearance
Reduce axial walls
Place axial grooves
Remove caries as necessary
Refine and finish margins
Determine draw
Dry and isolate site
Place cavity medication if needed
Retract gingiva
Obtain final and opposing impressions
Obtain bite registration
Fabricate and place temporary restoration
Postoperative instructions
Prepare case according to OSHA guidelines and prescription for laboratory

8 D

9 B

10 C

11 E

12 A The procedural steps for the cementation of a casting includes the following:
Disinfect the casting
Administer anesthetic if necessary
Remove temporary restoration and excess cement
Try in cast restoration
Assess stability
Check contacts
Check occlusion
Determine margin integrity
Make necessary adjustments
Finish margins
Complete final laboratory finish and polish
Disinfect cast restoration
Isolate tooth
Prepare final cement
Place thin film of cement on inner surface of casting
Cement cast restoration on tooth
Remove excess cement
Reevaluate occlusal contact and margins
Make final adjustments if necessary
Provide postoperative instructions

13 B Premedication such as an antibiotic may be prescribed to prevent any potential infection caused by bacteria invading the bloodstream. Additionally, anesthetic with a vasoconstrictor is contraindicated because it would constrict the flow of blood.

14 A See Nos. 3-7.

15 A Mould is the shape of the teeth. Tooth mould is determined by the shape of the patient's face. The four basic face forms are square, square tapering, tapering, and ovoid.

16 A Shade selection for denture teeth is based on the patient's hair and eye color as well as complexion.

17 A Border molding is the process of recording the denture border by manipulating the tissues adjacent to the borders. This process is completed on the tissue areas of partial dentures, such as the saddle or tuberosity areas.

18 B Dental compound is placed on the peripheral borders of a tray during border molding.

19 B A _clasp_ is an attachment on a partial denture that is applied to an abutment tooth to provide retention to the removable prosthesis; a _rest_ is a rigid extension of the partial denture that contacts a tooth to dissipate vertical and horizontal forces.

20 B See No. 2.

21 A When a tooth is lost, it is the beginning of future dental problems, including open contacts resulting in a potential for tooth drifting, hypereruption, periodontal trauma, ridge distortion, food impaction, loss of aesthetics, difficulty in mastication, and change in phonetics.

22 B Lingual bars are placed not on the maxillary arch but on the lingual of the mandibular arch as major connectors.

23 B Palatal bars on the maxilla are major connectors because this part of the device connects the sides of bases of a partial denture.

24 A A minor connector is a connecting link between the major connector or base and the other parts of the prosthesis, such as the clasps and rests.

25 B Stippling—the orange-peel, pebble-like appearance that exists in the natural attached gingiva—is re-created on the external portion of the denture base.

To enhance your understanding of the material in this chapter refer to the illustrations in Chapter 30 of Finkbeiner/Johnson: *Mosby's Comprehensive Dental Assisting: A Clinical Approach.*

CHAPTER 21

Temporary Restorations

OUTLINE

Types and Uses
Patient Education

Intracoronal Temporary
Restorations

Extracoronal Temporary
Restoration

KEY TERMS

Acrylic crown

Aluminum crown

Coping

Extracoronal dressing

Festoon

Interim dressing

Intracoronal dressing

Stainless steel crown

Temporary restoration

A primary responsibility of dental professionals is to provide relief, comfort, and a stable environment in the oral cavity. A temporary restoration placed in or on a tooth often fulfills this need. In some states the dental assistant who is educated in advanced functions is delegated the responsibility for providing a temporary restoration for the patient. In many states this task is delegated to the credentialed dental assistant or hygienist. This delegation usually occurs with a patient of record and is assigned to the team member under direct or general supervision of the dentist. The operator in the procedural examples discussed in this chapter could be the assistant, hygienist, or dentist. This delegated responsibility can increase productivity and efficiency in the dental practice and relieve the dentist of these duties.

TYPES AND USES

I. **Temporary restorations** are **interim dressings**—that is, fillings that are placed for a short time to protect the tooth until a permanent restoration can be placed.

II. These restorations are designed in two basic forms:
   A. **Intracoronal dressing** or restoration—dental material that is placed directly into the crown or a cavity preparation
      1. Used when a tooth is prepared for placement of an inlay.
      2. Used when a tooth has a deep carious lesion.
   B. An **extracoronal dressing** or restoration—dental material that surrounds a large portion or all of the crown of a tooth
      1. Used when teeth have been prepared for crown or bridge procedures.
      2. Usually a full-coverage temporary constructed from self-curing acrylic or designed from preformed plastic or metal crowns.

III. Temporary restorations perform the following functions:
   A. Aid in mastication

B. Prevent hypereruption of the prepared tooth and the opposing tooth until a permanent restoration is placed

C. Avoid further trauma to the tooth

D. Avoid mesial drift of the tooth and/or an abutment tooth

E. Maintain space for the permanent tooth eruption

F. Provide an aesthetic appearance

G. Relieve discomfort by creating an anodyne effect

H. Deter the decay process

PATIENT EDUCATION ▰▰▰▰▰▰

I. Patients must be advised that a temporary restoration is not final treatment for the specific tooth.

II. If the temporary restoration is lost during the interim treatment, the patient must return for the cementation appointment.

III. Patient education tips for temporary restorations should be provided, as follows:

A. Brush the temporary restoration as any other tooth.

B. Floss the teeth, but pull the floss through the contact toward the buccal (cheek) side to avoid disturbing the temporary restoration.

C. Temporary cement is weak, and the temporary restoration can easily be lost.

D. If the temporary is dislodged, call the dental office immediately to arrange to have it recemented to avoid mesial drift and hypereruption.

E. Mesial drift and hypereruption may result in the permanent restoration not fitting properly.

F. The temporized tooth may be sensitive to temperature.

G. Avoid sticky foods that may dislodge the temporary.

INTRACORONAL TEMPORARY RESTORATIONS ▰▰▰▰▰▰

I. Intracoronal temporary restorations are usually constructed of plastic or a temporary cement.

II. The acrylic or plastic temporary restoration is designed, contoured, and often cemented with a temporary zinc oxide-eugenol cement that can be easily removed.

III. The cement intracoronal temporary is fabricated of a zinc oxide-eugenol cement to provide an anodyne effect and for ease in the removal of cement at a later appointment.

IV. A permanent cement of greater strength—zinc phosphate—could be placed if the temporary res-

---

ARMAMENTARIUM FOR A CEMENT TEMPORARY

Dental cement (one of the following)	Ball burnisher
	Articulating paper
(Short-term cement)	2 × 2 gauze
ZOE, cavit	Cement spatula
(Long-term cement)	#1 amalgam condenser
zinc phosphate,	#2 amalgam condenser
polycarboxylate	Matrix band and retainer
Instruments	
Explorer	Wedge
Mirror	7C cleoid-discoid carver
Cotton pliers	#26 spoon excavator
Spoon excavator	Anatomic burnisher
FP1 plastic instrument	Cotton rolls
5C cleoid-discoid carver	Cotton pellets
Ward's C carver	Mixing pad

---

toration remains in place for more than 3 to 4 weeks.

V. The armamentarium for a cement temporary is listed (box above).

VI. The procedure for placement of a cement temporary is described (box on pages 352-353).

VII. The criteria for a properly contoured intracoronal temporary are listed (box on page 353).

VIII. The operator may prefer to place an intracoronal temporary made of acrylic instead of cement.

A. The armamentarium for this type of temporary is listed (box on page 353).

B. The procedure for preparation and placement of an intracoronal acrylic temporary is described (box on page 354).

IX. Criteria for a properly trimmed acrylic temporary are listed (box on page 355).

EXTRACORONAL TEMPORARY RESTORATION ▰▰▰▰▰▰

I. When excess amounts of tooth structure have been lost to decay, trauma, or the preparation procedure, the temporary restoration becomes extracoronal; that is, it covers the clinical crown that exists.

II. Extracoronal temporary restorations might include a pontic in the configuration of the temporary restoration to maintain the integrity of space that once was occupied by a tooth.

III. Types of extracoronal temporary restorations that are prefabricated and provide full-coverage protection include the following:

PROCEDURE FOR A CEMENT TEMPORARY

- Are all universal barrier techniques being used?
- Is all of the armamentarium available and prepared for use?
- Are the instruments arranged in order of use?
- Are you prepared for alternative treatment plans?
- Is the necessary equipment turned on and ready to operate?

UPDATE MEDICAL HISTORY

The medical history is especially important if the dentist considers providing the patient with medication to relieve the pain caused by treatment. All current medications and the overall physical well-being of the patient need to be considered to correctly prescribe any medication.

EXAMINATION OF THE TREATMENT SITE

The treatment site is examined if the operator is unsure about the integrity of the pulpal tissues. One option that demonstrates a conservative approach to treatment is to provide a temporary restoration, allowing time for the tooth to become asymptomatic or for evidence to appear that suggests the pulpal tissues are dying and endodontic treatment is necessary.

DETERMINATION OF OCCLUSAL RELATIONSHIP

The occlusal relationship must be determined before placement to aid in proper positioning and avoid occlusal disharmony in the temporary restoration.

PLACEMENT OF ISOLATION

Cotton rolls are placed in the buccal vestibule, sublingual area, and maxillary arch near the parotid gland.

MATRIX BAND, RETAINER, AND WEDGE PLACEMENT

The matrix band, retainer, and wedge are prepared, passed, and placed.

PLACEMENT OF THE CEMENT

A temporary cement is mixed to base consistency, cut into small increments, and passed to the operator along with a small condenser or other instrument of choice for placement. The operator places an increment of cement in the preparation, working it firmly into the opening. Each increment is added; the cement is condensed and formed against the tooth structure and the matrix band (if used).

A larger condenser may be used to complete the condensation. As the cement is placed, the operator occasionally places the end of the condensing instrument into extra cement powder on the pad. The cement powder on the instrument tip helps avoid the increments that stick to the instrument during condensation and prevents the material from being pulled out while increments are added.

INITIAL CARVING

The area is overfilled with cement, and the operator begins to carve the material to the correct shape of its original anatomy. In this procedure the material may be carved with various instruments, such as a 7C cleoid-discoid carver. The carver rests on the existing tooth structure, across the cavosurface margin, and onto the cement. The cement is refined with small carving movements. The carver is exchanged for the explorer to remove excess cement from the marginal ridge and matrix band.

REMOVAL OF MATRIX RETAINER, WEDGE, AND BAND

The wedge, retainer, and band are removed. Removal of the band may need to be delayed until the cement becomes hardened to avoid fractures.

PROCEDURE FOR A CEMENT TEMPORARY—cont'd

FINAL CARVING

The least accessible area, the interproximal space, must be carved as soon as the matrix band is removed. The operator may use a Ward's C carver or other smooth surface carvers to remove the smooth surface excess, contouring the cement to the tooth structure. Objectives of this step are the re-creation of the interdental space and the marginal ridge contact. The carver is exchanged for the explorer to examine the carved surface for smoothness and for removal of any cement from the sulcus.

An anatomic carver, such as the #5C carver, is used to create more refined occlusal anatomy in the cement. Placement of anatomic grooves and fissures and refinement of the marginal ridge are completed.

The cement temporary is burnished and finished for patient comfort and smoothness to the tongue. Burnishing and finishing can create a high level of shine and smoothness in dental cement.

REMOVAL OF COTTON ROLL ISOLATION

The assistant removes the cotton rolls with the cotton pliers.

CHECKING ARTICULATION

A complete mouth rinse is performed to remove all debris and refresh the patient's mouth. Articulation paper is attached to an articulating paper holder and positioned over the tooth that has been temporized with cement. The occlusion is checked by the operator and carved and burnished if necessary.

POSTOPERATIVE INSTRUCTIONS

The temporary restoration is not as strong as a permanent restoration. Fractures can occur easily from biting pressure and from routine hygiene procedures. The patient is given this information and asked to return to have the temporary restoration replaced with a permanent restoration.
- Are the appropriate universal barriers removed?
- Have all appropriate surfaces been cleaned and disinfected?
- Has all of the armamentarium been removed?
- Has all equipment been repositioned?
- Has all equipment been disinfected/sterilized according to OSHA guidelines?

CRITERIA FOR A PROPERLY CONTOURED INTRACORONAL TEMPORARY

Temporary cement is adapted to the margins.
Interproximal contact is established.
Marginal ridge is contoured to the same height as abutment tooth/teeth.
Interproximal contour is the same as natural tooth structure.
Occlusion is adjusted to allow proper articulation.
Excess cement is removed from all areas, especially the gingival sulcus.

ARMAMENTARIUM FOR AN INTRACORONAL ACRYLIC TEMPORARY

Temporary dental cement	Modified sickle/curet scaler
Acrylic material	Lubricant
Explorer	Articulating paper
Mirror	Cotton rolls
Cotton pliers	Cotton pellets
Spoon excavator	Mixing pad
FP1 plastic instrument	Floss
2 × 2 gauze	Finishing/polishing burs and disks
Cement spatula	Polishing wheel
Dappen dish	
Flour of pumice	

PROCEDURE FOR PREPARATION AND PLACEMENT OF AN INTRACORONAL ACRYLIC TEMPORARY

Most acrylics are provided by the manufacturer as liquid and powder, with various shades of color from which to select. The color selection is not as critical for an acrylic temporary that is to be placed in a posterior tooth.

Cotton rolls are placed to provide isolation. Acrylic powder is dispensed in a dappen dish or similar deep-welled device. Acrylic liquid is added until the powder no longer absorbs the liquid. The material may be mixed with a spatula or an FP1 instrument until it is homogeneous. The operator places lubricant on the abutment tooth; a small amount of lubricant can also be applied to the preparation.

The acrylic is pressed into the prepared tooth. Care is taken to ensure that the placement of the acrylic extends to all cavosurface margins. The acrylic can be molded by hand or with an instrument to form it in the preparation. If the acrylic extends beyond the cavosurface margin and is allowed to harden, it can be trimmed away with rotary instruments later. Most carving and refining of the anatomy is made after the material has set; however, excess material can be removed by carving it away with an instrument before it has set.

Some operators may like to remove the acrylic temporary before it reaches a final set, ensuring that the temporary is not trapped in undercuts. The operator may ask the patient to bite down on the acrylic before it has reached the final set. This provides guides as to how the opposing tooth/teeth occlude on the temporary and will aid in the finishing and trimming steps.

If the temporary is difficult to remove, a modified sickle scaler, curet scaler, or spoon excavator can be used against an edge of the acrylic to lift it out of the preparation. If the acrylic temporary is removed from the preparation too soon, a distortion may occur that will not allow the acrylic temporary to reseat. If this occurs, completion of the procedure is delayed so that another temporary can be fabricated.

TRIMMING THE ACRYLIC TEMPORARY

If the auxiliary is delegated to construct the temporary, the use of rotary instruments must be outside the patient's mouth or in a laboratory setting. The temporary will most likely need to be trimmed extensively to fit in the tooth. The trimming can be accomplished by the use of finishing stones, burs, and disks that vary in grit (from coarse to fine) and size.

As the rotary instrument is used, a fulcrum must be established to maintain complete control of the handpiece during the trimming of the acrylic. If a fulcrum is not maintained, the rotary instrument may wander from the desired position and remove acrylic from an incorrect area.

This position allows the operator to use the rotary instrument to feather or thin the cervical margin, removing bulk acrylic that causes gingival irritation that acts as a mechanical irritant. The feathering continues around the circumference of the tooth, reducing thickness throughout. The operator must be well acquainted with tooth anatomy to recreate the anatomy in restorations. The temporary is tried in the preparation many times during this adjustment phase of the procedure.

The temporary is placed in the preparation and the occlusion checked with the articulating paper. If marked heavily, the temporary is removed and adjusted. The temporary is placed again, and the operator runs floss through the proximal contact. The floss should slide through the contact without interruption. If the floss cannot be pulled through the contact, the temporary restoration is removed; the contact is adjusted by removing a slight amount of acrylic with a rotary instrument.

The temporary is polished with a slurry of pumice on a wetted polishing wheel that is placed on a lathe. A high luster on the acrylic can be achieved during this step.

CEMENTING THE ACRYLIC TEMPORARY

The preparation is dried and isolation is continued. It is beneficial to place lubricant on the exterior surfaces of the temporary before cementation. The layer of lubricant eliminates the cement adhering to the external surface of the acrylic temporary, thus making cement removal easier.

An even thickness of cement is placed on the interior surfaces of the temporary with an FP1 plastic instrument or with any instrument of choice. The patient is directed to bite firmly on a cotton roll that is placed on the occlusal of the temporary. Cement along the margins, in the gingival sulcus, and in all other areas must be removed. The cement-removal instrument—a spoon excavator, a scaler, or an explorer—is exchanged for floss that is passed through the interproximal and pulled to the buccal side of the mouth carrying cement through the contacts, rather than leaving it or forcing it into the sulcus further. The area is completely rinsed and dried.

The patient is directed to bite on the articulating paper; however, no excessive articulation markings should show on the temporary because articulation was checked earlier. If the temporary appears high or the patient occludes on the temporary more than on the other teeth, it can be adjusted in the oral cavity with a rotary instrument.

POSTOPERATIVE INSTRUCTIONS

The instructions are similar to those for any temporary restoration, but good oral hygiene must be maintained during this time.

CRITERIA FOR A PROPERLY TRIMMED ACRYLIC TEMPORARY

- Acrylic is adapted to the preparation margins.
- Interproximal contact is established.
- Marginal ridge is contoured to the same height as the abutment tooth/teeth.
- Interproximal contour is same as natural tooth structure.
- Occlusion is adjusted to allow proper articulation.
- Excess cement is removed from all areas, especially the gingival sulcus.

CRITERIA FOR A PROPERLY CONTOURED ACRYLIC CROWN

- Acrylic is adapted and trimmed to the margins.
- Interproximal contact is established.
- Interproximal contour is the same as natural tooth structure.
- Incisal length is adjusted to match adjacent teeth.
- Occlusion is adjusted to allow proper articulation.
- Excess cement is removed from all areas, especially the gingival sulcus.

    A. Stainless steel
    B. Aluminum
    C. Acrylic crown
    D. Acrylic is used to fabricate customized crowns and bridges.

IV. An acrylic crown can be used.
    A. For esthetics, an **aluminum crown** would not be acceptable in the anterior segment of a patient's mouth, so an **acrylic crown** is fabricated according to the criteria listed (box).
    B. The operator may select a preformed acrylic crown or construct a crown from a coping.
    C. A **coping** is a piece of plastic formed over a model of the tooth (or teeth) before the beginning of the preparation; it is created as follows:
        1. The first step is to recreate the anatomy of the tooth that was lost because of fracture.
        2. Fractured surfaces are replaced with wax that is heated and formed on the replica of the tooth in the study casts.
        3. A sheet of plastic approximately 5 inches by 5 inches is placed and secured in the hinged frame of the Omnivac machine.
        4. The frame holding the plastic sheet is positioned at a stop near the heating element.
        5. The study cast, with wax in place on the tooth, is placed on the vacuum plate base.
        6. The heating element is turned on, and the plastic begins to warm.
        7. As the plastic sheet is heated, it begins to lose its cloudiness and to droop.
        8. The edges of the plastic are not warmed, allowing the plastic to continue to be held in the frame.
        9. When the plastic sheet droops within 1 inch of the occlusals of the study cast, turn on the vacuum machine motor.
       10. Pull the frame that holds the melted plastic sheet down on top of the study cast.
       11. Allow the plastic to adapt closely over the form.
       12. Turn off the machine.
       13. The plastic can be removed from the model and three teeth—the tooth to be restored and adjacent teeth—are cut from the square of plastic with scissors or a scalpel.
       14. The cut extends approximately 1 to 2 mm below the cervical tissue line.
    D. The armamentarium for the placement of the acrylic coping temporary is listed (box on page 356).
    E. The procedure for preparation and placement of the acrylic temporary is described (box on page 356).

V. A metal temporary crown can be used.
    A. The three types of prefabricated metal crown forms can be placed in posterior crown preparations: aluminum crown, **stainless steel crown,** and tin crown forms.
    B. The aluminum and stainless steel crown forms are more anatomically correct than the tin crown forms and are used more often to provide the patient with anatomy that is normal to the mouth.
    C. The most common application for stainless steel crowns is in pediatric dentistry.
    D. The armamentarium for the placement of a metal temporary crown is listed (box on page 356).
    E. The procedure for a temporary aluminum crown is described (box on pages 357-358).
    F. Criteria for a properly contoured aluminum crown form are listed (box on page 357).

VI. Alternative temporary procedures can be performed.
    A. Polycarbonate crown forms

ARMAMENTARIUM FOR PLACING AN ACRYLIC COPING TEMPORARY

Explorer	Cotton rolls
Mirror	Acrylic
Spoon excavator	Temporary cement
Scaler	Acrylic burs
FP1 plastic instrument	Lubricant
Scissors	Polishing wheels
Temporary coping material	Flour of pumice
	Floss
Omnivac	2 × 2 cotton gauze

ARMAMENTARIUM FOR A METAL TEMPORARY CROWN

Explorer	Aluminum crown kit
Mirror	Temporary cement
Cotton pliers	Lubricant
Spoon excavator	Floss
FP1 plastic instrument	Cotton rolls
Ball burnisher	2 × 2 gauze
Contouring pliers	
Crown and collar scissors	

PROCEDURE FOR AN ACRYLIC COPING TEMPORARY

The patient returns for the preparation appointment, and the procedure for the temporization phase continues. The coping is tested on the teeth for fit before the tooth is prepared. The coping should cover the tooth and fit closely, forming itself around all anatomic structures.

FABRICATION OF THE ACRYLIC TEMPORARY

The selection of the acrylic powder color is important because the temporary will be visible in the oral cavity. Various shades are available and can be mixed to provide the patient with an esthetically pleasing temporary crown. A light covering of lubricant is placed. The acrylic is mixed as described for the intracoronal acrylic temporary, or the acrylic powder can be placed in the coping at the site and liquid added to it until it is completely wetted. An FP1 plastic instrument is used to reposition any acrylic that flows onto the adjacent teeth of the coping. The coping, with acrylic in it, is placed on the lubricated teeth in the mouth and allowed to set. Excess acrylic often exudes from the coping and is removed with an instrument, avoiding any injury to the gingiva.

TRIMMING AND POLISHING THE TEMPORARY

When the acrylic has set, the coping and acrylic form are removed from the mouth and the acrylic is removed from the coping. Excess material is trimmed away with rotary instruments, and the criteria for the temporary are as described for the previous acrylic temporary.

CEMENTATION OF THE TEMPORARY CROWN

The temporary crown form is cemented as are the other temporaries described. Excess cement is completely removed from all surfaces of the crown and in the sulcus area.

CHECKING ARTICULATION

Articulating paper is placed between the arches, and the patient is directed to bite down. If the patient occludes heavily on the temporary crown, the marked area is removed with a rotary instrument.

POSTOPERATIVE INSTRUCTIONS

The postoperative instructions are the same as for the other temporaries, except that *the patient should definitely not bite directly on the temporary* because it could fracture or be displaced.

---

1. Instead of a coping form, prefabricated stock acrylic crown form kits (also known as *polycarbonate crown forms*) are available.
2. A crown form is selected from a kit from a variety of teeth available in a shell of acrylic that fits over a prepared tooth structure.
3. Forms are anatomically correct, but length and width may need to be adjusted for a particular tooth.

CRITERIA FOR A PROPERLY CONTOURED ALUMINUM CROWN FORM

- The metal is adapted to margins of prepared tooth.
- Interproximal contact is established.
- Crown is in the plane of occlusion.
- Marginal ridge is contoured to the same height as abutment tooth/teeth.
- Interproximal contour is the same as natural tooth structure.
- Occlusion is adjusted to allow proper articulation.
- All areas of the crown are smooth, avoiding accumulation of debris.
- Excess cement is removed from all areas, especially the gingival sulcus.

PROCEDURE FOR A TEMPORARY ALUMINUM CROWN

The patient is scheduled to have tooth #4 prepared for a full-coverage cast alloy crown. The preparation and impression have been completed; temporization is the next step.

The operator is passed a temporary sizing device, which most aluminum crown form kits provide. The distance between the abutment teeth is measured by placing the device over the prepared occlusal surface of tooth #4 and measuring from distal to mesial. A number on each end of the measuring device correlates to the different lengths of prefabricated crowns. If the exact size is not available, select a crown form that is slightly larger to establish proximal contacts rather than selecting a smaller one with possibly light or no contacts.

The crown form is tried on the prepared tooth structure. Usually, if the initial placement of the crown form does not fit correctly, the goal is to determine whether the form will provide contact with the abutment teeth after it is trimmed. The form should not be placed back in the kit if it does not fit; it can be sterilized and replaced in the kit later if it has not been distorted.

The appropriate length of the crown is determined when the temporary tooth is placed. An explorer is held at the cervical margin, marking the exact location of the margin on the crown of the tooth. When the crown form is placed on the tooth and extends beyond this marked length, it is scored; this is accomplished by using the tip of the explorer to etch a line around the circumference of the crown at the location of the margin. The criterion for the length of the crown form is at or within 1 mm of the margin but not beyond the margin.

Another method can be used to determine the correct length of an aluminum crown form. When the crown is placed on a prepared tooth, the excess length on the form flairs out **festoons;** this flair of aluminum occurs at the site of the cervical margin, providing another guide to indicate the proper length to which the form should be trimmed. If the temporary crown is too long, the gingival tissues become irritated and inflamed, creating difficulties for the operator, who attempts to seat the permanent cast alloy restoration at a later appointment.

The operator uses the crown and collar scissors to trim the excess metal from the cervical area. The scissors are held parallel to the edge of the metal, and long, smooth strokes are used to cut around the circumference of the crown form. If the cuts are short and jerky, tags of aluminum are left, or the form may be distorted. As the cuts are made, the metal flairs out and the natural contour of the original form is not retained. The ball segment of the contouring pliers is placed inside the crown to contour the cervical of the form. The crown form is placed back on the tooth and the contouring is checked.

Cutting, contouring, and trying in the form may be done several times to ensure a correct fit. If at some point the proximal contact is open, it must be reestablished by placing the crown form occlusal side down on several 2 × 2 gauze sponges. A ball burnisher is positioned on the inside of the form at the marginal ridge area. Force is placed against the aluminum to press it out at the marginal ridge; this expands the aluminum crown and provides a marginal ridge contact for the form when it is placed on the tooth. The form is tried back on the tooth; if necessary, the step can be repeated until the ridge contact is reestablished.

Once the cervical margins and marginal ridge contact are correct, the occlusal contacts must be rechecked. If the contacts are high, the cervical margins must be recontoured to enable the form to be pushed down further on the tooth. The crown form is checked again, and once the objectives have been met, it is polished with a Cratex wheel, Burlew wheel, or other rotary instrument. Smoothing the metal surfaces eliminates areas of possible plaque accumulation on the crown form.

Continued.

PROCEDURE FOR A TEMPORARY ALUMINUM CROWN—cont'd

CEMENTATION OF THE TEMPORARY ALUMINUM CROWN

As with the acrylic intracoronal temporary, the lubricant is placed on the external surface of the crown form. The temporary cement is mixed and a thin layer placed inside the crown form, with some excess near the occlusal. The form is positioned, and a cotton roll is set on the occlusal surface; the patient is directed to close firmly, holding the cotton roll in place.

The operator checks the margins with an explorer to ensure proper placement of the form. If the form is short of the margins, the patient is directed to bite harder on the cotton roll, forcing the form to the cut length. Once the cement has set, the excess is removed with the instrument of choice—possibly a scaler, a spoon excavator, or an explorer. Floss is passed through both contacts and pulled to the lingual or buccal to avoid forcing any cement into the gingival sulcus or popping the temporary off the tooth. The articulation is checked again because the cementation may have left the crown form high. If this has happened, the operator can remove the high spot with a rotary instrument.

POSTOPERATIVE INSTRUCTIONS

After refinement of the temporary restoration is completed, the patient is given the following directions:
- Do not chew on that side of the mouth.
- Avoid sticky food as much as possible.
- Call the office if the crown becomes loose so that it can be recemented immediately, avoiding mesial drift and hypereruption and possible discomfort.

---

4. The forms are shells that can be customized to fit a tooth by using an acrylic wash inside the form and then positioning it over the prepared tooth.

5. Excess material is removed with rotary instruments and contoured as previously described.

6. Adaptation of the crown form with an acrylic wash provides a stronger and better adjusted temporary that fits more accurately.

B. Temporary restorations from study model impressions
   1. A temporary crown can be made with the study model impression that is taken before the preparation of a tooth.
   2. If the tooth is intact and not fractured or decayed substantially, the alginate impression is used to make a form for a temporary.
   3. The acrylic is placed in the impression over the prepared tooth, and the impression with the acrylic is placed back in the patient's mouth.
   4. The acrylic is allowed to set, and both impression and acrylic are removed.
   5. The acrylic is separated from the impression and is trimmed, contoured, and cemented in place.

C. Temporary bridges
   1. When teeth are being prepared for a bridge to replace a missing tooth (or teeth), a temporary bridge must be placed in the period between preparation of the abutment teeth and placement of the permanent bridge.
   2. Many of the techniques described can be used, but the need for the temporary restoration is similar to that for any other: provision for covering the teeth temporarily, maintaining space, aiding in mastication, and providing comfort and an esthetically pleasing appearance.

Questions

Temporary Restorations

1 Temporary bridges are used for
1. Aesthetics
2. 1 week or less
3. Mastication
4. Investing procedures
5. Lessened thermal sensitivity
a. 1, 2, and 3
b. 1, 3, and 5
c. 2, 3, and 4
d. 3, 4, and 5

2 The common reasons for placing a temporary restoration include all *except* which of the following?
   a. Prevent drifting
   b. Prevent hypereruption
   c. Aid in mastication
   d. Aid in creation of the permanent restoration
   e. Provide aesthetics

What type of temporary restoration could be used for the teeth involved in each of the situations listed in items 3-7?
   a. Full-coverage acrylic crown
   b. Full-coverage metal crown
   c. Intracoronal
   d. Acrylic bridge

   _____ **3** #3 to #5 are prepared for crowns
   _____ **4** #8 porcelain veneer crown
   _____ **5** #19^{MOD} inlay
   _____ **6** #28 porcelain veneer crown
   _____ **7** #31 full-coverage crown

8 Which of the following could be used as a temporary restoration for a posterior tooth that has been prepared for a full crown?
   1. Aluminum crown with acrylic wash
   2. Celluloid crown form with zinc phosphate cement
   3. Custom-made acrylic crown
   4. Intracoronal zinc oxide-eugenol
   5. Preformed aluminum crown
   a. 1 and 2
   b. 1 and 3
   c. 1, 3, and 4
   d. 1, 3, and 5

9 Trimming of the temporary crown margins to fit the prepared tooth is called
   a. Burnishing
   b. Border molding
   c. Festooning
   d. Crimping
   e. Contouring

10 On a properly trimmed temporary crown, the margins should fit the prepared tooth
   a. Subgingivally
   b. Supragingivally
   c. At or 1 mm short of the crown margins
   d. At or 1 mm beyond the crown margins

11 Complete removal of a temporary restoration from an inlay preparation is essential because the
   a. Cement will irritate the pulp
   b. Inlay will not seat completely
   c. Remaining cement will interfere with the set of the final cement
   d. Remaining cement will destroy the cavity varnish

12 Which of the following cements would be most appropriate for use when cementing a temporary crown?
   1. Zinc oxide-eugenol
   2. Glass ionomer
   3. Zinc phosphate
   4. Low-strength luting agent
   5. Zinc polycarboxylate
   a. 1 and 4

   b. 1, 2, and 5
   c. 1, 3, and 5
   d. All of the above

13 The advantages of using an acrylic wash in an aluminum temporary crown include which of the following?
   1. The wash provides an anodyne effect.
   2. Increased strength is provided.
   3. Removal is easier.
   4. Better retention is provided.
   5. The wash increases wear resistance.
   a. 1, 2, and 4
   b. 2 and 5
   c. 2, 3, and 4
   d. 2, 4, and 5

14 Which of the following would be appropriate as a temporary restoration on an anterior crown preparation?
   1. Zinc oxide-eugenol cement
   2. Celluloid crown form
   3. Polycarbonate crown form
   4. Aluminum preformed crown
   5. Custom-made acrylic crown
   a. 1 and 2
   b. 1 and 3
   c. 2 and 5
   d. 2, 3, and 5

15 Which of the following cements is ideal as an intracoronal temporary restoration?
   a. Zinc polycarboxylate
   b. Glass ionomer
   c. Zinc phosphate
   d. Zinc oxide-eugenol

16 Intracoronal temporary restorations can be inserted on which of the following preparations?
   1. Class I
   2. Class II
   3. Class III
   4. Class V
   5. Class VI (modified class II)
   a. 2 and 5
   b. 1, 2, and 5
   c. 1, 3, 4, and 5
   d. 1, 2, 3, 4, and 5

17 Which of the following describes clinically acceptable marginal ridges of an intracoronal temporary crown? They should
   1. Be cervical to the contact area
   2. Be at the same height as the adjacent tooth
   3. Be coronal to the contact area
   4. Follow the buccal and lingual contours of the tooth
   5. Be slightly higher than the adjacent tooth
   a. 2 and 4
   b. 1, 2, and 4
   c. 2, 3, and 4
   d. 2, 3, 4, and 5

18 If a properly trimmed aluminum crown flairs out at the cervical margin, you should do which of the following?
   1. Retrim the margins.
   2. Force the margins in with an explorer.

3. Cement and then contour the crown after the cement is set.
4. Use contouring pliers.
5. Check the margins with an explorer.
    a. 2 and 3
    b. 1 and 5
    c. 4 and 5
    d. 1, 4, and 5

19 Which of the following statements is true when referring to the placement of a temporary on a maxillary central incisor that has been prepared for a porcelain veneer crown?
    a. Full-coverage acrylic crown is seated with a secondary consistency of zinc oxide-eugenol.
    b. Full-coverage acrylic crown is seated with a primary consistency of zinc phosphate.
    c. Full-coverage acrylic crown is seated with a primary consistency of zinc oxide-eugenol.
    d. Intracoronal acrylic is seated with a primary consistency of zinc oxide-eugenol.
    e. Intracoronal temporary of zinc oxide-eugenol is mixed to secondary consistency placed directly into preparation.

20 To remove an intracoronal temporary, the choice of instrument would be which of the following?
    a. #2 bur on slow-speed handpiece
    b. #2 bur on high-speed handpiece
    c. Explorer
    d. Scaler

21 If a crown festoons, it should be
    a. Cut
    b. Contoured
    c. Cut and contoured
    d. Cemented immediately

22 If a metal crown does not abut to the cervical margin, the patient could experience which of the following?
    a. Nothing
    b. Gingival sensitivity
    c. Hypereruption
    d. Gingival and cold sensitivity

23 If a patient loosens a temporary crown a week prior to the seating appointment, the patient should be directed to do which of the following?
    1. Replace the crown on the tooth and wait for the appointment.
    2. Immediately come in for an appointment.
    3. Use a weak home glue to recement the crown.
    4. Avoid eating on that side of the mouth.
    5. Do nothing because the appointment is only a week away.
    a. 1 and 3
    b. 1, 3, and 4
    c. 2 and 4
    d. 2, 4, and 5

Place an A for *True* or a B for *False* for items 24 and 25.

_____ **24** It is important not to floss under a temporary bridge so that it is not accidently moved.

_____ **25** If a tooth is sensitive before the temporary crown

is cemented, it is advisable to cement it with a glass ionomer.

Rationales

Temporary Restorations

1 B Temporary bridges are used to maintain an esthetic appearance for the patient; they are usually in place for the time necessary to place the permanent bridge, and they assist the patient in mastication. A temporary bridge usually reduces thermal sensitivity for the prepared teeth while the patient is waiting for the permanent restorations.

2 D Temporary restorations prevent drifting and hypereruption and enhance the patient's ability to masticate. They reduce sensitivity, avoid further trauma to the tooth through injury or decay, and improve esthetic appearance.

3 D An acrylic three-unit bridge would be used on #3 and #5 with an acrylic pontic for #4 for protection and to avoid mesial drift.

4 A A full-coverage acrylic temporary would be placed on #8 for protection and esthetics.

5 C An intracoronal temporary constructed of acrylic or a cement mixed to secondary consistency are both options for temporary restorations.

6 A Because #28 is usually visible when a person smiles or talks, an acrylic temporary would likely be used to maintain esthetic value.

7 B #31 is a posterior tooth, and a full-coverage metal crown would likely be used. It is also possible to place an acrylic wash in the metal crown or create a full-coverage acrylic crown for this tooth according to operator preference.

8 D If the patient is not concerned about aesthetics in this area, an aluminum crown may be used. If the crown needs more of a customized fit and greater ability to withstand masticatory action, an acrylic wash may be used. However, if the patient is concerned about esthetics, an acrylic temporary would likely be constructed.

9 C When an aluminum crown is placed on a prepared tooth and the cervical edge extends beyond the crown margin, it flairs, or festoons. This flair must be removed and the cervical margin contoured to simulate the natural structure of the tooth.

10 C If the gingival margin of the temporary crown extends below the prepared margin of the tooth, it will cause gingival irritation and potential inflammation. If the crown is trimmed too short, it may not be retained on the tooth for the necessary time. A properly trimmed temporary crown should be at or 1 mm short of the gingival margins of the prepared tooth.

11 B Temporary cement left in a preparation that is to receive a cast restoration will interfere with the placement of the permanent restoration.

12 A A temporary crown is a restoration that will be removed in the near future. The choice of cement might be directed by the length of time the temporary is to remain in place (approximately 2-4 weeks). Zinc oxide-eugenol and low-strength luting cements are usually used to allow for easy removal during the cementation appointment for the permanent restoration.

13 D The placement of an acrylic wash in an aluminum crown increases the strength and resistance of the crown and customizes the fit, reducing the chance of the temporary being dislodged prematurely.

14 D See Nos. 4 and 13.

15 D Zinc oxide-eugenol cements are more easily removed from a cavity preparation than is zinc polycarboxylate, glass ionomer, or zinc phosphate cement. Zinc oxide-eugenol also offers an anodyne effect.

16 D Class I to Class VI cavity preparations are contained within the structure of the tooth and can accommodate intracoronal restorations.

17 C When a temporary restoration is created, it should reproduce tooth structure that previously existed or build the tooth to the ideal anatomic structure. This would include having the marginal ridge of the temporary restoration conform anatomically to the adjacent tooth, having the correct embrasure contact in the coronal areas, and maintaining continuity of the buccal and lingual planes in the quadrant.

18 D A crown that flairs at the cervical margin is too long and must be trimmed at or within 1 mm of the margins on the prepared crown. Once cut, the margins should be contoured to draw the margins of the temporary inward. Then the temporary should be replaced on the tooth and the margins checked with an explorer for length and smoothness.

19 C Usually in the anterior segment of the mouth a full-coverage acrylic crown is the temporary of choice and is cemented with a primary consistency of zinc oxide-eugenol so that it can be easily removed later.

20 D A scaler is an example of an instrument that may be used manually to remove an intracoronal temporary. If a temporary is removed with a rotary instrument, care must be taken to avoid removal of tooth structure.

21 C A festooned crown has excess length that should be cut to remove and recontoured to establish the correct fit of the temporary.

22 D If a cervical margin is open, the exposed tooth structure may be sensitive.

23 C If a temporary restoration is lost, the tooth may drift, be sensitive, or fracture; or it and the opposing tooth might hypererupt.

24 B The patient should be instructed as to proper flossing technique so that the temporary is not dislodged. Healthy tissue must be maintained; this includes flossing and brushing.

25 B A glass ionomer is not considered a temporary cement. Usually, a cement that decreases sensitivity is a zinc oxide-eugenol cement. A sensitive tooth might have a temporary for a longer time, or the operator may temporarily cement the permanent restoration to determine whether there are pulpal problems with the tooth prior to final cementation.

To enhance your understanding of the material in this chapter refer to the illustrations in Chapter 32 of Finkbeiner/Johnson: *Mosby's Comprehensive Dental Assisting: A Clinical Approach.*

Endodontics

To a patient, a referral or a visit to an endodontic practice indicates the need for root canal treatment. However, an endodontist provides many services beyond a root canal or pulpectomy. Although the pulpectomy— a complete removal of pulpal tissues—is one of the most common forms of treatment performed by this specialist, other procedures are performed as well, including pulpotomy, apicoectomy, root resections, replants, and bleaching of vital and nonvital teeth.

The endodontist must be concerned about the pulpal and periodontal tissues of the tooth. A symbiotic relationship exists between the pulp and periodontal ligament because of the existence of the apical foramen, dentinal tubules, lateral canals, and other accessory canals. It is possible to have a tooth with a primary endodontic lesion with secondary periodontal involvement (Fig. 22-1), likewise, a periodontally involved tooth may have secondary endodontic involvement. Clinical exami-

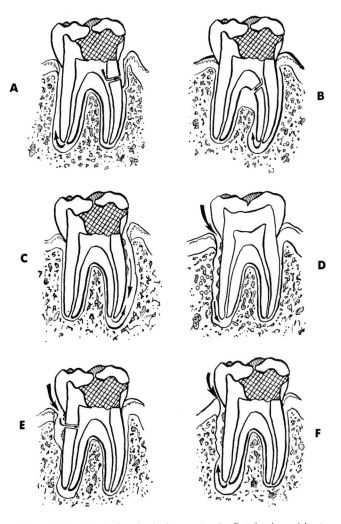

Fig. 22-1 Endodontic lesions: *A,* A fistula is evident through the periodontal ligament from the apex or from a lateral canal. *B,* Fistulation through the apex or a lateral canal, causing bifurcation involvement. *C,* Secondary periodontal involvement. With the passage of time the pathway through *A* will encounter plaque and calculus formation from the cervical line. Periodontal lesions. *D,* Progression of periodontitis to apical involvement, with vital pulp. *E,* Secondary endodontic involvement. The primary periodontal involvement at the cervical margin and the resultant pulpal necrosis, once the lateral canal is exposed to the oral environment, produce this condition. *F,* Combined lesions, coalescence. (From Cohen S, Burns RC: *Pathways of the pulp,* ed 6, St Louis, 1994, Mosby.)

nation of a tooth may indicate mobility; furcation or bone loss; sensitivity to percussion; or a draining sinus tract, canal, or passage that leads to an abscess in the gingival sulcus. Initially, the dentist may consider these symptoms an indication of periodontal disease, but to make a final diagnosis, the dentist must conduct a battery of tests to determine whether the tooth discomfort is due to an endodontic or a periodontic problem. The relation-

ship between these tissues also relates to the potential success or failure of endodontic treatment. For instance, a tooth that needs endodontic treatment but is supported by unhealthy periodontal tissues is not a good candidate for treatment unless the periodontal prognosis is good.

PULPAL PATHOSES

I.   Various diseases and injuries can cause the dental pulp to degenerate, resulting in the need for endodontic therapy.

II.   Table 22-1 outlines pulpal pathoses, symptoms, reactions to common diagnostic tests, and prognosis and treatment.

III. The following terms are commonly associated with pulpal pathoses:

A. **Hyperemia**—not a disease itself but the first stage of inflammation; indicated by an increased or excessive amount of blood in the pulpal tissue.

B. **Pulpitis**—inflammation of the pulpal tissue; like inflammation in any other body tissues, it is the response to an irritant that has injured the cells.

C. *Reversible pulpitis*—if pulpitis is treated in its early stages by removing the irritating factor and placing a sedative dressing before performing a permanent restoration, the prognosis is often good, and no further treatment may be needed. If untreated, the sequelae of pulpitis will include the following:

1. *Irreversible pulpitis*—inflammation of pulpal tissues progresses to an extent that no recovery is imminent.

2. **Granuloma**—pulpal inflammation progresses into the periapical tissues.

3. **Periodontal involvement**—pulpal disease can progress beyond the apical foramen and involve the periodontal ligament with the inflammation.

4. **Periapical abscess**—the inflammation process extends past the tooth apex and becomes a localized collection of exudate (pus); all tissue in the local area is destroyed in this highly acidic environment.

5. **Extraoral fistula**—this is a result of the body turning the abscess into a chronic lesion and creating a drainage to an outer or external surface.

6. **Cellulitis**—when the abscess spreads along facial planes, it can become a serious infection.

7. **Osteomyelitis**—a latent stage of the progression of a periapical infection, which re-

Table 22-1 Reactions to common endodontic diagnostic procedures

Symptoms	EPT/DPT	Heat	Cold	Percussion	Radiograph	Prognosis	Treatment
REVERSIBLE PULPITIS							
Acute pain, short duration, or clinically observed in dental radiograph	Positive	Normal, indicating vitality	Normal, indicating vitality	Negative	Caries invade dentin near pulp	Good—can return to normal, develop secondary dentin	Protection with sedative dressing; e.g., zinc oxide-eugenol cement
IRREVERSIBLE ACUTE PULPITIS							
Severe pain, increasing in duration and intensity. Analgesics often provide limited relief	Positive	Positive, may react more severely or be more prolonged than normal	Positive, may provide relief	Negative, unless inflammation spreads to periapical tissue	Negative for bone change	Pulp degeneration with a potential for recovery	Pulp extirpation/endodontic treatment
CHRONIC PULPITIS							
May be asymptomatic, often occurs in older patients in teeth that have been restored	Positive, may require more electric current to react	Excess amount needed to elicit reaction	Excess amount needed to elicit reaction	Negative	May note a resorption in canal; evidence of bone change	No recovery	Pulp extirpation/endodontic treatment; endodontic treatment or asymptomatic teeth as a prophylactic measure
ACUTE APICAL ABSCESS							
Severe pain; no relief from analgesics. Intraoral or extraoral swelling present. Possible draining sinus/fistula	Negative	No response	No response	Positive, often severe reactions	If early stage, no bone change; latent stage thickening of periodontal membrane	No recovery	(1) Establish drainage through occlusal/lingual, opening apex of tooth with file or incision of soft tissue (2) Prescribe antibiotic (3) Hot salt oral rinses

Symptoms	Test	Test	Test	Test	Radiographic	Recovery	Treatment
							(4) Medication for pain; narcotic optional (5) Treat endodontically at later date
NECROSES							
May be asymptomatic or may have had previous pain	Negative	No response	No response	Negative	No change evident	No recovery	Pulpectomy and endodontic treatment
CHRONIC APICAL PERIODONTITIS							
Mild degree of pain; sensitivity less than pulpitis. Tooth may feel high and discomfort is evident on biting or clenching teeth	Negative	No response	No response	Negative	Bone resorption evident; radiolucent lesion at apex	No recovery	Pulpal extirpation and endodontic treatment
ROOT FRACTURE							
May be asymptomatic; paresthesia may occur after traumatic blow; dull feeling	Negative	No response	No response	Painful	May indicate fracture, if extensive; hairline fractures may be blocked	No recovery	Extirpation and endodontic treatment; root removal or removal of tooth
CHRONIC APICAL SUPPURATIVE							
Draining sinus or gingival abscess is present; may be mild degree of pain	Negative	Negative	Negative	Negative	Radiolucent lesion at apex	No recovery	Pulpal extirpation and endodontic treatment

sults in the infection spreading into the bone.

8. **Actinomycosis**—this is a bacterial infection that spreads to the mouth, throat, and neck.

D. **Pulp stone**—a calcification that occurs in the coronal region of the pulp; typically, pulp stones have no clinical significance. However, they may increase in frequency and size with age or irritation; large pulp stones can complicate gaining access to a canal during root canal therapy.

INJURIES

I. Trauma to the teeth can generally be categorized as luxation injuries, avulsion injuries, alveolar fractures, or mechanical injuries to the pulp.

II. Luxation injuries
A. A tooth with luxation injury is generally sensitive to percussion and may have mobility.
B. A luxated tooth is one that has been moved from its normal physiologic position.
1. Extruded, displaced out of the socket, along its long axis
2. Intruded, forced into its socket in an axial or apical direction
3. Laterally luxated, rotated out of normal position from its long axis in a buccal, lingual, mesial, or distal direction
C. Depending on the extent of the injury, it may be necessary to reposition the teeth, splint the luxated teeth, or perform root canal treatment if evidence of irreversible pulpitis is apparent. Such injuries may require consultation with other specialists, including an orthodontist or oral maxillofacial surgeon.

III. Avulsion injuries
A. An avulsed tooth is one that has been knocked completely out of its socket.
B. The tooth can be **replanted;** however, time is crucial in the success of such treatment.
C. For immediate replantation the following instructions should be given to the patient or caregiver:
1. Rinse the tooth gently in tap water.
2. Do not scrub the tooth.
3. Gently place the tooth into the socket in as close to normal position as possible; the patient may bite down on a piece of soft fabric or handkerchief to help maintain the position.
4. See a dentist immediately.
D. If the tooth cannot be reinserted in the socket,

the following directions should be given to the person transporting the tooth:
1. Place a clean cloth over the site of the injury and ask the patient to bite on it.
2. Transport the patient and the tooth to the dental office immediately.
3. Transport the tooth in a liquid medium, such as saline, saliva, or milk; water is not considered a good medium for transport because it does not maintain the vitality of the periodontal ligament cells.
E. Time is the primary factor in the success of replantation; the patient should be brought to the office promptly and seen immediately upon arrival.
F. The procedure for replantation is provided (box on page 367).
G. Replantation of an avulsed deciduous tooth is not considered a primary treatment choice; however, if the tooth is to be retained for 1 to 2 years before natural exfoliation, the procedure may be an effective method of space maintenance.

IV. Alveolar fracture
A. During a traumatic blow an alveolar fracture may occur and pulpal **necrosis** may develop.
B. Typically, an oral maxillofacial surgeon sees the patient when a traumatic injury occurs, but the follow-up visit with the general practitioner or endodontist should include periodic radiographs and vitality tests to determine whether root canal treatment will be necessary.

V. Mechanical injury
A. This type of injury is usually the result of trauma from a handpiece.
1. When an area of decay is close to the pulp, mechanical exposure results.
2. Trauma may occur is the patient bites down on a handpiece, resulting in pulpal trauma.

DIAGNOSIS

I. The components of most endodontic procedures include the following:
A. Complete dental and medical history
B. Clinical evaluation
C. Diagnosis
D. Presentation of a treatment plan
E. Treatment procedure
F. Recall appointment for follow-up visit

II. Initially, the patient calls the dental office to report a problem. To determine whether a tooth has potential endodontic involvement, the following questions are beneficial:

REPLANTATION OF TEETH WITH LESS THAN 2 HOURS EXTRA-ALVEOLAR TIME

- Are all universal barrier techniques being used?
- Is all of the armamentarium available and prepared for use?
- Are the instruments arranged in order of use?
- Are you prepared for alternative treatment plans?
- Is the necessary equipment turned on and ready to operate?

The following procedure begins when the patient has arrived in the office with the avulsed tooth.

1. Place the tooth in a cup of saline.
2. Radiograph the area of injury; look for evidence of alveolar fracture.
3. Examine the avulsion site carefully for any loose bone fragments that can be removed.
4. Gently irrigate the socket with saline; it is not necessary to remove blood clots.
5. Remove the tooth from the cup of saline with extraction forceps to avoid handling the root surface.
6. Examine the tooth for debris, which, if present, can be removed with cotton pliers.
7. Reinsert the tooth into the socket; after partial insertion, using the forceps, the rest of the procedure can be accomplished by gentle finger pressure or letting the patient bite on a 2 × 2 gauze until the tooth is seated.
8. Check the tooth for proper alignment; avoid hyperocclusion.
9. Stabilize the tooth for 1 to 2 weeks with a nonrigid splint.
10. Prescribe antibiotics as needed for mild to moderate oral infections. A tetanus booster injection is recommended if the last one was administered more than 5 years earlier.
11. Supportive care includes a soft diet and mild analgesics as needed.

REPLANTATION OF TEETH WITH MORE THAN 2 HOURS EXTRA-ALVEOLAR TIME

The following procedure begins when the patient has arrived in the office with the avulsed tooth.

1. Examine the patient and the area of tooth avulsion; examine the radiographs for evidence of alveolar fractures.
2. Examine the tooth and remove debris and any pieces of soft tissue that may be adhering to the root surface.
3. Soak the tooth in a fluoride solution for at least 5 minutes.
4. Extirpate the pulp and fill the root canal while holding the tooth in a fluoride-soaked piece of gauze. Often, the root canal procedure can be accomplished from an apical direction if the tooth is not completely mature.
5. Carefully suction the alveolar socket; for this type of replantation, it is beneficial to remove blood clots. Irrigate the socket with saline (an anesthetic may be required first).
6. Gently replant the tooth into the socket; check for proper alignment and occlusal contact.
7. Stabilize the tooth for 1 to 2 weeks.

- Are the appropriate universal barrier techniques removed?
- Have all appropriate surfaces been cleaned and disinfected?
- Has all of the armamentarium been removed?
- Has all equipment been repositioned?
- Has all equipment been disinfected/sterilized according to OSHA guidelines?

A. Which tooth is causing the pain?

B. Describe the pain. When does it bother you? Does anything trigger the pain, such as hot or cold temperatures?

C. How long does the pain last?

D. Do you ever get any relief? If so, how?

E. Does the pain keep you awake at night?

DIAGNOSTIC TESTS

I. Medical/dental history

    A. Special attention is given to previous accidents or traumatic injuries that may now be the cause of a devital tooth.

    B. Complaints about a specific tooth over time may also aid in diagnosing the tooth in question.

II. Endodontic charting

    A. Endodontists use a specially designed chart to record pertinent findings.

III. Clinical examination

    A. External tissues are first observed to identify facial asymmetry and determine whether edema exists that may be caused by dental pathosis or trauma.

    B. An external fistula may indicate a draining sinus from intraoral tissues.

    C. During the intraoral examination attention should be given to the following:

1. *Discolored teeth*—teeth with necrotic pulp are often darker or less translucent than healthy teeth.
2. *Soft tissue lesions*—periapical or periodontal abscesses may be identified by areas of bony or soft tissue swelling; draining sinuses in the vestibular or palatal area may be traced to a chronic abscess.
3. *Fractured teeth*—hairline fractures of the enamel may go undetected and extend to the dentin, resulting in pulpal damage.
4. *Deep caries or extensive restoration*—caries that have extended to the pulp generally do irreparable damage to the pulpal tissue.
5. *Malocclusion*—constant traumatic occlusion may result in damage to the periapical and pulpal tissues.

IV. Radiographs
   A. Periapical, Panorex, and bitewing radiographs are valuable diagnostic tools in endodontics when used in conjunction with other diagnostic tests.
   B. Radiographs in the endodontic diagnosis have several limitations and should not alone be considered a conclusive diagnostic tool.
   C. Radiographs are only two dimensional, and a variety of angles may be needed to create a three-dimensional perspective.
   D. Pathologic changes in the early stages of pulpitis or periapical disease may not be visible on radiographs.
   E. Periapical lesions are noted in radiographs only as the inflammatory process spreads into its latent stages, when a break in the lamina dura or the presence of a granuloma is evident.
   F. Buccal object rule
      1. The **buccal object rule** defines the buccolingual relationship between two superimposed structures.
      2. To apply this rule, two radiographs are taken—the first using standard periapical technique.
      3. The second radiograph is made in the same way, except that the tube is shifted about 20 degrees in either the vertical or the horizontal angulation.
      4. When the two radiographs are compared, the buccal object appears to have moved in the opposite direction from the tube shift.
      5. The basic concept is *buccal opposite* when this rule is applied; thus, if a radiograph were taken of a mandibular molar and the vertical angulation increased by moving the beam down, the buccal object would appear to have moved superiorly on the film.
   G. Periapical radiographs in endodontic diagnosis indicate the following:
      1. Presence of radiolucent areas
      2. Internal or external resorption or calcification of the pulp chamber or root canal
      3. Involvement of disease in the periapical or periodontal tissues
      4. Presence of pulp stones
      5. Bone loss and furcation involvement
   H. Bitewing radiographs in endodontic diagnosis can determine the extent of dental caries and the level of bone loss
   I. Panoramic radiography in endodontic diagnosis can aid as follows:
      1. Determine conditions evident in a periapical radiograph
      2. Gain a broader perspective of the entire oral cavity
      3. Compare adjacent and opposing structures

V. Percussion test
   A. This test is frequently done by tapping the handle of a mirror on the symptomatic tooth.
   B. A tooth with a periapical lesion causes sharp pain or severe discomfort.
   C. A devital tooth or a fracture may result in a dull thudlike sound or no response at all.

VI. Bite test
   A. This test is similar to the percussion test.
   B. Ask the patient to bite normally, or place a cotton roll or a tongue blade wrapped with gauze over the suspected tooth and ask the patient to bite.
   C. If the patient indicates discomfort while biting on a specific tooth, additional tests can be conducted to verify the findings.

VII. Palpation test
   A. Similar to the percussion and bite tests, the palpation test helps determine the extent of inflammation in the periapical tissues.
   B. Pressure is applied with a gloved finger over the apical region of the suspected tooth.
   C. If the patient reacts to this pressure by indicating that pain is present, the inflammation evidently has invaded the periapical tissues and is present in the bone and mucosa of the apical region.
   D. Mobility of the tooth can also be determined at this time by using two gloved fingers to create lateral pressure on the tooth.
   E. If the mobility exceeds a Class III level, the tooth likely has little periodontal support and

may not be a candidate for successful endodontic treatment.

VIII. Thermal test

A. A *cold test* uses dry ice (CO_2), refrigerant (ethyl chloride), or regular ice that is made into an ice stick by freezing water in the non-injection end of a protective needle cover or in prefabricated ice sticks.

   1. The stick is held between the gloved fingers and placed on the labial or buccal surface.

   2. A vital tooth responds with a sharp pain that quickly disappears when the ice is removed.

   3. If the sharp pain increases in intensity and persists even after the ice is removed, an irreversible pulpitis probably exists in the tooth.

   4. In necrotic teeth no response occurs with cold stimulation.

B. A *heat test* is performed by placing a heated instrument (such as a ball burnisher) directly on the tooth, by heating gutta-percha in a Bunsen burner and applying it to the tooth, or by rotating a dry rubber prophylaxis cup on the tooth to create frictional heat.

   1. When heat is applied to the isolated tooth, the temperature gradually increases until pain is elicited.

   2. A sharp, nonlingering pain indicates a vital tooth; a sharp, nonsubsiding response generally indicates irreversible pulpitis.

   3. A lack of response indicates a necrotic pulp.

C. The suspected tooth and comparison teeth are isolated and dried with cotton pellets.

IX. Electronic pulp test (EPT)/digital pulp test (DPT)

A. Electronic pulp testers are powered by direct electric current or batteries, providing a high-frequency current that creates an electrical stimulus to generate a reaction in the tooth.

B. The difference between an EPT and a DPT is the method of providing the readout—the DPT provides a digital readout.

C. Both testers operate similarly.

   1. The tooth is isolated and dried and a saliva ejector is placed.

   2. A small amount of toothpaste or similar medium is placed on the tip of the electrode; the tip is then placed on the labial or buccal surface of the tooth.

   3. Care should be taken to place the tip on the natural tooth surface and not on a restored surface or on gingival tissue.

   4. As the test begins, the rheostat on the tester is slowly advanced to increase the amount of current until a response is indicated.

   5. The typical recording on most pulp testers is from 0 to 10; the higher the reading, the greater the amount of current needed to create the stimulus, indicating that the tooth is probably devital.

X. Periodontal probing

A. Aids in determining the periodontal status of the tooth

B. Lends credence to the prognosis for endodontic treatment

XI. **Transillumination**

A. This allows for a concentrated amount of intense light to pass through a tooth from the lingual to the labial surface.

B. In a necrotic tooth the outline of the pulp chamber is visible as a dark outline.

XII. Test cavity

A. This is the least common diagnostic test.

B. When no definitive diagnosis can be made, an opening is made (without anesthesia) in the occlusal or lingual surface of the tooth through the enamel or an existing restoration.

C. If, during this opening procedure, the patient indicates pain from the heat of the handpiece as the bur reaches the dentin, it can be determined that the tooth has vitality and can negate a previous devital diagnosis.

D. A permanent restoration can then be placed.

XIII. When endodontic treatment has been confirmed, a consent form must be reviewed with the patient and signed by the patient or responsible party.

ANESTHESIA

I. Anesthesia is an important component of endodontics.

II. Even in a tooth that is necrotic and has a periapical lesion, vital tissue exists in the apical region of the root canals.

III. Anesthesia is frequently used in the initial appointments, although it may not be necessary in the **obturation** appointment.

IV. Traditional anesthetic techniques used in endodontics include the following:

A. A maxillary division block can be used.

B. An inferior alveolar block can be used.

C. Intraligamentary injections can be administered.

D. An infiltration may also be used as the dentist attempts to block any accessory nerves that lead to the tooth.

E. An intrapulpal injection that is placed di-

BENEFITS OF RUBBER DAM ISOLATION FOR ENDODONTIC TREATMENT

- Improves visibility
- Reduces salivary leakage to promote a dry field
- Decreases exposure to cross-contamination
- Confines intracanal irrigants and medicaments to eliminate distaste to the patient
- Decreases interference of soft tissues
- Increases patient comfort
- Increases efficiency
- Improves standard of care (all U.S. dental schools require the use of rubber dam during endodontic procedures; its use obviously decreases potential negligence)

---

rectly into a vital and sensitive pulp may be needed.

V. Achieving profound anesthesia often is difficult in patients with highly inflammatory conditions.

ISOLATION

I. The isolation method of choice in endodontic treatment is the rubber dam.
  A. The benefits of rubber dam isolation are listed (box).
  B. Light-colored dam material is often chosen because it allows for greater illumination. Also, because it is somewhat transparent, the lighter color aids in film placement when radiographs are taken.
  C. A medium-weight dam is often chosen because it is relatively easy to apply and can eliminate salivary leakage.

II. The choice of frames is a concern.
  A. A metal frame is radiopaque and must be removed when the radiograph is taken.
  B. The Nygaard-Ostby and the Star Visi frames are radiolucent and need not be removed during radiographic exposure.

III. Clamps, metal or plastic, used in endodontics are the choice of each dentist or may not be used.

IV. Only one hole is required.

ENDODONTIC RADIOGRAPHY DURING TREATMENT

I. For diagnosis and treatment the film must not be bent, and the image must not be distorted.

II. Special film holders, including the Endo Ray, Easy Grip IIE, and the Snap-a-Ray, aid in positioning the film and preventing movement or bending of the film.

III. When the rubber dam is in place, a hemostat is used and the patient is asked to hold the film in place to avoid the interference of the beaks in the film.

IV. Position the film to provide a clear and complete view of the apex of the tooth.

V. Eliminate elongation and foreshortening.
  A. Such errors can distort length for the dentist during biomechanical preparation.
  B. Use the paralleling technique to avoid distortion and provide greater clarity in the film.

VI. Improperly processed film can make a diagnosis difficult.

VII. Radiographs can be used during treatment for the following purposes:
  A. Determine the shape, number, location, and direction of the root canals
  B. Determine the length of the canal before biomechanical preparation
  C. Verify working or trial length of files during biomechanical preparation
  D. Verify malpositioned or broken files
  E. Confirm location of **master cone**
  F. Examine final root canal filling
  G. Observe and evaluate surgical treatment site
  H. Evaluate tissue changes at recall appointment

VIII. Processing radiographs during endodontic treatment need to be processed quickly.
  A. During root canal therapy and endodontic surgical procedures, traditional processing time is prohibitive.
  B. Processing time can be decreased by increasing the strength of the developer and fixer; in some instances, the temperature of the solutions must be increased.
  C. The film is immersed in the developer for about 5 to 10 seconds, rinsed, and then placed in the fixer for about 15 to 20 seconds, until the film is clear.
  D. Specialized tanks can be purchased for endodontic use (such as the Chairside Darkroom).

STERILIZATION

I. Sterilization of endodontic instruments is similar to that of other dental instruments.

II. Two factors pose potential complications to successful treatment:
  A. Evidence of stress, fatigue, or damage to the fine delicate intracanal instruments is a factor. Small instruments (such as #8, #10, or #15) are disposable and are discarded after only one use.

B. Larger instruments can be reused for one or more cases after sterilization, but they lose cutting efficiency with reuse. Examine each instrument at the time of sterilization and again before it is inserted into a canal to ensure that it is free of stress or damage.

III. Steam and dry heat may be used for sterilization of endodontic instruments according to manufacturers' recommendations.
   A. If steam is used, the instruments must be protected with a protective emulsion to avoid damage.
   B. Some dentists prefer to avoid the emulsion and use dry heat instead.
   C. Dry heat poses potential damage to delicate instruments because of the high heat over a long period.

IV. At chairside, a small, rapid method of sterilization is often needed, which can be accomplished by using a salt sterilizer.

SPECIALIZED ENDODONTIC INSTRUMENTS ▬

I. Table 22-2 describes common endodontic instruments.

II. Endodontic instruments can be divided into the following basic categories:
   A. Examination and preparation
   B. Intracanal (Table 22-3)
   C. Cleansing
   D. Medicating
   E. Obturation
   F. Surgical
   G. Miscellaneous

INTRACANAL MEDICATIONS AND SOLUTIONS ▪

I. Irrigation solution
   A. An irrigating solution is used primarily as a biomechanical cleaning agent to flush the canal free of debris.
   B. It should be nontoxic, allow the instruments to slide freely into the canal, act as a disinfectant, be a tissue solvent when possible, and be relatively inexpensive.
   C. *Sodium hypochlorite (NaOCl)* (household bleach) is the most common biomechanical cleaner.

II. Dentin softeners
   A. Their function is to remove mineral deposits (such as calcium) from the dentin.
   B. These products, known as *chelators,* remove metallic ions (such as calcium and decalcifiers), which are chemicals that remove mineral salts in solution.

C. Two common chelators are ethylenediamine-tetra-acetic acid and dilute citric acid.

III. Lubricants
   A. These help the dentist gain access to the full length of the canal during filing.
   B. They can also help the dentist negotiate small constricted canals.
   C. These substances do not dissolve tissue.
   D. Glycerin is a sterile, inexpensive, and nontoxic substance that works effectively as a lubricant; it is water soluble and can be removed from the canal easily after its use.

IV. Canal medication
   A. This is considered significant in providing comfort and preventing pain after biomechanical preparation, providing antimicrobial action in the pulp and periapical tissues, and neutralizing the canal remnants to make them inert.
   B. Three medications are used in endodontics:
      1. Formocresol (FC)
      2. Camphorated monochlorophenol (CMCP)
      3. Calcium hydroxide (CaOH)
   C. Medicaments are applied with a small cotton pellet (the size of the access opening) that is saturated in the substance.
   D. The pellet is tapped dry on a sterile gauze and then placed into the coronal portion of the pulp chamber; it is then sealed in place with a temporary cement and remains until the next appointment (within 3 to 10 days).

PULPOTOMY ▬▬▬

I. A **pulpotomy** is indicated when trauma occurs to the pulp of a tooth in a young child—due to an accident or extensive dental caries. The apical constriction is probably not complete, and the root may have an open apex.

II. Two treatment alternatives include the following:
   A. **Apexification,** performed on a tooth with necrotic pulp, is the process of creating an environment within the root canal and periapical tissues to allow a calcified barrier to form across the open apex.
      1. It involves cleaning and shaping the root canal to remove toxic agents and bacteria, drying the canal with absorbent paper points that are inserted into the canal, and placing a radiopaque calcium hydroxide paste into the canal.
      2. The access opening is closed with a zinc oxide-eugenol cement and then a permanent cement.

Text continues on page 376.

Table 22-2   Common endodontic instruments

Instrument/device	Purpose	Distinguishing characteristics

GATES GLIDDEN DRILL	• Facilitates preparation of the canal
	• Aids in opening access to canal
	• Removes curvature of the orifice
	• Prepares tooth for a post
		• Long-shanked rotary device
		• Elliptically shaped with cutting end resembling a football
		• Used with latch-type, slow-speed handpiece
		• Rotates clockwise
		• Available in six sizes
		• #1 size = #50 K-style file
		• Scribed mark on side of shank indicates size: single indentation
		  = #1, double = #2, etc.
		• Designed as a safe tip instrument; a hole must be made before
		  instrument is used

PEESO REAMER	• Widens coronal access quickly • Opens the orifice • Aids in removing curvatures of the orifice • Used in canal in conjunction with enlarging instruments • Used intermittently with modern rotation	• Long-shanked rotary instrument with sharp parallel flutes • Tungsten carbide • Available in six sizes • #1 size = #70 K-style file • Scribed mark on side of shank indicates size: single indentation = #1, double = #2, etc.

ORIFICE BUR	• Used to roughly enlarge root canal after instrumentation is
	  complete
	• Excavation of root caries
	• Opens orifice or difficult bicuspid and molar root canal
	• Opens tooth to drain canal
		• Flame-shaped rotary device resembling Gates Glidden drill
		• Used on latch-type contra-angle
		• Available in only one or two sizes, commonly has 1.6 mm
		  diameter

ENDODONTIC EXPLORER	• Probes the chamber and canals • Identifies location of canals	• Long shank • Generally doubled ended • Common sizes are #2, #16, #17 (right angle at one end), and shepherd's hook
ENDODONTIC SPOON	• Aids in removing debris and other materials from chamber • Aids in placing temporary in canal	• Long shank • Spoonlike shape • Generally double ended
ENDODONTIC PLIERS	• Grasp instruments and points for transport to canals • Locking style permits transport without loss of material	• Central groove along axis • Available in locking or nonlocking • Commonly about 6 inches long

PLASTIC INSTRUMENT	• Used to place and pack temporary filling material into chamber
	  area
		• Many style available
		• Common styles include nib, paddle, ball, or condenserlike
		  working end

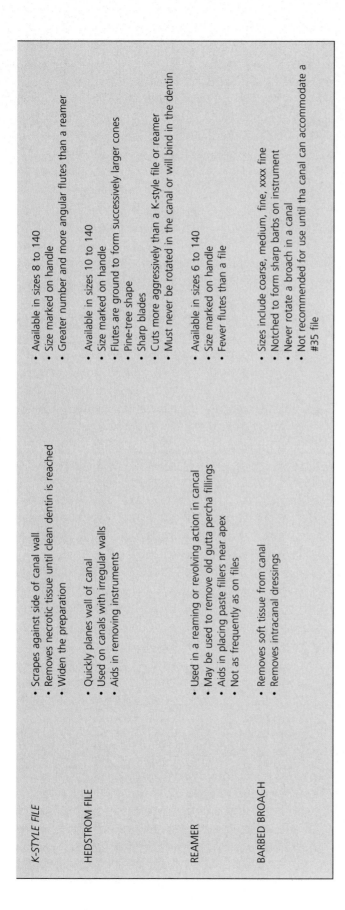

K-STYLE FILE

- Scrapes against side of canal wall
- Removes necrotic tissue until clean dentin is reached
- Widen the preparation

- Available in sizes 8 to 140
- Size marked on handle
- Greater number and more angular flutes than a reamer

HEDSTROM FILE

- Quickly planes wall of canal
- Used on canals with irregular walls
- Aids in removing instruments

- Available in sizes 10 to 140
- Size marked on handle
- Flutes are ground to form successively larger cones
- Pine-tree shape
- Sharp blades
- Cuts more aggressively than a K-style file or reamer
- Must never be rotated in the canal or will bind in the dentin

REAMER

- Used in a reaming or revolving action in cancal
- May be used to remove old gutta percha fillings
- Aids in placing paste fillers near apex
- Not as frequently as on files

- Available in sizes 6 to 140
- Size marked on handle
- Fewer flutes than a file

BARBED BROACH

- Removes soft tissue from canal
- Removes intracanal dressings

- Sizes include coarse, medium, fine, xxxx fine
- Notched to form sharp barbs on instrument
- Never rotate a broach in a canal
- Not recommended for use until tha canal can accommodate a #35 file

Table 22-2 Common endodontic instruments—cont'd

Instrument/device	Purpose	Distinguishing characteristics
LENTULO SPIRAL	• Carries and places root canal cement apically in clockwise rotation	• Delicate, flexible, strong, spring type • Used on latch-type contra-angle • Reverse spiral shape • Available in four to six sizes • Sizes range from 0.25 to 0.44 mm, smaller than most K-style files
FINGER PLUGGER	• Used with finger pressure for apical condensation of gutta percha	• Smooth, tapered with dull-tipped instrument shaped like a file with no flutes • Sizes from 15 to 40 consistent with standard file sizes
FINGER SPREADERS	• Used with finger pressure for lateral condensation of gutta percha	• Smooth, tapered, sharp-pointed instrument, shaped like a file with no flutes • Sizes from extra fine to medium
ENDODONTIC SPREADER	• Used manually for lateral condensation of gutta percha	• Long shank with pointed tips • Available in sizes equivalent to #25 to #40 K-style file • Single ended
ENDODONTIC PLUGGER	• Vertical condensation of gutta percha	• Long shank with dull tip • Single or double ended • Available in sizes equivalent to #25 to #85 K-type file
ROOT CANAL PLIERS	• Used to retrieve points, file, or other materials from canal • Transport and grasp materials for canals	• Grooved and serrated • May resemble hemostat or plier handle
ENDODONTIC UTILITY SCISSORS	• Used to cut gutta percha and paper points	• Typical scissor style • Delicate sharp beaks
RETRO MIRROR	• Used to observe retrograde filling at apex of tooth	• Small face • Angled shank to aid access
RETRO FILLING AMALGAM PLUGGERS	• Aid in placement of apical amalgam	• Resembles back action amalgam condenser • One end multiple angled, opposite end commonly at right angle • Small diameter of tip
RETRO AMALGAM CARRIER	• Transport small amount of amalgam to small retro fill preparations	• Carrier and diameter small: 3/64 to 5/64 inch • Delicate tip end • Resembles thumb forceps
MICROCONTRA-ANGLE	• Used for retrograde amalgam preparation	• Small head • Adjustable head

ENDO-HEAD CONTRA-ANGLE
- Aids in using specialized rotary devices
- Generally latch type
- Oscillating, quarter-turn movement
- Operates at speeds up to 3000 rpm
- Reduction-style contra-angles rotate at speeds between 500 and 1000 rpm
- Maintain high torque at low speeds

ENDODONTIC AMALGAM GUN
- To place apical amalgam
- Resembles anesthetic syringe
- Nozzles available, straight or angled
- Diameter of nozzle tips 1 to 1.5 mm

GUTTA PERCHA POINTS
- Used to obturate the canal
- Thermoplastic
- Compressible to adapt to shape of canal
- Radiopaque
- Dense, stiff, and unbreakable
- Soluble in chloroform
- Dimensionally stable when hardened
- Available in sizes equivalent to #15 to #140 K-style file

SILVER POINTS
- Used for obturation of canals
- Not frequently used today
- Rigid silver point
- Made of bactericidal silver
- Matched to sizes of standard K-style file #8 to #140
- Retains shape
- May be configured to fit curved canal

ABSORBENT PAPER POINTS
- Used to dry canals
- Introduce medication and sealers
- Culture canals
- Absorbent
- Made of high-quality bibulous paper
- Sterilized and nonsterilized available
- Can be sterilized
- Available in sizes equivalent to #15 to #140 K-style file

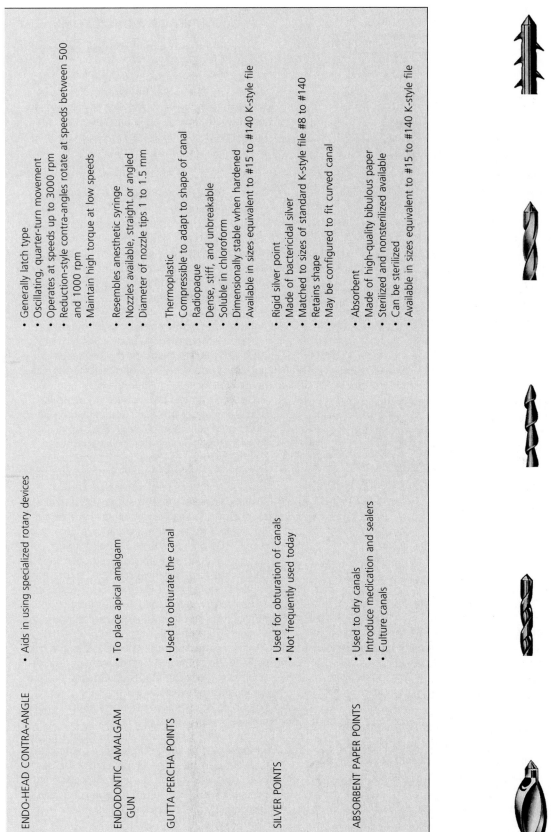

Gates Glidden drill

K-style file

Hedstrom

Reamer

Barbed broach

Table 22-3 Standardized sizes and handle colors of intracanal instruments

Size	Handle color code
08	Gray
10	Purple
15	White
20	Yellow
25	Red
30	Blue
35	Green
40	Black
45	White
50	Yellow
55	Red
60	Blue
70	Green
80	Black
90	White
100	Yellow
110	Red
120	Blue
130	Green
140	Black

ARMAMENTARIUM FOR A PULPOTOMY

Explorer
Mirror
Cotton pliers
Spoon excavator
Rubber dam setup
Sterile cotton pellets
Burs
   Opening: #34, #57, or other size
   Removing dentin and coronal pulp: #4 or #6
   (sterile)

Formocresol
Zinc oxide-eugenol
  cement
Permanent cement
Temporary crown setup

---

   3. The patient is recalled at a later date and the tooth is examined clinically and radiographically.
   4. If evidence of a calcified stop at the apex is apparent, routine root canal therapy can be performed.
  B. **Apexogenesis** is the treatment of a vital pulp by pulp capping or pulpotomy to permit continued closure of the open apex and growth of the root. This is the procedure of choice when possible.
III. The armamentarium for a pulpotomy is listed (box above).
IV. The procedure for a pulpotomy is provided (box).

PROCEDURE FOR A PULPOTOMY

1. The tooth is anesthetized, and the segment is isolated with a rubber dam.
2. The tooth is opened with a #34 bur on a high-speed handpiece, and the basic outline form is completed with a #57 bur. The cavity walls are extended to provide adequate access to the pulp chamber. The burs may need to be modified, depending on the amount of tooth structure previously lost to decay or the specific tooth involved.
3. A #4 or #6 round bur is used on the slow-speed handpiece to slowly remove the large carious lesion. A large spoon excavator may be used to aid in caries removal.
4. A round bur (#4, #6, or #8) is then used at low speed to remove the remaining dentin and expose the occlusal portion of the pulp chamber; this portion is **extirpated** to the level of the pulp canals.
5. With a sterile cotton pellet, pulpal debris is removed. Hemorrhaging is likely to occur, and the cotton pellets help control the bleeding. Do not use air because this will desiccate the pulpal tissue and contaminate the site.
6. Dip a sterile cotton pellet into formocresol and pass it to the dentist. The cotton pellet is placed in the pulp chamber for about 5 minutes.
7. After 5 minutes the cotton pellet is removed. The formocresol will have fixed or mummified the pulpal tissue that remains in the pulp canals. The pulpal stumps will appear dark brown.
8. A zinc oxide-eugenol cement is mixed, and a drop of formocresol is incorporated as part of the liquid. The cement is mixed to a secondary consistency and passed to the dentist with a cement plugger; the mix is placed over the pulpal stumps to a thickness of about 2 to 3 mm.
9. A permanent cement (such as zinc phosphate or polycarboxalate) could be inserted before the tooth is prepared for the stainless steel crown.
10. The final restoration may be placed at the dentist's discretion. If not placed, a temporary restoration is placed until it is determined that no postoperative complications exist.
11. The isolation is removed and the patient is dismissed.
12. The parent or caregiver for the patient should be instructed to contact the office immediately if severe discomfort develops. Before the patient leaves the office, the dentist provides instruction for pain medication (if needed) and explains any postoperative complications that might occur.

PULPECTOMY

I.   A **pulpectomy**—commonly called a *root canal*—is the complete removal of the pulp tissue from the pulp chamber to the dentinocemental junction at the apex of the root.

II.   This procedure can be done in a single appointment but commonly is done in two or three appointments (box below).

III. Stages of treatment include the following (Fig. 22-2):
   A. Opening
   B. Biomechanical preparation
   C. **Biomechanical cleansing**
   D. **Trial-point radiograph**
   E. Final cone radiograph
   F. Canal medication
   G. Temporization
   H. Obturation

IV.   Although it is possible to place a final restoration at the obturation appointment, a temporary will likely be placed.

V.   The armamentarium for the first appointment is listed (box on page 380).

VI.   The procedure for the first appointment is provided (box on page 380).

VII. The armamentarium for the second appointment is the same as for the first appointment; however, selection of the master cone may be added.

VIII. The procedure for the second appointment is provided (box on page 381).

IX.   The armamentarium for the obturation appointment is listed (box on page 381).

TYPICAL APPOINTMENT SEQUENCE FOR A PULPECTOMY	
INITIAL	
1. Anesthetize tooth if necessary.	9. Take trial-point radiograph.
2. Place rubber dam isolation.	10. Flush canals with NaOCl.
3. Disinfect treatment field.	11. Dry canals with sterile paper points.
4. Make occlusal opening for access.	12. Place intracanal medication.
5. Locate the root canals.	13. Place interim dressing in the occlusal opening and adjust occlusion.
6. Determine tooth length and set rubber stops for reference points.	14. Remove rubber dam.
7. Determine working length.	15. Provide patient with prescription for an antibiotic or analgesic if needed for inflammation or discomfort.
8. Complete biomechanical preparation of the canals.	
INTERIM	
1. Anesthetize tooth if necessary.	9. Flush the canal with NaOCl.
2. Place rubber dam isolation.	10. Dry the canal with absorbent paper points.
3. Disinfect treatment field.	11. Place intracanal medication.
4. Remove the interim dressing.	12. Place interim dressing in the occlusal opening and adjust occlusion.
5. Check for dryness of canals by placing a dry absorbent point in each canal.	13. Remove rubber dam.
6. Irrigate canals with NaOCl.	14. Provide patient with prescription for an antibiotic or analgesic if needed for inflammation or discomfort.
7. Complete the biomechanical preparation.	
8. Verify the length of the canal with a radiograph of the final size file in place.	
OBTURATION (FINAL)	
1. Anesthetize tooth if necessary.	8. Dry the canal with sterile absorbent points.
2. Place rubber dam isolation.	9. Select the master cone and adjust to final length.
3. Disinfect treatment field.	10. Take a trial-point radiograph with the master cone in place.
4. Remove the interim dressing.	11. Obturate the root canals.
5. Check for dryness of canals by placing a dry absorbent point in each canal.	12. Take a final radiograph.
6. Irrigate canals with NaOCl.	13. Place final or temporary restoration.
7. Place the final file to length to verify the canal length.	14. Remove rubber dam.

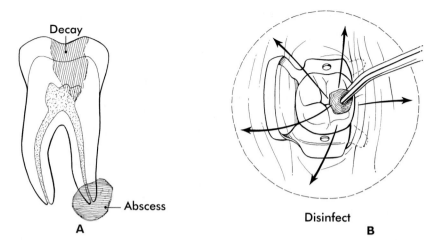

Decay

Abscess

A

Disinfect

B

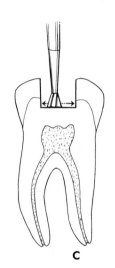

C

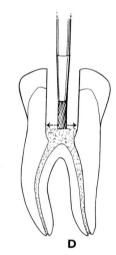

D

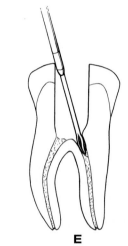

E

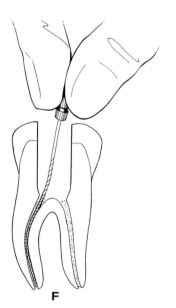

F

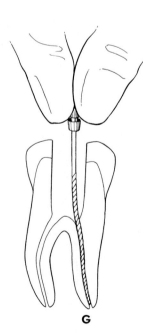

G

H

I

J

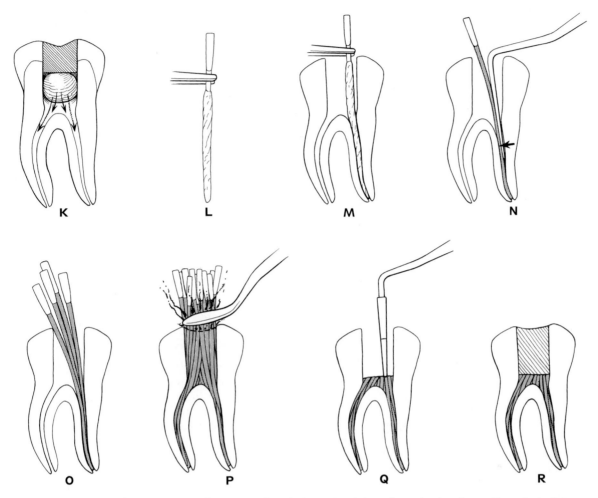

Fig. 22-2 Pulpectomy procedure. *A,* Carious lesion extends into the pulp chamber, with periapical involvement. *B,* Molar is isolated with rubber dam, and site is disinfected. *C,* Access to pulp chamber is accomplished with a round or inverted cone bur on high-speed handpiece. *D,* Enlargement and flaring of preparation are done with a fissure bur. *E,* Peeso reamer is used to gain access to canals. *F,* Intracanal instruments are angled to gain access to canals. *G,* Biomechanical preparation continues. During this phase the pulp chamber is flushed with sodium hypochlorite and the canals are shaped and cleaned. *H,* Radiographs are obtained to determine that the length of the files are not too long, *H,* are not too short, *I,* or are approximately 1 mm from the apical opening *J. K,* After the canals are flushed with sodium hypochlorite and dried with paper points, the tooth can be medicated with a cotton pellet that is saturated with formocresol or chlorbutanol, and a small amount of Cavit or ZOE cement can be placed over the pellet. *L,* Obturation will take place at a later appointment, with a gutta percha point that has been coated with a sealer. *M,* The master cone is placed into the canal, and laterally condensed, *N. O,* Auxiliary gutta percha cones are placed into the canal and laterally condensed. *P,* Both canals are filled, and the excess gutta percha is removed with a heated spatula. *Q,* A plastic instrument is used to condense the gutta percha in the coronal portion of the tooth. *R,* Temporary restoration is placed, and the patient is referred to the general dentist for a final restoration.

ARMAMENTARIUM FOR THE FIRST APPOINTMENT

Anesthesia setup
Rubber dam setup, with clamp for the appropriate tooth
Endodontic explorer
Mirror
Endodontic locking pliers
Endodontic excavator
Plastic instrument
Endodontic ruler
Irrigating syringe with NaOCl
Gauze sponges
Cotton pellets

Disinfectant
Cotton applicator (optional)
Endodontic tray with files, reamers, and broaches
File holder (optional)
Appropriate handpieces and contra-angles
HVE tips (standard and surgical)
Radiographic film
Film holder or hemostat
Temporary filling material

X. The procedure for the obturation appointment is provided (box on page 382).
XI. A recall appointment is scheduled.
  A. Follow-up on the patient who has had a pulpectomy is important.
  B. The appointment may be scheduled in 6 weeks and again in 3 to 6 months.
  C. The patient is seen at least every 6 months for the next 2 years.
  D. If the procedure was performed in a general-practice office, follow-up is often done at the patient's routine prophylaxis visit.
  E. At this recall appointment the intraoral tissues, tooth mobility, and tooth color are examined.
  F. Radiographs are taken to observe the periapical tissues.

PULPECTOMY: PROCEDURE FOR FIRST APPOINTMENT

1. The tooth is anesthetized if necessary.
2. Place the rubber dam isolation.
3. Disinfect the treatment field with a cotton applicator or cotton pellet that is dipped in disinfectant.
4. Make an occlusal opening for access to the canals. The assistant passes a high-speed handpiece with a #34 bur to the dentist and uses the HVE to evacuate fluid from the treatment site as it accumulates on the rubber dam. The dentist may exchange the #34 bur for a #57 or other bur to complete an outline form of the access opening.
5. Exchange the handpiece for an endodontic explorer to locate the root canals. *Do not blow air or spray water into the pulp chamber.* The dentist may wish to irrigate the site with NaOCL at this point. If so, pass the syringe; the assistant uses the HVE tip.
6. Pass a small file (usually a #10 or #15) to the dentist, who places the file into the canal to determine the length.
7. Determine tooth length and place the silicone stops on all files to be used. Pass the forceps periodically if the stop position needs to be adjusted.
8. Take a radiograph with the file in place, using the hemostat or film holder to position the film. After the length is determined, record it on the patient's record.
9. Biomechanical preparation of the canals is completed by passing files in numeric sequence, from smallest to largest, to the dentist. The dentist returns the used file; it is positioned on the tray or other holder while the dentist receives a new file. During the biomechanical preparation procedure the canal must always be kept moist with NaOCl.
10. Record the final file sizes to which the canal was filed. Other important information—such as unfound canals, file too short, or perforations—should be recorded on the patient's record.
11. The canal is flushed with NaOCl; the assistant removes any excess with the HVE.
12. Pass sterile paper points to the dentist to dry the canal. Two cotton forceps expedite this process.
13. The operator places the intracanal medication (foramocresol or chlorobutanol). Saturate the pellet with the medication, using a sterile forceps to enter the bottle. Tap the pellet dry on a sterile 2 × 2 gauze and pass it to the operator. Transfer a plugger or plastic instrument to push the pellet into place.
14. The plastic instrument can be used to insert the temporary cement. A small amount of Cavit or ZOE cement is prepared on the mixing pad and inserted into the occlusal opening. A small wet cotton pellet is used to smooth the occlusal surface of the material and secure the seal. This moist pellet also accelerates the material's setting time.
15. Remove the rubber dam and rinse the patient's mouth. Make certain the patient's face is clean and free of debris. The occlusion is checked with articulating paper. If adjustment is needed, a spoon excavator, a condenser, or an occlusal carver may be used.
16. Provide postoperative instructions.
17. Record any final instructions to the patient on the record and dismiss the patient.

PULPECTOMY: PROCEDURE FOR SECOND APPOINTMENT

1. Tooth is anesthetized if necessary.
2. Place rubber dam isolation.
3. Disinfect treatment field with a cotton applicator or a cotton pellet in forceps that is dipped in disinfectant.
4. Pass a spoon excavator to remove the interim dressing.
5. Pass sterile paper points to the operator to be inserted into each canal to check for dryness of canals or a purulent odor.
6. Pass the irrigating syringe to irrigate the canals.
7. Complete the biomechanical preparation.
8. Verify the length of the canal with a radiograph of the final size file in place.
9. Flush the canal with NaOCl.
10. Dry the canal with absorbent paper points.
11. Place intracanal medication.
12. Place interim dressing and adjust occlusion.
13. Remove rubber dam.
14. Provide patient with prescription for an antibiotic or analgesic if needed for inflammation or discomfort. If a prescription was given at the first appointment, instructions for completion of the prescription should be clarified.

ARMAMENTARIUM FOR THE OBTURATION APPOINTMENT

Rubber dam setup with clamp for the appropriate tooth
Endodontic explorer
Mirror
Endodontic locking pliers
Endodontic excavator
Plastic instrument
Endodontic spreader
Absorbent paper points
Heat source
Root canal pluggers
Master cone or filling material
Auxiliary cones as needed
Root canal sealer

SURGICAL ENDODONTICS

I. Drainage of an **apical abscess** is done to remove pressure and pain.
   A. The armamentarium for this procedure is listed (box on page 383).
   B. The procedure is provided (box on page 383).
   C. Written postoperative instructions are given to the patient (box on page 383).
II. A **hemisection** is the process of surgically removing a single root from a multirooted tooth, leaving the remaining root or roots intact.
III. Root amputation is not significantly different from a hemisection.
   A. It is more commonly done on maxillary than mandibular teeth.
   B. It involves the surgical removal of one or more roots on a multirooted tooth.
   C. The entire crown is left intact, and endodontic therapy is performed on the remaining root(s).

IV. **Bicuspidization** is a surgical procedure in which two premolars (bicuspids) are created from a mandibular molar. This procedure is used when severe bone loss is confined to the furcation area.
V. An **apicoectomy** is the surgical removal of the apex or apical portion of a root.
   A. It is indicated when traditional endodontic therapy has not been successful in the following situations:
      1. It is impossible to eliminate apical pathosis resulting from root perforation, root fracture, or recurring apical disease.
      2. It is impossible to debride and fill the entire root using the traditional coronal approach, such as in teeth with severe root curvatures or calcified canals.
      3. Treatment has failed because of broken instruments, apical perforation, or incomplete canal obturation.
   B. The procedure for an apicoectomy is provided (box on page 383).
   C. Written postoperative instructions are given to the patient (box on page 383).

BLEACHING

I. Teeth may become discolored for various reasons.
II. Natural or acquired stains are caused by pulpal necrosis; developmental defects in the enamel are caused by fluorosis, systemic drugs (such as tetracycline), or systemic diseases.
III. *Iatrogenic* or *inflicted* stains are often caused by chemicals or materials used in dentistry.

PULPECTOMY: PROCEDURE FOR OBTURATION APPOINTMENT

1. Anesthetize tooth if necessary.
2. Place the rubber dam isolation.
3. Disinfect the treatment field.
4. Pass the excavator to remove the interim dressing. Exchange the spoon for an explorer, if necessary, to remove the cotton pellet. Use the HVE to remove the debris from the opening. *Do not irrigate the canals.*
5. The canals are checked for dryness. Pass dry absorbent points to the dentist to place in each canal.
6. Pass the irrigating syringe to the dentist and place the HVE near the tooth that is to receive irrigating fluids.
7. Pass the final files on which silicone stops have been set to final working length. The files are placed in the canals to reorient the dentist and verify that the length is correct and the canals have been filed to completion. A radiograph may be taken.
8. Pass the irrigating syringe to the dentist for final irrigation, followed by a series of paper points to dry the canal. Use two cotton forceps to expedite this procedure.
9. The dentist will select the master cone and adjust it to final length; the assistant can then place the cone in a chairside sterilizer or petri dish filled with full-strength NaOCl. Allow the points to remain for at least 1 minute. Remove the master cone from the disinfectant and blot it dry on a sterile gauze or towel.
10. Pass the master cone to the dentist to insert into the appropriate canals. If the cone needs to be adjusted, pass a pair of curved crown and collar scissors to the dentist to cut off the excess.
11. Once the master cone is adjusted and seated in place, pass a cotton forceps to the dentist to check the cone seating for snugness of fit. Take a trial-point radiograph with the master cone in place. Develop the film and pass it to the dentist to verify the correct length. If the points are correct, proceed to the obturation step. However, steps 9 and 10 may need to be repeated if the master cone is not the correct length; it may even be necessary to return to the filing procedure. Be prepared to repeat any of the necessary steps.
12. The dentist removes the cone from the canal and passes it to the assistant. Place the points on a sterile towel or gauze. If multiple canals are being filled, place the points in a specific order that can be identified for each canal.
13. Place the final point and auxiliary points in the disinfectant solution. After 1 minute, remove them from the dish and dry them thoroughly on a dry towel.
14. Mix the root canal sealer on a sterile slab according to the manufacturer's directions. Select a file one or two sizes smaller than the final file size. Pass the file to the dentist and hold the mixing slab with the sealer in the passing zone. The dentist saturates the file with the sealer and places it in the canal, rotating the file counter clockwise with a pumping action. The objective is to coat the walls but not fill the canal with sealer.
15. Pass the master cone to the dentist, using the cotton forceps. Position the sealer nearby if the dentist prefers to dip the master cone tip in some of the sealer. The dentist then seats the master cone.
16. Pass the spreader to the dentist. Prepare to pass the auxiliary cones until the canal is filled. After each use, wipe the excess sealer off the spreader with a gauze sponge. If multiple canals are to be filled, this process is repeated for each canal.
17. Heat a plastic instrument or plugger in a flame until it is warm enough to melt the gutta percha inside the crown of the tooth. Pass it to the dentist to place the instrument into the crown of the tooth and remove the excess gutta percha. Use the HVE tip near the tooth to pick up any smoke that may be created. Wipe the end of the plugger with a piece of gauze. Repeat this procedure if necessary. The dentist may want to use the plugger again to pack the remaining gutta percha into the occlusal access opening. Often, a cold instrument is preferred.
18. Mix a temporary cement to cover the gutta percha filling. If this procedure is being done in a general practice office, the dentist may place the final restoration at this time, but often, a temporary restoration is placed to verify the comfort of the tooth.
19. Remove the rubber dam.
20. Take a final radiograph. This one is important because it will serve as a reference for follow-up appointments in future years.
21. Inform the patient about recall appointments every 6 months over the next 2 years.
22. Make certain the patient's face is clean and free of debris. Dismiss the patient.

NOTE: If a heat-softened gutta percha obturation technique is used, follow the manufacturer's directions.

ARMAMENTARIUM FOR DRAINAGE OF AN APICAL ABSCESS

Anesthetic setup	Periosteal elevator
Explorer	#11 or #15 scalpel
Mirror	Drain (rubber or iodo-
Cotton forceps	form)
2 × 2 gauze sponges	Hemostat
HVE tip	Irrigating syringe
	Sterile saline solution

PROCEDURE FOR DRAINAGE OF AN APICAL ABSCESS

1. The patient is anesthetized with a field or mandibular block. Infiltration anesthesia may prove painful and ineffective.
2. Once anesthesia is obtained, pass a #11 or #15 scalpel blade to the operator to make an incision directly into the edematous mass. Exudate generally flows out immediately, followed by some hemorrhaging. The dental assistant should keep the HVE tip near the site to remove all fluids.
3. Pass a closed small hemostat or needle holder to the operator to enlarge the opening, allowing additional drainage.
4. Pass the operator a 2 × 2 gauze to wipe the site free of hemorrhage or exudate.
5. If the site is to be irrigated, transfer sterile saline solution to the operator in an irrigating syringe. The assistant should hold the HVE tip nearby to collect fluids that drain from the site.
6. If a drain is to be placed, pass the drain in the forceps for insertion. This drain will be kept in place for 3 to 5 days.
7. Wipe the face clean of any debris, and dismiss the patient.
8. Tell the patient of the need to retain the drain in place. Record the treatment on the clinical chart and indicate if a prescription for an antibiotic or analgesic was given.
9. Provide the patient with written postoperative instructions. Tell the patient to notify the office in the event of severe discomfort or excessive drainage.

INSTRUCTIONS FOR PATIENT AFTER APICAL SURGERY

1. To minimize swelling, apply an ice bag with minimal pressure to the area, alternating 10 minutes on and 10 minutes off for the remainder of the day.
2. Brush the teeth in the normal manner, but be cautious at the site of the surgery.
3. If oozing of blood occurs, place a sterile moistened gauze over the site with finger pressure for 15 minutes. If the bleeding does not subside, call the office.
4. Avoid chewing hard foods. Eat a soft diet, but be sure to eat. Drink plenty of fluids.
5. Rinse the mouth with warm salt water tomorrow—this can be done every 3 hours. Avoid forceful rinsing.
6. Refrain from smoking or consuming alcoholic beverages for 24 hours.
7. Avoid lifting the lip to look at the area—the stitches may tear.
8. Some discomfort may occur—this is normal. If a prescription is given for a pain medication, take it according to the prescribed directions. If no prescription is given and discomfort occurs, take a nonprescription medication that you would normally take for pain.
9. If severe pain or excessive swelling or bleeding occurs, call the office.
10. Sutures need to be removed in 7 to 10 days. If a drain has been placed, it will be removed in 3 to 5 days.

PROCEDURE FOR APICOECTOMY

- Anesthetize the patient.
- Make a flap incision.
- Retract tissue flap.
- Gain access to the apex.
- Perform apical curettage.
- Perform apicoectomy.
- Complete retrograde preparation and restoration.
- Replace flap and suture.
- Give postoperative instructions.

A. These stains are commonly from metallic restorations, such as amalgam, which may turn the dentinal tissues gray over time.

B. Pulpal fragments left in the tooth during endodontic therapy can gradually become discolored.

C. The use of some obturating materials, such as root canal sealers that contain silver particles, are left in the coronal portion of the tooth and may come in contact with oral fluids through percolation, causing the tooth to darken.

IV. A patient may opt for **bleaching** the stained tooth

or having porcelain veneer, laminate, or full-coverage restorations placed.

V. Restorative methods are described in Chapters 20 and 21.

VI. Various bleaching techniques are available, including internal, external, and even home bleaching.

    A. Various oxidizing agents have been used for internal bleaching, including NaOCl, hydrogen peroxide, and sodium perforate.

    B. Methods of application for internal bleaching include the following:

       1. *Thermocatalytic technique,* which involves placing the chemical in the pulp chamber and then applying heat.

       2. *Walking bleach technique,* in which the affected teeth are isolated with a rubber dam and existing restorations and cement bases are removed; the pulpal chamber may be cleaned with a solvent. A paste of sodium perforate and water or anesthetic solution is mixed to the consistency of wet putty; the paste is placed in the chamber, and a temporary cement can then be placed. The patient is rescheduled for two or three similar appointments.

       3. *Light-activated technique,* in which an ultraviolet light beam is applied to the tooth after a cotton pellet saturated with a 30% to 35% hydrogen peroxide solution has been inserted into the chamber.

VII. *External* or *vital bleaching technique,* which is not dissimilar to vital or internal bleaching.

    A. Use hydrogen peroxide technique.

    B. Isolate the teeth.

    C. Apply a solution of 30% hydrogen peroxide to the enamel with a heat application.

    D. Benefits of this bleaching technique are not definitive, and the effect of the solution on the enamel and the potential damage of the heat on the pulp raise significant questions.

    E. An alternative vital bleaching technique involves mixing a paste of 35% hydrochloric acid with an equal volume of water to which flour of pumice is added.

Questions

Endodontics

1 The following are necessary for diagnosis and treatment planning in endodontic therapy:
1. Radiographs
2. Vitality of the tooth
3. Study models
4. Clinical examination
5. Centric relation
a. 1, 2, and 4
b. 2, 3, and 5
c. 2, 4, and 5
d. 3, 4, and 5

2 The rubber dam is used in endodontics to
a. Provide asepsis
b. Promote quadrant dentistry
c. Prevent the patient from seeing the instruments
d. Prevent the patient from breathing through the mouth

3 Endodontic files are used to
a. Enlarge the root canal
b. Remove the contents of the pulp chamber
c. Drain a periapical abscess
d. Reduce the occlusal forces on an endodontically treated tooth

4 Gutta percha is used to
a. Irrigate the root canal
b. Gain access to the root canal
c. Fill the root canal
d. Sterilize the root canal

5 At which of the following steps during endodontic therapy are radiographs taken?
1. At the beginning of each visit
2. At measurement
3. After the pulp is extirpated
4. At the fitting of the master point
5. After the final fill
a. 1, 2, and 4
b. 2, 3, and 4
c. 2, 4, and 5
d. 3, 4, and 5

6 Obtaining an accurate measurement of the root canal length is necessary to
a. Extend the final point 1 mm past the apex
b. Obtain a sterile root canal
c. Avoid creating periapical irritation near the apex

Items 7-15, place an **A** for *True* or a **B** for *False* in the space provided next to each statement.

_____ **7** A Young's frame is radiolucent.

_____ **8** CMCP is used during biomechanical cleansing.

_____ **9** Gutta percha cones are the usual final fill material.

_____ **10** An apicoectomy provides for an opening through the coronal portion of the tooth to control infection.

_____ **11** A trial-point radiograph is taken of the master cone to ensure that the cone fits 1.0 mm beyond the apical stop.

_____ **12** A barbed broach is used to enlarge a canal during biomechanical preparation.

_____ **13** The master gutta percha cone is seated during final filling, before placement of supplemental gutta-percha points.

_____ **14** A cotton pellet saturated with CMCP, FC, or NaOCl is placed during the interim appointment.

_____ **15** A Hedstrom file is the most abrasive of the intracanal instruments.

16 Bicuspidization is an optional treatment procedure for which of the following conditions?
a. Severe bone loss confined to the furcation area
b. Periapical abscess
c. Apexification
d. Internal resorption

17 A caregiver calls and reports that a 10-year-old child has just knocked out the maxillary right central incisor. This condition would be described as
a. Avulsed
b. Intruded
c. Laterally displaced
d. Luxated

18 For immediate replantation the caregiver should be instructed to take which of the following actions?
1. Rinse the tooth gently in tap water.
2. Scrub the tooth thoroughly.
3. Check to see that no pieces are missing.
4. Gently replace the tooth in its socket.
5. Wrap the tooth and bring it to the office.
a. 1 and 3
b. 2 and 4
c. 1, 3, and 4
d. 5 only

19 Replantation of this tooth is generally successful if done in

a. Less than 2 hours
b. More than 2 hours
c. More than 4 hours

20

Anesthesia	Plastic instrument
Rubber dam setup	Endodontic ruler
Endodontic explorer	Irrigating syringe
Mirror	Sponges
Locking pliers	Cotton pellets
Endodontic excavator	Disinfectant
Endodontic tray	HVE tips
Handpiece and angles	Radiographic film
Film holder or hemostat	Temporary filling material

If the instruments listed above are part of an endodontic tray setup the procedure will likely be which of the following?
a. Pulpotomy
b. Apicoectomy
c. Hemisection
d. Opening for a pulpectomy
e. Obturation for a pulpectomy

From the diagram of the tray setup, answer items 22–26.

21 Instrument #26 is a
a. Hemostat
b. Needle holder
c. Retrograde amalgam condenser
d. Bilateral scalpel with handle

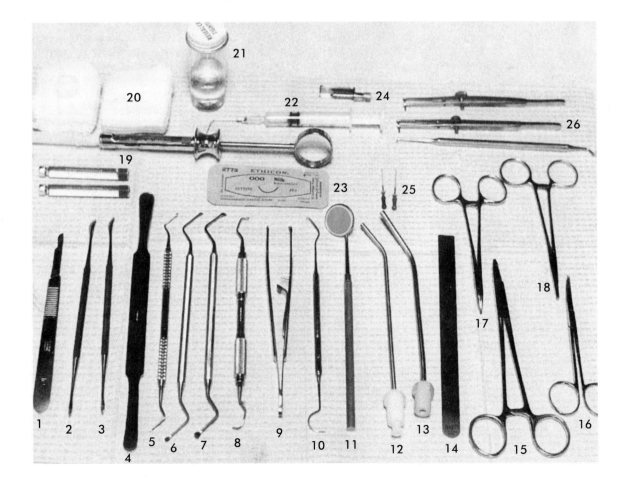

22 The tray setup would be used for a/an
   a. Drainage of an apical abscess
   b. Root amputation
   c. Pulpectomy obturation
   d. Apicoectomy

23 Instrument #9 is a
   a. Hemostat
   b. Locking pliers
   c. Needle holder
   d. Cotton plier

24 Instrument #12 is a/an
   a. Retractor
   b. HVE tip
   c. Aspirator tip

25 Instrument #7 is a/an
   a. Explorer
   b. Surgical curette
   c. Retractor
   d. Scaler

Rationales

Endodontics

1 A To determine the presence of pulpal pathoses, accurate periapical, panorex, or bitewing radiographs are required. The status of the tooth can also be determined by a variety of vitality tests and a thorough clinical examination.

2 A The primary function of the rubber dam is to maintain asepsis. The dam is placed over one tooth, and the dam and tooth are disinfected with a surface disinfectant.

3 A Files are the most common form of instruments used during preparation of the canal and are available as K-style files and Hedstrom files. The file is used in a scraping motion against the side of the canal wall to remove necrotic tissue while the root canal is enlarged.

4 C Gutta percha points are thermoplastic compressible points that adapt to the shape of the canal.

5 C To determine the length of the canal and set the stops on files, the canal must be measured. This is done with a periapical radiograph as the reference. Before the master point is placed, at the fitting appointment another radiograph is taken; once the point is seated, a final radiograph is taken. These radiographs provide the operator with continuous documentation that the file is properly located and the cone properly placed. The final radiograph can be a reference for follow-up radiographs to verify changes in the surrounding tissues.

6 C Tooth length is determined when the file reaches the apical constriction at the dentinocemental junction. If the canal is filed beyond the apical constriction, irritation of the periapical tissues can occur, resulting in discomfort during treatment and possible failure of the root canal.

7 B A Young's frame is made of metal and is radiopaque.

8 B CMCP and FC are canal medications. NaOCl is a biomechanical cleansing agent.

9 A Of the two choices for obturation—gutta percha cones or silver cones—gutta percha is more common.

10 B An apicoectomy is a surgical procedure whereby the apical portion of the root is removed, usually after the root canal filling has been completed without success and relief of pain.

11 B See No. 6.

12 B K-style files are used to enlarge the canal. A barbed broach is used to remove materials from the canal, such as cotton or paper points.

13 A The master cone is placed first in the canal and seated to the apical constriction. Supplemental gutta percha cones are then placed into the canal and laterally condensed until the canal is filled completely. Excess gutta percha is removed with a heated instrument; a plastic instrument is used to condense the gutta percha in the coronal portion of the tooth. A temporary restoration is then placed.

14 B See No. 8.

15 A A Hedstrom file is shaped like a pine tree and has sharp blades. It cuts more aggressively than a K-style file or reamer.

16 A Bicuspidization is a surgical procedure used when severe bone loss is confined to the furcation area. The process involves creating two premolars (bicuspids) from a mandibular molar. The severe bone loss in the furcal area requires that a pulpectomy be performed on both roots; the tooth is then cut in half with a bur in a high-speed handpiece. The furcal area is completely curettaged, and a full crown is placed over the two premolar teeth.

17 A An avulsed tooth is one that has been knocked completely out of the socket.

18 C For immediate replantation the following instructions can be given:
Rinse the tooth gently in tap water.
Do not scrub the tooth.
Gently place the tooth into the socket in as close to normal position as possible; the patient may bite down on a piece of soft fabric or handkerchief to help maintain the position.
See the dentist immediately.

19 A Time is the primary factor in the success of replantation. Therefore, the patient should be brought to the office promptly and seen immediately upon arrival. Success is more common in teeth replanted in less than 2 hours.

20 D None of the surgical instruments listed indicate a surgical procedure, and no filling materials are listed for an obturation. The temporary filling material and ruler indicate that this would likely be an opening or filing appointment.

21 C Instrument #26 is a retrograde amalgam condenser that is used to place amalgam at the apical opening during an apicoectomy procedure.

22 D   See No. 21.

23 B   Instrument #9 is a locking pliers that can be used to secure instruments or materials (such as paper points) during an endodontic procedure.

24 C   Instrument #12 is a surgical oral evacuator tip that is used in a site specific area during surgical endodontic treatment.

25 B   Instrument #7 is a surgical curette that may be used to curette an apical abscess during an apicoectomy.

To enhance your understanding of the material in this chapter refer to the illustrations in Chapter 33 of Finkbeiner/Johnson: *Mosby's Comprehensive Dental Assisting: A Clinical Approach.*

Oral and Maxillofacial Surgery

Oral and maxillofacial surgery is the dental specialty that deals with the diagnosis and surgical treatment of diseases, injuries, and deformities of the face and jaws. **Maxillofacial** refers to the portion of the face that includes the maxilla and mandible.

In addition to **extraction** of teeth (**exodontia),** the oral surgeon treats oral pathoses, facial injuries, and trauma (such as broken bones); practices preprosthetic surgery to prepare the mouth to receive prosthetic devices (such as dentures or implants); and performs **orthognathic surgery,** (surgery of the jaws to correct deformities, making the jaws more functional). Orthognathic surgery

is always performed in a hospital; the patient receives a general anesthetic that is administered by an **anesthesiologist,** a physician who administers medication that causes a loss of sensation with or without a loss in consciousness. Oral surgery performed in the dental office also can involve either general anesthesia or **conscious sedation.** In the office, however, the oral surgeon usually administers the anesthetic and performs the surgery.

An individual who wishes to specialize in oral surgery must first complete dental school and then usually spend an additional 4 years in a hospital residency program. This residency includes extra training in internal medicine, general surgery, anesthesia, and oral and maxillo-facial surgery. Some individuals spend 2 additional years to earn a doctor of medicine (MD) degree. After completing the residency, the individual must pass a state, regional, or national specialty board examination; practice is restricted to oral surgery. General dentists also practice oral surgery, but usually they restrict themselves to less involved cases and do not practice in the hospital setting.

ROLE OF THE DENTAL ASSISTANT

I.   Intraoral responsibilities
II. Patient management
III. Teaching
IV. Maintaining infection control standards

OFFICE DESIGN

I.   Design is similar to that of a general dental office, with special emphasis on the following aspects:
   A. The environment should be as soothing as possible.
   B. Soft music, subdued colors, rounded edges of counters and door frames, etc., can have a subtle calming effect.
II. The reception room and hallways must be comfortable and well lighted.
   A. Adequate seating should be provided for drivers who accompany oral surgery patients.
   B. Hallways should be wider than in the general dental office because many oral surgery patients are sedated for the procedures and must be supported when they leave the office.
III. Oral surgery treatment rooms must be designed as follows:
   A. They must be wider than general dental treatment rooms.
   B. Ideally, each room should have two entrances so that neither the operator nor the assistant is trapped in a corner.
   C. There should be room at the foot of the chair for an assistant to walk around if necessary.
   D. Counter space should be adequate to accommodate the various instruments used to monitor patient functions (such as BP, pulse, and respirations).
   E. There should be at least one sink, preferably two.
   F. Oxygen, **nitrous oxide,** and other gases (such as nitrogen) as well as suction should be plumbed into the wall directly behind the patient's head.
   G. A communication system must be available.
   H. The chair must have the following features:

     1. Must be adjustable to elevate high enough so that the surgeon does not have to stoop, if standing.
     2. Must have a flat arm that can easily support a sedated patient's arm with an **intravenous** (IV) apparatus in place.
     3. Must be equipped to function in emergencies, strong enough to withstand CPR compression, and able to be placed in the **Trendelenburg** position.
IV. Adjunct rooms are designed as follows:
   A. Sterilization area must be central to the treatment rooms and must provide adequate storage space.
   B. A radiography/Panorex area must be available.
   C. There must be recovery rooms where patients who have had conscious sedation or general anesthesia can wake up. These are often small rooms with a bed or cot, small sink, suction, and oxygen that is easily available to aid the patient as needed.
   D. A restroom and business office must be included.
   E. A separate private exit is advisable for patients who have just had surgery.

MEDICAL EVALUATION

I.   Detailed history and careful examination for safe and effective treatment
II. Separate appointment to review health questionnaire, obtain and evaluate radiographs, and examine patient
   A. At this appointment the informed consent can be discussed and the patient can ask questions.
   B. Other tests (such as blood studies) may need to be ordered, and the oral surgeon may want to consult the patient's physician regarding the patient's health or prior surgery.
III. Evaluating heart and lungs
   A. Physician consultation is always recommended for patients with significant medical problems.
   B. Special considerations for patients with significant medical conditions include the following:
     1. A patient who has had a heart attack within the past 6 months is not a candidate for elective surgery because the risk of further heart damage from secondary infections is significant.
     2. Patients with heart disease of any sort are

best handled in a low-stress environment, possibly with either oral or IV sedation. Appointments should be relatively short and are best scheduled in the morning. It is important to make sure that the patient takes all regularly scheduled medications on the morning of the appointment.

3. A patient with lung disease, such as asthma or tuberculosis, might best be treated with nasal oxygen during the procedure.

4. Preventive medication, such as nitroglycerine for patients with angina or inhalers for those with asthma, should be readily available during the procedure and in many cases should be given before the procedure for safety reasons.

C. Determine whether the patient has a heart murmur. Even a mild murmur can put the patient at risk for SBE if it goes unrecognized and untreated.

1. A heart murmur can indicate an underlying abnormality that can cause an irregular flow of blood through the heart.

2. The recommendation of the American Heart Association for antibiotic prophylaxis is to have the patient take 3 g of amoxicillin 1 hour before the dental procedure and 1 g 6 hours later.

IV. Hypertension

A. Patients with hypertension can be difficult to assess in the oral surgery office.

B. Anxiety and pain, which can increase a patient's blood pressure are often present in patients who need oral surgery.

C. A thorough evaluation of the patient history is necessary.

V. Systemic diseases

A. A history of kidney or liver disease can affect the way various drugs, including local anesthetics and antibiotics, are metabolized.

B. Patients with systemic disease should be evaluated carefully before surgery is performed.

C. A patient undergoing kidney dialysis needs special protocols to schedule antibiotic doses and surgery at the most opportune time relative to dialysis treatment.

D. Patients with kidney and liver diseases often have bleeding problems that must be taken into account when surgery is scheduled.

E. Often cardiac patients are taking a medication, such as coumadin, that thins the blood.

F. Patients who have a history of bleeding problems or are taking blood-thinning medication need several blood tests before surgery to ensure that the blood will clot after surgery.

G. Some medications may need to be discontinued 1 or 2 days before surgery.

H. Aspirin is probably the most likely drug to cause bleeding problems in the general dental population.

VI. Pregnancy

A. If possible, oral surgery should be postponed until the second trimester of pregnancy.

B. During the first trimester the risk of spontaneous abortion and birth defects is increased.

C. During the third trimester the stress of the procedure can bring about early labor.

D. In an emergency, such as severe infection or a fractured jaw, these guidelines cannot be followed.

E. The oral surgeon must work with the obstetrician to make the procedure as safe as possible for the woman and the fetus.

VII. Diabetes

A. Diabetic patients who receive daily insulin injections are particularly in need of evaluation before surgery.

B. The amount of insulin a person takes depends on the number of calories ingested. This presents a problem because individuals who need oral surgery are often asked to fast before the procedure and often don't eat normally afterward.

C. In this situation the patient is scheduled early in the morning and is asked to take one half of the normal morning dose of insulin and to eat a light breakfast. The blood sugar is unlikely to drop too low because only half of the insulin dose was given, and the patient may be able to eat soft food by lunchtime.

D. Insulin doses for the remainder of the day are determined by the blood glucose levels (checked with finger sticks).

E. Diabetic patients are more susceptible to infection than other patients, and many surgeons prefer to premedicate them with antibiotics.

F. Consultation with the patient's physician is necessary when change is made in a drug regimen.

VIII. Other drugs

A. The surgeon must carefully evaluate the list of medications and decide whether the drugs noted on the health questionnaire might interact with medications that will be used in surgery or anesthesia.

    B. The patient must be warned about any possible drug interactions.

    C. Alcohol and drug abuse can alter a patient's reaction to medications such as sedatives or even local anesthetics.

    D. Patients who are recovering alcoholics or chemical dependents who are currently free of drugs may prefer to avoid using any narcotic medication during or after surgery.

IX.   Allergies

    A. The surgeon must carefully question each patient about his or her allergies.

        1. Which ones are true allergies?

        2. Which ones cause sensitivities to the patient (such as an upset stomach)?

X.   Infectious patients

    A. Universal precautions should be practiced as in all dental offices.

    B. Patients with human immunodeficiency virus may be premedicated with an antibiotic to reduce the increased risk of other infection.

RADIOGRAPHIC EVALUATION

I.   At the preoperative appointment appropriate radiographs are obtained to evaluate the surgical area.

II.   The panoramic radiograph is the most effective.

III.   When a single tooth or small area is to be visualized, a periapical film can be used.

ANESTHESIA, PREMEDICATION, AND SEDATION

I.   Conventional anesthesia, premedication, and sedation are used to reduce anxiety.

II.   Sedation techniques can be divided into three general classes:

    A. Oral medications

    B. Inhaled gases

    C. IV medications

III.   Usually, local anesthetic is administered in conjunction with conscious sedation or general anesthesia. This is mandatory with conscious sedation because the patient would still be able to feel pain without the local anesthetic.

    A. Local anesthesia reduces the depth of general anesthesia necessary to make the patient comfortable.

    B. The epinephrine in the local anesthetic helps control bleeding, and as the patient recovers from the procedure, no sudden burst of pain occurs.

MONITORING VITAL SIGNS

I.   For safety, the patient's vital signs must be monitored regularly.

II.   Blood pressure must be assessed frequently throughout the procedure with an automatic blood pressure monitor.

    A. The automatic blood pressure cuff is applied as a manual blood pressure cuff.

    B. The wrist clips are applied.

    C. Small metal plates in the clips pick up an electrical signal from the patient's pulse and transmit it through the wires to the **electrocardiogram** (EKG) machine, where this electrical activity is displayed on a screen.

    D. Finger clips are available for hospital outpatient and office use.

    E. To ensure that a clear electrical signal is received, a conductive spray must be used to moisten the patient's wrists before the clips are placed.

    F. Reassure the patient that some of the movement seen on the ECG screen is caused by artifact or movement and does not indicate that the heart is malfunctioning.

III.   Respirations and the amount of oxygen in the patient's bloodstream must be evaluated throughout the procedure with a **pulse oximeter.**

IV.   It is helpful to have an ECG strip that runs throughout the procedure to warn of unusual heart action.

SURGICAL INSTRUMENTS

I.   A vast majority of instruments are unique to surgery and not other areas of dentistry.

    A. Most surgical instruments have polished working ends of stainless steel.

    B. The handles of the instruments are textured to enable the surgeon to maintain a firm grasp on the instrument during the procedure.

II.   Anesthetic syringes

    A. Aspirating syringes are commonly used to prevent injection of anesthetic into the blood vessels.

    B. If both long and short injection needles are used, it is helpful to have two syringes set up, one with each length of needle.

III.   HVE hosing and tips

    A. Surgical HVE tubing is lightweight and flexible and can be sterilized.

    B. The orifice of most **surgical HVE tips** is small, may be fabricated from metal or disposable plastic, and comes in a variety of sizes and shapes.

IV. Retractors
   A. Lip and cheek retractors provide clear vision for the surgeon.
   B. Various lip, cheek, tongue, and tissue retractors are available.
   C. A mouth prop may be needed when a patient is unable to cooperate.
V. Scalpel
   A. A **scalpel** is a thin, sharp blade that is used to make a cut or incision; it is common to most surgical tray setups.
   B. Most surgeons use reusable and sterilizable scalpel handles with disposable sterile scalpel blades.
   C. A scalpel blade remover is used to remove a scalpel blade safely.
   D. Four common blade sizes and shapes are #11, #12, #12B, and #15; the letter B beside the number denotes that both edges of the blade have a cutting surface.
VI. Elevator
   A. The **elevator** is the workhorse of the surgical extraction tray.
   B. The elevator is wedged between the tooth to be extracted and the adjacent bone; it is then rotated (the bone is used as a fulcrum), without pushing on the adjacent teeth, to compress the space between the tooth and the bone.
   C. It is often used rather than the mallet and chisel, to split teeth.
   D. Elevators can be divided into two major classes: straight and angled. The angled elevators are usually used as a pair (right and left).
   E. Root-tip elevators or root-tip picks are similar to dental elevators but usually are much thinner and finer.
      1. They are available in pairs (right and left).
      2. They are designed to tease fractured root tips out of sockets.
      3. They do not expand the bone as do the elevators.
VII. Periosteal elevator
   A. A **periosteal elevator** is used to reflect, pull away, or detach and lift the tissue (including the periosteum) from the bone.
   B. Most periosteal elevators have one sharp and one rounded end.
   C. Some oral surgeons also use the periosteal elevator to retract tissue.
VIII. Chisel
   A. A **chisel** is used to remove bone from around an impacted tooth.
   B. Chisels and mallets are also used to split teeth.
   C. Chisels can either be *single beveled,* with one flat side and one sharp angled side, or *bi-beveled,* with two sharp angled sides.
IX. Surgical curette
   A. The **surgical curette** is used to clear the socket of tissue fragments and infected material, such as abscesses.
   B. Surgical curettes are usually double ended and have a round tip that is used to scoop material out of dental sockets. The ends are polished steel and range from rather small to rather large.
X. Rongeur
   A. A **rongeur** is used to remove excess tissue from around the site of an extracted tooth, but it can also be used to remove or contour excess bone.
   B. It looks like a forceps, but the handle is usually spring loaded. The edges of the beaks are sharp and are used to tug tissue away from bone and to nip sharp edges of the bone to smooth it.
   C. It is useful in preparing the alveolar ridge for dentures after extractions.
XI. Bone files
   A. These are used after the rongeur to smooth the sharp edges of the alveolar ridge.
   B. Most bone files are double ended and usually are a different size on each end.
XII. Surgical scissors
   A. These are used routinely in oral surgery to cut sutures, undermine tissue, or spread tissue away from other tissue. They are also used (rather than a scalpel blade) to trim tissue.
   B. Surgical scissors are available in lengths of 4 to 7 inches.
   C. Tips can be blunt, sharp, curved, or straight or combinations of these.
XIII. Hemostats and needle holders
   A. These are often confused with each other.
   B. **Hemostats** are primarily used to grasp tissue and clamp off blood vessels; **needle holders** are used to hold **suture** needles.
   C. Hemostats can be curved or straight; needle holders are generally straight.
   D. Hemostats are usually narrower than the more blunted, heavier needle holders.
   E. The serrated portion of the beaks of the hemostat is longer than the same area on a needle holder.
   F. Many needle holders have a criss-cross pat-

tern on the internal portion of the beak or a slotted groove down the midline of the beak.

XIV. Tissue pliers
   A. **Tissue pliers** and forceps are used to hold tissue during surgery and suturing.
   B. Tissue pliers are similar to cotton pliers and are usually very fine instruments.
   C. Usually the ends have small teeth to aid in holding the tissue.
   D. They are designed to hold larger portions of tissue, such as a fragment for a **biopsy.**

XV. Surgical forceps
   A. **Surgical forceps** permit the surgeon to grasp the crown of the tooth beyond the cementoenamel junction and luxate the tooth for removal.
   B. Forceps are not always needed for extractions; when impacted teeth are removed, forceps are almost never used.
   C. The two major types of surgical forceps are *maxillary* and *mandibular.*
      1. The direction of the beaks of maxillary forceps parallels the direction of the handle.
      2. The direction of the beaks of mandibular forceps is usually at a right angle to the direction of the handle.
   D. *Universal forceps* can be used for incisors, cuspids, premolars, and roots; but they are not often used for molars.
   E. *Bayonet forceps* are commonly used in the maxilla for removing molar teeth.
   F. The *cowhorn forceps* have somewhat rounded, pointed beaks that resemble a cow's horns; they are usually used for the removal of mandibular molar teeth.

XVI. Basic instruments and their routine uses (Table 23-1)

XVII. Additional armamentarium
   A. Surgical dressings
   B. Surgical suture material
   C. Lubricant

PREPARATION FOR SURGICAL PROCEDURES ▪

I. Preset trays
   A. Less frequently used items (such as forceps) bagged separately can be stored on fixed cabinetry or in a nearby drawer.
   B. The surgical assistant must draw up any medications that may be needed for sedation or general anesthesia; sometimes these are placed on a separate smaller tray with all the items necessary for the anesthesia.

II. Barrier techniques
   A. Universal barrier techniques are essential.
   B. Sterility is vital; sterile surgical gloves rather than nonsterile gloves are required for each case.
   C. Additional protective coverings, such as hospital gowns, are used as directed by OSHA regulations.

III. Managing medical wastes
   A. The oral surgery office presents many opportunities for producing regulated wastes and hazardous materials, including extracted teeth, diseased tissues, needles, and scalpel blades.
   B. The policies for management of these wastes are regulated by OSHA Rule 29 CFR and by individual state regulations.

IV. Preparing the IV bag
   A. The assistant must prepare the IV bag and draw up the medications (box).
   B. IV bags come in several sizes; the most common are 250, 500, and 1000 ml.
   C. The assistant prepares the medication syringes. Some oral surgeons use manufactured prefilled syringes, but most use multidose vials and draw up set amounts of medications into each syringe.

PREPARING THE IV BAG

1. Open the overwrap and remove the sterile IV bag. With the port end of the bag held upside down so that the fluid cannot leak out, pull the seal from the neck of the bag.
2. Remove the protective cover from the pointed end of the drip chamber of the IV tubing set, and with a twisting motion insert it into the port of the IV bag.
3. Turn the bag so that the port and the IV tubing are at the bottom. Place the bag on the stand. Gently squeeze the drip chamber of the IV tubing, filling it about half full.
4. Remove the protective cover of the opposite end of the IV tubing and allow the fluid to flow through the tube. When the fluid reaches the end, tighten the adjustable clamp to stop the flow. Replace the protective cover over the end until the tubing is attached to the IV needle in the patient's arm.

Table 23-1 Basic surgical instruments and their routine uses

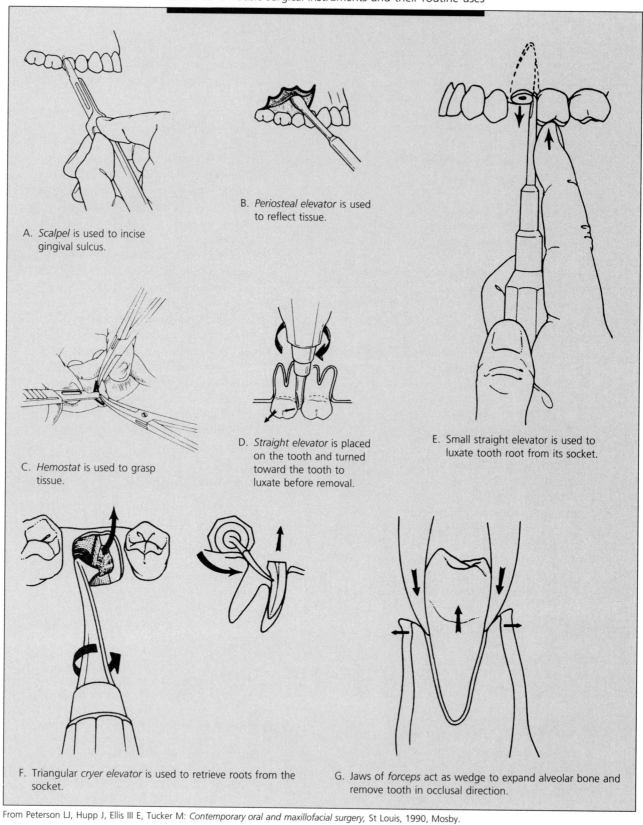

A. *Scalpel* is used to incise gingival sulcus.

B. *Periosteal elevator* is used to reflect tissue.

C. *Hemostat* is used to grasp tissue.

D. *Straight elevator* is placed on the tooth and turned toward the tooth to luxate before removal.

E. Small straight elevator is used to luxate tooth root from its socket.

F. Triangular *cryer elevator* is used to retrieve roots from the socket.

G. Jaws of *forceps* act as wedge to expand alveolar bone and remove tooth in occlusal direction.

From Peterson LJ, Hupp J, Ellis III E, Tucker M: *Contemporary oral and maxillofacial surgery,* St Louis, 1990, Mosby.

D. Each syringe must be labeled so that the medications are not incorrectly administered.

E. The syringes and medications should be kept in a locked cupboard for protection and when specified by law.

F. When a medication syringe is prepared, the assistant should first check the expiration date, read the label before filling the syringe, and recheck the label after filling the syringe to ensure that the proper medication has been prepared.

G. The procedure for preparing medication from a multidose vial is provided (box).

V. Patient preparation and monitors

PREPARING MEDICATION FROM A MULTIDOSE VIAL

1. Wipe the rubber diaphragm on the top of the vial with an alcohol sponge and dry it with a sterile sponge.
2. To withdraw liquid from the vial, which is under a vacuum, inject air into the vial. To accomplish this, pull back the plunger of the syringe until it reaches the specific graduation mark that indicates the proper amount of medication to be used. That is, if the syringe is to be filled with 3 cc of medication, withdraw the plunger to the 3-cc mark.
3. Hold the vial with the diaphragm facing the floor and remove the needle cap. Do not touch the sterile end of the needle. Pierce the rubber diaphragm.
4. After piercing the top of the vial with the needle, and with the vial still inverted, push down on the plunger, thus injecting 3 cc of air into the vial.
5. Pull back on the plunger again to withdraw the desired amount of medication to fill the syringe.
6. If bubbles enter the chamber, remove them by gently tapping the syringe with the needle end of the syringe pointing upward; this sends the bubbles to the top of the medication. Expel the bubbles by slightly pressing the plunger forward.
7. After the syringe is filled, withdraw the needle from the vial and place the cap back over the needle.
8. To avoid accidental needle sticks, use a recapping device or the one-handed scoop technique to assist in this process.
9. If additional medication is needed, repeat the process, filling a sterile syringe each time.

A. Preparatory steps before surgery are listed (box).

B. Assess the patient's vital signs.

C. In patients who are to have only local anesthetic, only the BP needs to be taken.

D. After the patient is connected to the monitors, the machines are started.
   1. Most machines can be set to record once each minute and up to once every 30 minutes. As long as a patient is stable, it is usually sufficient to monitor every 10 or 15 minutes.
   2. Data generated from these recordings can be attached to the patient record.

VI. General anesthesia and sedation

A. The surgeon usually converses with the patient to ensure that the patient has no further questions about the procedure or the consent form that has been signed.

B. The surgeon places the patient in a reclining position, applies the nitrous oxide rubber mask to the patient's nose, and tightens the cord so that the mask does not slip off.

C. The patient is allowed to breathe a fairly high

PREPARATORY STEPS BEFORE SURGERY

- Verify that the patient consent form is accurate and has been signed.
- Confirm that a driver is present for a sedated patient.
- Ask the patient to remove contact lenses if he or she is to be sedated or receive general anesthetic.
- Verify that any prescribed premedication has been taken.
- Confirm the patient's height and weight to determine anesthetic dosage.
- Review and confirm information on the health history form.
- Determine whether a female patient is pregnant or is taking a contraceptive.
- Determine the time of the last meal taken by a patient who is to be sedated or receive general anesthetic.
- Check and record the status of vital signs before and after the surgical procedure.
- Connect monitors, BP, EKG, and pulse oximeter.
- Provide an antimicrobial rinse before seating the patient.
- Use universal precautions.
- Assist with the administration of all forms of anesthetic.

rate of nitrous oxide/oxygen (60%/40%) for a few minutes; this helps reduce anxiety, reduces the discomfort of the venipuncture, and gives the surgeon a chance to evaluate the patient's reaction to an easily reversible analgesic.

D. The patient is told that in a few minutes he or she will notice a sweet smell from the nitrous oxide and will start to feel more relaxed.

E. The patient may also be aware of numbness or tingling in the extremities.

F. The patient must never be left alone once the nitrous oxide is introduced.

G. Once the nitrous oxide has had an effect, it is time to start the IV.

   1. If IV sedation is not being used, the next step is to administer a local anesthetic.

   2. Some surgeons do not use nitrous oxide and begin with an IV.

H. The procedure for starting the IV is provided (box).

VII. Local anesthesia

A. Every oral surgical procedure must include profound local anesthesia.

   1. It controls bleeding during surgery.

   2. It provides pain control immediately after the patient wakes up.

B. Usually, oral surgery requires the use of more local anesthetic than restorative dentistry because oral surgery involves a greater part of the mouth.

C. Local anesthesia must be more profound for oral surgery than for restorative dentistry.

D. Not only the teeth but also the soft tissue and bone around the teeth must be anesthetized.

STARTING THE IV

- Are all universal barrier techniques being used?
- Is all of the armamentarium available and prepared for use?
- Are the instruments arranged in order of use?
- Are you prepared for alternative treatment plans?
- Is the necessary equipment turned on and ready to operate?

1. Pass the tourniquet to the surgeon to place tightly above the patient's elbow. The patient is instructed to make a fist or is given an object to squeeze to make the veins protrude at the elbow or on the back of the hand.
2. Open the alcohol wipe packet. Hold the outside of the packet while the surgeon removes the alcohol wipe. Wipe the patient's arm with the alcohol to clean it before placing the IV.
3. Retrieve the used alcohol wipe and pass the surgeon a dry gauze to dry the area. (It is more uncomfortable for the patient if the IV puncture is made while the arm is still wet with alcohol.)
4. Take the butterfly needle (some surgeons use other types of needles and a slightly different technique), slightly loosening the plastic shield over the needle without touching the needle. Bend up the wings of the needle so that the surgeon can take the needle in the proper position for use. Hold the plastic shield as the surgeon slides the needle out.
5. As the surgeon inserts the needle into the patient's vein, take a piece of tape (which has already been laid out) and hand it to the surgeon to fasten the needle in place as soon as the needle is in the vein and blood can be seen in the small plastic tube that is attached to the needle.
6. The surgeon takes the cap off the end of the butterfly tubing, allowing blood to flow to the end of the tubing, and releases the tourniquet. Meanwhile, move to the IV stand, remove the cap from the end of the IV line, and hand the end to the surgeon to attach to the butterfly tubing.
7. Once the IV line is attached to the tubing, open the clamp on the IV line, allowing the contents to start flowing into the vein. A final piece of tape is then applied to the needle and tubing to hold everything in place during the procedure, and the patient's arm is secured to the chair to reduce the chance of dislodging the IV catheter.
8. If a high dose of nitrous oxide and oxygen has been used to provide anxiety control or mild analgesia during this portion of the procedure, the level of nitrous oxide is turned down to a maintenance dose (approximately 30% nitrous oxide and 70% oxygen).

- Are the appropriate universal barrier techniques removed?
- Have all appropriate surfaces been cleaned and disinfected?
- Has all of the armamentarium been removed?
- Has all equipment been repositioned?
- Has all equipment been disinfected/sterilized according to OSHA guidelines?

RESPONSIBILITIES OF THE DENTAL ASSISTANT DURING SURGERY

Transfer instruments in order of use
Observe changes in treatment site
Monitor patient's vital signs
Observe patient's nonverbal cues
Monitor patient's movements
Inform surgeon of changes in patient's status
Observe and retract tissues to avoid injury
Maintain a clear working field, free of blood and oral fluids
Keep instruments clean and free of debris
Clear HVE line frequently
Aid in irrigation
Keep track of amount of local anesthetic being used
Keep track of number of sutures placed
Dispose of medical wastes according to OSHA guidelines
Clean blood from patient's face
Accurately and thoroughly record treatment on the patient's record

ARMAMENTARIUM FOR VARIOUS SURGICAL PROCEDURES

BASIC SURGICAL PROCEDURE

Local anesthetic setup	Mirror
Anesthesia/patient monitor setup	3 × 3 gauze sponges
Nitrous oxide setup (optional)	Surgical HVE tip
	Lubricant
Oximeter	Cup with sterile water
Automatic BP cuff	Surgical curette
	Irrigating syringe

E. The dental assistant must record on the patient record the amount of anesthetic administered.

VIII. Responsibilities of the dental assistant during surgery (box at top of page)

SURGICAL PROCEDURES

I. Armamentarium for various surgical procedures is listed (box above).

This armamentarium is the same for each surgical procedure.

ROUTINE EXTRACTION SETUP

Periosteal elevator	Maxillary universal forceps
Retractor	Ronguer
Straight elevator	Surgicel (placed nearby)

SURGICAL EXTRACTION

Retractor	Appropriate forceps
Cotton pliers	Rongeur
Scalpel handle with blade (#11, #12, or #15)	Bone file
	Surgical burs with handpiece
Periosteal elevator	Suture (placed in sterile water to soften)
Straight elevator (#77)	
Root-tip elevators	Needle holder

SURGICAL EXTRACTIONS WITH IMMEDIATE DENTURE PLACEMENT

Retractor	Suture (placed in sterile water to soften)
Cotton pliers	
Scalpel handle with blade (#11, #12, or #15)	Needle holder
Periosteal elevator	Surgicel (placed nearby)
Straight elevator (#77)	
Assorted forceps (optional)	Root-tip elevators (optional)
Rongeur	
Bone file	Stent
Surgical burs with handpiece	Denture

SURGICAL REMOVAL OF THIRD MOLARS

Retractor
Cotton pliers
Scalpel handle with blade (#11, #12, or #15)
Periosteal elevator
Straight elevator (#77)
Assorted forceps (optional)
Maxillary universal forceps (#150)
Maxillary posterior bayonet forceps (#210S)
Maxillary right and left molar forceps (#53R and L)
Rongeur
Bone file
Surgical burs with handpiece
Suture (placed in sterile water to soften)
Needle holder
Surgicel (placed nearby)
Root-tip elevators (optional)
Bite block

EXPOSURE OF IMPACTED CANINE/CUSPID

Cotton pliers
Scalpel handle with blade
   (#11, #12, or #15)
Periosteal elevator
Bone chisel
Rongeur
Surgical burs with
   handpiece

Suture (placed in
   sterile water to
   soften)
Needle holder
Periodontal dressing
Root-tip elevators
   (optional)

FRENECTOMY

Tissue pliers
Tissue scissors
Straight hemostat
Scalpel handle with blade (#11, #12, or #15)
Suture (placed in sterile water to soften)
Needle holder

II. A team approach for routine extraction of maxillary right first premolar is provided (box at bottom of page).

III. Common surgical procedures used in specific cases are provided (boxes on pages 399 through 408).

IV. Postoperative instructions are given to the patient.

Text continues on page 409.

BIOPSY

Tissue pliers
Tissue scissors
Straight hemostat
Scalpel handle with blade
   (#11, #12, or #15)

Suture (placed in
   sterile water to
   soften)
Needle holder
Small bottle with
   10% formalin

ROUTINE EXTRACTION OF MAXILLARY RIGHT FIRST PREMOLAR: TEAM APPROACH

Before this procedure is begun, monitors are connected and anesthetic administered. When the patient is sufficiently anesthetized, the procedure is begun.

OPERATOR	ASSISTANT
	Pass curette or periosteal elevator.
Grasp instrument and detach periodontal ligament; return curette or periodontal elevator.	Exchange instrument for straight elevator.
Grasp elevator; place elevator on tooth; apply pressure and luxate tooth; return elevator.	Exchange elevator for universal maxillary forceps.
Receive forceps; grasp tooth; luxate.	Observe site; evacuate blood; keep HVE tip near site to pick up debris and tooth fragments; retract tissue as necessary.
Lift out tooth; examine apex of tooth; transfer forceps with tooth.	Grasp forceps with left hand; if root is not intact, pass root-tip elevator; transfer curette.
Grasp curette and remove granulation tissue or any abscess from socket.	Place HVE near site to withdraw debris and blood
Return curette.	
Grasp rongeur to remove tissue that has been loosened from bony socket.	Exchange curette for rongeur as elsewhere.
Return rongeur.	Wipe off tips of rongeur as needed; pass HVE over site to clean area.
Grasp curette and clean socket.	Exchange for curette.
Return curette.	Use HVE to clean site.
	Receive curette; transfer irrigating syringe with sterile saline.
Grasp irrigating syringe; ask patient to turn on side; irrigate the area.	Use HVE to collect fluids; fold 3 × 3 gauze into small pillow.
Return irrigating syringe.	Exchange syringe for folded gauze.
Place gauze over extraction site; ask patient to close on gauze.	Use moistened gauze to wipe blood from patient's lips and cheeks.
Remove gloves and other surgical attire as necessary.	
Sign prescriptions.	Provide postoperative instructions; enter clinical data on chart; dispose of medical waste according to OSHA standards.

CASE #1 ROUTINE EXTRACTION

PATIENT DATA:

65-year-old female in good health.
Some mild hypertension that is well controlled with routine blood-pressure medication.
Periodontally involved maxillary right first premolar to be removed.
The tooth has been abscessed several times in the past.
The patient is not apprehensive and prefers a local anesthetic.

PROCEDURE

1. Pass the surgeon a surgical curette or a periosteal elevator to detach the periodontal ligament from around the tooth.
2. Exchange this instrument for a straight (#77) elevator.
3. The surgeon places the elevator on the mesial side of the tooth and applies pressure in a distal direction. Because the tooth is already slightly mobile, a great deal of pressure is not needed.
4. The surgeon exchanges the elevator for a maxillary universal forceps (#150). This can be done with either a one- or two-handed transfer, whichever works best for the surgical team.
5. Observe the surgical site; using the HVE tip, remove excess blood as it accumulates, maintaining a clear field of operation for the surgeon.
6. The surgeon luxates the tooth with the forceps.
7. Watch closely and keep the HVE tip nearby. The tip can be used for tissue retraction and evacuation of debris, such as a fragment of tooth or amalgam that fractures when the forceps is placed firmly on the tooth. Clear the suction line with sterile water periodically to prevent clogging.
8. When the tooth is sufficiently mobile, the surgeon lifts the tooth out of the socket.
9. Receive the forceps from the surgeon. The surgeon holds the forceps by the handle. Take the working end of the forceps and the extracted tooth in the palm of the hand while transferring a surgical curette to the surgeon. The apex of the tooth must be observed to ensure that the root has not fractured. If the tooth is not intact, obtain root-tip elevators to retrieve the remainder of the root.
10. The surgeon uses the curette to remove granulation tissue and dental abscesses from the socket. Once the curette is passed to the surgeon, be ready to evacuate the surgical site.
11. Hold the rongeur in readiness for transfer to the surgeon as soon as the socket has been curetted. The rongeur is used to remove the tissue that was loosened from the base of the socket.
12. While the rongeur is being used, the surgeon periodically brings the instrument out of the patient's mouth because it holds tissue debris. Use a 3 × 3 gauze to efficiently remove the tissue from the rongeur without taking the instrument from the surgeon. Ideally, the surgeon's eyes should never leave the operating field.
13. When the surgeon has finished with the rongeur, make the curette available to exchange in case it is needed again.
14. Pass the HVE tip over the surgical site regularly during this procedure so that vision of the site is not impaired by bleeding.
15. Once the surgeon is satisfied that the socket is sufficiently clean, transfer an irrigating syringe to the surgeon to use at the site. Usually, a sterile saline (salt water) solution is used rather than tap water because the sterile saline is less damaging to the tissue.
16. While the area is being irrigated, ask the patient to turn to one side or the other so that the irrigation solution does not fill the back of the throat and cause choking. Because this is a relatively simple extraction, sutures are not needed to close the tissue.
17. Finally, fold a 3 × 3 gauze into a small pillow and either give it to the surgeon to place or place it directly over the surgical site.
18. Instruct the patient to apply firm biting pressure to the area to control the bleeding and aid in clot formation.
19. In this case, there was not an exceptional amount of bleeding during the procedure, so surgical dressing was not used.
20. Take a moistened piece of gauze and use it to wipe any blood from the patient's lips and cheeks.
21. The surgeon decides what type of pain medication to give the patient, signs the prescriptions, and moves on to the next patient.
22. Be certain that a description of the surgery, the type and amount of anesthetic administered, and the pain prescription given are entered on the patient record.
23. Dispose of medical wastes and barrier covers according to infection control policies.

CASE #2 SURGICAL EXTRACTION
PATIENT DATA:

70-year-old male.

Maxillary right first molar has had periodontal therapy, endodontic treatment, and a crown; the tooth is badly broken down and may fracture during removal.

The patient had rheumatic heart disease as a child.

The patient was premedicated with 3 g of amoxicillin 1 hour before his appointment.

PROCEDURE

1. Simultaneously, pass the retractor and the curette to the surgeon to assess the level of anesthesia. Because the patient feels only pressure and no sharp sensation when the area is checked, the surgeon hands the curette back to the assistant and begins the procedure.

2. Exchange the curette for the #77 elevator. The surgeon attempts to luxate the tooth, but as expected, it doesn't move easily. Rather than placing the forceps on the tooth, with the high probability of fracture, the surgeon decides to remove the tooth surgically.

3. The surgeon returns the elevator to the assistant in exchange for a scalpel with a #15 blade. Safety is important, and care must be taken whenever sharp instruments such as this are exchanged; it would be easy to cut oneself through a glove if careless.

4. The surgeon makes an incision along the margin of the gingiva and down to the bone. The incision usually extends the width of one tooth on either side of the tooth to be extracted. If the incision is less than or equal to the width of the tooth, vision will not be clear and the tissue may be torn. A sharp, clean incision heals more quickly than a jagged tear. When maxillary teeth are removed, a vertical releasing incision is usually added to one end or the other of the incision to add visibility (Fig. 23-12).

5. The surgeon uses a retractor in the left hand to keep the cheek out of the way, using the scalpel in the right hand. The assistant uses the HVE tip in the right hand to keep the surgical site clear, keeping the left hand free to exchange instruments. If this were an extraction in the mandibular right quadrant instead of the maxillary arch, the HVE tip might also be used as a retractor for the tongue. The surgical HVE tip does not need to be in the mouth at all times, but the assistant must keep a close watch on the surgical field to make sure that the area is as clean and dry as possible.

6. Once the incision has been made, exchange the surgeon's scalpel for a periosteal elevator. Usually, the pointed end of this instrument is used to start reflecting the mucoperiosteal flap (the full-thickness soft-tissue flap, including the top or mucosal layer and the inner layer, which covers the periosteum). Once the flap is partially reflected, the instrument can be turned and the flatter end used to complete the reflection. During this process the surgeon places a Minnesota retractor between the reflected tissue and the bone to see the site of operation.

7. The surgeon returns the periosteal elevator to the assistant. Some surgeons use this elevator as a retractor rather than one of the specific retractors; therefore, it is helpful to have two periosteal elevators on the tray—one for reflection and one for retraction. The surgeon receives from the assistant the surgical handpiece with a round bur.

8. Pick up the irrigating syringe. Some handpieces have a device that provides automatic irrigation during use so that the irrigating syringe is not needed. The surgeon uses the handpiece and the retractor while the assistant uses the irrigating syringe and the HVE tip. Whenever a handpiece is used to remove bone, the area must be irrigated simultaneously; this helps keep debris from the flutes of the bur, keeps the bone from desiccating (overheating and burning), and helps keep the area clean so that the surgeon has good visibility. A slight stream of water must be kept on the end of the bur.

9. Place the HVE nearby so that the mouth does not fill with water, but do not keep it so near that the liquid from the irrigating syringe goes directly into the HVE tip without touching the bur.

10. As the surgeon moves the handpiece and bur, follow closely, making sure that the water always stays on the end of the bur.

11. Occasionally, when bone relief or sectioning is done, the assistant will have to stop and refill the syringe. If the surgeon asks, it is helpful occasionally to irrigate and clean the entire surgical site and evacuate the patient's mouth. During this point in the procedure, the surgeon's goal is to remove enough bone (usually a small amount) to be able to visualize the roots of the tooth and divide them.

12. In this situation the roots are exposed and the two buccal roots are divided from the rest of the tooth. To accomplish this, a groove is made part of the way through the roots of the tooth. At this point some surgeons prefer to switch to a different bur, such as a straight fissure bur.

CASE #2 SURGICAL EXTRACTION—cont'd

13. Pass the surgeon a straight elevator to complete the split from the rest of the tooth.
14. Sometimes the roots come out easily at this point; at other times a root tip elevator (#2 or #3) is needed to lift the roots from the socket. The common sequence is to remove the buccal root tips and the rest of the tooth; the palatal root can be luxated and removed as a single-rooted tooth.
15. Pass the root-tip or cryer elevators individually to the surgeon to loosen the root tips.
16. Transfer forceps, such as the rongeur, to the surgeon for removal of the root tips. Occasionally, the tips may be removed by the assistant with the surgical HVE tip. Care should be taken to clear the HVE tip.
17. After these root tips are removed, the rest of the tooth and the palatal root can be luxated and removed almost as a single-rooted tooth.
18. The surgeon then takes the bayonet forceps (#210S) and removes the rest of the tooth. The assistant takes the tooth and the forceps together in the palm of the left hand and simultaneously hands the surgeon a curette to check for abscess formation (as described for the routine extraction).
19. When a tooth is removed surgically, sharp bony edges must often be smoothed. After the surgeon has finished with the curette, the instrument is exchanged for a double-ended bone file. If only one tooth has been removed, the smaller end of the bone file usually is used; if multiple teeth have been removed, the larger end is often used. The sharp edges of the instrument are passed along the edge of the bone to smooth it.
20. When either the curette or the bone file is handed back to the assistant, the HVE tip or a gauze sponge should be used to clean the end of the instrument to make it ready for use again; this also helps minimize instrument cleaning later because blood and bone fragments are more difficult to remove after they have dried.
21. When the surgeon decides that the bone is sufficiently smooth and the socket is clean, the bone file is exchanged for an irrigation syringe and the entire area is irrigated. All bone fragments and tooth debris must be removed from the area; otherwise they may cause an infection. The assistant may find it easier to have the patient turn to one side to gain access to the fluid in the mouth.

SUTURE PLACEMENT

1. Hand the surgeon the needle holder with the needle attached, having placed the needle into the holder so that the needle points in the proper direction to pass through the tissue. The position of the needle should enable it to pass through the tissue from the most mobile tissue (the reflected flap) to the least mobile tissue (the unreflected soft tissue), with the tip of the holder grasping the needle at right angles and approximately two thirds of the way from the tip. One surgical knot is placed in each interproximal area. At least one additional knot is placed in the vertical extension.
2. When the surgeon has passed the suture through both sides of the tissue, the suture is tied. The surgeon needs both hands to tie the knot, so the assistant must retract the tissue. This may be done with the HVE tip, a mirror, or a retractor or by hand. The assistant needs to reach around the back of the patient's head to retract the cheek on the right side of the mouth to avoid obstructing the surgeon's view. At times the assistant may need to retract both cheek and tongue, such as in the mandibular right quadrant.
3. After the knot is tied, the suture must be cut. This is usually done by the assistant, although some dentists prefer to cut the suture themselves.
4. Hold the scissors with the thumb and the fourth (ring) finger. This technique provides more stability than holding the scissors with the thumb and the third finger. Most surgeons use suture scissors that are slightly curved. The assistant brings the scissors into the oral cavity with the beaks closed and the tips pointing away from the alveolar ridge. This prevents the assistant from inadvertently cutting the patient.
5. The suture should be cut with the tips of the scissors, and the assistant must watch carefully when cutting so as to protect the patient. The length of the suture ends should be approximately 2 mm, although this depends on the preference of the surgeon. Silk sutures that must be removed usually are left with longer tails than resorbable sutures, which dissolve and come out on their own.

During the extraction the assistant must keep the tray neat and orderly, returning used instruments to their original position. A basin or bag should be available for trash (such as empty suture packets and used gauze). Used sharps must be kept separate. Trash must not cover the tray, impeding easy access to the instruments. Some surgeons may request that the used anesthetic carpules be kept separate from the rest of the trash, so that the carpules can easily be accounted for.

CASE #3 MULTIPLE EXTRACTIONS WITH IMMEDIATE DENTURE PLACEMENT
PATIENT DATA:
55-year-old male. Heavy decay and periodontal disease are present. The prosthodontist has already made the denture.
PROCEDURE

1. Hand the curette and retractor to the surgeon. When the areas are evaluated for adequate anesthesia, the patient's response indicates that several spots are painful.
2. Return the curette and retractor to the tray and pass the syringe to the surgeon to administer more anesthetic.
3. Once the level of anesthesia is adequate, hand the scalpel to the surgeon to make an incision through the soft tissue in the mandibular right quadrant (this is an arbitrary place to begin surgery; each surgeon initiates the procedure at the preferred area).
4. Exchange the scalpel for a periosteal elevator; the surgeon reflects a small mucoperiosteal flap to allow access to the teeth.
5. Retrieve the periosteal elevator and pass a straight elevator to the surgeon to luxate the teeth.
6. The surgeon removes the remaining teeth with forceps as described for the extraction procedures.
7. After all teeth in this quadrant have been removed, hand the curette to the surgeon for removal of any pathosis in the alveolus. Throughout this procedure use the HVE to maintain a clear field of operation for the surgeon. Extractions of periodontally involved teeth can be quite bloody, and the need for the HVE tip must be anticipated.
8. Exchange the curette for rongeur to be used in removing any tenacious bits of tissue that are clinging to the bone. At this point the surgeon looks at the overall shape of the arch. The arch must be free of sharp edges, and undercuts should be kept to a minimum. The patient has one area of especially prominent bone over the edge of the mandibular right first premolar.
9. The surgeon uses the rongeur to remove most of this excessive bone. Each time the surgeon removes a piece of bone with the rongeur, hold out a gauze square and wipe the beaks of the instrument free of debris.
10. When the surgeon is satisfied with the shape of the bone, exchange the rongeur for a bone file. In this case the large end of the bone file is used because there is a lot of bone to smooth.
11. When the ridge is smooth, exchange the file for the irrigating syringe. The surgeon irrigates the site while the assistant evacuates. Suturing, which would ordinarily be done at this point, is delayed until the entire procedure is completed.

Attention now turns to the mandibular left quadrant. The procedure is identical to the one performed on the mandibular right quadrant. However, during the extraction of tooth #19, the mesial root fractures. Because a flap has already been reflected, it is relatively easy to remove the root tip.

12. The surgeon can handle a fractured mesial root in the following manner:
   a. Forceps are used on the root tip if it is accessible.
   b. Because roots usually aren't accessible enough, bone is removed to make the roots accessible; a medium-sized root pick (#2 or #3) is used to lift the root out of the socket, using the palatal portion of the socket as a fulcrum; in this case the root tip is located toward the buccal area.
13. The surgeon makes a small perforation through the bone at the apex of the root tip with the handpiece and uses the root elevator to ease the root tip out.
14. The remainder of this procedure, including the extraction of the six anterior teeth, proceeds as described for case #2. Often, the cuspids usually are strong teeth with excellent bone support, making them difficult to remove.

STENT TRY-IN/DENTURE INSERTION

When all of the teeth are removed, the ridge is prepared, and before suturing begins, the plastic stent is tried in. A **stent** is a clear plastic denture base that is made on the same model as the denture. The surgeon can see through the stent to the arch beneath to identify areas that impinge on the stent.

1. Pass the stent to the surgeon to try in. The stent does not seat correctly; the surgeon can see that the area already trimmed is the problem area.
2. The surgeon passes the stent back and removes more bone from this area, using the handpiece with a bone-trimming bur.
3. After the area is irrigated, the denture is tried in again. This time it fits. If a stent had not been used, it probably would have been more difficult to identify interferences that were causing the denture not to seat properly.

CASE #3 MULTIPLE EXTRACTIONS WITH IMMEDIATE DENTURE PLACEMENT—cont'd

SUTURE PLACEMENT

Now that the denture fits, the soft tissue is sutured. The surgeon decides whether to use individual knots or a continuous suture. With a continuous suture, a traditional knot is tied at one end of the arch. Only the short end of the knot is trimmed, and the long end is used to sew the tissue closed. Usually a knot is tied in the midline and a second suture is started from the other end. When it is time to tie the second knot, the needle is passed through the tissue; however, the last loop of suture is not pulled tight. Instead, it is used to make a knot with the remainder of the suture that is attached to the needle.

CASE #4 THIRD MOLAR EXTRACTIONS

PATIENT DATA:

18-year-old female.
The patient has insulin-dependent diabetes but no other health-related contraindications.

PROCEDURE
ANESTHETIC ADMINISTRATION

Because the patient is diabetic, the assistant asks her about her last meal. The patient reports that she ate a light breakfast approximately 1 hour before coming to the office and took half of her normal morning dose of insulin. The primary care physician and the surgeon had recommended that the patient be premedicated with an antibiotic to lessen the possibility of postoperative infection.

The patient is to have a combination of nitrous oxide and IV sedation. The surgeon comes in, reclines the chair, and places the nitrous oxide mask on the patient's nose. The level is set at 60% nitrous oxide and 40% oxygen. The patient is advised that soon she will begin to feel tingling in her hands and feet. As the nitrous oxide begins to take effect, the surgeon and the assistant place the IV (described in procedures earlier in this chapter). In this case, Versed and Demerol will be used. First, meperidine is administered and the patient is warned that stinging occasionally occurs in the area where the IV has been placed but goes away quickly. The Versed is **titrated** in slowly. The patient is told that she will start to feel as if she is floating, the lights will appear to be moving, it will become difficult for her to talk, and she will not remember anything of the procedure. The patient must be informed of the effect of the sedative.

Using nitrous oxide in addition to the IV sedation gives the surgeon more control over the anesthesia than if sedation alone were used. The nitrous oxide potentiates the sedation, making it more effective at lower doses. Therefore, the patient is relaxed and comfortable throughout the procedure and recovers quickly after the surgery. The extra oxygen supplied to the patient helps with sedation; it eases breathing and reduces anxiety during recovery.

Local anesthetic is administered. Approximately 1 1/4 carpules are used for each third molar; one is used to infiltrate the mucosa next to the maxillary third or to block half of the mandible, and approximately 1/4 carpule is used to infiltrate the palatal and the long buccal nerves; the technique for this is identical to that described earlier in this chapter.

EXTRACTION PROCEDURE

Maxillary left third molar

1. Pass the retractor and the curette to the surgeon. Assess the soft tissue posterior to tooth #15 for patient reaction. When the patient indicates there is no pain when the curette is used, the procedure continues.
2. Exchange the curette for a scalpel; the surgeon makes an incision through the tissue in the posterior left maxilla. Using the HVE tip on the tissue before the first incision is made keeps saliva to a minimum, and optimum vision is maintained. The incision parallels the ridge posterior to the second molar tooth, follows the gingival crevice around the second molar to the papilla, and is extended vertically up into the vestibule.
3. Exchange the scalpel for the periosteal elevator, passing the latter to the surgeon with the pointed end available for immediate use. The surgeon uses the retractor in the left hand to hold the patient's cheek out of the way and elevates the mucoperiosteal flap with the periosteal elevator in the right hand. Once some of the tissue is reflected, the surgeon places the retractor between the tissue and bone to continue to facilitate vision.

Continued.

CASE #4 THIRD MOLAR EXTRACTIONS—cont'd

4. When the flap is completely reflected, the surgeon returns the periosteal elevator and receives a chisel or a bone bur in a surgical handpiece. Surgeons vary the technique based on the amount and density of the bone to be removed.

5. When using a surgical handpiece, follow the technique for removing an erupted tooth. Hold the HVE tip in the right hand and the irrigation syringe in the left hand. Drip a slow, steady stream of sterile water or saline solution onto the bur to prevent heat generation. Use the HVE tip to keep the surgical site clear.

6. When this procedure is used for maxillary teeth, the mandibular arch and posterior pillar region must be evacuated occasionally. Be alert to the patient's needs because the patient's gag reflex is diminished when he or she is sedated.

7. Once an adequate amount of bone has been removed from the buccal surface of the tooth, the surgeon exchanges the handpiece for a #77 elevator (or other preferred elevator).

8. The surgeon positions the elevator between the tooth and the edge of the bone and pushes the impacted third molar distally out of the socket, using the bone as the fulcrum. Support the patient's head as needed during this step because a sedated patient has lost muscle strength and will move along with the pressure of the elevator. When the head is supported, the pressure from the elevator is more effective.

9. If the tooth does not move easily, the elevator is exchanged for the handpiece to remove more bone.

10. Once the tooth has been elevated from the socket, the surgeon exchanges the elevator for a bayonet forceps. The angle on the end of the forceps allows the instrument to be placed in a small area.

11. If the elevator dislodges the tooth, the surgeon may ask for a rongeur or forceps to remove the loosened tooth from the mouth. Sometimes it can be brought out with the elevator, or it can be removed with the HVE tip.

12. Keep the HVE tip in place until the tooth is removed from the mouth. Teeth can be quite slippery, and occasionally a tooth may pop out of the socket and into the patient's mouth, where it could be swallowed or aspirated, so position the HVE tip between the tooth and the throat as a precautionary measure.

13. Once the tooth has been removed, assess the roots of the tooth for fractures.

14. If one or more of the root tips is sharp or appears to be fractured, notify the surgeon. Many surgeons examine extracted teeth themselves. In case #4 all of the root tips came out intact.

15. The surgeon receives the curette from the assistant and uses it to remove the *dental follicle*—a sac of slightly thickened membrane—from the socket; this occurs routinely when third molars are removed from young patients. The follicle is part of the developing tooth. With age, the follicle shrinks and eventually disappears. It is important to remove the follicle, however; if it remains, it might develop into a cyst.

16. Exchange the curette for the rongeur, and while the surgeon is removing tissue from the socket, prepare a gauze sponge to remove any tissue from the ends of the rongeur.

17. When the surgeon is finished with the rongeur, it is returned.

18. Once the socket has been cleaned, pass the bone file to the surgeon, who smoothes the edge of the socket. Occasionally, the surgeon might extend the bone file toward you to clean the end of it with the HVE.

19. The surgeon exchanges the file for the irrigating syringe. Evacuate the entire surgical site as it is irrigated with sterile saline or water. The surgeon returns the syringe.

20. Pass the needle holder with the suture needle placed so that the surgeon can suture from posterior to anterior.

21. When the surgeon is ready to tie the suture, retract the oral tissues so that the surgeon can use both hands to tie the suture.

22. In the maxillary and mandibular left quadrants, with a right-handed surgeon, you can cut the suture; however, often it is difficult for the assistant to see well enough to do this on the right side of the patient's mouth. In this case the surgeon cuts the suture. Usually, three sutures are needed to close the third molar incision: one interproximally, one posteriorly, and one in the vertical extension of the incision.

23. If a removable suture is used, record on the patient chart the number of sutures used in each area.

24. After this extraction has been completed, put a folded gauze sponge over the extraction site.

Maxillary right third molar

1. Turn the patient's head to the left and adjust the light to shine on the maxillary right quadrant.

2. The surgeon receives the retractor and the curette and begins the procedure again. Tooth #1 is removed in the same fashion as #16.

3. Once the extraction of #1 has been completed, raise the patient to a semisitting position. Readjust the patient's head to the right and adjust the light.

CASE #4 THIRD MOLAR EXTRACTIONS—cont'd

Between each of these procedures, the assistant should reorganize the tray, discarding any used sponges appropriately and repositioning the instruments. The assistant checks the length of the remaining suture to make sure there is enough to continue (this may be a problem when suturing after the last tooth has been extracted). Some surgeons may want the scalpel blade to be changed at this point. The surgeon also assesses the patient's state of relaxation. In this case the patient had started to awaken, so more of the sedative drug midazolam was administered. Refill the irrigation syringe and prepare more gauze sponges for later use. Once the procedure begins, it is vital to keep the chair time to a minimum.

Mandibular right third molar

The procedure for removing the mandibular third molars is similar to that for removing the maxillary third molars, with several important differences.

1. Ask the patient to open the mouth wide. Remove any gauze sponges that are present.
2. Because the patient is drowsy and has difficulty keeping the mouth open, place a rubber bite block on the right side of the mouth. This helps stabilize the jaw and protects against closing down on the bur or scalpel and possibly causing pain.
3. The surgeon assesses the anesthesia with the curette as before. In this case the patient did not react to the curette but did react slightly when the incision was extended to the interproximal space between teeth #18 and #19. This indicated that the anesthesia from the long buccal injection (which covered the area directly over the third molar area) was adequate, but the mandibular block was not completely successful. This block controls anesthesia of the tooth, bone, and soft tissue from the interproximal forward.
4. Exchange the scalpel for the anesthetic syringe. The surgeon administers another mandibular block to provide complete anesthesia.
5. Once the anesthesia is adequate, pass the scalpel to the surgeon to make an incision.
6. Exchange the scalpel for a periosteal elevator for the surgeon to begin the reflection of the flap. The surgeon makes an angled incision over the soft tissue that lies immediately over the third molar and extends this incision forward along the gingival margin and through the interproximal papilla. In this flap design a vertical extension is not used, although some surgeons use one routinely.
7. Often, during reflection of this flap, the surgeon and the assistant must alternate the scalpel and the periosteal elevator several times. Keep the scalpel ready for reuse until the surgeon indicates that it is no longer needed. On the patient's left side, help retract the patient's cheek with the HVE tip. On the patient's right side, help retract the patient's tongue with the HVE tip. In the mandibular arch, gravity tends to direct the saliva, irrigation, and blood into and over the surgical site, so use the HVE tip efficiently.
8. The surgeon finishes with the periosteal elevator and returns it. In this case, however, the surgeon is not satisfied with the exposure achieved with the periosteal elevator alone.
9. Transfer the scissors to the surgeon to place in the posterior portion of the incision, between the bone and periosteum and with the beaks closed and the tip curved toward the bone and away from the tissue. The surgeon then opens the beaks of the scissors, stretching the tissue and improving visibility.
10. This opening and closing may need to be done several times before the surgeon is ready to exchange the scissors for the periosteal elevator to make the final reflection of the flap.
11. The surgeon receives the rongeur and removes some fibrous material from over the tooth.
12. After removing this bone, the surgeon can opt to use a handpiece with a bur or a mallet and chisel. Most surgeons today use the handpiece.
13. The surgeon holds the retractor in the left hand and the handpiece in the right hand. Hold the HVE in the right hand for both evacuating and retracting, and hold the irrigation syringe in the left hand. Use the single-handed instrument transfer to retract in the mandibular arch. That way, one hand is always free.
14. The surgeon removes bone from the surgical site until the tooth is exposed and follows the outline of the tooth with the bur to expose as much of the crown of the tooth as possible. Always warn the surgeon when the end of the water supply is near. Another assistant may need to fill the sterile water supply. Do not leave chairside to obtain more solution.
15. Once the tooth is exposed, the surgeon might ask for an elevator to luxate the tooth. In this case, however, the tooth cannot be lifted out in one piece, so the surgeon asks the assistant to refill the irrigation syringe. The next task is to divide the roots of the tooth.

Continued.

CASE #4 THIRD MOLAR EXTRACTIONS—cont'd

16. The surgeon makes a vertical groove along the central groove of the buccal surface of the tooth. A straight fissure bur may be used to extend the groove about halfway through the tooth. Then exchange the handpiece for a #77 elevator.
17. The surgeon places the elevator into the groove in the tooth and rotates it distally. This completes the crack through the crown of the tooth. Now that the fragments are loosened, the elevator can be used to remove them.
18. Completion of this extraction is almost identical to that of the maxillary third molar. The only difference is that the surgeon may decide to place a medicated dressing made of tetracycline and an absorbable gelatin sponge (Gelfoam) in the socket.
19. In earlier preparations a dappen dish with tetracycline powder was placed on the tray. Mix this with sterile saline to make a slurry paste.
20. Dip a piece of the gelatin sponge into the solution with a cotton forceps.
21. Transfer this to the surgeon after the suture has been placed for the last stitch but before the knot is tied.
22. The surgeon places the gelatin sponge in the socket, returns the cotton pliers, and finishes tying the suture knot.
23. Remove the bite block, evacuate the patient's mouth, and allow the patient to close the mouth and rest for a moment before the last tooth is removed.
24. Inspect and reorganize the tray and refill the irrigating syringe.

Mandibular left third molar

1. The surgeon asks the patient to turn to the right and open the mouth wide.
2. Place the bite block and adjust the light before the procedure begins again.
3. The procedure is identical to the previous extraction, with one exception. On this side, after the crown of the tooth is sectioned, both halves of the crown are removed, but the root tips fracture. Slightly more bone is removed to expose the root tips, which are edged out with a fine root-tip pick.

CASE #5 EXPOSURE OF IMPACTED CUSPID

PATIENT DATA:

11-year-old female.
The patient was referred by her orthodontist for exposure of the impacted right maxillary cuspid.

PROCEDURE
ANESTHETIC ADMINISTRATION

The patient is quite anxious about having this procedure done because she has never had local anesthetic. As a result, her mother has given permission for her to be sedated. The procedure is much the same as those previously described, except that the surgical team has the additional responsibility of managing child behavior by encouraging the child to trust them. In this case, all of the equipment was demonstrated at the preoperative visit to reduce the patient's anxiety. At this appointment the patient is still a little nervous, so nitrous oxide and oxygen are used to help her relax before insertion of the IV needle. Once the IV is placed and flowing, the patient is sedated. Patient positioning is important for this procedure. Most of the work will be done on the patient's palate, and she is placed in a complete supine position or even slightly beyond supine position, so that the surgeon's vision is as unobstructed as possible. The light is adjusted so that it shines on the palate without being blocked by the surgeon's or the assistant's head. The local anesthetic is administered, and the nitrous oxide is discontinued. After 5 minutes on 100% oxygen, the mask is removed (it would press on the lip and interfere with the surgeon's view). In this case, local anesthetic is infiltrated on both buccal and palatal sides of the arch from just posterior to tooth #6 to the midline.

EXPOSURE PROCEDURE

1. Pass a curette to the surgeon to assess anesthesia.
2. If the anesthesia is adequate, exchange the curette for a scalpel; the surgeon makes an incision on the palatal side of the involved area.

CASE #5 EXPOSURE OF IMPACTED CUSPID—cont'd

3. The surgeon alternates the scalpel with the periosteal elevator while reflecting the flap because palatal tissue is fibrous and can be difficult to reflect.
4. The surgeon removes a thin layer of bone that overlies the impacted tooth. The surgeon must be careful during this procedure because the tooth must not be scarred. Often, when the bone gets to be quite thin, the surgeon completes the remainder of the bone relief by using a bone chisel. Use caution during irrigation to prevent water from entering the posterior of the mouth.
5. Once the surgeon exposes the crown of the tooth, there is usually a fairly good-sized follicle that must be removed. Exchange either the handpiece or the chisel for a curette. Often the surgeon uses a periodontal curette, which is more useful in removing a follicle.
6. Be ready with the rongeur—once the follicle is loosened, the surgeon will want to use the rongeur to remove any loose tissue.
7. After the follicle is removed and the tooth is clearly exposed, the surgeon returns the curette and the rongeur to the assistant and prepares to irrigate the site.
8. Receive the irrigating syringe and any retractors that the surgeon has used. Transfer a tissue pliers and either a scalpel or a tissue scissors to the surgeon to trim the tissue so that the tooth can be clearly seen.
9. The surgeon passes the excised tissue to the assistant. Transfer the suture setup and the needle holder; the surgeon places one suture in each interproximal area.
10. When the flaps are repositioned and sutured, place some gauze sponges in the patient's mouth to keep the area as dry as possible.

DRESSING PLACEMENT

1. Mix a periodontal dressing to cover and protect the area while it is healing.
2. Give the surgeon some lubricant to prevent the gloves from sticking to the dressing.
3. When the dressing begins to stiffen, pass the material to the surgeon.
4. Pass the surgeon a plastic instrument to place the dressing around the surgical site while you retract the tissues.
5. Remove debris from the plastic instrument when necessary.
6. The surgeon asks the patient to tap the teeth together a few times to make sure that the dressing does not interfere with the occlusion. If the dressing is marked by tooth marks, it must be adjusted so that the dressing will not be dislodged by chewing.
7. Tell the patient to eat only soft foods for the next week and not to chew gum until the dressing is removed 1 week later at the follow-up appointment.

CASE #6 FRENECTOMY

PATIENT DATA:

Edentulous 47-year-old patient.
Thick, fibrous frenum on the maxillary that interferes with prosthesis placement.

PROCEDURE
ANESTHETIC ADMINISTRATION

The patient is prepared and anesthetized in the usual fashion.

FRENECTOMY PROCEDURE

1. The surgeon assesses for adequate local anesthesia by pinching tissue with a tissue pliers. The patient indicates that this does not feel sharp.
2. The surgeon everts and exposes the frenal attachment area. Exchange a straight hemostat for the tissue pliers. The hemostat is used to grasp the tissue of the frenum. The surgeon locks the hemostat closed and uses it as a handle for the tissue.
3. Pass the surgeon a scalpel and retract the lip. The surgeon runs the scalpel down each side of the hemostat, removing a thin section of tissue along with the hemostat. When the lip is relaxed, this leaves a diamond-shaped incision.
4. The surgeon then takes the sharp tissue scissors, undermines the tissue, and irrigates the area.
5. The surgeon closes the incision with three or four sutures, leaving a vertical incision.
6. At the follow-up appointment 3 months later, the area is healing.

CASE #7 BIOPSY/CYTOLOGY SMEAR

PATIENT DATA:

64-year-old male who has been a smoker during his adult life.
An ulcer that would not heal was discovered on the inside mandibular lip about a month ago.
The ulcer is about 2 cm in diameter; the surgeon plans an incisional biopsy.
Further treatment is planned after the pathologist reports a diagnosis.

BIOPSY PROCEDURE

The area is anesthetized by infiltrating local anesthetic around the lesion.
1. Transfer the scalpel to the surgeon to make a wedge-shaped incision through the edge of the lesion.
2. Pass the surgeon a tissue forceps to hold the biopsy specimen while it is released from the underlying tissue. (Two dental assistants are needed for this type of procedures.) Retract the lip, holding it out with fingers on each side of the lesion. The lip is pinched tightly to help control the bleeding. The second assistant passes instruments and evacuates in the usual fashion; during the biopsy, simply blotting the surgical site frequently with gauze is more effective than using suction on the soft tissue.
3. After the surgeon has removed the wedge of tissue, provide a small bottle of 10% formalin into which the specimen is dropped. Tightly close the lid and then irrigate the surgical site. The surgeon closes the incision.
4. Prepare the specimen with the necessary data (patient's name, date, site of the biopsy, history of the lesion, and tentative diagnosis). Send the specimen to the laboratory for analysis.
5. Give the patient an appointment to return in 1 week for the results.

A. The patient is given written instructions for later reference (box on page 409).
B. In addition, the assistant explains the prescriptions and the schedule for taking the medication.
C. If the patient is older and possibly forgetful, is a child, or has been sedated, the assistant invites the person who has accompanied the patient into the treatment room to listen to the instructions.
D. Before the patient is discharged, demonstrate how to change the gauze; give the patient some extra gauze to take home.
E. If the procedure is difficult, give the patient an ice pack.
F. When the patient has no more questions, walk with him or her to the business desk.
V. Place a follow-up call later in the day or early the next morning to verify the patient's progress.
VI. The procedure for suture removal is provided (box on page 410).

HOSPITAL DENTISTRY

I. Many surgical procedures, especially anesthetic administration, may be performed in a hospital setting.
II. Many hospitals include operating suites that are completely equipped to perform clinical dentistry—both restorative and surgical.
III. A dentist who frequently practices hospital dentistry may use the services of his or her own dental assistant.
IV. The protocol of the particular hospital is followed to meet the appropriate credentials, staffing, scheduling, and facility use.
V. Many hospitalized patients require dental treatment because of illness or traumatic injury.
VI. Most hospital dental patients are admitted specifically for dental treatment, including the following:
A. Medically compromised patients who have a systemic disease and thus are at greater risk than normal for treatment in the general practice office.
B. Disabled patients who are unable to tolerate care in the private dental office, because of their physical or emotional disability. Those with Down syndrome, severe arthritis, or Parkinson's disease may be unable to control motions and may present potential safety complications during treatment.
C. Trauma patients with jaw fractures or head and neck injuries who may not be able to be transferred to a dental chair.
D. Patients needing extensive oral procedures, such as multiple extractions, alveoloplasty, or other full-mouth construction.
E. Individuals who have been hospitalized for

GENERAL INSTRUCTIONS*

1. Keep the pressure gauze firmly over the surgery site for 30 to 45 minutes unless instructed otherwise. After this it may be discarded.
2. Do not rinse your mouth or spit forcefully the day of surgery. Starting the next evening it may be beneficial to use a warm saltwater rinse (1/3 teaspoon salt to a full glass of warm water) gently twice a day, or use chlorhexidine gluconate (Peridex) rinse if it has been prescribed.
3. Do not brush your teeth in the area of surgery the day your teeth are removed. After that, gentle brushing is recommended until the area is healed.
4. If it is more comfortable, or if you are instructed to do so, eat soft or liquid foods but *not not stop taking nourishment*. Do not drink through a straw. Change to a regular diet as soon as possible, but do not skip a meal.
5. Do not smoke for at least 24 hours.

PRESCRIPTION SCHEDULE

1. **PAIN** Start taking the pain medication that is prescribed for you before the anesthetic wears off. Follow the instructions written on the bottle—do not take more medication than you are instructed to take. If the medication does not give you sufficient relief, please call the office. All pain medication should be taken with milk, yogurt, or food to prevent nausea.
2. **BLEEDING** Slight oozing of blood may occur the first day and night after surgery. If it seems excessive, place a pad of gauze folded so that it is at least an inch thick directly over the surgery site and close your teeth together firmly. (Do not use absorbent cotton or paper tissues.) If no gauze is available, a small, clean handkerchief or a tea bag will do. Do not get excited. Sit quietly and put pressure on the gauze for 30 minutes. If bleeding persists, take a fresh gauze pad and apply pressure for 30 minutes more. If you are still concerned about the bleeding, call the office.
3. **SWELLING** Temporary swelling of the cheeks after surgery is common. An ice pack placed on the cheek for 30 minutes of each hour for the first 12 to 24 hours after surgery will help keep the swelling to a minimum. Any swelling that develops will subside in 4 to 6 days.
4. **JAW STIFFNESS** Like the swelling, this stiffness is a natural reaction of your body to surgery and should disappear within 4 to 6 days. Starting 72 hours after the surgery you may use warm, moist towels; a hot water bottle; or an electric heating pad to help reduce the swelling or stiffness. Make sure the heat is not excessive—extreme heat can cause painful skin burns.
5. **FACIAL DISCOLORATION** A day or so after the surgery you may notice a yellow, blue, or brown color on the skin of the face adjacent to the surgery area. This, too, is temporary and will disappear after a few days.
6. **SUTURES** Sutures (stitches) May be placed at the time of your surgery. These will dissolve within 4 to 6 days. You do not need to return to have these removed.
7. **OTHER** If you have any questions or concerns, please call the office (try to call during office hours unless it is an emergency).

Note:
   On the day of surgery please follow the schedule provided below. On the day after surgery try taking the Motrin only. If you need the Tylox/Zydone, take it; however, because it is a narcotic, please stop taking it as soon as you no longer need it.

Today:
   Tylox/Zydone ____   ____   ____   ____   ____
   Motrin: ____   ____   ____   ____
   Other: ____   ____   ____

Tomorrow:
   Try taking Motrin only.
   If an antibiotic has been prescribed, continue taking it as directed until all the tablets are gone.

Tomorrow evening:
   Start Peridex/saltwater rinses and continue as prescribed for 1 to 2 weeks.

*(Courtesy Helen Zylman, DDS, Ann Arbor, Michigan.)

PROCEDURE FOR SUTURE REMOVAL

- In some states suture removal is delegated to a qualified assistant. Typically, removable sutures are left in place 5 to 7 days. If they remain longer, they may increase the contamination of the underlying tissues. Suture removal involves the following steps:
1. Examine the patient's record to determine the type and number of sutures that were previously placed.
2. Clean surface debris from the site with a cotton-tipped applicator that has been soaked in peroxide, iodophor, or other antiseptic solution.
3. Cut the suture with a sharp, pointed, or specially designed suture scissors. If the suture was continuous, a single suture is cut at a time.
4. With a cotton pliers, remove the suture by pulling it toward the incision line—not away from the suture line. However, if the suture knot is positioned on the incisional side, the suture is removed from the knot side.
5. Wipe the area with a piece of cotton gauze.
6. Record on the patient's record the appearance of the tissue and the number of sutures removed

cancer treatment and are to receive radiation treatment before hospital release.

    F. Patients who seek hospital dental care for convenience, because of irrational fear, or because the dental care is in conjunction with other head-and-neck surgical procedures.

VII. The environment and number of team members may change.

VIII. Constant monitoring of the patient is necessary.

IX. Sterile techniques must be used.

X. Medical wastes must be managed safely and according to policy requirements.

Questions

Oral and Maxillofacial Surgery

1 A biopsy is the
  a. Existence of a lesion in the oral cavity
  b. Surgical removal of an abscessed tooth
  c. Removal of tissue for diagnostic purposes
  d. Radical removal of a cancerous lesion

2 An impaction is a
  a. Succedaneous tooth
  b. Tooth that will not erupt fully
  c. Tooth that is ankylosed
  d. Tooth that never fully develops

3 A cyst is
  a. Found in the pulp of primary teeth
  b. A cell-lined sac
  c. A passageway for nerves
  d. Always connected to an abscess

4 To stop bleeding after an extraction, the best technique is to
  a. Medicate with antibiotics
  b. Apply indirect pressure
  c. Apply direct pressure
  d. Place a drain in the extraction socket

5 Which of the following groups of instruments should the dental assistant prepare for the removal and smoothing of sharp projections of bone on a patient's mandibular ridge during oral surgery?
  a. Rongeur, chisel, straight elevator, forceps, and bone file
  b. Chisel, bone file, and rongeur
  c. Straight elevator, forceps, and bone file
  d. Rongeur, chisel, straight elevator, and forceps

6 Which is not a major area of treatment for an oral surgeon?
  a. Temporomandibular surgery
  b. Cleft palate repair
  c. Pulpectomy
  d. Pathology

7 Which is not a minor area of treatment for an oral surgeon?
  a. Apicoectomy
  b. Extractions
  c. Biopsy
  d. Preprosthetic

8 Nitrous oxide is used
  a. With no other medication
  b. In conjunction with inhaled gases
  c. With injected agents
  d. All of the above

9 To prepare a medication from a multidose vial, the assistant must
  1. Recap the syringe after drawing the medication
  2. Draw the fluid with the vial diaphragm facing the floor
  3. Draw the fluid with the vial diaphragm facing upward
  4. Inject air into the vial
  5. Cleanse the vial diaphragm
  6. Remove bubbles from the syringe after the needle is removed from the vial
  a. 1, 2, and 4
  b. 1, 3, 5, and 6
  c. 1, 2, 4, and 5
  d. 1, 2, 4, 5, and 6

10 Which instrument is used primarily to reflect and lift the periosteum?
  a. Cryer
  b. Periosteal elevator
  c. Root-tip elevator
  d. Hemostat

11 Which instrument is used primarily to luxate a tooth from the socket?

a. Periosteal elevator
b. Root-tip elevator
c. Straight elevator
d. Forceps

12 Postoperative surgical instructions include
  1. Use a heat pack for the first 12 to 24 hours to reduce swelling.
  2. Maintain pressure over the surgical site with gauze for approximately 45 minutes.
  3. Begin eating only when food is comfortable in the mouth.
  4. Take pain medication with food to avoid nausea.
  5. Rinse with warm saltwater the day after surgery.

a. 1, 2 and 3
b. 1, 3 and 4
c. 1, 2, 3, 4 and 5
d. 2, 4, and 5

For items 13-15, select the instrument commonly used for each of the following procedures.

_____ **13** Which instrument is used to remove granulation tissue after an extraction?

_____ **14** Which instrument is used to contour the alveolar process?

_____ **15** Which instrument is used to remove roots of a mandibular molar when the crown is missing?

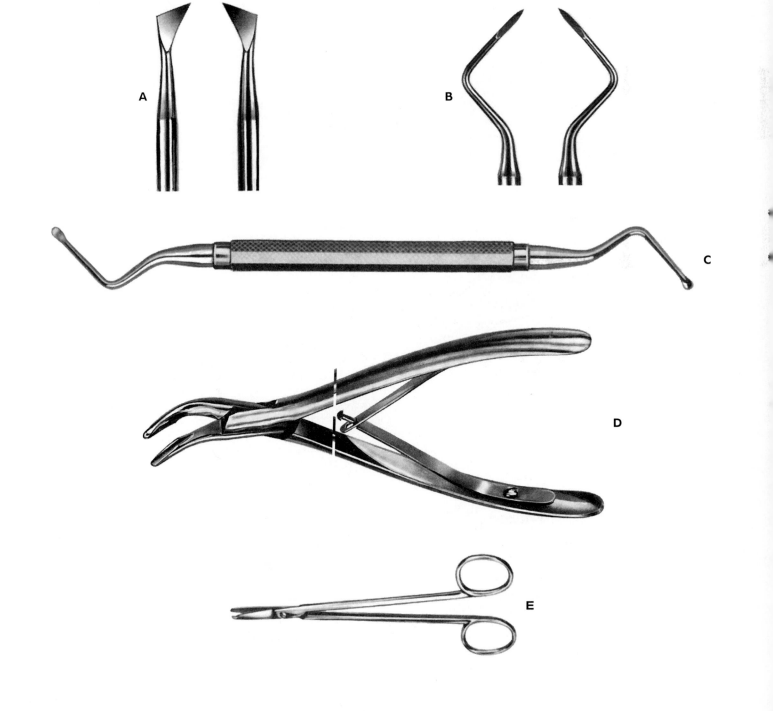

For items 16-18, select the instrument commonly used for each of the following procedures.

_____ **16** To remove the maxillary lateral incisor the following instrument is used.

_____ **17** To remove a maxillary right first molar the following instrument is used.

_____ **18** To remove a mandibular anterior tooth the following instrument is used.

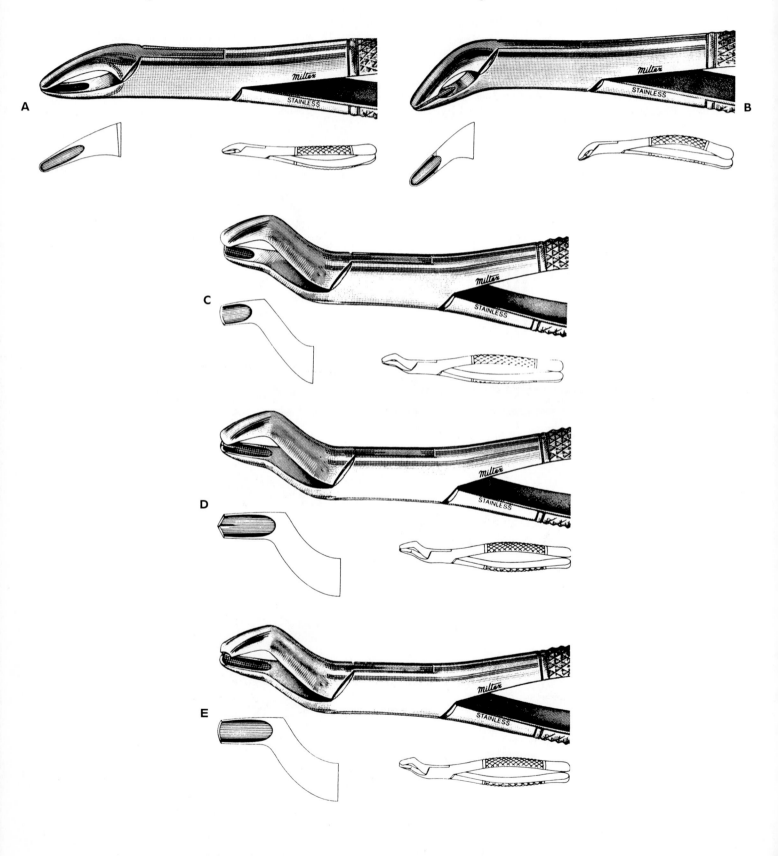

For items 19 and 20, select the instrument commonly used for each of the following procedures.

_____ **19** This instrument may be used for the apical portion of a root fracture during an extraction.

_____ **20** To release the periosteum prior to the extraction of a mandibular molar, this instrument would be used.

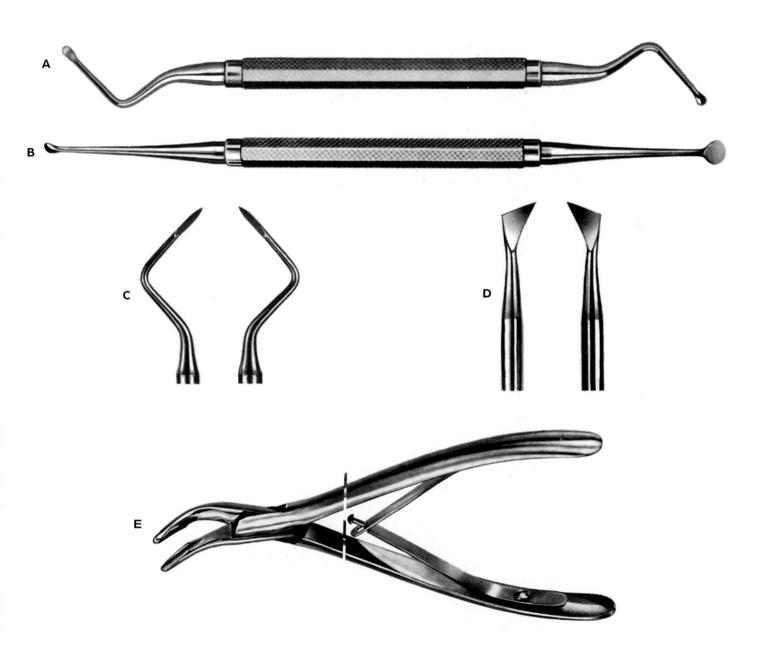

21 An osteoplasty is the
   a. Recontouring of gingival tissue
   b. Recontouring of bony defects
   c. Implanting of bone
   d. Treatment of choice for gingivitis

22 Electrosurgery is used to
   a. Cut tooth structure
   b. Cut bone
   c. Plate dies with copper

   d. Remove gingival tissue

23 An instrument used to hold a tissue flap away from the operating field is a(n)
   a. Pick
   b. Retractor
   c. Elevator
   d. Hemostat

24 An abscess is the
   a. Collection of serous fluid

b. Pathway for fluid drainage
c. Localized collection of pus
d. Infrabony process
25 A drain is placed to
    a. Create a pathway by which fluid can leave the body
    b. Hold bone fractures together
    c. Treat acute necrotizing ulcerative gingivitis
    d. Treat drug sockets

Rationales

Oral and Maxillofacial Surgery

1 C   A biopsy is a surgical diagnostic procedure. A biopsy may be incisional (only a small section of the lesion is removed, along with some normal tissue) or excisional (the entire lesion is removed, plus some normal tissue around the edge).

2 B   An impacted tooth is one that will not fully erupt. The position of the tooth in relation to other structures is such that other tissue impedes its full eruption.

3 B   A cyst is a pathologic space in bone or soft tissue that contains fluid or semifluid material, generally lined by epithelium.

4 C   Stopping bleeding in the oral cavity is not unlike doing so at any site in the body. Pressure must be applied. This is commonly done by folding a gauze pad and asking the patient to bite on it.

5 B   A combination of instruments could be used to remove a smooth projection of bone. The surgical chisel could be used alone for a small area or in conjunction with a mallet if a larger segment of bone needed to be removed. The rongeur would be used to remove sharp projections of bone. After bone removal the bone file would be used to smooth the site.

6 C   A pulpectomy is the removal of nerve tissue from the tooth. This procedure is performed by a general dentist or an endodontist.

7 A   An apicoectomy is an endodontic surgical procedure that involves removing the apex of the tooth and any necrotic tissue at the site. An amalgam restoration is then placed at the apical opening of the tooth.

8 D   Nitrous oxide is the most common anesthetic gas used in the dental office. It can be used as an analgesic gas alone or in conjunction with other inhaled or injected agents.

9 D   The procedure for preparing medication from a multidose vial involves the following steps:
- Wipe the diaphragm on top of the vial with an alcohol sponge and dry it with a sterile sponge.
- Inject into the vial the amount of air equal to the amount of medication to be used.
- Hold the vial with the diaphragm facing the floor and remove the needle cap. Pierce the rubber diaphragm.
- Push down on the plunger, injecting air into the vial.
- Pull back on the plunger again to withdraw the desired amount of medication to fill the syringe.
- If bubbles enter the syringe, remove them by gently tapping the syringe, sending the bubbles to the top of the medication at the needle end.
- Expel the bubbles by slightly pressing the plunger forward.
- After the syringe is filled, withdraw the needle from the vial and place the cap back over the needle again using the single-hand scoop method or a recapping device.
- If additional medication is needed, repeat the process, filling a sterile syringe each time.

10 B   The dental elevator is the workhorse of the surgical extraction tray. The periosteal elevator differs from the traditional elevator in that it is a double-ended instrument and is less bulky. Its primary function is to reflect, pull away, or detach and lift the tissue (including the periosteum) from the bone.

11 C   A straight elevator is the most common elevator used to luxate or loosen erupted teeth. The periosteal elevator was described in item 10; the root-tip elevator is reserved for use in the socket to remove fractured root tips.

12 D   General postoperative instructions for the patient include the following:
- Keep pressure gauze firmly over the surgery site for 30 to 45 minutes.
- Do not rinse the mouth or spit forcefully the day of surgery.
- Use warm saltwater as a gentle rinse the evening after surgery.
- Do not brush your teeth in the area of the surgery the day of the surgery.
- Eat soft foods or liquids if it is more comfortable. *Do not stop taking nourishment.*
- Do not smoke for 24 hours.
- Take prescribed medication as directed.

13 C   This is a surgical curette that is used to debride the socket and remove granulation tissue after a surgical procedure.

14 D   This is a rongeur used to cut and contour bone. After using it, a bone file may be used to smooth the area.

15 A   These are cryer elevators. The triangular beaks enable the operator to gain access to the furcation area and luxate the remaining tooth structure.

16 A   This maxillary universal forceps can be used to remove any of the maxillary anterior teeth. When placed on the tooth, the beaks are parallel to the long axis of the tooth, enabling the operator to grasp the tooth and remove it.

17 D   The beaks on a maxillary molar forceps are configured to grasp the single buccal root and the double lingual roots. In this forceps the groove on the buccal beak is placed between the two roots, and the flat beak is placed on the single lingual root. When positioned properly, the beaks are parallel to the long axis of the maxillary molar tooth.

18 B This universal mandibular anterior forceps is designed with the beaks nearly at a right angle to the handle. The small beaks can be placed around the tooth and, when in position, allow the operator to grasp and remove the tooth.

19 C The delicate blade of these root-tip picks or elevators allow the operator to access the alveolar socket and gently tease the root tip from the apical region.

20 A In addition to the periosteal elevator, the curette is sometimes used to release soft tissue from the site of a surgical procedure.

21 B Osseous surgery is the sculpting and contouring of the alveolar bone height. It may include the addition of bone or bone substitute.

22 D During this process an electrosurgery unit (a high-frequency electrical source) is used to cut or alter tissues in the oral cavity.

23 B Lip and cheek retractors provide clear vision for the oral surgeon. Some oral surgeons use a periosteal elevator for delicate tissue retraction, but most use delicate tissue retractors that are designed for this procedure.

24 C An abscess is a localized accumulation of pus in a cavity formed by tissue disintegration. Two common oral abscesses are periapical and periodontal.

25 A To allow exudate or pus to drain from a lesion, an oral surgeon may place a small tube into the drainage tract to allow fluid to escape from the site.

To enhance your understanding of the material in this chapter refer to the illustrations in Chapter 34 of Finkbeiner/Johnson: *Mosby's Comprehensive Dental Assisting: A Clinical Approach.*

CHAPTER 24

Orthodontics

OUTLINE

Malocclusion

Causes of Malocclusion

Timing of Orthodontic Treatment

Orthodontic Records

Treatment Planning

Mechanism of Tooth Movement

Orthodontic Appliances

Instruments and Procedures

Oral Hygiene

KEY TERMS

Angle's classification of
  malocclusion

  Class I

  Class II

  Class III

Archwire

Bracket

Corrective treatment

Crossbite

Elastic bands

Fixed appliance

Functional appliance

Headgear

Interceptive treatment

Ligature tie

Malocclusion

Orthodontic band

Overbite

Overjet

Prognathic

Removable appliance

Retrognathic

Separator

Orthodontics is the specialty of dentistry that involves the diagnosis, prevention, and treatment of dental and facial irregularities. An orthodontist must receive at least 2 additional years of formal education in an accredited university after attaining a dental degree; to become certified or licensed as an orthodontic specialist, he or she must pass a specialty examination administered by the state or regional board of dentistry. Membership in the American Association of Orthodontists denotes that the individual has met these standards of education and experience.

Although the orthodontic specialist provides most of the orthodontic treatment today, a number of family or pediatric dentists perform orthodontic treatment of an interceptive or a corrective nature in less involved cases.

Most state laws allow the dental assistant to perform many of the tasks involved, such as sizing and placing bands and placing ligature ties and separators. These procedures may be carried out independently with the patient; thus, assisting in orthodontics involves more one-to-one patient interaction and less four-handed dentistry than in other dental disciplines. The dental assistant not only may perform tasks related to the placement of the appliances, but also may be responsible for the education and motivation of patients in the use and care of their appliances. Working directly with the orthodontic patient can be challenging from the standpoint of patient management and employing procedures unique to this specialty. With a basic knowledge of orthodontic diagnostic and treatment procedures and with practice, these skills may soon be mastered.

MALOCCLUSION ▬▬▬▬▬▬

I. The orthodontists's primary role is the correction of malocclusion.

II. **Malocclusion** literally means *bad closure* and refers to irregularities in the positions of teeth and the bite relationships.

III. Most malocclusions result from irregularities, including the following:
   A. Positions of the teeth
   B. Facial bones
   C. Oral musculature

IV. In the ideal occlusal relationship the cusps of the maxillary posterior teeth fit neatly into the embrasures or grooves of the mandibular posterior teeth.
   A. The mesiobuccal cusp of the maxillary first permanent molar coincides with the buccal groove of the mandibular first permanent molar.
   B. The maxillary cuspid fits neatly into the embrasure between the mandibular cuspid and first premolar.
   C. The maxillary teeth overlap the mandibular teeth slightly in both a horizontal and a vertical direction in the anterior and posterior segments of the dentition.

V. Horizontal overlap of the incisor teeth is referred to as **overjet**
   A. Overjet is measured as the distance from the labial surface of the mandibular central incisors to the labial surface of the maxillary central incisors.
   B. The ideal occlusion is in the range of 2 to 3 mm.

VI. The extent to which the maxillary incisors overlap the mandibular incisors in a vertical direction is referred to as the **overbite.** The ideal overbite is 2 to 3 mm.

VII. Dr. Edward Angle in 1899 introduced a classification of malocclusion based on the relationship of the maxillary and mandibular first permanent molars. This system is known as **Angle's Classification of Malocclusion.**
   A. Class I
      1. In the Class I malocclusion, the mesiobuccal cusp of the maxillary first molar occludes in the buccal groove of the mandibular first molar.
      2. The occlusal relationships of the cuspids and premolars may also be taken into account to determine the classification of occlusion.
   B. Class II
      1. In the Class II malocclusion, the mesio-
buccal cusp of the maxillary first molar occludes anteriorly to the buccal groove of the mandibular first molar. The mandible is retruded, thus **retrognathic;** the mandible has a distal relationship with the maxilla.
      2. This classification is further divided into two types—divisions 1 and 2—based upon the positions of the incisor teeth.
         (a) In the Class II, division 1 malocclusion, the maxillary incisors are all inclined and protrude anteriorly, resulting in a large overjet.
         (b) In the Class II, division 2 malocclusion, the maxillary central incisors are inclined posteriorly, and the maxillary lateral incisors are frequently tipped labially.
   C. Class III
      1. In the Class III malocclusion, the mesiobuccal cusp of the maxillary first molar occludes posteriorly to the buccal groove of the mandibular first molar.
      2. In this type of malocclusion the maxillary incisors are occluding lingually to the mandibular incisors, resulting in negative overjet.
      3. The mandible is protruded, thus **prognathic.**
      4. The mandible has a mesial relationship with the maxilla.

VIII. Dental irregularities in malocclusion may be found within the dental arch (e.g., crowding) or may describe a variation from the normal relationship between the maxillary and mandibular dental arches upon closure.
   A. Crowding
      1. Crowding occurs when the teeth are too large for the perimeter of the dental arch.
      2. This results in rotation, tipping, and displacement in the positions of individual teeth within the dental arch.
   B. Spacing
      1. Spacing may result when the teeth are too small in comparison to the dental arch.
      2. Both crowding and spacing problems are caused primarily by hereditary factors.
   C. Deep overbite
      1. A deep overbite refers to excessive vertical overlap of the incisors upon closure; this type of relationship may be functionally unhealthy for the dentition. In extreme cases, the mandibular incisors may occlude

on the palatal gingiva, resulting in an im-pinging overbite.
b. If left untreated, this type of discrepancy may result in periodontal problems and eventual loss of the anterior teeth.
D. Open bite
1. The opposite of a deep overbite is an open bite, which occurs when, upon closure, there is no vertical overlap and no contact between certain maxillary and mandibular teeth.
2. Open bites occur most frequently in the an-terior region and are commonly associated with an oral habit such as thumb sucking or tongue thrusting.
3. Posterior open bites also occur, although they are much less common and may be associated with lateral tongue thrusting or ankylosis of primary molars.
E. **Crossbite**
1. A crossbite refers to an abnormal bucco-lingual relationship of the teeth. Posterior crossbite may exist when the buccal cusps of the maxillary molars or premolars oc-clude lingually to the buccal cusps of the mandibular posterior teeth.
2. Crossbite may occur on just one side or both sides of the mouth and may involve one tooth or several teeth.
3. In an anterior crossbite, the maxillary in-cisors may occlude lingually to the man-dibular anteriors; this is frequently associ-ated with a Class III malocclusion when it involves several teeth, or it may be just an isolated problem when the displacement of a single tooth is involved.

CAUSES OF MALOCCLUSION ■■■■■■

I. The two major causes of malocclusion are genetic and environmental factors.
A. Genetic factors
1. The most common cause of malocclusion is heredity.
2. Genetic factors may result in an imbalance in the size of the teeth compared with the size of the jaws, as in crowding.
3. Disharmony in the size and relationship of the maxilla and mandible may also be ge-netic, resulting in hereditary Class II or Class III malocclusions.
B. Environmental factors
1. Premature or delayed loss of primary teeth may cause displacement or impaction of the permanent successors.

> ### DENTAL DISCREPANCIES ASSOCIATED WITH LONG-TERM THUMB SUCKING
>
> - Protrusion of the maxillary incisors
> - Excessive overjet
> - Open bite
> - Posterior crossbite

2. Presence of supernumerary teeth or con-genital absence of teeth may result in mal-occlusion.
3. Oral habits such as thumb sucking can dis-tort the dental arches, affecting the posi-tions of the teeth and the occlusion (box above).
4. Tongue thrusting is a deviation from the normal pattern of swallowing, in which the tongue is pushed anteriorly between or against the maxillary and mandibular an-terior teeth upon swallowing.
a. This action inhibits the alveolar bone growth and development in the arch of the thrust and usually results in an open bite.
b. Tongue thrusting may be secondary to the open bite created by thumb sucking and may be retained even after elimi-nation of the thumb-sucking habit, re-sulting in a permanent deformity.
5. Mouth breathing is another oral habit that may affect the growth of the dentofacial complex.
II. Discrepancies in an occlusion often affect the long-term health of the dentition and the surround-ing oral structures.
A. Many problems that are left untreated tend to gradually worsen.
B. Teeth that are crowded may have a greater risk of tooth decay and periodontal disease, with possible subsequent tooth loss.
C. Malocclusion may result in excessive and un-even wear on the enamel surfaces of the den-tition.
D. Incorrect bites may cause stress on the jaw muscles and joints and become a contributing factor in temporomandibular joint (TMJ) dys-function.

TIMING OF ORTHODONTIC TREATMENT ■■■■

I. The American Association of Orthodontists has recommended that a child's first visit to the ortho-dontist take place at 7 years of age.

A. This age frequently corresponds with the eruption of the permanent incisors and first molars—a time when many orthodontic problems are first noted.

B. The child's general or pediatric dentist is instrumental in the diagnosis of these early signs of malocclusion.

II. Although many malocclusions are amenable to treatment at any age, there is usually an optimal age at which to achieve the correction. The decision regarding when to start treatment is based on the following factors:

A. Level of dental development

B. Timing of skeletal growth

C. Nature of the problem

III. The goal of early orthodontic treatment (during the mixed dentition) is to improve the environment for dental development so as to reduce or minimize future orthodontic needs.

IV. Early treatment may be divided into two categories:

A. **Interceptive treatment** has the following purposes:

1. Head off certain problems before they can have a negative effect on the developing dentition.

2. Control deleterious oral habits such as thumb sucking and tongue thrusting.

B. **Corrective treatment** occurs at various stages:

1. During early to midmixed stage of dentition development, the goal is to improve existing problems. Correction of anterior and posterior crossbites may be undertaken at this stage.

2. In cases of severe skeletal imbalances, as in Class II and Class III malocclusions, early treatment may be initiated to improve the relationships of the jaws and reduce the amount of orthodontic treatment that may be needed in the future.

3. Removable devices called **functional appliances** are frequently used at this stage for this purpose.

4. Most orthodontic treatment is initiated in the late mixed or early permanent dentition development.

5. When most of the permanent teeth are present, the orthodontist has control over the development of the final occlusion.

6. Patients in the late stage are undergoing a pubertal growth spurt, and this is an excellent time to correct most dental and skeletal discrepancies.

7. Comprehensive **fixed appliance** therapy is the most common treatment modality in this adolescent group.

V. Adult treatment

A. Adults make up approximately 25% of all active orthodontic patients in the United States.

B. Many adult patients seek orthodontic treatment for esthetic reasons when it was not available to them as adolescents; others require treatment for corrective reasons, such as the enhancement of restorative dentistry or periodontic or TMJ therapy.

C. Lack of growth in adult patients may present some limitations and compromises in the treatment goals.

D. A combination of orthodontics and orthognathic surgery is often necessary to resolve severe skeletal imbalances in adult patients.

ORTHODONTIC RECORDS

I. Medical history

A. A variety of conditions and medications may affect the movement of the teeth, the growth of the jaws, or the patient's ability to cope with the treatment.

B. Children with a history of heart murmur or rheumatic fever may be at risk for life-threatening infections and are treated with SBE prophylaxis.

C. Severe infections and rapid periodontal breakdown may also occur with routine orthodontic care during the active phases of leukemia, sickle cell anemia, or uncontrolled diabetes.

D. Juvenile onset of rheumatoid arthritis may affect the growth sites of the mandible, resulting in deficient bone growth and malocclusion.

E. Medications used to control seizures may lead to gingival hyperplasia, interfering with tooth movement.

F. The patient's medical status may change rapidly; thus the medical history must be updated periodically.

II. Dental history

A. The dental history may provide insight into the nature and cause of the orthodontic problem.

B. Family traits can be determined.

C. Presence of deleterious oral habits may be confirmed.

D. The patient's attitude toward dental treatment can be determined.

III. Clinical examination

A. The patient's teeth and jaw relationships are

evaluated, as are the surrounding oral and facial soft tissues.

B. The stage of dental development may be recorded by charting the primary and permanent teeth that are present.

C. Abnormalities in the shape, size, color, and position of the teeth are noted.

D. Angle's Classification of Malocclusion is determined on both the right and left sides of the mouth.

E. Deviation in the occlusion, such as a crossbite, is recorded.

F. Overjet, overbite, and the amount of crowding or spacing are measured precisely.

G. Abnormal, functional, and neuromuscular patterns may be noted.

IV. Panoramic radiographs

A. These are commonly used to determine the positions of the teeth.

B. They also aid in assessing the health of the dentition and supporting structures.

V. Cephalometric radiograph and tracing

A. This allows the orthodontist to more accurately determine the specific areas of imbalance, measure the degree of discrepancy, and project the future growth of the bones of the face.

B. Future cephalograms can be superimposed and compared with the original, allowing the orthodontist to observe growth that has occurred and the effects of the treatment upon the skeletal and dental development.

C. Tracing the cephalogram on acetate tracing paper facilitates measurement of the positions of the teeth and jaws.

D. Measurements may be compared with various cephalometric standards, which are based upon good dentoskeletal balance.

VI. Intraoral and extraoral radiographs

A. These include periapical and occlusal radiographs.

B. They may give a close-up view of any irregularity noted on the panoramic radiograph.

VII. Study models

A. These reproduce the teeth and occlusion to provide an invaluable aid in the diagnostic procedure.

B. The teeth and the alveolar mucosa to the depth of the buccal and lingual vestibule must be recorded accurately.

VIII. Additional radiographs as needed

A. These might include TMJ, periapical, and occlusal radiographs.

B. These may indicate whether a more accurate view of the TMJ is necessary.

IX. Diagnostic photographs

A. Intraoral photographs are taken of the teeth in frontal, left and right lateral, and maxillary and mandibular occlusal views.

B. Extraoral photographs are taken of the patient's head in frontal and lateral views.

C. These photographs serve as a visual record of the dentition before orthodontic treatment and as a record of the progress of treatment.

TREATMENT PLANNING

I. Once the nature of the malocclusion has been clarified, the orthodontist must determine the appropriate timing and implement the treatment.

II. Phases of treatment include the following:

A. For patients with severe skeletal imbalances or dental discrepancies, early interceptive or corrective treatment may be initiated before comprehensive treatment with fixed appliances is begun (phase 1).

B. When comprehensive fixed appliances are placed in the permanent dentition (phase 2), the patient is usually seen at monthly intervals for adjustments of the appliance.

C. Most malocclusions require about 24 months of active treatment, but this can vary depending on the patient's age, the rate of growth, and the complexity of the problem.

D. Once the functional and esthetic goals of treatment have been achieved, the fixed appliances are removed and the retention phase (phase 3) of treatment begins.

   1. During this phase, removable appliances are used to further stabilize the teeth, bones, and oral musculature.

   2. The patient is frequently monitored for several years during the retention phase.

MECHANISM OF TOOTH MOVEMENT

I. When continuous gentle pressure is applied to a tooth, changes occur in the alveolar bone that surrounds the root, allowing the tooth to move.

II. A force applied to a tooth results in an area of compression of the periodontal ligament on one side of the root and an area of tension in the periodontal ligament on the opposite side.

A. The body reacts by sending specialized bone cells (osteoclasts) to the area under compression. The osteoclasts dissolve or resorb the alveolar bone, creating freedom for tooth movement in that direction.

B. On the tension side, osteoblasts deposit new bone into the area from which the tooth has moved. The efficiency of tooth movement may depend on the magnitude, duration, and direction of the force.

ORTHODONTIC APPLIANCES

I. An orthodontic appliance is a device that is used to produce changes in the relationships of the teeth and the skeletal structures.

II. Removable appliances

A. A **removable appliance** can be inserted into the mouth and removed by the patient. A **headgear** is a removable appliance that can be used in conjunction with fixed appliances.

B. Functional appliances are removable devices that are frequently used in phase 1 before the placement of fixed appliances.

1. Functional appliances are used to effect changes in the differential growth rate of the jaws when a skeletal imbalance is present.

2. Examples of functional appliances are the Fränkel appliance, the Bionator, and the Herbst appliance.

C. Retainers are removable appliances that hold (retain) the alignment of the teeth after fixed appliance therapy.

D. A removable appliance called a *positioner* may also be used to retain the teeth after the active phase of orthodontic treatment.

E. Removable appliances are worn from 12 to 24 hours a day to produce the desired effects.

III. Fixed appliances

A. Fixed appliances are cemented to the teeth and cannot be removed by the patient; they consist of several important parts.

B. **Orthodontic bands** are stainless steel rings that encircle the tooth and are cemented with zinc phosphate or glass ionomer cement. They come in a variety of sizes.

1. Each tooth must be individually sized and fitted before cementation.

2. Bands are most commonly used on molar and premolar teeth because these teeth are strong enough to withstand the heavy occlusal forces in the posterior segments of the dentition.

3. Each band has a **bracket** or tube that is welded to the facial surface and serves as a means of attachment for the **archwires.**

4. Orthodontic brackets are usually bonded directly on the enamel surface of the anterior teeth with an acid etch technique and acrylic bonding resin.

5. Orthodontic brackets are made of stainless steel, translucent ceramic, or acrylic.

6. Forces are applied to the dentition through the archwire.

7. Archwires fit into the horizontal slot in the brackets or slide into the buccal tubes on the molar teeth.

8. Archwires come in a variety of diameters and compositions, which affect the magnitude of the force that is applied to the teeth.

9. The archwires are secured into the brackets with **ligature ties;** the ligatures may be made of thin wire or tiny **elastic bands.**

10. Removable auxiliary attachments may be attached to the fixed appliances to provide additional support for the desired tooth movements.

INSTRUMENTS AND PROCEDURES

I. Placement of separators

A. For patient comfort and ease of placement, a slight amount of space must exist between the teeth to fit the orthodontic bands.

B. This space is provided through the use of orthodontic **separators,** which are usually placed 1 week before the banding appointment.

C. The procedure for placement and removal of separators is provided (box on page 422).

II. Sizing and fitting of orthodontic bands

A. Orthodontic bands come in a large range of sizes and may be precontoured to fit specific teeth.

B. The size, arch, and right or left designation are imprinted on each band for ease of identification.

C. The procedure for trial sizing and fitting the bands is described (box on page 423).

D. A properly adapted band should fit tightly around the tooth, with no space visible between the edges of the band and the tooth.

E. The occlusal edges of the band should be positioned approximately 1 mm cervical to the marginal ridges of the tooth; the band should not rock back and forth when buccal or lingual pressure is applied.

F. Unused bands that were tried on but not selected are sterilized, sorted, and returned to the box for future use.

PLACEMENT AND REMOVAL OF SEPARATORS

- Are all universal barrier techniques being used?
- Is all of the armamentarium available and prepared for use?
- Are the instruments arranged in order of use?
- Are you prepared for alternative treatment plans?
- Is the necessary equipment turned on and ready to operate?

PLACEMENT OF SEPARATORS USING SEPARATING PLIERS

1. Engage a separator on the tips of the separating pliers and squeeze the handles gently to slightly stretch the elastic band.
2. Place the separator on the embrasure area between the teeth where separation is desired.
3. Using a back-and-forth sawing motion (as used in flossing), work down one side of the separator through the interproximal contact until it rests completely beneath the contact. The occlusal portion of the separator should remain in the embrasure between the teeth, resting above the proximal contact.
4. Once the separator is properly positioned, release the tension on the plier handles and remove the separating pliers. This procedure is repeated at each interproximal contact where future orthodontic band placement is anticipated.

PLACEMENT OF SEPARATORS USING DENTAL FLOSS

1. Insert two strands of dental floss through the lumen of the separator.
2. Double over the ends of the floss, wrapping it around the middle finger of each hand. Stretch the separator slightly.
3. Insert the separator in a manner similar to flossing; pass one side of the separator through the proximal contact area between the teeth.
4. Once the separator is properly positioned, with one side of the elastic ring below the contact area and the other side above the contact, remove the strands of floss by pulling one end of each piece.

REMOVAL OF SEPARATORS

1. Before the orthodontic bands are placed, the separators must be removed. For removal, hook one end of a scaler or explorer beneath the occlusal aspect of the separator.
2. Place the index finger of the opposite hand over the top of the separator to prevent injury to the patient in case the elastic band should snap.
3. Pull gently on the instrument in an occlusal direction to disengage the separator.

- Are the appropriate universal barriers removed?
- Have all appropriate surfaces been cleaned and disinfected?
- Has all of the armamentarium been removed?
- Has all equipment been repositioned?
- Has all equipment been disinfected/sterilized according to OSHA guidelines?

III. Cementation of orthodontic bands
    A. A permanent cement, such as a zinc phosphate or glass ionomer, is used to cement the bands.
    B. The procedure for cementing orthodontic bands is provided (box on page 423).

IV. Direct bonding of orthodontic brackets
    A. The bonding of orthodontic brackets directly to the enamel surfaces allows for improved patient comfort and oral hygiene.
    B. Individual brackets are specific for each tooth in the arch.

    C. The procedure for bonding requires careful preparation of the tooth surface, which is critical to the adhesion of the bracket.
    D. The procedure is provided (box on page 423).
    E. Cementation of the appliances is generally done by the orthodontist except in states where this is a legally delegated duty for the assistant; however, the assistant may perform many of the sizing, fitting, and tooth preparation tasks.

V. Placement and removal of archwires and ligatures (box on page 424)

SIZING AND FITTING ORTHODONTIC BANDS

1. Estimate the size of the band by placing it on the tooth on the patient's study model.
2. Use finger pressure in the patient's mouth and push down the preselected band over the tooth. If the band slides down too easily, it is probably too large, and a smaller size is needed. If the band cannot be pushed down at all, it is too small, and a larger size is needed.
3. Place the serrated end of the Schure instrument or band adaptor on the edges of the band at the mesial and distal marginal ridges. Apply pressure in an attempt to push the band further in a cervical direction.
4. Use the band biter for the final seating of the band onto the tooth. Place the serrated metal tip of the instrument on the edges of the band; ask the patient to bite down on the plastic handle to produce the desired force. Pressure frequently needs to be applied alternately at several areas on the band to ensure complete seating. The best area for the application of biting pressure to seat a maxillary band is on the lingual surface, whereas the best area to seat a mandibular band is on the buccal surface.
5. Use the Schure instrument or band adaptor to contour the band into the grooves and around the marginal ridges by pressing the band material toward the tooth for a close fit. Because substantial pressure is applied, use extreme care to avoid patient injury.

CEMENTATION OF ORTHODONTIC BANDS

1. Place the plastic tip of the band-removing pliers on the occlusal surface of the tooth, while the opposing metal tip grasps the cervical edge of the band. With gentle pressure on the plier handles, lift the band from the tooth. As in band seating, mandibular bands are most easily removed by placing the tip of the pliers on the buccal surface, whereas removal of the maxillary bands is most easily approached from the lingual surface.
2. Prepare the bands for cementation by rinsing and drying, and fill the brackets and tubes with soft beeswax to prevent them from getting filled with cement.
3. Polish the teeth with pumice; then rinse, dry, and isolate with cotton rolls.
4. Slowly mix zinc phosphate cement on a refrigerated slab to increase the working time. The proper consistency of the cement is slightly thicker than the primary consistency used to cement inlays and crowns.
5. Place the cement inside the band and seat the band onto the tooth, using finger pressure, the band adaptor, and the band biter in the same sequence as used previously.
6. Once the cement has completely set, carefully remove the excess by using the scaler end of the Schure instrument.

DIRECT BONDING OF ORTHODONTIC BRACKETS

1. Arrange the brackets on an adhesive pad next to the tooth number corresponding to the specific bracket. The brackets are color coded for each quadrant with a small dot on the distogingival corner of the bracket face.
2. Polish the teeth to be bonded with pumice; then rinse and dry. Prophylaxis paste should not be used because some of the additives interfere with the bonding.
3. Isolate the areas to be bonded with cheek retractors, saliva ejector, and cotton rolls to retain a dry field.
4. Apply phosphoric acid etching gel to the enamel surfaces where the brackets will be attached. Allow the etching gel to remain on the teeth for 30 to 60 seconds.
5. Thoroughly rinse and dry the teeth. This is one of the most critical steps—an inadequate rinse or moisture contamination may cause the bonding agent not to adhere properly.
6. Apply the bonding agent to the enamel surface. Mix and apply the bonding agent to the back of the bracket according to the manufacturer's specifications.
7. Use special forceps to place the bracket on the tooth. The cement reaches its initial set within approximately 30 seconds. Repeat the last two steps for each of the brackets to be bonded.
8. Remove excess cement with a scaler before the resin has polymerized. Allow the cement to set for at least 5 minutes before the isolation is removed.

PLACEMENT AND REMOVAL OF ARCHWIRES AND LIGATURES

1. Select the appropriate wire.
2. Estimate the length of the wire on the study models and cut off the excess with the wire cutters.
3. Use the Weingart pliers to insert the wire into the buccal tubes of the molar bands. Take care not to injure the soft tissues with the sharp wire ends during insertion and removal. The Weingart pliers may also be used to fit the wire into the horizontal slots in the brackets.
4. If excess wire still remains distal to the ends of the buccal tubes on the molar bands, remove it or cut it with the distal-end cutting pliers.

WIRE LIGATURES

Placement

1. It may help to bend the loop at a slight angle before placement. Slide the preformed wire loops horizontally around the bracket so that one side of the loop rests under the gingival tie wings on the bracket and the other side rests under the occlusal tie wings.
2. Cross the ends of the ligature wire over the top of the archwire at the side of the bracket.
3. Place the ligature tying pliers on the tie wire crossing 4 to 6 mm from the bracket. Squeeze the handles of the pliers to engage the wire and to lock the pliers.
4. Rotate the pliers several times so that the wires are twisted tightly.
5. Squeeze the handles of the pliers to disengage the wires.
6. Use the ligature cutting pliers to cut the excess ligature wire, leaving a 3-mm *pigtail* of twisted wire next to the bracket.
7. The serrated tip of the Schure instrument may be used to tuck the sharp twisted end of the tie underneath the archwire, where it will not irritate the lips or buccal mucosa.

Removal

The ligature ties are removed at each appointment when the archwire is changed.
1. Place the ligature cutter at the mesial or the distal side of the bracket on the ligature wire. The cutting edges may be nearly parallel to the archwire.
2. Grasp the cut ligature with the ligature cutters and gently release it from the tie wings of the bracket.
3. Take care when handling the cut ligature wires because the sharp ends can easily penetrate oral mucosa as well as latex treatment gloves and fingers.

ELASTIC LIGATURES

Placement

1. Use the hemostat to grasp elastic ligatures and remove them from the holder.
2. Carefully stretch the ligature around the gingival tie wings of the bracket, over the archwire, and around the occlusal tie wings.
3. Release the hemostat, leaving the ligature securely encircling the bracket. The procedure is repeated until all brackets have been ligated to the archwire.

Removal

The elastic ligature ties are removed by inserting the tip of the scaler beneath the tie and between the occlusal tie wings, gently releasing it from the bracket.

ORAL HYGIENE

I. People who wear orthodontic appliances are susceptible to dental decay around the bands and brackets because food trapped in these areas can lead to the buildup of plaque.

II. If the plaque is not removed frequently, it may dissolve the enamel of the teeth underneath the surrounding brackets, resulting in permanent decalcification or decay.

III. The orthodontic patient must spend additional time brushing and using special techniques to thoroughly remove plaque from around the fixed appliances.

IV. An orthodontic toothbrush is frequently recommended because it has rows of bristles that are specially contoured to fit around the brackets more easily.

V.   A critical area to brush is the facial aspect of the teeth between the bracket and the gingival margin.

VI. Instruct the patient to place the toothbrush in this area with the bristles at about a 45-degree angle, with the ends pointing toward the brackets. A small circular motion should be used, starting at one side of the arch and continuing around to the other side and to the lingual and opposite arch.

VII. Flossing is also an important part of oral hygiene.

VIII. The orthodontic patient should brush after every meal and perform one session of complete flossing and brushing once a day.

IX. Oral irrigation devices may also be used as an adjunct to oral hygiene.

Questions

Orthodontics

1 Orthodontic appliances move teeth because
a. Bone is elastic
b. Roots dissolve
c. Bone resorbs under tension
d. New bone forms under tension and dissolves under pressure

2 A headgear
a. Is a removable appliance
b. Uses the muscles of mastication to produce force
c. Can only be inserted and removed by an orthodontist
d. Should be worn no more than 4 to 6 hours per day

3 A retainer is
a. Used during the active phase of treatment to align the teeth
b. Commonly used before fixed appliances are placed
c. Usually worn full time for several months, and then wearing time is gradually reduced
d. An example of a fixed appliance

4 An orthodontic bracket is not
a. The means by which forces are applied to the teeth
b. Part of a removable appliance
c. Held on a tooth by bands or direct bonding
d. Used to attach the archwires to the tooth

5 Which of the following statements regarding the orthodontic patient's eating habits is false?
a. Poor eating habits can loosen bands.
b. Poor eating habits can cause distorted archwires.
c. Extremely hard and sticky foods must be avoided.
d. High-sugar foods are not of concern because the bands cover much of the teeth.

6 A space maintainer may be classified as which of the following types of treatment?
a. Interceptive
b. Corrective
c. Maintenance

7 Which of the following is not a diagnostic tool in orthodontics?
a. Study model
b. Vitalometer
c. Panorex
d. Intraoral photograph
e. Extraoral photograph

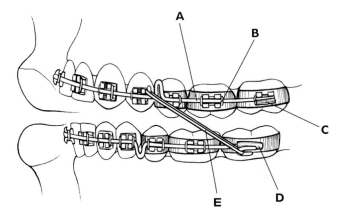

Use the diagram above to identify the following:

_____   **8** Archwire
_____   **9** Buccal tube
_____ **10** Ligature wire
_____ **11** Elastic

12 Which of the following dental discrepancies is not associated with a long-term thumb-sucking habit?
a. Prognathism
b. Open bite
c. Excessive overjet
d. Posterior crossbite
e. Protrusion of maxillary incisors

13 Which of the following statements is *not* likely in reference to a deep overbite?
a. It is excessive vertical overlap of the incisor on closure.
b. It may be functionally unhealthy.
c. The mandibular incisors may occlude on the palatal gingiva.
d. The maxillary incisors may occlude on the lingual gingiva.

14 Which of the following statements are true as they relate to elastic posterior separators?
1. The separators are placed to create temporary space between teeth, allowing room for bands.
2. The separator must completely surround the contact area.
3. Elastic separating pliers are used for placement.
4. Separators, like dental floss, are stretched and see-sawed through the contacts.
5. The number of separators that are placed is noted on patient's record.
a. 1, 2, and 3
b. 3 and 4
c. 1, 2, 3, and 4
d. 1, 2, 3, 4, and 5

15 When orthodontic bands are being sized for mandibular premolars and molars, the band is first seated on the _____ aspect.
a. Buccal
b. Lingual
c. Mesial
d. Distal

16 Which of the following statements are true for sizing orthodontic bands?
1. The gingival edge of the band goes over the tooth first.
2. The occlusal edge of the band goes over the tooth first.
3. A mallet and band driver may be used in seating the band.
4. Bands are preformed stainless steel rings.
5. Band sizes are universal, and bands can be adapted to fit any tooth.
a. 1 and 3
b. 1, 3, and 4
c. 1, 3, and 5
d. 2, 3, and 4

17 Ligature wires are secured in place by
a. Bonding
b. Elastic separators
c. Cementing with zinc phosphate
d. Twisting them to a length of 4 to 5 mm

18 Which of the following describe(s) a Class III malocclusion?
1. Mandibular first molar is retruded in relationship to the maxillary first molar.
2. Mandibular first molar is protruded in relationship to the maxillary first molar.
3. Mesiobuccal cusp of the maxillary first molar is in the mesiobuccal groove of the mandibular first molar.
4. Convex facial profile
5. Concave facial profile
a. 2 only
b. 1 and 4
c. 2 and 5
d. 3 and 5

19 Which of the following statements is *not* true regarding toothbrushing for orthodontic patients?
a. The patient must concentrate on the area between the band the gingival tissue.
b. Bands and wires become dull and tarnished from oral fluids, which is not indicative of poor toothbrushing.
c. Teeth that are blocked out and rotated require special attention when brushing.
d. Patients who are unable to brush after eating should rinse vigorously with water.

20 In which of the illustrations below is a Class II, division I malocclusion?

A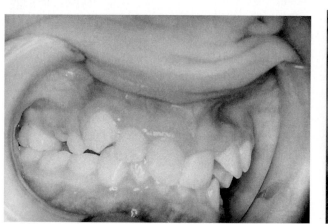

B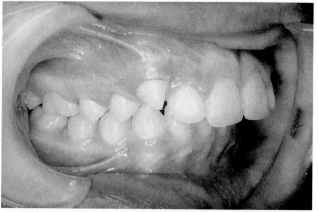

C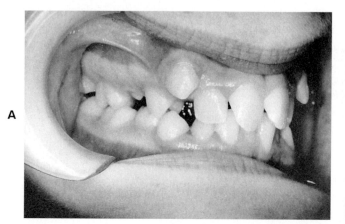

D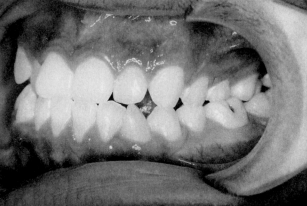

21 Which of the following is an impinging overbite?

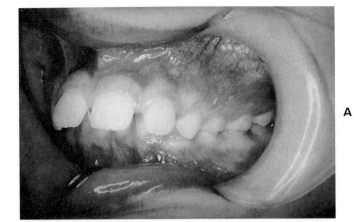

A

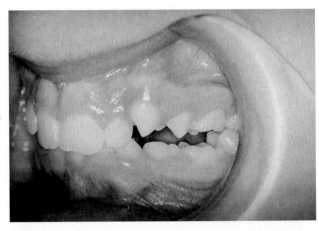

B

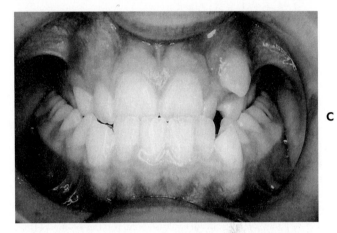

C

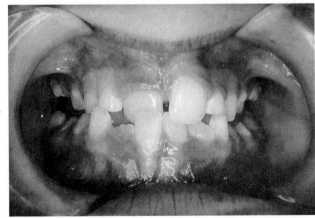

D

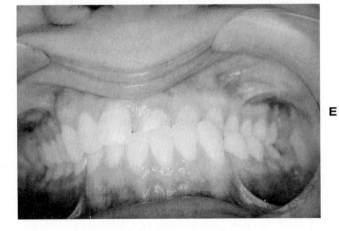

E

22 Which of the following is the correct sequence for sizing and fitting orthodontic bands?
1. Use the band biter.
2. Use the Shure instrument or band adaptor to contour.
3. Apply finger pressure to push the band over the tooth.
4. Size the band.
5. Slide the band with light pressure over the mesial and distal areas.

a. 1, 2, 3, 4, and 5
b. 2, 3, 4, 5, and 1
c. 3, 4, 5, 1, and 2
d. 4, 3, 5, 1, and 2
e. 5, 4, 3, 2, and 1

23 Which of the following is *not* used for placement of bonding material?
a. Skube

b. Cotton pledget
c. Explorer
d. Disposable brush

24 Which of the following is the correct sequence for direct bonding brackets?
1. Apply bonding agent.
2. Arrange brackets.
3. Polish teeth.
4. Rinse and dry teeth.
5. Place bracket on tooth.
6. Isolate.
7. Remove cement.
8. Apply etchant.
a. 1, 3, 4, 8, 6, 2, 5, and 7
b. 2, 3, 6, 8, 4, 1, 5, and 7
c. 2, 4, 5, 1, 8, 3, 7, and 3
d. 3, 2, 6, 1, 8, 4, 7, and 5

25 A distal-end cutter is primarily used to
a. Trim the archwire
b. Contour an appliance
c. Cut and contour a bracket
d. Cut the archwire between the brackets

Rationales

Orthodontics

1 D When continuous gentle pressure is applied to a tooth, changes occur in the alveolar bone that surround the root, allowing the tooth to move. A force applied to a tooth results in an area of compression of the periodontal ligament on one side of the root and an area of tension in the periodontal ligament on the opposite side. The body reacts by sending specialized bone cells (osteoclasts) to the area under compression. The osteoclasts dissolve or resorb the alveolar bone, creating freedom for tooth movement in that direction. On the tension side, osteoblasts deposit new bone into the area from which the tooth has moved.

2 B A headgear is a removable appliance that can be used in conjunction with fixed appliances to obtain movement.

3 C Retainers are removable appliances that hold or retain the alignment of the teeth after fixed appliance therapy.

4 D An orthodontic bracket is a small metal or plastic attachment fixed to a band for the purpose of fastening the arch wire to the orthodontic band.

5 D A, B, and C can all occur in an orthodontic patient's mouth if care is not exercised. High-sugar foods must be avoided because people who wear orthodontic appliances are more susceptible to dental decay around the bands and brackets. Food trapped in these areas can lead to the buildup of plaque.

6 A A space maintainer is an example of interceptive orthodontic treatment that may be used when a primary tooth has been lost prematurely. Placement of the space maintainer prevents drifting of the adjacent teeth into the edentulous area, which would subsequently result in impaction or displacement of the permanent successor.

7 B A vitalometer is not an orthodontic diagnostic tool but an electronic device used in endodontics to determine the vitality of a tooth. The remaining devices are all directly related to making a diagnosis.

8 A Archwire This is a wire that is applied to two or more teeth through fixed attachments to cause or guide tooth movement.

9 D Buccal tube This is a device on a molar band that allows archwires to be placed into the horizontal slot.

10 B Ligature wire This is a wire or threadlike substance used to tie a tooth to an orthodontic appliance.

11 E Elastic This is a rubber band used to apply force to the tooth during orthodontic treatment.

12 A Thumb sucking would create a discrepancy in the maxillary arch or between arches. Prognathism refers to a protruded mandible. The mandible has a mesial relationship with the maxilla.

13 D Deep overbite refers to excessive vertical overlap of the incisors upon closure. This type of relationship may be functionally unhealthy for the dentition. In extreme cases the mandibular incisors may occlude on the palatal gingiva.

14 D For patient comfort and ease in placing orthodontic bands, a slight amount of space must exist between the teeth. This space is provided by the placement of separators about a week prior to band placement.

The separators encircle the proximal contact and provide a gentle force, which moves the teeth apart over a period of days. Elastic separating pliers are used for placement. Separators, like dental floss, are stretched and see-sawed through the contacts. The separator must completely surround contact area.

At the end of the procedure the number of separators that are placed is noted on the patient's record. Sometimes the separator is lost before the next appointment because the separator becomes loose as the contact between the teeth opens.

15 B It is recommended that the band be seated on the lingual aspect first because this area is more difficult to visualize.

16 B An orthodontic band is a preformed stainless steel device that resembles the anatomic contour of the tooth. Therefore, to properly align the band, the gingival edge must go over the tooth first. With hand pressure, adaptation can begin, but a mallet and band driver or a band adapter such as a Shure instrument must be used to ensure complete seating.

17 D A ligature tying pliers can be used to secure wires. The pliers are squeezed to engage the wire and lock the pliers. The pliers are rotated several times so that the wires are twisted tightly. The pliers are disengaged, and a ligature cutting pliers is used to cut the excess wire. The end is safely secured.

18 C A Class III malocclusion results in a negative overjet, or a prognathic mandible. The visual effect is a concave facial profile. The mesiobuccal cusp of the maxillary first molar occludes posteriorly to the buccal groove of the mandibular first molar.

19 B Oral hygiene care is vitally important to orthodontic patients. People who wear orthodontic appliances are more susceptible to dental decay and must spend additional time brushing and using special techniques to thoroughly remove plaque from around fixed appliances. Regardless of the condition of the mouth, however, it is not common for bands and wires to become dull and tarnished from oral fluids.

20 B This relationship denotes that the mesiobuccal cusp of the maxillary first molar occludes anteriorly to the buccal groove of the mandibular first molar and that the maxillary incisors are inclined and protrude anteriorly.

21 A An impinging overbite results from a deep overbite that occurs when the mandibular incisors occlude on the palatal gingiva.

22 D The band is first sized as described in item 16. Seat the band onto the tooth. Using finger pressure or a band adaptor, slide the band over the mesial and distal areas. The band biter and Shure instrument can be used to contour the band.

23 C Use of the explorer is contraindicated in a bonding application because it will etch the surface.

24 B The brackets are arranged on an adhesive pad next to the tooth number corresponding to the specific bracket. The teeth to be bonded are polished with pumice, rinsed, and dried. The area is isolated with cheek retractors and cotton rolls. The tooth is etched with phosphoric acid etching gel where the brackets will be attached. The etchant remains on the teeth for 30 to 60 seconds. The teeth are rinsed and dried. The bonding agent is applied to the enamel surface. Bonding agent is applied to the back of the bracket and special forceps are used to place the bracket on the tooth. Excess cement is removed with a scaler before the resin has polymerized.

25 A When excess wire remains distal to the ends of the buccal tubes on the molar bands, it is removed or cut with a distal-end cutter.

To enhance your understanding of the material in this chapter refer to the illustrations in Chapter 35 of Finkbeiner/Johnson: *Mosby's Comprehensive Dental Assisting: A Clinical Approach.*

Pediatric Dentistry

KEY TERMS

Behavior modification techniques
Behavior patterns
Flooding

Hand-over-mouth
Modeling
Papoose board

Pediatric dentistry
Show-and-tell
Validation

Pediatric dentistry, one of the eight recognized specialties of dentistry, involves the delivery of dental treatment to children from birth through the age of mixed dentition. The focus of pediatric dentistry has changed to meet the needs of today's children.

The scope of pediatric dentistry today allows the practitioner to devote more time to new concepts that meet the needs of the patient, which include greater emphasis on diagnosis and prevention and on increased involvement in the correction of malocclusion. But often, the foremost need in the delivery of dental treatment to children is the ability to understand and manage the patient's needs, fears, and individual emotional variations.

BEHAVIOR MANAGEMENT

I.   It is important to understand that a child is not just a small adult.
II. Each year brings changes and new experiences to children's mental and physical development, and the dental staff must communicate at their level without being demeaning.
III. One of the more difficult situations confronting dental staff in the treatment of children is the potential for behavior management problems.
IV. Pediatric dental patients vary in physical age, emotional age, and level of maturity.

CHILDHOOD DEVELOPMENT

I.   Certain levels of emotional, chronologic, and intellectual growth can be expected at particular ages.
II. Common levels of development for each age-group can be described as follows:
   A. Birth to 2 years
      1. Children begin to develop trust in surroundings as nurturing needs are met through food, sucking, and general care.
      2. They are not able to respond rationally to questions that relate to dental needs.

3. The caregiver must be informed of the treatment and any postoperative instructions.
B. 2 years
   1. These children are rapidly developing physically, emotionally, and intellectually.
   2. They normally become toilet trained during this year and gain a sense of pride in achievement and independence from the caregiver.
   3. Vocabulary increases, both in usage and comprehension.
   4. They rely on feelings for understanding and depend on tone of voice and facial expression to completely understand certain situations.
   5. Sudden movements and sounds sometimes frighten them; thus, their dental experience must be handled with great care.
   6. Each sound and activity must be explained so that they are less fearful of the dental experience.
C. 3 years
   1. They are developing socially, with increased vocabulary skills and greater outside experiences through separation from parents.
   2. They may have had the opportunity to interact with preschool and outside authoritative figures and consequently are more willing to be left alone in a treatment room with another person.
D. 4 years
   1. They may be less cooperative and may be assertive, aggressive, and even resistant to any direction.
   2. They fear the unknown but are less fearful of strangers because of increased social experiences.
   3. They may understand but may respond negatively to minor pain incurred in dental treatment.
   4. Take every precaution possible to avoid or eliminate any discomfort for these patients.
E. 5 years
   1. They accept separation from caregivers.
   2. They are capable of interacting socially through verbal and physical activity and are usually interested in discussions of accomplishments, possessions, and themselves.
F. 6 years
   1. They are embarking on a major change in experiences as they begin first grade in school.
   2. Peer groups greatly influence children at this age.
   3. Interaction with peers and authority figures helps in developing self-esteem.
   4. They are more responsive to directions from adults other than the primary caregiver; this allows the dental team to direct these children toward a positive response to dental treatment.
G. 7 to 12 years
   1. They are physically and intellectually more capable of dealing with situations that might create anxiety.
   2. The maturity level of these children reflects a knowledge of the reality of having to deal with unpleasant situations, which is the way they may view the dental visit.

BEHAVIOR PATTERNS

I. The dental team must be able to recognize and respond appropriately to any **behavior pattern** (a repeated response or reaction to a stimulus) demonstrated by a child before or during treatment.
II. Once a child has succeeded in getting his or her own way in a dental office through the use of a particular behavior pattern, that behavior will be repeated at a later date to accomplish the same goal.
III. The following categories describe behavior often encountered when children are treated in a pediatric or a general dental practice.
   A. Most children are cooperative. They are willing to accept well-defined explanations, and they respond positively to directions.
   B. Children who lack the ability to cooperate are unable to understand explanations of procedures or to communicate their inability. These children usually are very young or mentally or physically disabled, with restricted communication levels and skills.
   C. Potentially uncooperative behavior can be exhibited by any pediatric dental patient.
      1. Usually fear is the stimulus for the uncooperative behavior.
      2. This behavior may be due to past negative dental experiences or discussions of negative dental experiences with parents, peers, or siblings.
      3. A child might demonstrate uncontrolled, defiant, timid, tense, cooperative, whining, or stoic behavior.

PARENT/CAREGIVER ATTITUDES

I. Many behavior patterns may depend on the interaction between a child and the primary caregiver.

II. Talking with and observing a caregiver's interaction with the child provides information regarding parental attitudes.

III. If a caregiver is overprotective, the child is limited in experiencing different lessons of life.
   A. A child of an overprotective caregiver is often shy, is afraid of new experiences, and may lack self-confidence and self-esteem.
   B. The caregiver may have had a negative dental experience and imparted these fears and anxieties to the child.

IV. An overindulgent caregiver creates in the child a sense of being able to make demands and expect reactions to his or her wishes.
   A. This attitude can result in disruptive behavior of the child.
   B. A child who does not get his or her own way may have a temper tantrum.
   C. The dental team may have to disrupt a pattern of care to address this problem.

V. Children of overauthoritative caregivers are expected to act an age other than their own. These children are overly criticized and may resent people with authority giving direction, including the dentist.

VI. Underaffectionate caregivers can display a range of attitudes toward their children.
   A. They may show a lack of interest in or obvious rejection of the child or may be physically abusive.
   B. Such a child exhibits low self-esteem, is stoic, and may even be nonresponsive; however, the child may be loud and aggressive in an attempt to seek attention.

BEHAVIOR MANAGEMENT TECHNIQUES

I. Communication is the primary means of response to a behavior management situation.

II. Children have specific interests, needs, desires, and personality characteristics.

III. Meet children with a friendly greeting and direct eye contact.

IV. The dentist should ask children about their interests and establish a line of communication.

V. An atmosphere that relaxes children is conducive to achieving a positive relationship.
   A. The reception area should be designed to entertain and educate the children as they wait for treatment.
   B. The reception area should be colorful and full of activities for children of various age levels.
   C. Uniforms should be colorful and attractive to relieve the anxiety that may be associated with white coats but still comply with OSHA uniform guidelines.

VI. Dental semantics must be explained at a level that the patient can understand.
   A. Avoid using baby talk, but use terms appropriate to the child's level, such as the following:
      1. Anesthesia—makes a sleepy tooth that will feel fat
      2. Rubber dam—looks like a raincoat and is placed on the tooth to keep it dry
      3. HVE—a vacuum cleaner for the mouth
      4. Explorer—a tooth feeler
   B. Allowing children to feel items such as the HVE and the rubber cup for polishing helps allay their fears.

VII. An authoritative figure is necessary for the child to respond positively.
   A. The dentist usually takes the lead in providing a child patient with directions and instructions.
   B. This way a child can focus on what one person is saying and not become confused by directions given by two people.

VIII. Validation techniques assist in obtaining cooperative behavior.
   A. When fear of an unfamiliar situation is evident, behavior may become uncooperative.
   B. When this happens, the child's fear must not be denied, but through **validation** the dentist should acknowledge and confirm the child's feelings, indicate that being afraid is all right, and explain the treatment to the child again.
   C. Denying the child's fear creates a feeling of distrust.

IX. Voice control may be necessary to gain a child's attention.
   A. Children who are uncomfortable will try to delay treatment by being overly talkative and trying to tell the dentist everything about himself or herself, having the need to visit the bathroom several times, or claiming to be ill.
   B. Dramatic change in the dentist's tone of voice directing the child to ''be quiet and open your mouth'' gains the child's attention.

X. **Modeling** refers to using a child who exhibits good behavior in a dental office as the model for a child who may pose a problem or has exhibited inappropriate behavior.

A. The dentist may use an open-bay design for the treatment room to allow children to see another child during treatment.

B. This concept promotes an opportunity to use peer pressure to help the child respond in a positive manner.

XI. A child who visits a dental office with fears may have to be desensitized through a **show-and-tell** technique.

A. The child is allowed to touch and feel equipment before it is placed in the mouth, allowing the child to experience its use.

XII. **Flooding** refers to steps taken in behavior therapy to reduce anxiety that is associated with phobias.

A. The following **behavior modification techniques** need to be discussed with the primary caregiver before implementation because these actions are more drastic.

1. The **hand-over-mouth** technique is usually used on children aged 3 years and older who are not physically disabled or mentally compromised.

2. A child who is uncooperative (screaming, biting, or kicking) must be dealt with immediately. The child must be told that this behavior is unacceptable, prolongs treatment time, and will not be tolerated.

3. The child is held in the chair; the dental assistant holds the arms and legs as the dentist firmly places a hand over the mouth and whispers in the child's ear, ''I want to talk with you. I will take my hand away when you are quiet and are holding still. Do you understand?''

4. As the dentist makes eye contact and the child agrees to the dentist's request, the child is thanked for cooperating.

5. If the technique must be repeated, the child must not see anger on the part of the dental team.

6. The child may need only to be physically restrained with a **papoose board** to gain cooperation.

7. Restraint ranges from holding a child's hands to completely immobilizing the child through the use of a body restraint or papoose board. The least amount of restraint is the most preferable.

XIII. Premedication is used for some children to restrict anxiety and pain related to dental procedures.

A. Various types and dosages of medication are given, each based on the weight and height of the child.

B. Barbiturates and tranquilizers are two of the most common types of medication given to relieve anxiety. Each would be used in conjunction with local anesthesia (nitrous oxide) and general anesthesia.

XIV. Information on office policy regarding the caregiver's presence in the treatment room and the recommended responses for the caregiver during treatment is helpful.

A. Often the caregiver must accompany the child into the treatment room.

1. Ideally, the caregiver sits quietly within the child's view.

2. If the child will not sit quietly in the dental chair, it may be necessary to have the caregiver and the dentist hold the child.

3. At times, the caregiver being in the treatment room causes anxiety, and the child begins to cry.

4. The dental team must provide treatment for the child and educate the caregiver before any treatment is begun.

COMMON TREATMENT PROCEDURES ▬

I. Several specific procedures are performed predominantly for pediatric patients (box below).

II. Certain treatment is provided for children in different age-groups, including preventive oral hygiene procedures (box below).

A. The preventive procedures used for children are similar to those used for adults.

COMMON TREATMENT PROCEDURES

Placement of stainless steel crowns
Placement of space maintainers
Treatment of fractured teeth
Pulp therapy
Manufacture of mouth guards

PREVENTIVE PROCEDURES

Oral examination
Prophylaxis
Pit and fissure sealants
Fluoride treatments
Restorative and surgical procedures as needed

B. It is vital to educate caregivers and children and encourage them to adopt the concept of keeping their teeth for a lifetime.

C. The primary teeth aid in mastication, speaking, and appearance; affect the health and development of the permanent dentition; and act as a guide for the permanent dentition.

III. The typical sequence of visits in a pediatric office may include the following (box below):

A. Initial visit
   1. Creates a sense of comfort and relaxation when a child is first exposed to the dental office (can be a nontreatment appointment)
   2. Introductory visit to meet the staff and see the equipment

B. Oral diagnosis
   1. Medical/dental history
   2. Oral examination
   3. Dental radiographs
   4. Oral hygiene instructions
   5. Study models

C. Patient education
   1. Determine whether the child is obtaining an adequate amount of fluoride.
   2. Instruct the caregiver in the techniques to avoid nursing-bottle syndrome (box at bottom right).
   3. Provide the caregiver with instructions on diet and nutrition.
   4. Explain the deleterious effect of medications such as tetracycline on teeth.
   5. Explain the concept of maintaining teeth for a lifetime.
   6. Describe the importance of restoring and/or retaining primary teeth.
   7. Describe the importance of wearing a mouth guard when participating in contact sports.

URGENT CARE NEEDS

I. Trauma

A. Statistics indicate that most traumatic injuries to the head and mouth occur in children, with the possible exception of those incurred in auto accidents.

B. Common conditions in children who come to the dental office include intruded, avulsed, or fractured teeth and lacerated lips, tongue, or mucosa.

II. Fractured teeth

A. Tooth fracture usually results from a blow that often affects the crown of the tooth.

B. The anterior segment of the oral cavity is usually affected in tooth-fracture accidents. Vitality of an injured tooth must be determined to develop a course of treatment.

C. A crown fracture may occur in primary or permanent teeth.

D. The Ellis classification system describes the extent of tooth structure lost.
   1. In a class I fracture, enamel is lost. Treatment involves smoothing the fractured surfaces for the patient's comfort.
   2. In a class II fracture, dentin as well as enamel is lost. Treatment involves placement of a bonding agent and a composite resin layer to restore the tooth to normal.
   3. In a class III fracture, enamel and dentin are lost, and the fracture encroaches on the pulpal tissues. The extent of the pulpal exposure may be minimal—a pinpoint exposure—requiring a direct pulp cap, or extensive, requiring a pulpotomy or pulpectomy.

E. Partially developed teeth
   1. Teeth may not be fully developed when they are traumatized, which can result in additional problems.
   2. Apexogenesis and apexification are treatments that involve the status of the root development.

F. Pediatric surgery
   1. Trauma may result in the need for pediatric oral surgery.

FIRST APPOINTMENTS

Complete and thorough medical and dental history (obtained from caregiver)
Radiographs
Intraoral and extraoral examination
Study casts
Prophylaxis
Possible fluoride treatment and/or placement of pit and fissure sealants

---

INSTRUCTIONS FOR CAREGIVER TO AVOID NURSING-BOTTLE SYNDROME

- Provide only water in the child's bottle.
- Wipe the alveolar ridge and erupted teeth with a small towel to remove debris.
- Do not allow the child to have a bottle.

2. An extensively fractured tooth, in which only a minor portion of the root is left in the socket, requires removal through a surgical procedure.

G. Luxation
1. The tooth may be intruded or extruded, with a degree of movement out of the socket.
2. Treatment for luxated teeth depends on whether primary or permanent teeth are involved.

H. Avulsed tooth
1. An avulsed tooth is one that has been completely removed from the mouth as a result of a traumatic injury.
2. An avulsed primary tooth usually is not replaced within the alveolus because of the possibility of periodontal infection.
3. A permanent tooth that is avulsed must be replanted immediately, followed by stabilization until the tooth is secure (approximately 7 to 10 days).
4. Directions for replantation are provided in Chapter 22.

I. Loosened primary tooth
1. The child may not want to remove the tooth or allow the caregiver to remove the tooth.
2. Primary teeth with resorbed roots may be attached only through soft tissue.
3. Tissue attachments can be extremely sensitive and painful, and any movement of the tooth may cause discomfort.

CHILD ABUSE

I. Statistics indicate alarming increases in suspected and reported cases of child abuse.
II. Several types of child abuse can be evident, including the following:
   A. Shaking
   B. Slapping
   C. Choking and squeezing
   D. Lacerations
   E. Genital trauma
   F. Bone fractures
   G. Burns and scalds
   H. Life-threatening injuries to the intraabdominal area, eyes, and cranium
   I. Bitemarks
   J. Bruising (in various stages of healing)
III. If child abuse is suspected, it is more than the health care professional's responsibility to notify the appropriate authorities—it is a legal mandate.

A. Responsible agencies—such as social service departments, child care institutions, and law enforcement agencies in every state—are able to respond to suspected incidents of abuse or neglect.
B. Have readily available the telephone number of the appropriate agency to contact if child abuse is encountered.
C. Some states also have provided good-faith protection clauses to conceal the identity of and protect the individual who submitted the abuse case to the authorities.
D. Once the case is submitted, the social service department notifies law enforcement agencies.

RESTORATIVE PROCEDURES

I. Restorative procedures for children are similar to those for adults.
II. Variations in the procedures usually involve the size of the instruments and the approach taken.
   A. Dental handpiece and burs
   B. Matrices
   C. Rubber dam clamps
III. Rubber dam isolation is common in pediatric dentistry.
IV. Explain to the child the procedure and the materials that are to be used.
V. Amalgam and composite resin restorations are placed on primary and permanent teeth; the procedures are the same as for adults.
VI. Placing temporary crowns in pediatric dentistry is an interim measure to retain primary teeth before the natural exfoliation process begins (until the permanent teeth erupt).
   A. Temporary crowns are placed on pediatric patients for various reasons (box below).
   B. The type of temporary crown is determined by the location of the tooth.
   C. A custom composite resin crown or polycarbonate crown is placed in areas visible under normal circumstances, and a stainless steel or aluminum crown is selected for the posterior areas of the mouth.

REASONS FOR PLACING TEMPORARY CROWNS

Trauma to a tooth that results in fracture
Extensive decay to the point that the restoration cannot be retained by the tooth
Systemic deformation of the tooth during formation
Tooth receiving endodontic treatment

PLACEMENT OF STAINLESS STEEL CROWNS

- Use a temporary sizing device to measure the distance between abutment teeth.
- The measured distance should coincide with a number on the end of the measuring device, which represents the width for a crown within the set of stainless steel crowns.
- Select the appropriate crown form.
- Try the crown form on the prepared tooth for fit.
- Determine the proper length for the crown; score the length with an explorer.
- Remove the excess length with crown and collar scissors; shape the cut edge with contouring pliers.
- Try the crown form on the tooth again, check the length, and establish the articulation of the crown and the contact with the abutment teeth.
- If necessary, adjust the length again and make any needed contact adjustments for a proper fit.
- The marginal ridge height should be similar to that of the abutment teeth. The interproximal contact should be maintained, and the occlusal contact should be uniform across the occlusal surface of the crown form.
- The stainless steel crown form can be smoothed with rotary instruments.
- Mix and place the cement of the operator's choice in the crown form and pass it to the operator to place on the prepared tooth.
- The type of cement used may be determined by the expected length of time the crown is to be left on a tooth and whether a cement that has an anodyne effect is needed.
- Examine the placement for contacts at the marginal ridge and the articulation; as the cement reaches its initial set, remove the excess with an explorer, a scaler, a spoon excavator, and floss.
- Reexamine the articulation and make adjustments with a rotary instrument as needed.

VII. Stainless steel crowns are usually selected for placement on posterior teeth in cases of extensive decay or as a result of trauma or decay. The procedure is provided (box above).

Questions

Pediatric Dentistry

1 Exfoliation of a primary tooth occurs by
   a. Resorption of the root of the primary tooth
   b. Extraction of the primary tooth
   c. Pushing of the primary tooth by the permanent tooth
   d. Bacterial degeneration of the primary tooth

2 Abuse is defined as an act of
   a. Commission
   b. Omission

3 Neglect is defined as an act of
   a. Commission
   b. Omission

4 Which of the following indicates neglect?
   a. Physically beating a child
   b. Failure to have badly decayed teeth treated
   c. Sexually molesting a child

5 Which technique can be used to allay a child's fear?
   a. Stop the child from breathing.
   b. Separate the child from the parent/caregiver.
   c. Cover the child's eyes.
   d. Tell, show, and do.

6 Which of the following techniques are used to alleviate a child's fear of dental treatment?
   1. Permitting the child to participate
   2. Threatening the child
   3. Offering to reward the child for good behavior
   4. Giving the child some control
   5. Presedating the child
   a. 1, 2, and 3
   b. 1, 4, and 5
   c. 2, 4, and 5
   d. 3, 4, and 5

7 A piece of equipment common to both pediatric dentistry and orthodontics is a(n)
   a. Face bow
   b. Spot welder
   c. Archwire
   d. Bead sterilizer

8 Full coverage of a deciduous molar usually indicates that which of the following be used?
   a. Amalgam crown
   b. Acrylic crown
   c. Stainless steel crown
   d. Amalgam core

9 Which of the following are tasks that the dental assistant may perform in a pediatric practice if delegated by state dental practice law?
   1. Permanent cementation of stainless steel crowns
   2. Providing fluoride treatment
   3. Obtaining radiographs
   4. Placing pit and fissure sealants
   5. Assisting on all procedures
   6. Mouth mirror inspection
   a. 1 and 3
   b. 2, 3, and 5
   c. 1, 2, 3, 4, and 5
   d. 2, 3, 4, 5, and 6
   e. 1, 2, 3, 4, 5, and 6

10 Which of the following manifestations observed during a clinical examination might indicate an abused child?
   1. Extremely shy behavior when questioned about bruises

2. Arms and legs completely covered during hot summer months
3. Falling down stairs given as an excuse
4. Fear of contact with certain gender of health care worker
5. Concerned about parent/caregiver being in treatment room
   a. 1 and 2
   b. 2 and 3
   c. 3, 4, and 5
   d. 1, 2, 3, and 4
   e. 1, 2, 3, 4, and 5

11 Which of the following is *not* considered a behavior management technique for dealing with the child patient?
   a. Hand-over-mouth
   b. Flooding
   c. Modeling
   d. All of the above

12 Which types of dental treatment are commonly performed on the pediatric patient?
   1. Pit and fissure sealants
   2. Prophylaxis
   3. Full-cast metal crowns
   4. Stainless steel crowns
   5. Amalgam restorations
   a. 1, 2, and 3
   b. 2, 4, and 5
   c. 1, 2, 4, and 5
   d. All of the above

13 A child is seen in the pediatric office over a 6-month period; the following details are observed during that time.
   1. Bruises on the child's head and neck area are evident on the front and the back surfaces. The back of the legs are often bruised.
   2. Bruise color ranges from bright blue to green to yellow.
   3. Even in warm weather the child often wears long pants and long-sleeved shirts; there does not appear to be a cultural reason for this type of dress.
   4. The child is shy and withdrawn.

   How should the dental team respond?
   a. Contact a social worker.
   b. Contact the parent/caregiver.
   c. Call the police.

For items 14-25, place an A for *True* or a B for *False* in the space provided next to each statement.

_____ **14** Drug therapy as a behavior management technique is an acceptable course of action for treatment of the child patient.

_____ **15** Stainless steel crowns are placed as a protective crown in the mouth of a pediatric patient.

_____ **16** If a child is not behaving appropriately during dental treatment, it is advisable to bring the parent/caregiver into the treatment room.

_____ **17** A pulpectomy is commonly performed on teeth of a pediatric patient.

_____ **18** Rubber dam isolation is not likely to be used in pediatric dentistry.

_____ **19** It is not necessary to use universal barrier techniques with a pediatric patient because these patients do not fall into one of the high-risk categories.

_____ **20** Space maintainers are placed in the oral cavity to gain space lost by movement of teeth.

_____ **21** It is primarily the responsibility of the dentist, not the dental assistant, to observe signs of child abuse.

_____ **22** Nursing-bottle mouth is seen only in children who are allowed to have a carbonated beverage in their bottle.

_____ **23** It is not necessary to have signed informed consent for a pediatric patient if a parent brought the child in for care.

_____ **24** It is recommended that a mask not be worn during treatment because it might frighten the child.

_____ **25** If a child loses a primary tooth at the age of 3 years, no treatment needs to be considered.

Rationales

Pediatric Dentistry

1 A Exfoliation is the natural loss of the primary teeth as the permanent teeth erupt. This occurs as the primary tooth develops in the alveolar process and the root of the primary tooth resorbs for easier loss.

2 A An act of commission is actually and cognitively committing the event.

3 B Neglect is a form of abuse committed by not completing an act, such as not taking a child for dental care and allowing the teeth to decay.

4 B See item 3.

5 D The technique of tell, show, and do involves explaining the procedure, such as a prophylaxis, to a child, then showing the child how the procedure will be done by letting him or her feel the A/W syringe flow and the rubber cup on the handpiece. Then complete the procedure that was explained.

6 B If a child is allowed to participate in the dental treatment and understand the care to be received, the child will be more cooperative. Allowing the child to ask questions at certain times or hold a device to "help" in the procedure will also assist in alleviating fear. If the previously described techniques do not work, it may be necessary to presedate the child to ensure a positive experience. On subsequent visits presedation may not be necessary.

7 B A spot welder is used to create a matrix band for primary teeth that fits a specific tooth. This device is often used in stabilizing orthodontic devices.

8 C Stainless steel crowns are used because they are more resistant to wear than acrylic crowns. An amalgam core does not provide full coverage and protection.

9 E In certain states all of the tasks listed may be performed in accordance with the state dental practice act.

To know which of these or other tasks are delegated to the assistant, contact the governing agency in your state.

10 E Usually an abused child is very reserved and unwilling to answer questions regarding injuries. The abuser may clothe the child to cover bruises. Children, if they answer any questions, often offer excuses for the injuries. If the child becomes more reserved or even frightened when a certain gender of dental health care worker has contact, a red flag may appear. The child may be frightened of a male because the abuser is a male (the same applies for a female). Some abused children will not want the parent/caregiver to be in the treatment room or may even be concerned about the parent leaving the room. Without the parent in the room, the child may think questions will be asked that will be difficult to answer.

11 A Usually placing a hand over the mouth of a child is unacceptable and may be considered assault in some situations.

12 C Usually, permanent full-cast metal crowns are not placed on primary teeth because these teeth are exfoliated. Stainless steel crowns, the restoration of choice, offer some of the benefits of cast metal crowns and are more cost-effective.

13 C Reporting child abuse or suspected child abuse is the responsibility of every health care worker and the legal obligation of the dentist.

14 A Sometimes noninvasive techniques of behavior management are not successful, and drug therapy is necessary.

15 A See No. 12.

16 B Usually children act out more when the parent/care-giver is brought into the treatment room. The child may feel he or she can control the parent more than the dental health care worker and try to manipulate the situation.

17 B A pulpectomy is usually performed on adults and a pulpotomy on children. Two alternative treatments are available: apexification (for a tooth with necrotic pulp) and apexogenesis (for a tooth with vital pulp).

18 B Rubber dam is often used in pediatric dentistry to increase patient comfort, allow the operator a clear treatment site, and aid in patient management.

19 B All patients are considered potentially infectious and should be treated with universal precautions.

20 B Space maintainers maintain the space that exists after a tooth is lost. This space is maintained for the permanent tooth or until a later time when a bridge is placed.

21 B All health care workers are responsible for observing and reporting child abuse.

22 B The only recommended beverage for bottles at night is water. Juices, milk, and carbonated beverages contain sugar, which will aid in the cause of nursing-bottle mouth.

23 B All patients must sign an informed-consent sheet. Parents must be made aware of proposed treatment and give consent for treatment.

24 B See No. 19.

25 B A space maintainer should be placed (see item 20).

To enhance your understanding of the material in this chapter refer to the illustrations in Chapter 36 of Finkbeiner/Johnson: *Mosby's Comprehensive Dental Assisting: A Clinical Approach.*

Periodontics

KEY TERMS

Attachment width

Bone swaging

Coronaplasty

Crevicular fluid

Curettage

Debridement

Digitized radiography

Donor tissue

Excise

False pocket

Festoon

Flap surgery

Furcation involvement

Gingivectomy

Gingivoplasty

Graft

Granulation tissue

Incise

Index

Infrabony pocket

Irrigation

Keyes technique

Mucogingival surgery

Mucoperiosteal flap

Mucosal flap

Occlusal equilibration

Osseous surgery

Oxygenating agent

Periodontal dressing

Periodontal surgery

Physiologic contour

Recession

Recipient tissue

Reflect

Resection

Root planing

Splint

Subtraction radiography

Sulcular fluid

Sulcus temperature gauge

Suprabony pocket

This chapter examines periodontal disease (what it is and how it is described and treated); discusses the role and responsibilities of the dental assistant; and describes periodontal examinations, instruments, and procedures. It concludes with specific directions for the technical procedures that dental assistants commonly perform.

PERIODONTAL DISEASE

I. Periodontal disease is an episodic, site-specific infection of the dental supporting tissues.

II. The American Academy of Periodontology estimates that three out of every four adults will acquire some form of this disease during their lifetime; adults are also more likely to lose teeth as a result of periodontal disease than caries.

III. Children do not develop periodontal disease at the same rate as adults, but they do contract it, and some juvenile forms are severe and progress rapidly.

IV. Gingivitis and periodontitis are two basic types of periodontal disease.
   A. Gingivitis is confined to the gingiva.
   B. Periodontitis extends into the periodontal ligament, cementum, and/or alveolar bone.
   C. Disease in a patient is described on the basis of extent, severity, resistance to treatment, age of onset, duration, speed of progression, and etiologic agent, if known.
   D. Table 26-1 lists the forms of periodontal disease and the terms (and their meanings) most commonly used to characterize each form.

THE PERIODONTICS TEAM

I. The periodontics team consists of the patient and selected dentists, dental assistants, and dental hygienists who work as a group to help the patient achieve and maintain good periodontal health.

II. Each team member has a specific role and responsibilities that contribute to treatment success.

III. Good human relations are vital to the success of periodontal treatment.
   A. The dentists and their staff must coordinate the treatment between the two practices (specialty and referring general practitioner) to provide comprehensive care to the patient.
   B. Periodontal treatment may extend over several months, and the goal of therapy must be maintained indefinitely.
   C. To avoid error and misunderstanding, everyone involved must maintain the three Cs: consultation, communication, and coordination.

THE PERIODONTAL THERAPY PROCESS

I. Periodontal therapy involves the following basic steps:
   A. Developing rapport
   B. Obtaining the history and performing the examination
   C. Evaluation
   D. Case presentation
   E. Treatment
   F. Continuing care

II. Coordination of periodontal care with restorative, surgical, and reconstructive care occurs at the treatment stage.

PERIODONTAL EXAMINATION

I. Table 26-2 lists signs of periodontal disease and what they mean; Table 26-3 lists the major contributing factors and how they assist in disease development.

II. Signs and contributing factors considered together

Table 26-1   Forms of periodontal disease

Characteristic	Description	Meaning
Extent	Localized	In small area
	Generalized	Over large area
Severity	Mild	Gingivitis
	Moderate	Progressing to periodontitis
	Severe	Significant tissue loss
Resistance to treatment	Refractory	Resistant
Age of onset	Juvenile	Childhood
	Prepubertal	Preteen years
	Adult	After teenage years
Duration	Acute	Short, rapid
	Chronic	Long, slow
Speed of progression	Rapid	Swiftly progresses to periodontitis
	Slow	Varying progression
Etiologic agent	Infection	Microorganisms; often complicated by poor tissue contour, functional trauma, improper diet, systemic disorder, or genetics

Table 26-2 Signs of periodontal disease

Sign	Appearance	Significance
Inflammation	Red, swollen	Indicates current infection
Bleeding on probing	Blood present	Early sign of inflammation
Changes in gingiva		
Color	Red	Inflammation is acute
	Purple	Circulation is stagnant
	White	Tissue is fibrotic
Contour	Swollen	Edema is present
	Papillae rounded, flattened, or rolled	Impairs self-cleaning
	Cleft	Traps food, debris, microorganisms
Consistency	Soft	Extra fluid present (blood, tissue fluid and/or pus)
	Hard	Infection is chronic
		Reparative fibers have grown into connective tissue
Texture	Smooth surface	Fibers are losing their elasticity
	Shiny surface	Epithelium is thin
Pocketing	Gingival	Sulcus enlarged
		Traps plaque, debris, toxins
	Suprabony	Loss of attachment
	Infrabony	Difficult to debride
Decrease in attachment width	Possibly normal	Loss of fiber attachment
	Possible root exposure	
Bone loss	Ragged or cupped alveolar crest	Beginning of bone loss
	Localized	Loss of tooth support
	Generalized	
Mobility	Too much tooth movement	Anchoring ligament fibers weakened
		Inadequate bone support remaining
		May be infection at root end

Table 26-3 Factors contributing to periodontal disease

Contributing factor	Mechanism of action	Result
Plaque	Harbors microorganisms	Produces toxins, enzymes
Calculus	Surface rough, irregular	Harbors debris, toxins
	Hard composition	Cannot be removed by brushing
	Securely attached	Difficult to debride
	Forms along tooth roots, furcations	Interferes with oral hygiene procedures
Malocclusion	Poor distribution of occlusal forces	Bone may resorb
		Mobility may develop
Missing teeth	Ligament fibers not present to exercise tendon on bone	Bone loss, hypereruption; adjacent tooth drifting
Frenum pull	Tension on soft tissue	Gingival recession
Improper diet		
Too soft	Food sticks between and around teeth	Gingival irritation
Too hard	Gingival trauma	Laceration
Deficient in essential nutrients	Unknown	Tissue integrity impaired
Systemic disease		
Diabetes	Impaired immune response	Poor healing
AIDS	Unknown	Severe, rapidly progressing periodontal disease
Heredity		
Poor host response	Unknown	Difficulty in controlling periodontal disease
Gene structure	Unknown	Development of juvenile forms of disease

give the clinician a picture of the disease process in a patient.

III. Treatment is planned to eliminate or control the disease and contributing factors.

IV. The examination procedure is as follows:

A. The operator observes, measures, evaluates, and announces the conditions present while the dental assistant transfers or operates the instruments, maintains excellent visibility of and access to the examination site, accurately records the conditions observed, monitors the patient's reactions, and assists the patient with physical needs or psychologic comfort as indicated.

B. Accuracy in recording is essential; if you do not hear or understand the conditions that are dictated, ask for clarification.

V. Examination instrumentation involves the following:

A. Manual examination instruments
1. Mirror
2. Explorer
3. Periodontal probe
4. Air/water syringe
5. Dental floss
6. Articulating paper/forceps

B. Automated instruments
1. **Sulcus temperature gauge**—To measure the temperature of **crevicular fluid** (an altered serum fluid in the sulcus) a handpiece sensor tip is placed under the tongue to obtain a baseline oral temperature. Then each sulcus is probed by positioning the sensor in the sulcus and activating a foot switch.

2. Automated bite recorder—Bite force can be measured by computer. Identifying data are programmed into the machine, a preformed bite sheet with disposable cover is inserted into the patient's mouth, and the patient is asked to bite slowly but firmly and carefully and hold this position for a short time. Sensors relay occlusal loads of the various teeth to the computer, which creates a three-dimensional image of bite forces throughout the dentition. This graphic is relayed to a monitor and may be printed as well.

3. Peri-optik probe—This instrument may be used to improve field visualization at the examination site. It consists of a fiberoptic wand large enough to use as a tissue retractor. Light shines out the ends of the fi-

bers, and air and water sprays can be activated. Enhanced vision, retraction, flushing, and drying of an area can thus be accomplished as needed, using only one hand.

4. Voice-activated data recording system— This system electronically records any data observed on examination. Before using it on a patient, the operator records a series of words that will be used to describe conditions seen. For example, the operator might indicate normal, numbers from 1 to 32, millimeters, and red. During the examination the operator wears a headset and speaks into its microphone. The examination is completed in a standard order. As the operator speaks, the machine recognizes the words that were recorded earlier and converts them to data records. For example, saying ''Number 1; 3, 4, 4'' would indicate pocket depths of 3, 4, and 4 mm for the distobuccal, buccal, and mesiobuccal surfaces of tooth #1. Data are stored electronically and can be printed in chart form.

VI. Radiography is an important diagnostic aid.

A. Paralleled bitewings and periapicals are the radiographs of choice for routine applications in periodontics.

B. Parallel vertical bitewings and periapicals provide the most accurate and complete view of the ligament space and interdental bone.

C. Criteria for radiograph assessment include the following:

1. Alveolar bone should follow the contour of the cementoenamel junction and be slightly apical to it; the alveolar crest and lamina dura should be clearly defined lines.

2. A widened periodontal ligament space indicates that inflammation has extended into bone.

3. An indistinct lamina dura or a ragged or cupped out alveolar crest indicates early bone loss.

4. Apically angled bone adjacent to the tooth indicates bone resorption in a particular area; it is often associated with tooth malposition and resulting traumatic occlusion.

5. Decrease in the height of bone around several teeth or an entire arch indicates a more generalized loss and is likely to be associated with generalized inflammation.

6. **Furcation involvement,** which concerns

the area where the root divides, indicates advanced disease.

7. A radiolucent area next to the tooth may indicate the presence of a periodontal abscess or cyst.

D. **Digitized radiography** is similar to conventional radiography except that no film is used, and the image may be manipulated to suit operator preferences before it is finalized.

1. A small camera is covered with a disposable plastic sheath and placed lingual to the teeth of interest just as a film would be.

2. A lead apron is not used.

3. The image is recorded electronically and projected on a small screen at the control console.

4. The operator can then alter the density or contrast or zoom in on a close-up view of a specific area.

5. A button is pressed to obtain a hard paper copy; only the image on the screen can be printed. Once printed, an image is not retained in digital form.

E. **Subtraction radiography** involves a series of radiographs taken over time to visualize areas of bone loss.

1. Either a conventional or a digitized system may be used.

2. The finished films or paper prints are placed in an image digitizer and compared electronically. Unchanged areas are subtracted from the image so that only the changed areas remain.

3. The final view, composed only of areas of loss, is printed as a positive image.

VII. Charting involves the following:

A. There are many variations of periodontal charts, but most include lines across and small boxes above and below the tooth roots.

B. The lines are used as guides for drawing in the height of the gingival margin and the alveolar bone.

C. The boxes are used to record measurements made of the depth of the sulcus and the width of the attached gingiva.

D. Common periodontal symbols are explained (box on page 444).

VIII. Evaluation involves the following:

A. The dentist analyzes and evaluates the data to arrive at a diagnosis and treatment plan.

B. The treatment plan should include a sequence in which the treatment tasks are to be performed, the time allocated for each task, in-

terim appointment times, and procedure fees.

C. The case presentation includes full information regarding examination findings, diagnosis, goals of treatment, recommended treatment procedures, available alternatives, time and discomfort involved, fees, insurance coverage, and available payment options.

PERIODONTAL TREATMENT

I. Periodontal therapy is individualized to meet the patient's needs.

II. A typical sequence of therapy is provided (box below).

III. Initial periodontal treatment includes the following:

A. Initial periodontal treatment extends over a series of appointments.

B. Initial treatment is conservative (non-surgical).

C. Procedures used include scaling, root planing, irrigation, Keyes technique, splinting, occlusal equilibration, and patient education and home care.

IV. *Scaling* involves **debridement** of plaque and calculus deposits from tooth surfaces.

A. *Calculus* is hardened plaque; its surface is rough and pitted (like a cement sidewalk); this roughness collects debris, more plaque, and microorganisms.

B. Microorganisms in the plaque release tissue toxins into the sulcus and sometimes enter and infect the tissue itself.

TYPICAL SEQUENCE OF PERIODONTAL THERAPY

Initial debridement of plaque and calculus—to eliminate periodontal infection and promote healthy tissue

Endodontic treatment—to eliminate dental infection

Oral and maxillofacial surgery—to eliminate hard- and soft-tissue infection and to prepare for implants if necessary

Restoration of carious teeth—to eliminate dental infection

Orthodontic treatment—to establish physiologic jaw and tooth alignment and establish major outline of bone and soft tissue

Periodontal surgery—to complete calculus debridement and establish fine bone and soft-tissue contour

Prosthetic procedures completed to newly established tissue contours—to promote ease of oral hygiene

---

COMMON PERIODONTAL SYMBOLS

PD = POCKET DEPTH: DISTANCE IN MILLIMETERS FROM GINGIVAL MARGIN TO BASE OF POCKET

Important facts about pocket depth:

Normal sulcus depth is 0.5 to 3 mm.

Epithelial attachment migrates apically in periodontal disease.

Resulting deepened sulcus is termed a *pocket.*

Pockets may be false, suprabony, or infrabony.

False pocket is gingival swelling without apical migration of attachment.

Suprabony pocket has apical migration of attachment and base above the alveolar crest.

Infrabony pocket has apical migration of attachment and base below the alveolar crest.

PD measurement indicates how deep the pocket has become.

Six measurements are taken: mesiofacial, facial, distofacial, mesiolingual, lingual, and distolingual.

Measurements are entered in order in boxes above facial and below lingual of each maxillary tooth and below facial and above lingual of each mandibular tooth.

AW = ATTACHMENT WIDTH: DISTANCE IN MILLIMETERS FROM THE BASE OF THE POCKET TO THE MUCOGINGIVAL LINE

Important facts about attachment width:

It indicates the amount of attached gingiva remaining.

AW measurement is the total gingiva minus pocket depth.

Measurements are made at same points and placed in boxes in same manner as for pocket depth.

M = MOBILITY: DISTANCE BEYOND NORMAL THE TOOTH MOVES IN ITS SOCKET

Important facts about mobility:

The tooth is rocked between clinician's index fingers or between one finger and the instrument handle.

The resulting motion is assigned one of the following classes:

N: Normal

Class 1: <1 mm

Class 2: 1 to 2 mm

Class 3: >2 mm

If the class is normal, mobility is *not* considered to be present.

OH = ORAL HYGIENE: NUMBER (SCORE) DESCRIBING THE ORAL HYGIENE CONDITION OF A SINGLE TOOTH OR ALL TEETH IN THE MOUTH

Important facts about an oral hygiene score:

It indicates the average amount of debris on a tooth.

Each tooth assigned a single score; the larger the score, the more the debris.

The scoring system is termed an **index.**

Many scoring systems and indices are available; the assistant should learn the index preferred for the periodontics practice in which he or she is employed.

C. Removal of calculus on root surfaces is essential to disease control.

D. Scalers are used to remove plaque and calculus.

V. Root planing involves the following:

A. Rough and diseased cementum is removed, and the root surface is smoothed until it feels as smooth as glass.

B. Studies have shown that sulcus epithelium reattaches more easily to a smooth, disease-free surface.

C. Curette scalers are used for root planing.

D. Repeated small scaling strokes are made in several directions on the root surface. This removes small bits of calculus, embedded or calcified periodontal ligament fiber ends, and a thin layer of the cementum itself to expose healthy cementum and produce the desired smoothness.

E. This procedure is repeated until all rough areas and diseased cementum have been removed and the underlying healthy tissue is completely smooth.

F. Root planing takes a considerable amount of time and can be painful; local anesthesia is typically used.

VI. Table 26-4 lists instruments and devices commonly used in periodontal therapy.

VII. **Irrigation** involves the use of a syringe or nozzle to flush a pocket clean of debris or place medication within it.

A. **Sulcular fluid** is fluid that has flowed from the sulcular epithelium. Its precise mechanism of formation is not completely known, but the selective barrier concept is believed to apply.

B. It often is more effective to place the medication directly into the sulcus to ensure that it reaches the pathogenic microorganisms there.

C. Various medications are used depending on the specific needs of the patient.

D. The sulcular fluid is cultured to determine what types of microorganisms are infecting the area.

E. An antibiotic, an **oxygenating agent** (a chemical containing oxygen), or another drug can be prescribed to target those organisms.

F. Both manual and automated irrigating devices are available.

G. Manual syringes include a root canal irrigating syringe (with the tip removed), a surgical irrigating syringe, and a bulb irrigator.

H. Automated systems include a small electric system with a single fluid reservoir, a delivery tube and several interchangeable nozzles, and a larger system that permits tube and nozzle delivery of a choice of several premixed solutions activated by a foot switch.

VIII. The **Keyes technique** involves cleaning the teeth with sulcus brushing and a paste of baking soda, salt, and hydrogen peroxide.

A. Baking soda is a basic substance, salt is hypertonic, and hydrogen peroxide liberates oxygen.

B. The chemical ingredients of the paste are thus antimicrobial, and some studies have found that using it regularly significantly reduces the bacterial population of the sulcus.

C. The taste of the paste may be objectionable; adding a drop or two of peppermint or wintergreen oil improves the flavor greatly and increases most patients' willingness to adhere to the regimen.

IX. A **splint** is a device that fits over or is bonded to teeth to broaden the area over which biting forces are distributed.

A. It may cover the occlusal or incisal surfaces of a few teeth or a whole arch, or it may connect adjacent portions of lingual tooth surfaces of single teeth.

B. There are two basic types of splints:

1. *Full-arch acrylic splints* are processed extraorally and are removable. They are used to relieve the pain and mobility associated with temporomandibular joint dysfunction.

2. *Small-area composite splints* are processed intraorally. They are made by etching the lingual surfaces of the recipient teeth and bonding plastic material to them. They are used to control mobility from trauma or periodontal disease long enough to permit strong fiber reattachment in the area.

C. The armamentarium used for preparing splints is listed (boxes on page 448).

D. The procedure for fabricating an extraoral full-arch acrylic splint is provided (box on page 448).

E. The procedure for fabricating an intraoral small-area composite splint is provided (box on page 448).

X. Oral hygiene aids include floss, interdental brushes, interdental tips, implant cleaners, therapeutic mouthwashes, and preventive toothpastes.

XI. **Occlusal equilibration,** also termed **coronaplasty,** involves reshaping the occlusal or incisal surfaces of selected teeth to improve the bite.

A. Carbide burs and occlusal registration paper are used for equilibration.

B. The periodontist uses the handpiece like a paintbrush to *draw* the new shape of the cusp or incisal surface and then checks the result with bite registration paper.

XII. Patient education is the backbone of successful periodontal treatment.

A. No amount of scaling, root planing, or other treatment is effective for long if the patient does not appreciate and maintain the gains achieved through treatment.

B. The patient must understand what has been done, why it was done, and what needs to be done to keep the supporting structures healthy.

C. Education works best when it is related to conditions in the patient's mouth, is couched in language the patient understands, and is delivered as an ongoing part of the treatment process.

D. Each patient should learn the following:

1. The definition of periodontal disease

2. The status and appearance of his or her periodontal disease

3. What normal healthy periodontal conditions are and how they appear

Table 26-4 Periodontal instruments

Instrument/use	Design characteristics
HAND EXAMINATION INSTRUMENTS	

Mirror
  Vision
  Retraction
	Reflecting surface

Explorer Detect hard deposits, caries, roughness	Small, thin, flexible tip

Periodontal probe
  Locate pockets
  Measure pocket depth, attachment width, size of lesions
	Thin, may be round or flat, tip blunt, often tapered, usually marked in millimeters

A/W syringe Increase visibility	Three-way: air, water, spray

Dental floss
  Detect overhangs, tight contacts
  Remove debris
	Operator's preference for waxed or unwaxed, floss or tape

SCALERS	

Sickle
  Remove supragingival deposits
  Three types: curved (universal), straight (for anterior surfaces), modified (for posterior proximals)
	Two cutting edges converge to pointed tip
	Triangular in cross section

Curette
  Remove subgingival deposits
  Two types: universal (all surfaces), area-specific (specified surfaces)
	Spoon-shaped blade with rounded tip
	
	Two cutting edges of same length; both edges used
	Two cutting edges, one longer; only longer edge used

Hoe Remove heavy supragingival deposits	Similar to small garden hoe Blade may be straight or curved
Chisel Remove deposits from exposed proximal surfaces of anteriors	Blade flat, beveled at 45-degree angle with shank Cutting edge slightly curved

File
  Crush calculus deposits
  Smooth restoration margins
	Multiple cutting edges
	Blades appear as series of small cutting edges on oval or round base

Sonic scaler Remove stain, hard deposits, and restoration overhangs	Air powered Rapid tip oscillation Several interchangeable tips

Ultrasonic scaler
  Remove stain, hard deposits, and restoration overhangs
  Flush sulcus
	Electric powered
	Uses water spray
	Very rapid tip oscillation
	Several interchangeable tips

Diamond file	Wedge-shaped rotary instrument Gingival side smooth Working side diamond or aluminum dust
POLISHING/SMOOTHING INSTRUMENTS	

Prophylaxis angle
  Remove stain
  Polish surfaces
	Small, right/contra-angle, slow speed; sterilizable or disposable

Porte polisher
  Remove stain
  Polish surfaces
  Massage gingiva
  Apply medication
	Manual instrument handle
	Uses disposable orangewood points

Air polisher Remove heavy stain	Air powered Spurts water/sodium bicarbonate slurry through nozzle

Polishing cap
  Remove light stain
  Polish surfaces
	Rubber rotary instrument, round with flexible edges

Table 26-4 Periodontal instruments—cont'd

Instrument/use	Design characteristics
POLISHING/SMOOTHING INSTRUMENTS—cont'd	
Cleaning brushes	Rotary instrument
Remove moderate stain	Hard black or soft white bristles
Amalgam knife	Straight sickle-shaped blade
Contour amalgam restorations	
Enamel file	Coarse, medium, or fine file on straight or oval base
Smooth enamel/restoration margins	Rounded end
HAND SURGICAL INSTRUMENTS	
Pocket marker	Similar to cotton pliers except has sharp triangular projection
Mark level of pocket base	on one arm
Scalpel	Single, sharp, beveled edge
Incise soft tissue	Several blade shapes
Periodontal knife	Kidney-shaped blade
Incise gingiva	
Interdental knife	Triangular with two beveled blades
Incise interdental gingiva	
Electrosurgery	Powered by high-frequency current
Cut soft tissue and seal circulatory vessels	Wand with interchangeable tips
Soft-tissue scissors	Pointed ends, curved blades
Cut and contour soft tissue	
Nippers	Small spring-loaded clippers
Clip tissue tags	
Remove bone spicules	
Surgical scalers and currettes	Similar to regular scalers except larger and with longer shanks
Remove hard deposits	
Burs	Many shapes
Cut, contour, and smooth bone	Often large and low speed
Surgical chisel	Similar to chisel scaler
Remove exostoses	May have slightly curved blade
Surgical currette	Similar to currette scaler but larger
Remove necrotic bone	
File	Round or oval base with multiple blades
Contour and smooth bone	
Periosteal elevator	Paddle or claw ends
Reflect incised soft tissue	
Suture needle/thread	Small, curved, usually prethreaded, disposable
Sew wound edges in position	
Needle holder	Similar to scissors except has blunt nose, ratchet handle
Position need for use	
Suture scissors	Blunt nose
Cut suture thread	One arm has half-moon cutout

4. How to achieve and maintain the healthiest conditions possible in his or her mouth

SURGICAL TREATMENT

I. The need for **periodontal surgery** is usually determined after initial therapy has been completed.

II. Conditions such as deep or inaccessible pockets, irregular bone contour, furcation involvement, mucogingival defects, and persistent inflammation might not be successfully treated without the high quality of deposit removal, tissue debridement, and recontour afforded by surgical treatment.

III. Not every patient is a good candidate for surgical treatment.

   A. Some patients are medically compromised, are mentally or physically unable or unwilling to cooperate in the surgical process, do not have

---

ARMAMENTARIUM FOR PREPARING AN EXTRAORAL FULL-ARCH ACRYLIC SPLINT

Alginate impression tray, impression material, and powder measure

Rubber bowl and alginate spatula

Water and alginate water measure

Dental stone, graduated cylinder, and water

Plaster spatula

Separator (petroleum jelly)

Acrylic powder and liquid

Disposable paper cup

Cement spatula

Reinforcing wire, bending pliers, and cutting pliers

Quartz, rag, and chamois wheels for lathe

Acrylic polishing compound

ARMAMENTARIUM FOR PREPARING AN INTRAORAL SMALL-AREA COMPOSITE SPLINT

Cotton rolls

Acid etch and application brush

Timing device

Light-cured bonding agent and application brush

Light-cured composite and plastic instrument

Curing light

Reinforcing wire and cutting pliers

Small wax spatula

Composite finishing disks

Abrasive polishing paste

Contra-angle and rubber cup

Dental floss

PROCEDURE FOR FABRICATING AN EXTRAORAL FULL-ARCH ACRYLIC SPLINT*

1. Obtain and disinfect alginate impression.
2. Pour impression in class II stone and allow to harden.
3. Trim excess stone from model to gain access to the anatomy.
4. Block out undercuts on model with wax and coat with a thin layer of petroleum jelly.
5. Bend and cut wire to fit lingual curve of arch.
6. Mix acrylic powder and liquid according to manufacturer's directions.
7. Adapt thin layer of soft acrylic to model and place wire cervical to occlusal surface on lingual portion of acrylic layer.
8. Adapt second layer of acrylic over wire, blend with first layer, and allow to set.
9. Remove splint from model; trim rough edges with quartz wheel.
10. Smooth splint with rag wheel and polishing compound; buff splint with chamois wheel.

*Follow OSHA guidelines as they apply.

PROCEDURE FOR FABRICATING AN INTRAORAL SMALL-AREA COMPOSITE SPLINT

1. Cut short piece of wire to act as ligature.
2. Isolate teeth and paint with acid etch according to manufacturer's directions.
3. Flush, dry, and check for chalky appearance.
4. Reisolate tooth and dry thoroughly.
5. Paint with bonding agent and cure.
6. Place composite to form small bridge between adjacent tooth surfaces and embed ends of wire in uncured composite.
7. Smooth composite to desired shape and cure.
8. Polish composite with disks, abrasive paste, and cup.
9. Pass dental floss through interproximal area to be sure that the area can be satisfactorily cleaned.

---

enough bone remaining to justify periodontal treatment, or decide not to make the necessary financial investment.

B. The dentist considers the whole patient—including periodontal condition, local and systemic contributing factors, and patient cooperation—before recommending surgery.

C. The patient makes the final decision.

IV. The overall objective of periodontal surgery is to eliminate the conditions that predispose a person to periodontal disease: poor tissue contour, pockets, and plaque accumulation.

V. Periodontal surgery procedures (Table 26-5) are performed on both hard and soft tissues.

CURETTAGE

I. **Curettage** is the surgical removal of diseased soft tissue that lines the sulcus.

II. It is preceded by scaling and **root planing** and is performed to eliminate inflamed epithelial tissue and **granulation tissue**—highly vascular tissue that forms in response to inflammation, edema, and **suprabony pockets** (pockets with a base above the level of the alveolar crest).

III. When these local factors are removed, swelling

Table 26-5 Periodontal surgery procedures

Procedure	Definition	Indications
Curettage	Removal of diseased soft tissue lining the pocket wall	Inflammation and edema of suprabony pockets
Gingivectomy	Removal of marginal and interdental gingiva	Suprapockets
		Periodontal abscesses
		Gingival enlargements
Gingivoplasty	Reshaping of gingiva	Gingival defects
Free gingival graft	Transfer of small piece of mucosal tissue from one site to another	Gingival recession
		Exposed roots
Flap surgery	Surgical separation of all or part of soft tissue in an area from underlying tissues, completion of other procedures, followed by return of soft tissue to same or adjacent area	Inaccessible root deposits
		Diseased hard and soft tissue
		Infrabony pockets
Osseous surgery	Sculpting of alveolar bone height and contour by addition or removal of bone or bone substitute	Bone roughness
		Bone defects or loss
		Infrabony pockets
		Exostoses
Root resection	Amputation of one root of a multirooted tooth	Extensive furcation involvement

subsides, pocket depth is reduced, and **physiologic contour** is reestablished.

IV. If the curettage has been extended subgingivally, new fiber attachment occurs at a more apical level on the root.

V. There are two types of curettage:
   A. *Closed curettage* takes place in a closed field; the gingival tissue remains in position around the tooth. In this instance a curette is turned around so that the blade faces the soft tissue rather than the root surface.
   B. *Open curettage* is done in an open field after a flap (a section of soft tissue) has been **incised** and pushed back to expose underlying tissues.
      1. **Reflecting** the flap improves visibility and access to the site.
      2. The remaining calculus is removed, root planing is done, diseased soft tissue is cut away, the flap is sutured back into position, and a **periodontal dressing** is placed.
      3. Healing takes approximately 6 weeks.

GINGIVOPLASTY

I. **Gingivoplasty** involves shaping the gingival tissue to the correct physiologic contour. Gingival aberrations—such as hyperplasia, clefts, craters, **festoons,** poor contour, and bulbous or misshapen papillae—are sculpted into correct forms by the use of soft-tissue cutting instruments and then repositioned and sutured as indicated.

II. Healing time depends on the type and extent of the wound.

FLAP SURGERY

I. **Flap surgery** consists of lifting a section of gingiva and/or mucosa from the underlying tissue, completing other procedures in conditions of good visibility and access while the flap is elevated, and repositioning and suturing the flap.

II. Some flaps are repositioned in the same area and some are displaced laterally, apically, or coronally.

III. There are two basic classes of flaps: **mucoperiosteal** (full-thickness) and **mucosal** (split-thickness).
   A. All soft tissues in an area—epithelium, connective tissue, and periosteum—are incised and elevated for a full-thickness flap.
   B. Only epithelium and part of the underlying connective tissue are elevated for a split-thickness flap, which leaves the bone covered with periosteum and a layer of connective tissue. This is the flap of choice when apical repositioning occurs.

IV. Apical repositioning is a widely used technique in surgery for pocket elimination because it helps increase the width of the gingiva.

V. Healing takes 4 to 8 weeks.

MUCOGINGIVAL SURGERY

I. **Mucogingival surgery** is plastic surgery of the gingiva and/or mucosa.

II. It is performed to correct mucogingival defects that help maintain or exacerbate periodontal disease.

III. Various procedures are used to increase the width of the attached gingiva, cover exposed tooth roots, reduce frenum or muscle attachment pull of soft tissue away from the tooth, and widen or deepen the vestibule.

LATERAL FLAP DISPLACEMENT

I. A laterally displaced flap is used to cover isolated areas of exposed root, such as those created by deep clefts, **recession**, retraction of tissues, or frenum pull.
II. Gingiva in the recipient (affected) site is **excised** (cut away or removed) and resected down to the periosteum.
III. The root surface is scaled and planed.
IV. **Donor tissue** is obtained by creating a partial-thickness flap in the laterally adjacent soft tissue. The open end of the flap is then moved sideways, adapted to cover the exposed area, and sutured into position.
V. The area is covered with a periodontal dressing.
VI. Healing takes 2 to 3 weeks.

GINGIVECTOMY

I. **Gingivectomy** is the cutting away of gingiva.
II. It is done to provide visibility and access for scaling and root planing, excise enlargements, and eliminate suprabony pockets or periodontal abscesses.
III. Cutting may be done with periodontal knives, electrosurgery, or chemicals.
IV. The depth of the pocket is measured, and the measurement is transposed to the gingival surface.
   A. A pocket marker is used to mark the base of each pocket on the outside of the gingiva.
   B. The resulting line of dots is then connected with incisions.
   C. A flap is reflected with an elevator.
   D. A surgical hoe or curette scaler is used to remove the incised marginal and interdental gingiva, the area is washed with water, granulation tissue and remaining root surface deposits are removed, and rough areas on the root surface are planed.
   E. The area is thoroughly flushed and then blotted with a gauze sponge until hemorrhage is controlled and a clot has formed.
   F. The flap is repositioned over the wound and may be protected with sutures and a periodontal dressing.
   G. Healing takes nearly 2 months.

GINGIVAL GRAFTING

I. A **graft** is the moving of tissue from one area to another.

II. A gingival graft is done to increase attached gingiva.
III. Pocket walls in the area are cut away, and root surfaces are scaled and planed.
IV. The **recipient tissue** is prepared by surgically creating a connective tissue bed in which to place the graft.
V. Donor tissue may be either gingiva or thick mucosa.
VI. A template of the prepared bed is made and used as a pattern for excising the graft.
VII. The graft is placed in the recipient bed, sutured into position, and protected with a periodontal dressing.
VIII. Healing takes about 2 weeks.

OSSEOUS SURGERY

I. **Osseous surgery,** or bone surgery, can be either augmentive or resective.
   A. *Augmentive surgery* is the addition of bone or bone substitute to fill bony defects.
   B. *Resective surgery* may be either bone or root resection involving removal of hard tissue.
II. Bone augmentation
   A. Augmentive procedures are performed to add bone or bone substitute to fill in bony defects.
   B. Bone may be added in the form of a bone graft from a different site in the same patient or from a different patient.
   C. Bone from the same patient is well tolerated but involves creating two wounds in the same patient. Two surgical procedures separated by days or weeks are required.
   D. Using bone from a different person raises questions of tissue compatibility and possible rejection of the graft.
III. Bone resection
   A. **Resection** is the process of removing tissue.
   B. Bone resection procedures are done to remove bone; they involve chiseling, clipping, filing, cutting, and smoothing to create the most physiologically accurate bone contour possible for a given patient.
   C. In general, steps proceed from gross to fine removal, followed by contouring and smoothing.
   D. After any type of bone surgery, covering soft tissue is contoured and sutured into place.
      1. The area is gently irrigated and blotted with 2 × 2 gauze squares to ensure that the sutures are well placed and a clot is beginning to form.

2. A periodontal pack is used to protect small areas or those with poor soft-tissue coverage.

3. Large sutured areas with adequate soft-tissue coverage may not be dressed.

IV Root resection

A. When periodontal disease in a multirooted tooth has caused extensive bone loss around one root but adequate bone remains around the other(s), the seriously involved root may be amputated.

B. Root resection is performed to eliminate furcation involvement and bony defects and to promote ease of cleaning.

C. A full-thickness flap is elevated, and a bur is used to amputate the root. The root stump is smoothed and contoured with diamond points, remaining roots are scaled and planed, the area is washed, the flap is repositioned and sutured, and the wound is covered with a periodontal pack.

D. Soft-tissue repair is completed in about 2 months; bone fill-in occurs in approximately 6 months.

SURGICAL INSTRUMENTS ■■■■■■

I. A typical armamentarium used for periodontal surgery is listed (box in the next column).

II. The periodontal surgery sequence is listed (box in the next column).

III. The procedure for periodontal surgery is provided (box on page 452).

IV. The team approach to periodontal surgery is provided (box on page 453).

V. Sutures may or may not be placed. Care of a surgical site with or without sutures is described (box on page 453).

VI. Periodontal dressings are used to protect surgical sites by covering the areas to avoid additional trauma during healing.

A. There are two types of dressings: eugenol and noneugenol.

B. Dressings are mixed, placed, contoured to physiologic form while soft, allowed to harden, and left in place for 1 week to 10 days.

C. The armamentarium for placement of a paste dressing is listed (box on page 454).

D. The patient returns to have the dressing removed and the healing assessed.

E. Dressings are removed less than 1 week after surgery, left in position for more than 10 days,

---

ARMAMENTARIUM FOR PERIODONTAL SURGERY

Anesthesia setup	Rongeur
Knives	Surgical curette
Mirrors	Tissue nippers
Cotton forceps	Surgical scissors
Pocket marker	Hemostat
Periodontal probe	Needle holder
Explorers	2 × 2 gauze
Scalpel with handle and blades	Dressing material and armamentarium
Specialized scalpels	Suture setup
Periosteal elevators	Surgical HVE tip
Specialized curets	Sterile saline solution
Sharpening stones	Irrigation syringes and cups
Chisels/scalers	Antibiotic ointment
Burs and stones	Lubricant
Interproximal files	

PERIODONTAL SURGERY SEQUENCE

Anesthetize site.
Examine and mark pockets.
Incise and reflect soft tissue.
Scale and root plane.
Debride site of diseased bone and tissue.
Smooth and contour hard and soft tissue.
Flush site.
Place sutures to close wound.
Place protective dressing.
Record procedure.
Give postoperative instructions.

---

or removed and replaced one or more times. The dentist determines when the dressings are to be removed, based on the healing assessment.

F. Noneugenol dressings are more widely used than eugenol because they are less irritating to the tissue, cause fewer allergic reactions, and take less time to prepare. They are available in two-paste and light-cured systems.

G. Mixing and placing eugenol and noneugenol dressings is described (box on page 454).

H. Placement of light-cured material is described (box on page 454).

I. Clinical criteria for evaluating the placement of a periodontal dressing are provided (box on page 454).

PROCEDURE FOR PERIODONTAL SURGERY

- Are all universal barrier techniques being used?
- Is all of the armamentarium available and prepared for use?
- Are the instruments arranged in order of use?
- Are you prepared for alternative treatment plans?
- Is the necessary equipment turned on and ready to operate?
  1. Anesthetize the patient.
  2. Pass the explorer to the dentist to examine the site. Exchange the explorer for a periodontal probe for examination of the periodontium.
  3. Pass the pocket marker to the dentist to mark the base of the pocket.
  4. After this is done, exchange the instrument for a periodontal knife. Some dentists may prefer to use a standard scalpel, such as a #12B, to detach the periodontal ligament before using the periodontal knife.
  5. Use the surgical HVE tip close to the surgical site to remove oral fluids and blood. Hold a 2 × 2 gauze sponge in the passing zone for the operator to pass cut tissue and for the assistant to clear the instrument tip.
  6. Exchange the scalpel intermittently for surgical scissors to cut the tissue. Use a forceps or hemostat to grasp the tissue, making it easier for the dentist to cut the tissue. Grasping the tissue permits it to be easily removed without using the HVE tip, which could clog the tip.
  7. The operator may use a surgical bur to cut a window in the bone when necessary to access the surgical site.
  8. After the soft tissue is removed, exchange a variety of scalers and periodontal files. During this debridement and root-planing procedure, flush the site with sterile water using an irrigating syringe. Constant use of the HVE tip and 2 × 2 sponges is necessary to clear the instruments and the site.
  9. If a suture is to be placed, pass it and prepare to cut the suture as the operator indicates.
  10. Place either a eugenol or a noneugenol dressing according to the manufacturer's directions.
  11. Place the dressing so that it meets the criteria used in the team approach (box on page 453).
  12. Provide postoperative instructions.
  13. Make entries on the patient record, including the type of sutures and dressing placed, patient reactions, and additional notations.
- Have the appropriate universal barrier techniques been removed?
- Have all appropriate surfaces been cleaned and disinfected?
- Has all of the armamentarium been removed?
- Has all equipment been repositioned?
- Has all equipment been disinfected/sterilized according to OSHA guidelines?

J. Postoperative instructions for periodontal dressings are given to the patient (box on page 455).

K. Removal of a periodontal dressing is described (box on page 455).

L. The armamentarium for removal of a periodontal dressing is listed (box on page 455).

CONTINUING CARE AFTER PERIODONTAL THERAPY

I. Patients who have received periodontal therapy must receive continuing care.

II. Studies consistently show that patients who practice thorough daily oral hygiene procedures and return to the dentist at prescribed intervals are most likely to maintain the status of periodontal health achieved in treatment.

III. Continuing care begins during treatment. As each phase is completed, the patient is taught about the new conditions in the mouth and is helped to master necessary cleaning techniques.

IV. When therapy is complete, the patient begins a maintenance program.

A. Maintenance appointments are a monitoring and early warning system; they consist of a standard series that can be readily adapted to the needs of each patient.

B. At each maintenance appointment the periodontal condition is reexamined and reevaluated, the patient is informed of the results and is educated and encouraged to perform any indicated home care procedures, routine scaling and root planing are done, and arrangements are made to treat any recurrent disease while it is still manageable.

PERIODONTAL SURGERY PROCEDURE: TEAM APPROACH

OPERATOR	ASSISTANT
Anesthetize patient.	Assist with anesthetic administration.
	Pass the explorer.
Grasp explorer; examine site.	
Return explorer; receive periodontal probe, and examine periodontium.	Exchange the explorer for a periodontal probe.
Return periodontal probe.	Receive periodontal probe and pass the pocket marker.
Receive marker and mark the base of the pocket.	
Return pocket marker.	Exchange marker for periodontal knife or scalpel.
Receive scalpel and make a flap/incision at marked site.	Place surgical HVE tip close to the surgical site to remove oral fluid and blood.
	Hold a 2 × 2 gauze sponge in the passing zone for the operator to pass cut tissue and to clear the instrument tip.
Return scalpel.	Receive scalpel; pass surgical scissors or burs if needed to cut gingival tissues or bone; retract tissues as needed; transfer and exchange a variety of scalers and periodontal files; wipe tips of instruments with gauze sponge; keep HVE tip near surgical site; flush site with sterile saline solution as needed.
Scale and plane exposed areas.	
Return scalers and files.	Receive scalers and files; prepare suture needle and pass if needed.
Receive needle and place sutures.	Retract tissues; evacuate site.
Return suture needle.	Receive suture needle; prepare dressing; pass lubricant to operator; pass dressing.
Receive dressing, place dressing, and adapt dressing to site.	Pass placement instrument and dressing material; wipe instrument as needed.
Return placement instrument.	Receive instrument.
	Clean patient's face; provide postoperative instructions; dismiss patient; record treatment.

CARE OF A SURGICAL SITE WITHOUT SUTURES (INSTRUCTIONS FOR PATIENT)

Bite on a folded gauze square for the next 30 minutes.
Slight bleeding may occur for the next 24 hours.
Do not eat or drink for 2 hours.
Avoid rinsing or brushing the area for 24 hours. After that time you should brush as usual.
Avoid hot, spicy, and hard foods for the next few days.
Take the medications(s) prescribed by the dentist according to the directions on the package.
Call the office if you have heavy bleeding, severe pain, or any unexpected symptom. (Office or clinic phone number should be provided.)
Make an appointment to return for the dentist to observe the area in_____ . (Fill in the blank with the appropriate number of days or weeks for the patient.)

PATIENTS WITH SUTURES

These patients receive the same directions as those above, with the following additions:
They are informed of the type of sutures they received (resorbable or nonresorbable) and whether they must return to have them removed.
Patients who must return are told the time interval for their return, and an appointment is made.
Patients are also told that some of the sutures may loosen and be lost. They should not be concerned unless bleeding returns after the loss.

ARMAMENTARIUM FOR PLACEMENT OF A PASTE DRESSING

Lubricant

Dressing base and catalyst

Paper pad and tongue depressor

Disposable cup of cold water

Mirror

Cotton pliers

Spoon excavator

Curette scaler

Plastic instrument

Crown and collar scissors

2 × 2 gauze sponges

PLACEMENT OF LIGHT-CURED MATERIAL

1. Prepare all necessary armamentarium.
2. Isolate and dry the surgical site.
3. Lubricate gloves.
4. Dispense material on a mixing pad; with a lightly lubricated finger, roll the ribbon of dispensed material off the pad and onto the surgical site.
5. Muscle-trim the material through manipulation of the lips and cheeks.
6. Contour the material.
7. Expose each area of the dressing, four teeth at a time, for at least 40 seconds under the curing light.
8. Curing must be done on the lingual as well as the buccal or facial surfaces.
9. If the dressing interferes with the occlusion or is uncomfortable for the patient, after hardening it can be contoured with a finishing bur on a slow-speed handpiece (see clinical criteria).

CLINICAL CRITERIA FOR EVALUATING THE PLACEMENT OF A PERIODONTAL DRESSING

Dressing material should have the following characteristics:

Be firm but not tacky (unless light-cured)

Have smooth edges and surfaces

Extend 3 mm beyond the margins of cut soft tissue

Cover the cervical third of any teeth adjacent to the wound

Follow the contours of the teeth and interdental gingiva

Attach securely

Lack excessive thickness or shelflike projections

Feel comfortable to the patient

MIXING AND PLACING EUGENOL AND NONEUGENOL DRESSINGS

1. Coat the patient's lips with a thin layer of lubricant.
2. Dispense proper proportions of the dressing as directed by the manufacturer.
3. Incorporate catalyst into the base using the tip of the tongue depressor with circular strokes until the mass is streaked in color.
4. Switch to the side of the depressor and complete the mix with figure-eight motions; the mix is complete when the color is homogeneous.
5. Gather the mix on the tongue depressor and place it in cold water until it can be easily handled.
6. Once the material becomes tacky, coat your gloves with a thin layer of lubricant.
7. Roll the mass into a thin piece of rope the length of the wound and approximately 3 mm in diameter.
8. Pinch the rope into two halves and shape one half to fit the lingual side of the surgical site.
9. Isolate the surgical site with cotton rolls or gauze sponges; dry and maintain the area by blotting gently with sterile gauze.
10. Using gentle finger pressure, adapt the lingual half of the dressing to fit the material into the interdental spaces.
11. Adapt the other half to the facial area in the same manner.
12. Gently press the two halves into interproximal areas until they meet; lock the two pieces together.
13. Remove excess material with a plastic instrument or scaler.
14. Use the back of the beaks of the cotton pliers to adapt the material into the interdental space more accurately.
15. Muscle-trim the material through the manipulation of the lips and cheek to ensure that the material does not impinge on movement; remove any excess with the scaler.
16. Smooth the cut edges and contour the material around the teeth using a spoon excavator.
17. Contour the material on the tooth surface (not to exceed one third the length of the tooth) to prevent interference with occlusion.
18. Create a smooth and even thickness of material.
19. Wet a gauze sponge and gently massage the dressing material to increase the smoothness (see clinical criteria).

REMOVAL OF A PERIODONTAL DRESSING

1. Irrigate the area with warm water.
2. Remove facial portion first by **working gently and carefully** to place the instrument under the distoapical margin of the dressing and work forward.
3. Pry the dressing loose.
4. If the sutures are embedded in the dressing, cut the dressing into sections with an instrument blade, work loose one section at a time, and cut the sutures that prevent a section from loosening easily.
5. Remove interproximal debris with an explorer or with floss that has a single knot tied in it.
6. Irrigate the site with antiseptic solution.
7. Grasp the free end of each remaining suture above and close to the knot with cotton pliers.
8. **Gently** elevate the knot.
9. Slip one blade of the scissors under the suture and cut the thread near the tissue.
10. Pull the cut thread **(never the knot)** through the tissue; save removed sutures on a gauze square; **count to verify that all have been removed.**
11. Irrigate the area with sterile water.
12. Verify that all dressing fragments, debris, and suture ends have been removed.
13. Have the patient rinse with mouthwash.
14. **Record removal on the patient's record; include the suture count.**
15. Have the dentist examine the healing area.
16. Transfer the mirror and gauze sponge for healing examination.

ARMAMENTARIUM FOR REMOVAL OF A PERIODONTAL DRESSING

Mirror
Explorer
Cotton pliers
Spoon excavator
Curette scaler or plastic instrument
Delicate suture scissors
Irrigating syringe with tip removed

Antiseptic irrigating solution (commercial or hydrogen peroxide in water)
HVE tip
Floss
2 × 2 gauze sponges
Cup and diluted mouthwash

POSTOPERATIVE PATIENT INSTRUCTIONS FOR PERIODONTAL DRESSINGS

Dressing should remain in place for 7 to 10 days or as directed by the operator.
Brushing should be done as usual.
Avoid hot, spicy, and hard foods.
Small pieces of the dressing may crumble and fall off; do not be alarmed.
If large pieces of the dressing (or the entire dressing) are lost, call the office to arrange for replacement or removal as indicated.
Make an appointment for observation and probable dressing removal in 7 to 10 days.

Questions

Periodontics

In numbers 1-4, place the correct surgical steps from a-e in the spaces provided.

a. Make incision.
b. Flush site.
c. Determine depth of involved site.
d. Cut window.
e. Debride site.

_____ **1** Surgical suction tip
_____ **2** Pocket marker
_____ **3** 12B
_____ **4** Saline solution

In items 5-9, place in correct order, in the space provided, the steps in a-e for placing a periodontal dressing.

a. Do not exceed one third the length of the tooth.
b. Using cotton pliers, adapt the material into the interdental space.
c. Roll mass into rope the length of the wound.
d. Use gentle finger pressure in the interdental space.
e. Muscle-trim the material.

_____ **5**
_____ **6**
_____ **7**
_____ **8**
_____ **9**

10 The most important factor in the reduction of hypersensitivity is
   a. Use of fluoride at home
   b. Minimized removal of tooth structure during root planing
   c. Professionally applied fluoride treatments
   d. Daily removal of all plaque from the mouth

11 A gingivectomy is the
   a. Surgical removal of the mucogingival junction
   b. Surgical removal of the apex of the tooth
   c. Replacement of inflamed gingival tissue
   d. Surgical elimination of the gingival pocket

12 A periodontal dressing is analogous to
   a. Cleaning teeth
   b. Suturing
   c. An oral bandage
   d. Protecting the periodontium from plaque

13 Which of the following groups of instruments would be used during a soft-tissue curettage?
   a. Mouth mirror, periosteal elevator, and curette scaler
   b. Explorer, scalpel, and periosteal elevator
   c. Anesthetic syringe, diamond stone, scalpel, and curette scaler
   d. Anesthetic syringe, HVE tip, and curette scaler

14 A modified sickle scaler is primarily used on the
   a. Interproximal surfaces of anterior teeth
   b. Interproximal surfaces of posterior teeth
   c. Interproximal surfaces of anterior and posterior teeth
   d. Lingual and buccal surfaces

15 Which of the following is true of the straight sickle scaler? It
   a. Is considered a universal scaler
   b. Should not be used to remove subgingival calculus on mandibular anterior teeth
   c. Should not be used to remove supragingival calculus on mandibular anterior teeth
   d. Is used to remove posterior interproximal calculus

16 The removal of calculus and portions of cementum to create a smooth, hard root surface is referred to as
   a. Supragingival scaling
   b. Subgingival scaling
   c. Gross scaling
   d. Root planing

17 The design shape of a curette scaler is similar to a(n)
   a. Ovoid
   b. Triangle
   c. Half-moon
   d. Rhomboid

18 Air may be used to deflect the free gingival margin to detect
   a. Inflammation
   b. Subgingival calculus
   c. Supragingival calculus
   d. Smooth root surfaces

19 The primary function of a periodontal file is to
   a. Remove supragingival calculus
   b. Perform root planing
   c. Fracture heavy, tenacious calculus

20 An ultrasonic scaler should not remain on tooth structure very long because it will
   a. Cause trauma to the gingival tissues
   b. Damage the tooth surface
   c. Cause the tip of the scaler to stop vibrating
   d. None of the above

21 After an ultrasonic scaler is used, a manual scaler must be used
   a. As a follow-up
   b. Only when directed by the dentist
   c. Only if scaling was difficult
   d. None of the above

22 A sharp dental instrument increases efficiency by
   1. Allowing the use of more lateral pressure
   2. Enhancing tactile sense
   3. Reducing trauma
   4. Decreasing the number of strokes that are necessary
   a. 1 and 3
   b. 2 and 4
   c. 2, 3, and 4
   d. 4 only

23 Which of the following procedures should be performed as part of the initial therapy phase of periodontal treatment?
   1. Oral hygiene instruction
   2. Temporary stabilization
   3. Removal of overhanging restorations
   4. Periodontal surgery
   5. Presurgical evaluation
   a. 1, 2, and 4
   b. 1, 2, 3, and 5
   c. 2, 3, 4, and 5
   d. 1, 2, 3, 4, and 5

24 Periodontal dressings are primarily used to
   1. Maintain the position of soft tissue
   2. Protect soft tissue during flossing
   3. Promote healing
   4. Protect tooth structure from temperature changes
   5. Provide an aesthetic appearance for the patient
   a. 1, 2, and 4
   b. 1, 3, and 4
   c. 2, 3, 4, and 5
   d. 1, 2, 3, 4, and 5

25 Which of the following diets would be acceptable for a patient after periodontal surgery?
   1. Normal, with care given to eating habits
   2. Soft
   3. Crumbly, for easier chewing
   4. Bland
   5. Nonirritative
   a. 1 and 2
   b. 1, 3, and 4
   c. 2, 4, and 5
   d. 1, 2, 4, and 5

Rationales

Periodontics

1 E   The surgical suction tip is smaller than the conventional HVE tip and allows more access to the surgical site.

2 C   A pocket marker has a tip that is at a right angle to the beak and allows the operator to make an indentation in the tissue on the buccal or lingual at the depth of the pocket.

3 A   A 12B scalpel has a two-sided cutting surface and is curved. It is often the scalpel selected for the incision.

4 B Saline solution is used to flush the surgical site to maintain a clear and clean working field.

5 C After surgery has been completed a periodontal dressing may be placed to protect the site. After the material is mixed it is rolled into one or two masses depending on the amount mixed and the length of the wound.

6 D Finger pressure forces the material into the interdental space to connect the buccal and lingual pieces of dressing and to form over the shape of the alveolar process.

7 B The interdental areas can be contoured with the beaks of cotton pliers or another instrument of choice. The contouring occurs on both the buccal and lingual surfaces.

8 E When contouring is completed, the patient's lip should be manipulated over the dressing to ensure that it does not impair movement or impinge on the vestibular area. Excess material should be removed.

9 A As the material is adapted over the wound, it should not extend to exceed a height of one third the crown of the teeth. If left longer, it may impinge on the patient's bite.

10 D The removal of plaque from the teeth reduces the sensitivity the patient may have from the exposed root surfaces.

11 D A gingivectomy is the surgical removal of infected and diseased gingival tissue to stop periodontal disease. The removal of this tissue also involves excision of the gingival pockets, which are areas the patient has had difficulty keeping healthy.

12 C A periodontal dressing covers the surgical wound, stabilizes the tissue, protects the wound from trauma and spicy foods, and increases comfort.

13 D The syringe is used to anesthetize the treatment site, and the HVE tip removes debris that the curette scaler dislodges during the scaling process.

14 B The modified sickle scaler, with the working end at a right angle to the shank, provides the operator access to the interproximal surfaces of posterior teeth. A straight sickle scaler, without the extra angle, is used similarly in the anterior segment of the mouth.

15 B A straight sickle scaler is used primarily to remove supragingival calculus in the anterior segment of the mouth on the interproximal surfaces.

16 D Calculus may be removed from the crown of the tooth, but when subgingival calculus is removed, it is often on the root of the tooth. To remove deposits and obtain a smooth surface, root planing is performed.

17 C The curette scaler is shaped like a half-moon to allow positioning on the contours of the tooth surfaces to remove calculus.

18 D When gingivitis and periodontal disease exist in the mouth, pockets are present. The gingival tissue surrounding the diseased areas is less taut than healthy tissue and can be deflected from the normal position with a blast of air to allow the operator to see the root surfaces.

19 C A periodontal file, with its grooved surfaces, allows for fracture of heavy, thick calculus. The operator can remove the fractured calculus with a scaler to smooth the surface.

20 B An ultrasonic scaler is used with intermittent contact to avoid damage to the tooth. A constant spray of water helps increase visibility.

21 A An ultrasonic scaler may not be as effective as a manual scaler in obtaining a smooth surface, so its use is usually followed by the use of a manual scaler for the smoothest surface.

22 C Sharp instruments are tantamount to efficient and effective dental treatment. The operator can remove calculus more quickly, with less effort and trauma to the patient.

23 B Periodontal treatment will not be effective in the long run if the patient has not committed to maintaining good oral hygiene. Successful periodontal treatment is predicated on stabilizing mobile teeth, removing overhanging restorations that cause inflammation, and extensive presurgical evaluation.

24 B See item 12.

25 C After periodontal surgery a patient usually does not want and should not have a diet that contains hard foods that can cause trauma, is spicy, or may irritate the surgical site. The patient must realize the importance of following an adequate diet to maintain good health but may be cautioned to eat softer foods.

To enhance your understanding of the material in this chapter refer to the illustrations in Chapter 37 of Finkbeiner/Johnson: *Mosby's Comprehensive Dental Assisting: A Clinical Approach.*

Forensic Dentistry

KEY TERMS

Adjudication

Antemortem

Assailant

Coroner

Forensic anthropologist

Forensic odontology

Identification

Litigation

Mass disaster

Medical examiner

Perpetrator

Postmortem

FORENSIC ODONTOLOGY

I. **Forensic odontology** is the science of dentistry as it relates to civil and criminal law.

II. Forensic dentistry can be divided into five major areas:
   A. Identification of human remains
   B. Mass disasters
   C. Bite- and tooth-mark recognition and case management
   D. Child-abuse
   E. Battered-adult recognition

III. Dentists who practice forensic odontology are often required to testify as expert witnesses regarding dental evidence in civil and criminal **litigation** (a legal contest by judicial process).

IV. Although forensic odontology is not a recognized dental specialty, it requires training and expertise beyond that of the general dental practitioner or the dental specialist.

V. The American Board of Forensic Odontology certifies dentists who have demonstrated expertise in forensic odontology by examination as diplomates.

VI. Forensic dentistry is not practiced in the traditional office setting, and the role of the dental assistant may be limited.

VII. **Identification** means providing proof of identity for human remains. This process is usually conducted in morgues, offices of medical examiners or coroners, or funeral homes.

VIII. Bite-mark evidence may be collected in hospitals or law enforcement facilities.

IX. The dental assistant can play a significant role in two areas:
   A. Record keeping—The dental assistant may ensure that patient records are kept as legible, accurate, and complete as possible.

B. Reporting abuse—The dental assistant may observe evidence of abuse in patients seen in the dental office and report it to the dentist, who is mandated by law to report it to the appropriate authorities.

IDENTIFICATION OF HUMAN REMAINS

I. No two individuals, including identical twins, have exactly the same dentition.

II. Teeth withstand both fire and decomposition and can be used in identifying bodies if accurate **antemortem** dental records are available for comparison.

III. In bodies that are burned beyond visual recognition, much of the dentition usually remains intact.

IV. Unprotected anterior teeth are often charred, but posterior dentition is protected by the cheeks and usually remains intact.

V. The bodies of drowning victims are frequently distorted, preventing positive visual identification.

VI. Decomposed and even skeletal remains can be positively identified by comparing **postmortem** and antemortem dental data.

VII. If the dentition is not intact because of decomposition, dismemberment, or fire, the area where the body was found should be carefully searched for teeth and other dental evidence.

VIII. Age, race, and sex of decomposed bodies or skeletal remains can be determined in conjunction with a **forensic anthropologist.**

POSTMORTEM DATA COLLECTION

I. Unless the body is to be prepared for viewing, the jaws are usually resected to allow better access for charting and radiographs.

II. The dentition of the postmortem remains is visually charted tooth by tooth to include the following:
A. All dental restorations (and their types)
B. Apparent caries
C. Anomalies
D. Abrasions
E. Erosion
F. Implants
G. Prostheses
H. Missing teeth (Teeth that are missing after death that were apparently present before death are noted as *missing postmortem* to distinguish them from those teeth that were missing antemortem.)
I. Periodontal condition, when possible
J. Occlusal relationships, when possible

III. Periapical and bitewing radiographs are obtained for comparison with antemortem films.

IV. Photographs of the oral structures may be helpful.

V. The body of a homicide victim is examined for evidence of bite and tooth marks. This evidence should be documented because it may be needed to identify the **assailant** (the aggressor in a confrontation between two individuals) or the **perpetrator** (the individual who committed the crime in question).

ANTEMORTEM DATA COLLECTION

I. An antemortem charting is compiled from the dental records and supporting information obtained from the dentist of record for the individual in question.

II. To facilitate comparison, similar forms are used for antemortem and postmortem charting.

COMPARISON OF POSTMORTEM AND ANTEMORTEM DATA

I. If the remains are suspected to be those of a particular individual, the postmortem and antemortem data are compared for similarities.

II. The following are used for comparison:
A. Restorations
B. Crown and root morphologies
C. Pulp-chamber morphology
D. Sinuses
E. Trabecular bone patterns

III. If sufficient consistency is present with no discrepancy, a positive identification can be made.

IV. The remains of an unknown individual can be compared with available records of missing persons for possible identification.

V. Records of missing persons may be supplied by the National Crime Information Center.

VI. If the available evidence is not sufficient to allow the dentist to form a conclusion, no identification can be made.

MASS DISASTERS

I. Identification of remains
A. This requires a team effort and is coordinated through the Office of the Medical Examiner/ Coroner within whose jurisdiction the **mass disaster** occurs.
B. The **medical examiner** is an appointed public official who makes postmortem examinations to determine the cause and manner of death.
C. The **coroner** is an elected official who inquires by inquest into the cause of any death

in which there is reason to suspect that death is not due to natural causes.

    D. Forensic odontologists work with forensic pathologists and anthropologists, the Federal Bureau of Investigation, and supporting personnel to identify the victims of the disaster.

    E. Dental assistants and hygienists may work with dentists in recording antemortem and postmortem data and obtaining postmortem radiographs.

II.   Forensic dental identification team

    A. The team should have a leader certified in forensic odontology to coordinate the team's efforts and act as the liaison between the team and the Office of the Medical Examiner or other agency in charge.

    B. Forensic dental teams are typically divided into four sections:

       1. Postmortem

       2. Photography and radiography

       3. Antemortem

       4. Comparison

    C. Each section should have a leader or supervisor who is responsible for coordinating the section's efforts and conveying the results to the team leader.

III. Postmortem section, photography and radiography section

    A. The remains are transported to a designated location.

    B. In airline disasters the designated location often is an available hangar.

    C. Refrigerated trucks can be used as holding facilities.

    D. Personal effects, fingerprints, identifying marks, and pertinent anthropologic data are documented by the appropriate individuals as belonging to the corpse, which is assigned an identifying number.

    E. Dental data are collected as described above.

    F. Forms are completed accurately, using standard designations.

    G. Photographs and radiographs are taken.

IV. Antemortem section

    A. Dental and medical records of individuals who were likely to have been involved in the disaster are requested (in writing) from the dentist on record, by either the responsible agency or its designee.

    B. Upon receipt, these must be cataloged.

    C. Medical records may be cataloged in the antemortem dental section and made available to the medical examiner.

ARMAMENTARIUM FOR MASS DISASTER FORENSIC IDENTIFICATION

Staplers	Mallets
Marking pens	Chisels
Zip-lock plastic bags	Long-handled pruning
Modeling clay	shears
Plastic buckets	Scissors
Dental x-ray film	Tissue forceps
Cotton rolls	Portable x-ray units
Toothbrushes	Automatic developers
Mouth mirrors	X-ray view boxes
Explorers	Personal protective
Scalers	equipment
Scalpels	

    D. To facilitate comparison, dental data are recorded on a standardized form similar to that used for recording postmortem data.

    E. Inaccurate, illegible records frequently make this task difficult or even impossible.

    F. The necessity for accurate, legible records cannot be overemphasized.

V.   Comparison section

    A. After all postmortem data are recorded and the antemortem data compiled, the process of comparison can begin.

    B. Postmortem and antemortem data can be entered into a database; possible matches can be obtained by comparing each postmortem record with each antemortem record.

VI. Armamentarium (box above)

VII. Marking dental prostheses (Some states require that all newly fabricated removable dental prostheses and appliances contain identifying marks, such as the name and social security number of the individual for whom the device is made.)

BITE- AND TOOTH-MARK RECOGNITION AND CASE MANAGEMENT

I.   Bite- and tooth-mark evidence is recognized by the courts and may be important in criminal and civil litigation that result in **adjudication** (a judicial decision or sentence).

II.   Initial recognition of bite and tooth marks, followed by proper recording and documentation of the lesion, is critical as trace evidence.

III. Tooth-pattern injuries can be seen in victims of sexual assault (heterosexual or homosexual), nonsexual assault, homicide, and child-abuse and battered-adult cases.

IV.   Any victim of an assault may have been bitten.

V.   Conscious victims should be questioned regarding the possibility of having been bitten or of having bitten an assailant.

VI.   Unconscious or deceased victims should be examined thoroughly because any part of the body may show evidence of bite and tooth marks.

VII.   Bite- and tooth-mark injuries can show brush/rub or bruiselike patterns, laceration, avulsion of tissue, or a combination of any or all of these.

VIII.   The primary concern of the health care professional must be the care of the victim/patient; the collection of bite-mark evidence must never interfere with timely treatment.

IX.   Whenever possible, authorization for collecting evidence should be received before any procedures are performed.

X.   The collection of evidence should follow a routine procedure once the bite mark has been recognized and recorded in the medical and dental records.

XI.   The bite-mark protocol is as follows:
A.   Photographs should include both orientation and close-up views.
B.   Whenever possible, these photographs should be taken before the area is sutured.
C.   Trace salivary evidence should be collected by swabbing the wounds.
   1.   Approximately 80% of the general population secretes blood-type proteins in the saliva.
   2.   These laboratory data can be used as evidence in implicating the perpetrator.
D.   Impressions of the wound pattern are useful if dimensional changes occur in the area after the bite.
E.   Wound-pattern impressions can be obtained from living or deceased victims.
F.   Follow-up photography may be used to detect wound patterns at a later date.
G.   Infrared and ultraviolet photography can be used to visualize old wound patterns that cannot be detected with routine procedures.

XII.   The forensic dental work-up of the suspect involves the following:
A.   Dental data must be collected from the suspected assailant when a victim presents with a bite or tooth mark.
B.   A search warrant that describes all procedures necessary for documentation must be obtained.
C.   Saliva and blood samples are taken for comparison with the salivary evidence.
D.   A complete oral examination is performed, and intraoral and extraoral photographs, dental impressions, and bite registrations are obtained by the forensic dentist.
E.   The dentist takes photographs and makes impressions of any marks on the suspect that might be relevant to the case.

XIII.   Bite- and tooth-mark evidence is evaluated only by a trained forensic odontologist.

CHILD ABUSE

I.   Child abuse may be classified as follows:
A.   Physical
B.   Sexual
C.   Emotional
D.   Overall neglect

II.   Abuse occurs at all educational, economic, and social levels.

III.   Health professionals are mandated by law to report suspected abuse in all states, and in most states they are given immunity from civil or criminal liability when they make the report in good faith.

IV.   Reporting suspected abuse may prevent additional suffering and possible death of a child.

V.   Dentists are faced with child abuse in two ways:
A.   Postmortem bite or tooth marks on a child
B.   Patients who may be victims of child abuse

VI.   Characteristics of child abuse include the following:
A.   A child may show signs of overall poor care and neglect.
B.   A child may be unduly aggressive or withdrawn.
C.   A child may bear signs of previous injuries.
D.   A child may exhibit atypical fear of the dental visit or withdraw and become silent or otherwise inhibited in the presence of the parent/s (the possible perpetrator/s).
E.   A child may manifest various neuroses, encephalopathies, autism, or childhood schizophrenia.
F.   Psychotic withdrawal in abused children is characterized by a shuffling gait, with eyes focused on the floor and unresponsiveness to the environment.
G.   Abusive parents are frequently distrustful of others and reluctant to give information regarding the child's injuries.
   1.   They may be overly critical of the child or may totally ignore the child.
   2.   They may refuse to cooperate with the suggested treatment and fail to keep follow-up appointments.

VII. The child should be interviewed without the parents present.

    A. The extraoral and intraoral examination should include both visual and palpable examination of the head, neck, and all oral structures.

    B. Exposed body parts should be examined for scars, keloids, lacerations, bruises, possible bite and tooth marks, and other signs of injury.

    C. The intraoral examination may reveal findings that suggest abuse, such as untreated fractures of teeth; discolored or devital teeth; fistulous tracts; oral burns; and lacerations of the lip, frenum, or uvula.

    D. A torn labial frenum is common in children learning to walk but should prompt suspicion when observed in infants or children who walk freely.

    E. Bite and tooth marks may be found on any area of the body.

        1. Most commonly these are seen on the cheek, shoulders, chest, abdomen, arms, legs, and buttocks.

        2. Bite marks may be single or multiple.

        3. Bite marks may appear as bruising, suck-like marks; incised marks with bruising lacerations; and even avulsion of tissue.

        4. Ask the child about being bitten; a sibling may be the aggressor when other signs of abuse are not apparent.

        5. Marks made by belts, belt buckles, cords, wires, and other tools may be seen.

VIII. Injuries should be documented in the medical and dental records.

    A. Photographs with a reference scale should be taken.

    B. Parental consent is usually not necessary for photographs of visible areas or radiographs that are taken to document suspected abuse.

    C. Reports of suspected abuse should be made to the state or county Social Services Office, Bureau of Child Welfare, or Department of Family Services or the local police department.

    D. In most states, failure to report suspected abuse is a misdemeanor.

BATTERED ADULTS ▬▬▬▬▬▬

    A. Adults, particularly those who are dependent on others, may be victims of abuse.

    B. The dental team should be aware of the possibility of abuse in adults who present with traumatic injuries, especially when the stated cause is inconsistent with the injury, dental injuries are repeated, or evidence of bruising or biting.

    C. Most often, victims are women and older adults.

    D. If the perpetrator brings the patient to the dental office, he or she may be reluctant to allow the patient to be alone with dental office personnel.

    E. If abuse of a competent adult is suspected, the dentist should provide the patient with the phone numbers of social service agencies that might be of assistance.

    F. Documentation should be placed in the patient record.

    G. If the patient is mentally challenged or otherwise incompetent, the dentist should notify the appropriate authorities of suspected abuse.

Questions

Forensic Dentistry

1 Which of the following is not a major area in which forensic dentistry plays a major role?
    a. Abuse recognition
    b. Mass disasters
    c. Identification of human remains
    d. Bite-mark recognition and case management
    e. Operative dentistry

2 Which of the following is not an area in which the dental assistant assumes responsibility in forensic dentistry?
    a. Maintaining complete and accurate patient records
    b. Evaluating abuse
    c. Observing evidence of abuse in patients

3 Which of the following is not likely to be considered a reason to suspect child abuse?
    a. Lacerations of the lip, frenum, or uvula
    b. Torn labial frenum of child learning to walk
    c. Untreated fractures of teeth
    d. Oral burns

4 Which of the following might suggest child abuse?
    1. Marks of belts, belt buckles, cords, or wires
    2. Bite and tooth marks on various areas of the body
    3. Bruises of assorted colors on dorsal aspect of legs and neck
    4. Bruises of a single color on the knees
    5. Lacerations on face and neck
    a. 1 and 3
    b. 2 and 4
    c. 1, 2, 3, and 4
    d. 1, 2, 3, and 5

In items 5-22, place an A for *True* and a B for *False* in the space provided for each statement.

_____ **5** Forensic dentistry relates only to criminal law.

_____ **6** Identification applies only to human remains.

_____ **7** Forensic dentistry is a recognized specialty of the American Dental Association.

_____ **8** No two people, including identical twins, have the same dentition.

_____ **9** Paul Revere made the first recorded dental identification in the United States.

_____ **10** The forensic anthropologist studies the science of human beings.

_____ **11** The Office of the Medical Examiner is responsible for coordinating the forensic team's investigation.

_____ **12** One of the largest mass disasters occurred at Waco, Texas.

_____ **13** Every state requires that all newly fabricated removable prostheses contain identifying marks.

_____ **14** Health professionals in all states are mandated by law to report suspected abuse.

_____ **15** Reporting suspected abuse may prevent additional suffering and possible death of an innocent person.

_____ **16** Failure to report child abuse may be considered a misdemeanor.

_____ **17** Tooth marks are recognized by the courts as proof of the assailant's identity.

_____ **18** Antemortem charting is completed before death.

_____ **19** Teeth missing postmortem were present after death.

_____ **20** Antemortem and postmortem records are compared for similarities.

_____ **21** Tooth imprints on a piece of cheese constituted the first use of bite-mark evidence in a court case.

_____ **22** An identification mark is sometimes placed on dental prostheses or appliances.

23 The forensic identification team includes which of the following?
1. Forensic odontologist
2. Medical examiner
3. Postmortem section
4. Radiography
5. Antemortem section
6. Comparison section
   a. 1, 2, 4, and 5
   b. 1, 3, 4, and 5
   c. 1, 3, 4, 5, and 6
   d. 2, 3, 4, 5, and 6

24 The process of comparison can begin when
   a. Antemortem records are complete
   b. Postmortem records are complete
   c. Antemortem and postmortem records are complete

25 Which of the following is *not* part of bite-mark protocol?
   a. Saliva samples
   b. Wound-pattern impressions
   c. Photographs of the victim
   d. Bite-mark patterns of the victim

Rationales

Forensic Dentistry

1 E Forensic odontology is the art and science of dentistry as it relates to civil and criminal law. It involves identification of human remains, mass disasters, bite- and tooth-mark recognition and case management, and child-abuse and battered-adult recognition.

2 B Dental assistants may observe evidence of child abuse in patients seen in the dental office and report it to the dentist, who is mandated by law to report it to the appropriate authority or agency.

3 B It is common for a child learning to walk to fall forward and tear a frenum. It is not likely, however, for lacerations in the posterior of the mouth to be caused by a fall. Untreated fractures of teeth indicate neglect, and oral burns are evidence of abuse.

4 D Bruises of various colors on dorsal areas of the body indicate a cause other than a normal fall. If the bruises are a single color, it means they occurred at one time, but if they range from bright blue to yellow to green, they occurred at various times. Lacerations on the neck are seldom self-inflicted. Bite marks and evidence of belt marks are indications of abuse.

5 B See item 1.

6 A In forensic odontology, identification applies only to human remains.

7 B This specialized area is not one of the eight recognized specialties of the American Dental Association. The American Board of Forensic Odontology certifies dentists who have demonstrated expertise in forensic odontology by examination as diplomates.

8 A According to genetic studies, there is no evidence that any two people have the same dentition.

9 A Early history indicates that Paul Revere identified the body of General Joseph Warren on the basis of a dental prosthesis that Revere had made for him.

10 A The age, race, and sex of decomposed bodies or skeletal remains can be determined by a forensic anthropologist who studies the science of human beings.

11 A The medical examiner in a geographic region is responsible for coordinating activities of identification.

12 B Many mass disasters have occurred throughout the world; however, the Waco, Texas, incident was not nearly the largest.

13 B Identification of a body through markings in a dental prosthesis is an excellent identification technique. However, not all states have made this a requirement.

14 A Each state requires health professionals to report suspected abuse. In most states, failure to report suspected abuse is a misdemeanor.

15 A To terminate continued abuse, intervention must occur. Reporting suspected abuse may save a life.

16 A See item 14.

17 A Clear plastic overlays can be used to trace tooth patterns from photographs (ratio 1 : 1) of the bite or tooth mark and the dentition of the suspect.

18 A The prefix *ante-* means *before*. Therefore, antemortem records refer to dental charts that were completed before death.

19 B Teeth missing postmortem were missing after death. They may have been lost during the trauma of death.

20 A Antemortem and postmortem records are compared to establish similarities of the oral conditions before and after death.

21 A History relates that tooth imprints left on a piece of cheese at the scene of a burglary in England were used to convict one of two suspects. This was the first use of bite-mark evidence in a court case.

22 A See item 13.

23 C All persons and groups listed are part of the forensic examination team except for the medical examiner, who coordinates the action of the team.

24 C Only when the antemortem and postmortem records are complete is it possible to compare both records to complete the identification of a body.

25 D It is not likely that the bite-mark patterns are from the victim; therefore, this option would not be considered. Saliva samples from the suspect and victim as well as wound-pattern impressions and photographs of the victim can be used for comparison.

To enhance your understanding of the material in this chapter refer to the illustrations in Chapter 38 of Finkbeiner/Johnson: *Mosby's Comprehensive Dental Assisting: A Clinical Approach.*

Dental Laboratory Procedures

The laboratory in a dental office presents an opportunity for an assistant to become acquainted with equipment not found in the dental treatment room. Many laboratory procedures are performed in a commercial laboratory, but basic tasks may be performed by an assistant within the office. Perhaps the most common of these tasks are pouring impressions, trimming diagnostic models, and constructing custom-made trays. Baseplates, mouth guards, copings, and even waxed patterns for investment and casting procedures may be done in the office. Accessibility to a commercial laboratory, cost-effectiveness, staff skills, and the personal interests of the dentist dictate the extent to which various laboratory duties may be delegated to the assistant.

RULES FOR SAFETY IN THE DENTAL LABORATORY ▬▬▬▬▬▬▬

I.   Do not smoke—many flammable agents are used in this area.

II.   Wear safety glasses when operating any rotary equipment, using the Bunsen burner, and chipping away plaster or stone from models.

III. Wear hair pulled back and secured.

IV. Do not wear hanging jewelry or clothing.

V. Do not lean over a Bunsen burner or a torch.

VI. If a handpiece with an engine belt is used, change the belt frequently to avoid unexpected breaks in the belt.

VII. Keep electrical cords out of areas where water is used.

VIII. Turn off lathes, handpieces, model trimmers, and other rotary devices when not in use.

IX. Use acceptable ventilation and exhaust systems when working with dental materials such as acrylic or when grinding on the lathe.

X. Follow OSHA guidelines for handling laboratory materials and substances.

INFECTION CONTROL IN THE DENTAL LABORATORY

I. In both commercial and office laboratories, infection control guidelines must meet OSHA requirements.

II. Transferring a patient case to a commercial laboratory involves the following:

A. Before dental materials are transferred to a commercial dental laboratory, they should be rinsed and disinfected (or sterilized, if appropriate). Materials include impressions, bite records, and preliminary denture setups.

B. A **laboratory prescription** or work authorization form must accompany all laboratory cases and should be placed in a plastic bag to avoid contamination.

C. After disinfection or sterilization the materials should be placed in a plastic bag and heat-sealed.

D. The infection-control protocol for transferring laboratory cases is listed (box).

III. Guidelines for preventing disease transmission in the general work and production areas include the following:

A. Clean and disinfect work benches daily.

B. Disinfect work pans as soon as possible after removing an appliance to ensure that the pans have been decontaminated before being used again.

C. Do not eat or drink at laboratory workstations.

D. Do not use the same pumice for new work and repair work. For repair work, premeasure pumice in small amounts and discard it after each use.

E. Discard pumice that is used for new work at least once a week.

> ### INFECTION-CONTROL PROTOCOL FOR TRANSFERRING LABORATORY CASES
>
> - Do not give wet impressions to an ungloved delivery person or technician.
> - Do not contaminate the delivery package; the laboratory staff may have to throw it away, which will increase laboratory costs.
> - Explain to the dental technicians the infection-control procedures that are followed in the office. Identify the types of infection control materials that are used.
> - To avoid cross-contamination, repeat the infection-control procedures each time the case is returned to the original laboratory or dental office for a try-in or an adjustment.

F. Wet pumice with a mixture of disinfectant and bacteriostatic soap. Do not use water alone.

G. Soak brush wheels and rag wheels in a disinfectant for 10 minutes and allow to air-dry overnight.

H. After pumice is used on a repair, disinfect the appliance for 10 minutes. These materials are surface disinfectants only, and when the material is cut or broken, the appliance must be disinfected again.

I. Use universal precautions, masks, glasses or face shield, and gloves when operating mechanical devices. Use dust-mist face masks in the laboratory; all face masks used in the dental laboratory should be approved by National Institute of Occupational Safety and Health.

J. Use an effective suction or vacuum system when an appliance is adjusted.

K. Keep disinfectant solutions readily available in the laboratory.

L. In states where denturism is legal, the denturist is responsible for following the same infection control procedures used in the dental treatment room regarding contact with patient secretions.

MATERIAL SAFETY DATA SHEETS

I. The OSHA Hazard Communication Standard, Title 29 Code of Federal Regulations 1910.1200, requires that all dental professionals take certain steps to comply with the standard. Compliance instruction includes a training program that involves a review of a list of hazardous chemicals, collection and maintenance of material safety data sheets (MSDS), and proper labeling of all chemicals on site.

II.   Hazardous chemicals are found in many areas of the dental laboratory.
  A.   Products that contain hazardous chemicals vary with each dental office and with the types of materials kept in each facility.
  B.   Product labels provide information about the substances contained in the product that are considered to be hazardous.
  C.   This form of labeling is required of the dental manufacturers for products containing a hazardous chemical.
  D.   The other source of information regarding hazardous chemicals is provided on the MSDS. All manufacturers of products containing hazardous chemicals are legally obligated to provide the MSDS for each product when it is shipped to the purchaser.
  E.   A simple form that lists all hazardous chemicals in the dental office can be developed and made available to all dental personnel. This form can be set up as shown:

Chemical	Product	Manufacturing company	Generic area	MSDS on file
Mercury	Tytin	Kerr/Sybron Mfg.	Amalgam	Yes

III. Precautions that should be taken to minimize the risk from hazardous chemicals to dental personnel include the following:
  A.   Handle the chemical properly in accordance with the manufacturer's or supplier's instructions.
  B.   Avoid skin contact.
  C.   Minimize the chemical vapors in the air.
  D.   Never leave bottles of flammable chemicals open or use them near open flames.
  E.   Do not smoke or consume food in areas where chemicals are used.
  F.   When appropriate, use protective eyewear and masks.
  G.   Dispose of all hazardous chemicals in accordance with MSDS instructions and applicable local, state, and federal regulations.

IV.   OSHA requires that MSDS include the following information:
  A.   Product or chemical identity used on the label
  B.   Manufacturer's or supplier's name and address
  C.   Chemical and common names of each hazardous ingredient

D.   Name, address, and phone number for hazard and emergency information
E.   Preparation or revision date of MSDS
F.   Physical and chemical characteristics (such as vapor pressure and flashpoint) of the hazardous chemical
G.   Physical hazards, including the potential for fire, explosion, and reactivity
H.   Known health hazards
I.   OSHA-permissible exposure limit (PEL), American Conference of Government Industrial Hygienists threshold limit value (ACGIH), threshold limit values (TLV), or other exposure limits
J.   Emergency and first-aid procedures
K.   Whether OSHA, National Toxicology Program, or International Agency for Research on Cancer lists the ingredient as a carcinogen
L.   Precautions for safe handling and use
M.   Required control measures, such as engineering controls, work practices, hygienic practices, and personal protective equipment
N.   Primary routes of entry
O.   Procedure for spills, leaks, and cleanup

V.   The Hazard Communication Standard requires labeling of all hazardous products.
  A.   Certain products regulated by the Food and Drug Administration are exempt from the Hazard Communication Standard.
  B.   Labels affixed to containers holding hazardous chemicals must not be removed for any reason.
  C.   Chemicals transferred from the original container to a smaller container for use in the dental office should be labeled with the original label information, including the following:
    1.   Identity of the hazardous chemical
    2.   Proper hazard warnings
    3.   Name and address of the manufacturer, importer, or other responsible party.

VI.   Dental office employers are required by OSHA to provide a written hazard communication program that includes specific information regarding meeting requirements for handling labeling and other forms of warning, MSDS, and employee information and training schedules.
  A.   Employers are required to provide employees with information and training on all hazardous chemicals found in the dental office at any given time.

B. Training regarding new substances must be provided.

C. Employees are entitled to know about the data reflected in the Hazard Communication Standard, work areas that contain hazardous chemicals, and location of the written information regarding the program, lists of chemicals, and MSDS.

D. The training session for employees should include the means to determine the following:

1. Presence of a hazardous chemical in the work area.
2. Physical and health hazards of chemicals.
3. How employees can protect themselves.
4. Specific details of the hazard communication program of that office

DENTAL LABORATORY EQUIPMENT

I. **Dental lathe**
   A. The dental lathe is used to polish dentures, crowns, bridges, inlays, and other prostheses.
   B. Most lathes come with a right and left chuck onto which a variety of attachments can be placed, such as rag or chamois wheels, brushes, and burs.
   C. A splash hood (with or without a light), shield, and some form of exhaust must be included to collect the debris created by the lathe.

II. **Bunsen burner**
   A. This is used to warm waxes and heat materials and solutions.
   B. It provides an adjustable flame.
   C. A small tripod may be needed to hold a crucible when a solution is warmed; this may be placed over the Bunsen burner.

III. **Alcohol lamp** (to provide a small flame)

IV. Air and gas outlets
   A. An air outlet is frequently used to dry impressions and other materials.
   B. A gas line is needed for the **gas torch** or Bunsen burner.
   C. A gas torch may be used in some offices to provide a hot flame for casting or soldering procedures.

V. **Vacuum machine**
   A. This is used to construct baseplates, **custom-made trays,** mouth guards, bruxism splints, temporary splints, and copings.
   B. It provides a heating element to warm the material to be used and a vacuum device that aids in adapting the material to a model.

C. An automatic vacuum machine is available.

VI. **Vacuum mixing and investing machine** (for mixing stone, plaster, and **investment** materials under a vacuum to give a smooth, dense finished product).

VII. **Model trimmer**
   A. Its primary use is for trimming casts for both diagnostic and working models.
   B. Elaborate trimmers provide calibrated tables to permit trimming models at desired angles.

VIII. Small **vibrator**
   A. This is used for pouring impressions.
   B. Larger units can be purchased for heavier use.

IX. **Dental engine**
   A. A high-speed engine with a triple section arm is a standard version; a compact engine with a single arm is also available.
   B. It is used for various extraoral duties, including cutting, trimming, and polishing.

X. Plaster/**gypsum bins** and laboratory benches
   A. Plaster storage bins ensure a dry storage area for all gypsum products.
   B. Laboratory benches come in different heights to accommodate standing, sitting, and wheelchairs and may be installed with a variety of different types of countertops.

XI. Exhaust system (central or countertop)

XII. **Articulator**
   A. It is used to articulate models for fixed prosthodontics, analyze a case, or mount denture setups for specialized relationships.
   B. A plain articulator allows for basic movements of opening and closing and for lateral movement.
   C. A complex articulator allows the dentist to achieve special condylar movement and more precise alignment of the arches.

XIII. **Sandblaster**
   A. This provides a current of air to spray sand at a high velocity to etch or clean metal or hard surfaces.
   B. It is used in a dental laboratory with a silica medium to clean castings or etch the internal surface of a casting to aid in the identification of undercuts.

XIV. Waxing unit (to melt the wax to a specific temperature and maintain the molten wax in this state)

XV. **Casting machine**
   A. This is used in offices in which the dentists or laboratory technicians frequently make their own castings.
   B. It includes an assortment of sprue bases, ring flasks, and tongs.

C. Safety regulations require that the casting machine be embedded in a well so that it is not on the counter.

D. An automatic casting machine and **casting oven** eliminate the manual steps required in the centrifugal casting machine.

XVI. Assorted knives and spatulas

A. Laboratory spatulas may be flexible or rigid depending on the materials to be mixed.

B. Wax spatulas, including the commonly used #7 spatula, are used universally in waxing patterns and in many repairs.

C. Carvers are also widely used in the laboratory to carve wax and prepare other devices.

XVII. Heavy-duty shears or nippers (to cut bulky materials)

XVIII. Rubber bowl

A. This is used for many functions, including mixing plaster, alginate, and a variety of other materials.

B. Flexible bowls come in various sizes.

DIAGNOSTIC MODELS

I. **Diagnostic models** are replicas of a patient's mouth that are studied to determine a diagnosis.

II. A set of diagnostic models has two basic parts:

A. The **anatomic portion,** which includes all of the dental arch and alveolar processes

B. The **art portion,** which provides a **base** for the models

III. Constructing a set of diagnostic models includes the following steps:

A. Assembling the armamentarium

B. Mixing the plaster and/or stone

C. Pouring the impression

D. Pouring the bases

E. Removing the impression from the models

F. Trimming the models

G. Finishing the models

H. Labeling the models

IV. The purposes of diagnostic models are listed (box at top of next column).

CONSTRUCTION OF DIAGNOSTIC MODELS

I. Before a set of diagnostic models can be produced, an alginate impression of the maxillary and mandibular arches must be obtained.

A. The impressions are a negative reproduction of the intraoral anatomy.

B. The set of diagnostic models is a positive reproduction.

C. Diagnostic models are typically poured in plaster, but stone may be used for the anatomic portion to increase strength.

PURPOSES OF DIAGNOSTIC MODELS

1. Record the occlusal relationship of both dental arches in centric relation for present and future treatment
2. Provide three-dimensional study of the relationship of the alveolar processes
3. Allow study of tooth and occlusal relationships from the lingual aspect
4. Allow study of tooth positioning, dental arch form, and occlusal relationships with the patient not present
5. Use as teaching aids in case presentations and patient education
6. Demonstrate changes that occur during and after treatment
7. Provide reproduction of an actual arch for use in constructing auxiliary devices, such as custom-made trays and copings
8. Function as legal records for insurance, malpractice suits, and forensic purposes
9. Study asymmetries in the dental arches

ARMAMENTARIUM FOR POURING AN IMPRESSION

Model plaster or snow white plaster	Plaster spatula
	Vibrator
White stone or cast stone (optional)	Base formers (optional)
	#7 wax spatula
Scale (to weigh powder)	Maxillary and mandibular alginate impression
Graduated cylinder (100 ml)	
	Waxed paper or glass slab
Rubber bowls	

D. The impressions are taken, rinsed, sprayed with a disinfectant, wrapped in a paper towel, and placed in a plastic bag for 15 minutes.

II. The armamentarium for pouring an impression is listed (box above).

A. The impressions are rinsed and air dried with compressed air before pouring.

B. The anatomic portions of the models are poured in white rapid stone; the base portions are poured in white model plaster in the following proportions:

1. Dental stone: 30 ml of water to 100 g of powder

2. Model plaster: 50 ml of water to 100 g of powder

C. Prepare a mix of white stone using the proper water-to-powder ratio; approximately 200 g of dental stone powder and 60 ml of water is sufficient to pour the anatomic portion of both impressions.

D. When the mix is smooth and homogeneous, hold the bowl firmly on the vibrator until all the bubbles come to the surface.

III. The impression can be poured separately from the base.

A. Place the mandibular impression on the vibrator.

B. Using the #7 spatula, place a small amount of stone at one heel and allow the material to flow slowly toward the anterior of the arch.

C. Vibrate the first portion of stone in the impression by tilting the tray until the stone flows to the heel on the opposite side; as the material flows to the opposite side, allow it to flow into all of the embrasures.

D. Continue adding small increments to cover all occlusal surfaces; this helps eliminate voids and bubbles on the teeth of the model.

E. More stone can then be added with the plaster spatula until the impression is filled to the top.

F. Place the impression on the vibrator intermittently to prevent possible overflow onto the outside of the impression.

G. Do not try to smooth the surface; leave it rough for greater attachment to the base.

H. Set the filled mandibular impression out of the way of the vibrator to prevent movement in the poured stone.

I. Pour the maxillary arch in the same manner; begin in the tuberosity area and continue, making certain the palate is thoroughly covered.

IV. The base of an impression becomes the art portion of the model.

A. Prepare a mix of model plaster using the proper water-to-powder ratio; usually a separate mix of plaster is needed to fill each model base former. In most cases, 250 g of model plaster powder and 125 ml of water provides a large enough mix to fill a base former or provide an adequate mass to create a base. For a firmer mass, use less water.

B. Spatulate and vibrate the plaster mix until it is free of bubbles and lumps.

C. When the mix is smooth and homogeneous, hold the bowl firmly on the vibrator until all the bubbles come to the surface.

D. Place the base former on the vibrator and pour from the rubber bowl slowly and directly into the base former so that bubbles rise to the surface.

E. Immediately after the model former is filled, invert the stone-filled impressions onto the freshly poured plaster surfaces.

F. Gently work the stone-filled impressions slightly down into the plaster of the base former. A continuous union between the stone and the plaster must be formed; avoid embedding the tray in the plaster mass.

G. Center the impression over the plaster base former and position it on the plaster base so that the occlusal plane will be parallel to the bottom of the base in the final model.

H. Fill in voids at the posterior to ensure that the posterior areas, the heels of the mandibular, and the tuberosity areas of the maxillary model are well supported by plaster.

I. Smooth the open tongue space.

J. Repeat this process for the opposing impression.

K. Allow the poured models to remain undisturbed until the plaster and stone are hard.

V. An alternative method for pouring a base is accomplished without the use of a former.

A. Prepare the mix; spatulate and vibrate the plaster.

B. Form a mound of the plaster on waxed paper or a large glass slab. The shape of the mass should resemble the shape of the impression tray—wider at the posterior and narrower at the anterior.

C. Gently place the stone-filled impression onto this mass, forming a continuous union between the stone and plaster. Pay special attention to the posterior, heels, tuberosity, and tongue areas.

D. Center the impression in the mass and position it so that the occlusal plane is parallel to the slab or countertop, making certain not to embed the tray in the base plaster.

E. Smooth the outer edges of the plaster base, leaving not more than 1 inch of plaster around the outer edge of the tray.

F. Allow the model to remain undisturbed until the plaster or stone is hard.

VI. After the gypsum material has set, the impression can be removed from the model.

A. Gently lift the impression from the model, using a laboratory knife to carefully break any undercuts and push up on the impression, dislodging it from the stone model.

B. Do not force the impression—teeth can be fractured during this process.

C. If the impression is not removed in a timely manner, syneresis will occur in the alginate impression. This makes it more difficult to remove the dried impression from the model and thus creates a potential for fracture of the teeth as the impression is removed.

D. Once the models have been separated, the alginate impression material can be discarded.

E. The trays are cleaned, sterilized, and returned to the storage area for future use.

F. The criteria for poured models are listed (box below).

VII. Diagnostic models are trimmed to create symmetry and **parallelism** in the bases.

A. Several methods are used to trim models.

B. Regardless of the technique that is used, the maxillary model is trimmed first, and the mandibular model is trimmed in occlusion with the maxillary model to meet the criteria listed (box at top of next column).

C. Assemble the armamentarium listed (box at bottom of next column).

D. Figs. 28-1 through 28-3 illustrate the procedure for one method of model trimming.

E. Remove any bubbles or imperfections with a #7 wax spatula.

F. Type labels for both models; include the patient's name, age at the time of the impression in years and months (10-2 indicates 10

CRITERIA FOR POURED MODELS

1. All plaster and stone surfaces must be free of voids and bubbles.
2. The union between the stone in the anatomic portion of the cast (dental arch and alveolar process) and the art portion (plaster base) should be continuous and free of voids.
3. The anatomic portion must be centered on the plaster base to provide adequate plaster on all sides for proper trimming.
4. The occlusal plane of the dental arch should be parallel to the bottom of the rapid stone base.
5. The base must be thick enough to provide adequate plaster for trimming the casts to the proper height.
6. The anatomic portion must have sufficient vestibular and posterior extension to allow for proper depth of model trimming.
7. The tongue area on the mandibular model should be free of excess plaster or stone.

CRITERIA FOR TRIMMED DIAGNOSTIC MODELS

1. The backs of the models must be located posterior to the maxillary tuberosity and posterior to the most posterior mandibular tooth.
2. The backs of the maxillary and mandibular models must be in the same plane.
3. When articulated in occlusion, the backs of the models should sit flush on a flat surface with no movement of the occlusion.
4. The bases of the maxillary and mandibular models should be parallel to each other.
5. All of the angles should be symmetric from side to side.
6. All of the trimmed sides opposite each other should be the same height.
7. The art portion of the maxillary model should be one third the total height of the model.
8. When articulated together, the models should be double the height of the maxillary model when the maxillary occlusal plane is parallel to a flat surface.
9. The occlusal plane should be between 0 and 5 degrees to the bases.
10. The occlusal plane should be centered in the total height of the model.
11. The midline of the maxillary model should be established at the posterior two thirds of maxillary palatal raphe.
12. Flat cuts and angles should be symmetric with the midline.
13. Vertical cut lines should be parallel to each other and at a 90-degree angle to the base.
14. Sides should be trimmed to the greatest depth of the vestibule without destruction of anatomic structure.
15. Models should be finished with the following:
    Smooth sides and bases
    Bubbles and voids removed or filled
    Sharp line angles
    Smooth tongue space
16. Type labels for both models; include the patient's name and age and the date of the impression.

ARMAMENTARIUM FOR TRIMMING DIAGNOSTIC MODELS

Model trimmer	Miter square or **angle**
Plastic protractor	**former**
Flexible millimeter ruler	Laboratory knife
Pencils (graphite and	#7 wax spatula
colored)	Wet-and-dry sandpaper
Dividers	

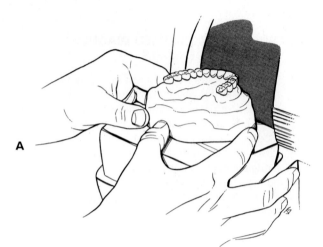

A,

Fig. 28-1 **A,** The base of the maxillary model is placed on the table of the model trimmer. **B,** The water is turned on to a moderate volume. The sides of the model are pressed onto the blade and trimmed until smooth. The base is also trimmed until smooth. **C,** The posterior two thirds of the maxillary midline is marked with a colored pencil. A protractor is used to draw a line for the posterior of the upper model at a 90-degree angle to the midline. **D,** If the second or third molars are not present, the assistant moves anterior to the most aligned teeth and establishes a measurement that would extend distal to the location where the normal anatomy would have existed. **E,** To ensure that there is enough space on the posterior, articulate the models together. *Continued*

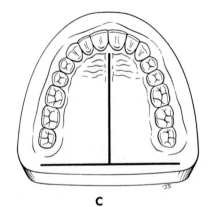

B,

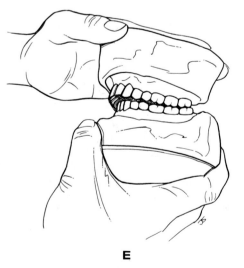

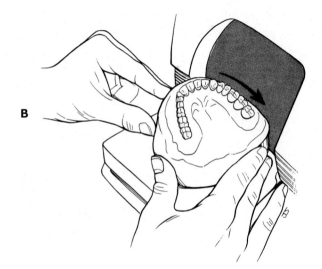

C

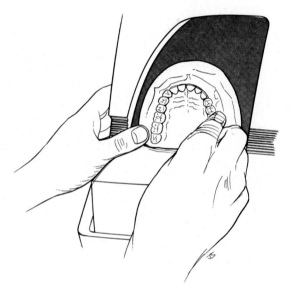

D

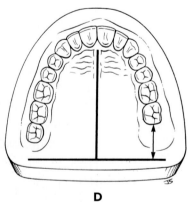

E

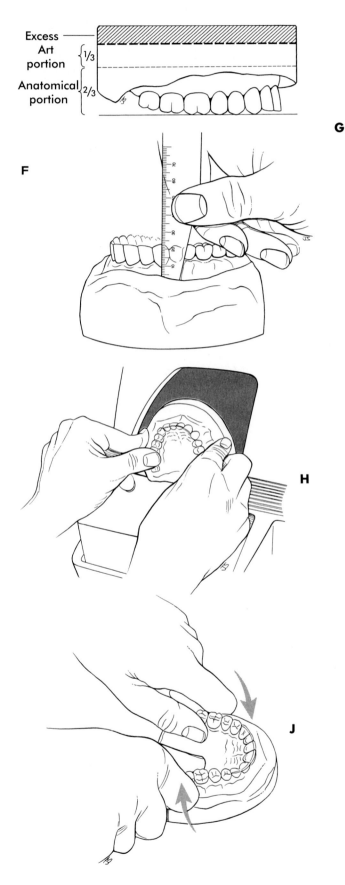

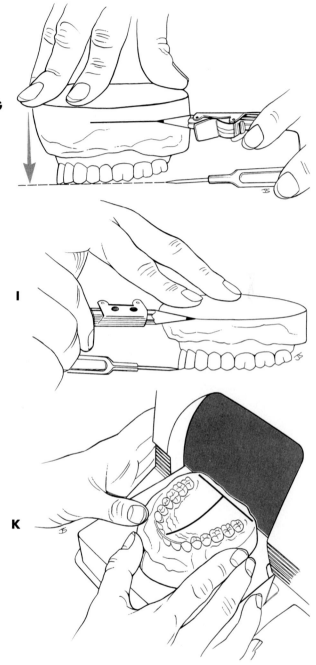

Fig. 28-1 cont'd   F, A millimeter ruler is placed into the mucolabial fold to the cusp tip of the cuspid on both sides, and the height is determined. **G,** The model is placed on a flat surface and rocked forward toward the central incisors; a line is drawn with the dividers around the base of the model. **H,** The base of the model is trimmed down to the pencil line. **I,** The height of the model is assessed by placing it on the lab bench, rocking it forward, and measuring the height with the dividers. **J,** Bevels on the base are assessed by placing the base on the lab bench and rocking it laterally. **K,** The base surface of the maxillary model is placed on the model trimmer table and trimmed to the pencil line that was drawn perpendicular to the palatal midline. *Continued*

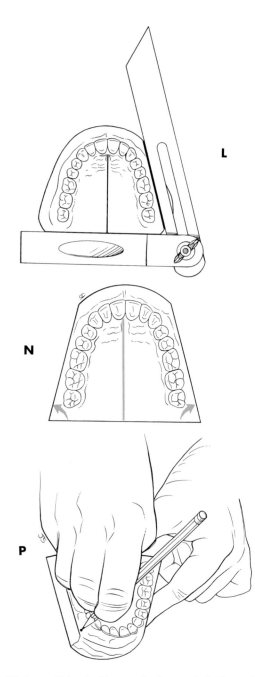

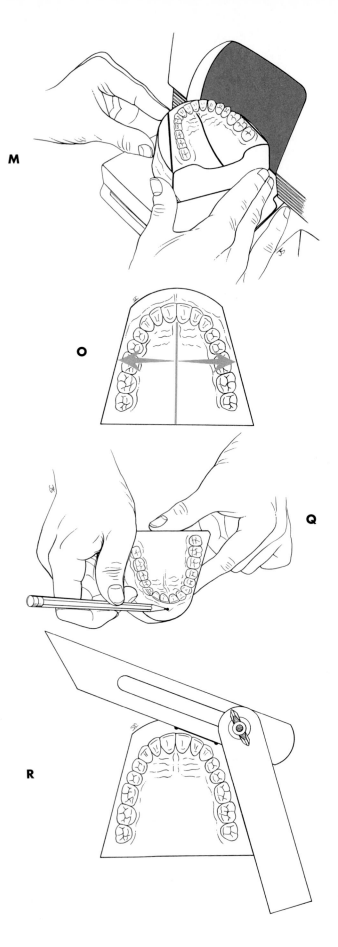

Fig. 28-1 cont'd **L,** The angle former is laid parallel to the buccal plane of one side and marked with a line along the greatest depth of the buccal vestibule, which is approximately 5 mm from the buccal surface of the teeth. The angle former is turned over to the opposite side and the side of the model is marked in the same manner. **M,** The model base is placed on the table and trimmed to the pencil lines on both sides. **N,** Both trimmed sides should be at the same angle to the back of the model. **O,** The sides of the model should be an equal distance away from the palatal midline. **P,** The maxillary model is marked at the deepest point of the buccal vestibule at the most normally positioned cuspid. **Q,** The midline of the maxillary cast is marked on the anterior vestibule at about 5 mm from the labial of the central incisors. **R,** Using the angle former a line is drawn from the cuspid mark to the midline and then the same line is drawn on the opposite side. *Continued*

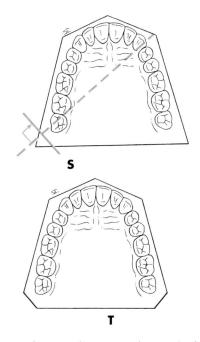

S

T

Fig. 28-1 cont'd S, A line at 90 degrees is drawn to a bi-sector of the cuspid angle of the side and front cuts. This is done on both sides and is trimmed to the pencil line. **T,** The heel cuts should be symmetric in length from side to side (3/8 inch to 5/8 inch wide) and at the same angle to the back.

years, 2 months), and the date of the impression (next to the patient's age).

VIII.   Some models require modifications in trimming, such as in those with missing teeth, severe malocclusion, or an asymmetric arch.

    A. Keep in mind the criteria for acceptable models and attempt to meet as many of them as possible.

    B. When a crossbite or other types of malocclusion are present, always articulate the models together to anticipate the need to extend a buccal or anterior cut line.

CONSTRUCTION OF CUSTOM-MADE ACRYLIC TRAYS

I.   The basic goal is to fabricate a tray that will accurately fit the patient's dental arches regardless of their configuration.

II.   Custom-made trays have several advantages (box at top of next column).

III.   Trays are constructed for the specific types of treatment, as follows:

    A. *Quadrant trays* are used for a final impression for a single crown, inlay, or small fixed bridge.

ADVANTAGES OF CUSTOM-MADE TRAYS

Improved accuracy in the impression ensures a better fit of the tray.

Uniform thickness of the impression between the tissues and tray walls eliminates a potential for voids.

Use of stops prevents the tray from resting on occlusal or incisal surfaces and consequently prevents *burn-through* on dentulous trays.

Less impression material is required to fill a custom-made tray than a ready-made tray.

Tray design can be altered to compensate for missing teeth, unusual arch form, tori, or small mouth openings.

ARMAMENTARIUM FOR CONSTRUCTING CUSTOM-MADE TRAYS

Study models	Unwaxed cup
Acrylic powder and liquid	Nonasbestos casting liner or baseplate wax
Devices for measuring powder and liquid	Tongue blade
Rubber bowl (with water)	Bunsen burner
Scissors	Wooden roller and board
Colored pencil	Lubricant

    B. *Full-arch trays* are used for a final impression for single or multiple crowns, inlays, bridges, or partial dentures.

    C. *Full-arch edentulous trays* are used for final impressions for a complete denture.

    D. *Segment trays* may be used for final impressions for anterior crowns, bridges, or laminates.

IV.   Construction of a custom-made acrylic tray involves the following steps:

    A. Preparing the model

    B. Adapting the spacer

    C. Mixing the material

    D. Adapting the material to the spacer

    E. Removing the tray from the model

    F. Finishing the tray

V.   The armamentarium for constructing custom-made trays is listed (box above).

VI.   Preparing the model

    A. With a colored or indelible pencil, mark the model for the location of the periphery of the tray.

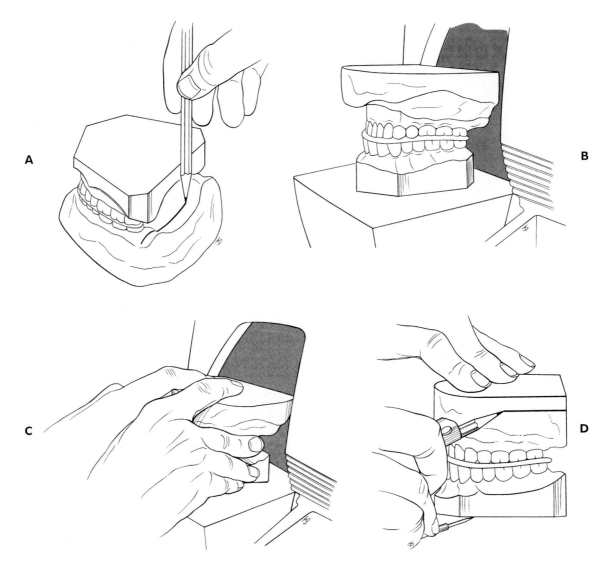

Fig. 28-2 **A,** The mandibular cast is marked parallel to the maxillary cast. **B,** The casts are occluded and the wax bite is placed. **C,** With the maxillary model on the bottom, the back of the mandibular model is trimmed just short of the line drawn on the mandibular model. **D,** With the top of the maxillary model flat on the bench and the models articulated, a line twice the height of the maxillary model is drawn. *Continued.*

B. On dentulous models, the mark should be 2 to 3 mm below the cervical margin of the tooth on the buccal and lingual sides.

C. On edentulous mandibular models, the line should be drawn at the greatest depth of the vestibule on the buccal side, extending posterior to the retromolar area, and continuing on the lingual side at the same depth as the buccal.

D. On edentulous maxillary models, the line should be drawn at the greatest depth of the vestibule on the buccal side; on the posterior side the line should connect the hamular notch to the fovea.

E. Soak the model for 5 minutes.

VII. Adapting the spacer

A. The **spacer** is used to control the amount of impression material that will ultimately occupy the space between the teeth and the tray walls. It acts as a guide for adapting the acrylic to the model.

B. The amount of space between the tray and teeth is determined by the thickness of the material used as a spacer.

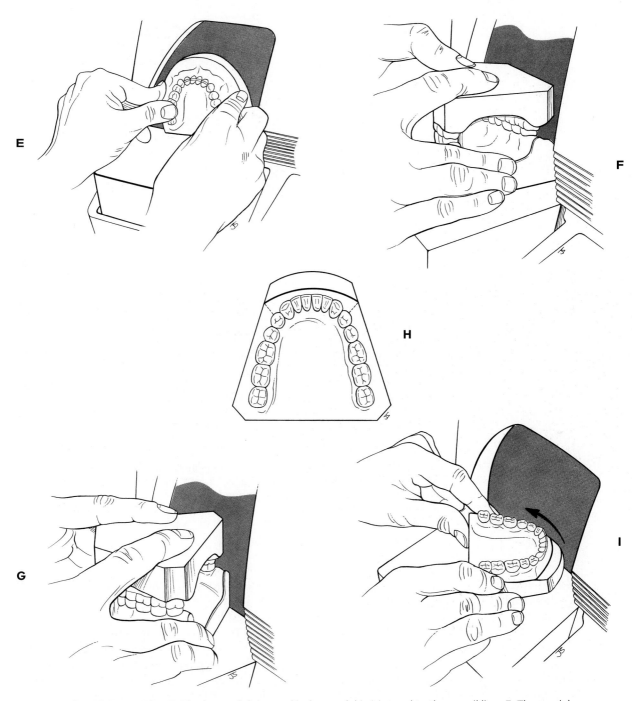

Fig. 28-2 cont'd   E, The base of the mandibular model is trimmed to the pencil line. **F,** The models are articulated together again; the back and then the sides are trimmed flush with the maxillary model. **G,** The heels of the mandibular cast are trimmed even with the maxillary cast. **H,** The models are separated, and an arc is marked on the mandibular model at the deepest point of the vestibule, from the midline of the first premolar to the midline of the opposite premolar. **I,** The mandibular model is trimmed in an arc.

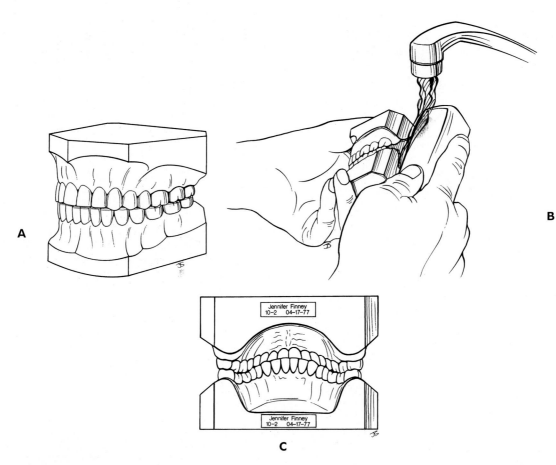

Fig. 28-3 **A,** The top of the maxillary model and the base of the mandibular model are trimmed as needed to establish an accurate final height. The occlusal plane should be centered between both models. **B,** After a laboratory knife is used to trim the tongue space flat and smooth, all flat surfaces are smoothed under running water with a block wrapped in wet-and-dry sandpaper. Keep all line angles sharp and parallel. **C,** Labels are typed for both models.

C. A well-adapted spacer should meet the following criteria:
 1. Provide uniform thickness of the spacer material
 2. Extend to the site of the tray periphery marked on the model
 3. Be contoured to compensate for malalignment of teeth or structures, such as a torus
 4. Be designed to eliminate potential undercuts

VIII. Constructing the custom tray
 A. A self-curing or heat activated acrylic should be used to construct the tray.
 B. A disposable nonwaxed cup should be used for mixing.

IX. The criteria for a clinically acceptable custom-made acrylic tray are listed (box on page 479).

X. Special considerations
 A. Sometimes a model on which an acrylic tray is to be constructed has special anomalies.
 B. Teeth may be missing or rotated, or a torus may be present, making it necessary to block out undercuts with the spacer material.

CONSTRUCTION OF MOUTH-GUARDS

I. A **mouth guard** is made of resilient plastic that is prepared directly from a cast of the patient's mouth.

II. A mouth guard can prevent many injuries during contact sports; its functions are listed (box on page 479).

III. Several options are available to the patient:
 A. Purchase a preformed mouth guard at a

CRITERIA FOR A CLINICALLY ACCEPTABLE CUSTOM-MADE ACRYLIC TRAY

- It is free from voids and wrinkles.
- It has uniform thickness.
- Its peripheral borders are smooth and even.
- It is free from lateral rocking.
- Stops are well defined.
- The dentulous tray extends 2 to 3 mm below the cervical border.
- The border of the edentulous tray extends to the greatest depth of the vestibule.
- The full-arch tray extends posterior to the maxillary tuberosity or the retromolar pad.
- A tray with full palatal coverage does not extend distal to the fovea area.
- Handles are at least ½ inch but no more than ¾ inch long and are placed at an angle to provide easy removal from the mouth.
- Stops are marked on the exterior.
- The interior surface is free from debris.

ARMAMENTARIUM FOR CONSTRUCTING A CUSTOM-MADE MOUTH GUARD

Maxillary model of patient's mouth
Laboratory engine
Large acrylic/cutting bur
Vacuum machine
Mouth-guard material
Alcohol torch
Laboratory knife or scalpel
Laboratory shears
Bowl of water
Finishing bur
Chamois wheel

CRITERIA FOR A CLINICALLY ACCEPTABLE MOUTH GUARD

Closely adapted to anatomic structures
Uniform thickness throughout
Smooth peripheral borders
Extends to the maxillary tuberosity
Does not impinge on vestibular or gingival tissue
Does not impinge on frena

FUNCTIONS OF A MOUTH GUARD

1. Prevents tooth injury by absorbing and deflecting blows to the teeth.
2. Prevents jaw fractures by creating a cushion between the teeth during the impact of a blow.
3. Shields the lips, tongue, and gingival tissues from laceration.
4. Reduces potential temporomandibular joint disorders by cushioning the lower jaw.
5. Prevents potential concussions by absorbing the shock of a blow to the mandible.

PROCEDURE FOR REPAIRING A FRACTURED DENTURE

1. Clean debris and food from the broken edges.
2. Hold the two parts together with the use of sticky wax and a toothpick or old bur.
3. Lightly lubricate the inner surface of the denture and gently vibrate plaster into this area.
4. Remove the denture from the cast and cut away acrylic resin from each side of the fracture.
5. Replace the denture onto the cast.
6. Paint the edges of the fracture with acrylic resin monomer and mix the repair acrylic resin.
7. Flow the acrylic into the cutaway space until the area is overfilled. The extra material will be needed to allow for finishing.
8. When the repair resin has been polymerized, excess material can be removed with large acrylic burs and finished as a denture base.
9. The plaster is removed and the inner surface finished.
10. The denture is polished and disinfected.

pharmacy or sports store and follow the directions for adapting it to the mouth.
  B. Have the dentist adapt a preformed mouth guard to the patient's mouth.
  C. Have the dentist prepare a custom-made mouth guard, which is adapted to a model made from an impression of the patient's mouth.
IV. The armamentarium for constructing a custom-made mouth guard is listed (box at the top of next column).
V. The criteria for a clinically acceptable mouth guard are listed (middle box in next column).

DENTURE REPAIR

I.   If the fracture is minor or a single acrylic tooth has been lost or broken, repair can be accomplished at the dental office.

II. The use of cold-curing resin simplifies the repair process.

III. The procedure for repairing a fractured denture is listed (box on page 479).

Questions

Laboratory Procedures

In items 1-3, match the term in column B with the appropriate description in column A.

	Column A	Column B
_____	**1** May be used with a rag wheel to polish a denture	a. Alcohol lamp
_____	**2** May be belt and pulley	b. Dental lathe
_____	**3** Available in quadrant, full-arch, or condylar styles	c. Gas torch
		d. Articulator
		e. Dental engine

In items 4-6, match the term in column B with the appropriate description in column A.

	Column A	Column B
_____	**4** Heats a ring from which a metal crown can be made	a. Dental lathe
_____	**5** Provides a source of heat to melt metal for a casting	b. Dental engine
		c. Casting machine
		d. Casting oven
_____	**6** A source of energy for a handpiece and various rotary instruments	e. Gas torch

Select the term from column B that best defines the cut or angle described in each statement in Column A.

	Column A	Column B
_____	**7** Anterior of mandibular model	a. Symmetric
_____	**8** Backs of articulated models	b. Parallel
_____	**9** Angle of the heels of maxillary model	c. Curved
_____	**10** Angle of the sides of both models	
_____	**11** Anterior cuts of maxillary model	

The following refers to items 12-14: A set of models is trimmed for a patient. The length of the anatomic portion from the tip of the cuspid to the base of the mucolabial fold is 25 mm on the right side and 23 mm on the left side.

12 The total height of the maxillary model will be
a. 24 mm
b. 32 mm
c. 36 mm
d. 42 mm

13 The art portion of the maxillary model will be
a. 8 mm
b. 12 mm
c. 24 mm
d. 36 mm

14 When articulated, the total height of the finished models will be
a. 48 mm
b. 64 mm
c. 72 mm
d. 84 mm

15 All of the following statements are true about a custom-made acrylic tray *except*
a. It may be made with chemically cured material.
b. Exothermic heat may be created during construction.
c. It decreases the need for additional impression material.
d. It increases the need for additional impression material.

16 After mixing the monomer and polymer together, acrylic is ready to be used
a. When the material is shiny
b. When the material loses its gloss
c. When a spatula cuts through the center of mass and the mass does not flow back together
d. When the material first becomes tacky
e. B and C

17 The spacer for a dentulous custom-made tray should
1. Have stop openings
2. Be made of nonasbestos material
3. Easily adapt to the model
4. Create space for impression material
5. Help establish a more accurate tray fit
a. 1 and 2
b. 1, 2, and 4
c. 3, 4, and 5
d. 1, 2, 3, 4, and 5

18 The setting time for dental plaster is decreased by using
1. Cold water
2. Warm water
3. Less water
4. Distilled water
a. 1 and 3
b. 2 and 3
c. 2 and 4
d. 4 only

19 Which of the following is *not* a safety rule that should be practiced when working in the laboratory?
a. Hair should be pulled back and secured.
b. Safety glasses must be worn when operating rotary devices.
c. Food may be eaten as long as it is kept away from contaminated objects.
d. Ventilation and exhaust systems should be used when working with acrylic materials.

20 Which of the following steps should be taken to prevent the transmission of disease from the laboratory to the office?
1. Rag wheels should be soaked in disinfectant.

2. An effective vacuum system should be used for grinding an appliance.
3. Pumice with a disinfectant mixture and water may be reused.
4. Appliances should be disinfected for at least 10 minutes.
5. Work pans do not need to be disinfected.
   a. 1 and 2
   b. 1 and 3
   c. 1, 2, and 4
   d. 2, 3, and 5

21 Which of the following is *not* a common duty a dental assistant might perform in the laboratory in the dental office?
   a. Construct copings
   b. Cast metal restorations
   c. Write the laboratory prescription
   d. Sign the laboratory prescription

22 Information required by OSHA to appear on MSDS include all of the following *except*
   a. Preparer of MSDS
   b. Physical hazards of substances
   c. Telephone number to call to find out if hazard is carcinogenic
   d. Procedure for spill and directions for cleanup

23 To promote the flow of dental stone into the impression,
   1. A large bulk of stone is placed into the impression
   2. The tray is placed firmly on the vibrator
   3. Small increments of the mix are placed into the impression
   a. 1 only
   b. 1 and 2
   c. 2 and 3
   d. 1, 2, and 3

24 A mouth guard worn during contact sports participation can do all of the following *except*
   a. Prevent tooth injury by absorbing and deflecting blows to the teeth
   b. Prevent jaw fractures by creating a cushion between the teeth during the impact of the blow
   c. Reduce potential temporomandibular joint disorders by cushioning the upper jaw
   d. Prevent potential concussions by absorbing the shock of a blow to the mandible

25 Buccal cuts on a maxillary model should begin at the
   a. Midline of the arch
   b. Center of the canine
   c. Distal of the canine
   d. Center of the first premolar
   e. Distal of the first premolar

Rationales

Laboratory Procedures

1 B A dental lathe is a common piece of laboratory equipment that is used to polish dentures, crowns, bridges, and inlays. Most lathes come with a left and right chuck onto which a variety of attachments can be placed, such as rag or chamois wheels, brushes, and burs.

2 E Dental engines constitute a major category of laboratory equipment. A high-speed engine with a single arm or a belt and pulley may be used for various extraoral functions. This device provides the energy to activate a handpiece used for extraoral laboratory work.

3 D Articulators are used to articulate models for fixed prosthodontics, analyze a case, or mount denture set-ups for specialized relationships. Styles vary from a plain articulator to complex condylar styles with more precise alignment of the arches.

4 D A casting oven is an insulated device that reaches temperatures compatible with various types of molten metals. This oven may be a separate unit or designed in conjunction with a casting machine.

5 E A gas torch that combines air and gas to reach temperatures sufficient to melt metal is used in conjunction with a casting machine and oven.

6 B See item 2.

7 C An arc is cut on the anterior portion of the mandibular model that extends from the midline of the first premolar to the midline of the opposite premolar. This cut differs from the anterior cut on the maxillary model.

8 B When articulated, the backs of the maxillary and mandibular models should be flush or parallel with each other when the backs are placed on a flat surface.

9 A The angle of each cut should be symmetric with the same cut on the opposite side of the model.

10 A See item 9.

11 A See item 9.

12 C The total height of a model is divided into two parts: the anatomic portion, which is two thirds the total height, and the art portion, which is one third the total height. In this problem the average between the right and left anatomic portion of the model is 24 mm. Therefore, 24 mm is two thirds the total model height. The art portion will be 12 mm. Combined, the total height of the maxillary model will be 36 mm.

13 B See item 12.

14 C If each model is 36 mm high, then when articulated, the models will be 72 mm high.

15 D A custom-made acrylic tray is commonly made with a chemically cured material that produces heat during the curing process. A custom-made tray is designed to fit a particular patient's mouth and adapt closely to anatomic structures, thus reducing the amount of impression material needed.

16 E When the monomer and polymer are mixed, the material becomes shiny and flows. As the material begins to set, the gloss is lost and the material becomes firmer, so that when it is cut through the midline of the mass, it will not flow back together.

17 D All the responses are correct. A spacer allows for the creation of space into which impression material can be placed. The spacer material may be a nonasbestos liner or wax that can easily be adapted to the working cast. When small openings are placed in the spacer material, the acrylic can make contact with the tooth on the model. This enables the operator to firmly seat the tray in place when the impression is taken, thus ensuring a more accurate tray fit.

18 B An increase in water temperature decreases the setting time of a gypsum product. An increase in the amount of the water increases the setting time, whereas less water decreases the time.

19 C Safety rules that apply to working in the dental laboratory include the following:
- Do not smoke.
- Wear safety glasses.
- Pull back and secure hair.
- Do not wear hanging jewelry or clothing.
- Do not lean over a Bunsen burner or torch.
- Change engine belts frequently, if used.
- Keep electrical cords out of areas where water is used.
- Turn off lathes, handpieces, model trimmers, and other rotary devices when not in use.
- Use acceptable ventilation and exhaust systems.
- Follow OSHA guidelines for handling materials and substances.
- Do not eat in a treatment or patient work area.

20 C General guidelines for infection control in the dental laboratory/production area include the following:
- Clean and disinfect workbenches daily.
- Disinfect work pans as soon as possible after removing an appliance to ensure that they have been decontaminated before being used again.
- Do not eat or drink at laboratory workstations.
- Do not use the same pumice for new work and repair work. For repair work, premeasure pumice in small amounts and discard it after each use.
- Discard pumice that is used for new work at least once a week.
- Soak brush wheels and rag wheels in disinfectant for 10 minutes and allow to air-dry overnight.
- After pumice is used on a repair, disinfect the appliance for 10 minutes. The disinfectants are surface disinfectants only, and when the material is cut or broken, the appliance must be disinfected again.

21 D Legally, the dentist's signature or a signature stamp (preapproved by the laboratory) must be used on a laboratory requisition when applicable.

22 C MSDS are required to be provided by the manufacturers/suppliers of hazardous chemicals. It is the manufacturer's responsibility to provide accurate and proper information and for the employer to ensure that the information on the sheet is complete. The responses include only three of the criteria required of an MSDS. However, no telephone number is provided on the sheet to call to find out if the substance is carcinogenic.

23 C An impression is placed on a vibrator, and small increments of the dental stone are poured into the impression at the same site until all anatomic areas are well covered. This technique ensures that air is forced out of the impression. Small additions of stone prevent bubbles and voids.

24 D Mouth guards may prevent oral lacerations, tooth injury, jaw fractures, and temporomandibular joint trauma but not potential concussion.

25 B The buccal or side cuts of a maxillary model begin at the center of the canine and continue posteriorly. This cut generally aligns near the buccal frenum.

To enhance your understanding of the material in this chapter refer to the illustrations in Chapter 40 of Finkbeiner/Johnson: *Mosby's Comprehensive Dental Assisting: A Clinical Approach.*

Common Medical/Dental Abbreviations

A amp
@ at
āā of each (F. ana)
a.c. before meals (L., *ante cibum*)
ad Latin preposition, -to, up to
a.d. alternating days (L., *alternis diebus*)
ad lib at pleasure, as needed or desired (L., *ad libitum*)
adm admission
Ag silver (L., *argentum*)
alt. dieb. every other day (L., *alternis diebus*)
alt. hor. every other hour (L., *alternis horis*)
alt. noct. every other night (L., *alternis noctibus*)
a, am, ag amalgam
AM, a.m., A.M. before noon (L., *ante meridiem*)
amp ampule
amt amount
anat anatomy, anatomic
anes anesthesia
ant anterior
AP anteroposterior
appl applicable, application, appliance
approx approximate
aq water (L., *aqua*)
av average
bact bacterium (-ia)
BF bone fragment
bib drink (L., *bibe*)
b.i.d. twice a day (L., *bis in die*)
biol biologic, biology
BP blood pressure
Br Bridge
BS blood sugar
BW bite-wing radiograph
Bx biopsy
C centigrade
C one hundred (L., *centum*)
c̄ with (L., *cum*)
CA cardiac arrest
CA chronologic age
Ca calcium

Ca carcinoma
cal calorie
caps capsules
carbo carbocaine
cav cavity
CBC complete blood count
CC chief complaint
cc cubic centimeter
CDA or **C.D.A.** Certified Dental Assistant
cent centigrade
CHD childhood disease
CHF congestive heart failure
chr chronic
CM Cast metal
cm centimeter
c.m. tomorrow morning (L., *cras mane*)
CO₂ carbon dioxide
comp compound
conc concentrated
cond condition
CP centric position
cpd compound
CSX complete series x-rays
Cu copper (L., *cuprum*)
cu cubic
cur curettage
CV cardiovascular
CVA cerebrovascular accident
Cx convex
CY calendar year
d dose (L., *dosis*)
D or **DV** devital
D, dist distal
dbl double
dc direct current
DDS or **D.D.S.** Doctor of Dental Surgery/Science
DEF defective
deg degree
dev develop, development
Dg or **Dx** diagnosis

diag diagnosis
dil dilute (L., *dilue*)
dis disease
disp dispensary
dist distal
DM diagnostic models
DMF decayed, missing, and filled (teeth)
DO Distoocclusal
DOA dead on arrival
DOB date of birth
doz dozen
Dr. doctor
d.t.d. give of such a dose (L., *datur talis dosis*)
dwt pennyweight
Dx diagnosis
EAC external auditory canal
ed effective dose
EDDA expanded duties dental assistant (auxiliary)
EENT ears, eyes, nose, and throat
EFDA expanded (extended) functions dental assistant (auxiliary)
e.g. for example (L., *exempli gratia*)
EKG (ECG) elektrokardiogram (German)
emerg emergency
EMT emergency medical treatment
ENT ears, nose, and throat
epith epithelial
equiv equivalent
esp especially
est estimate, estimation
et and, Latin conjunction
et al. and others (L., *et alii*)
etc. and so on, and so forth, and others (L., *et cetera*)
evac evacuate, evacuation
eval evaluate, evaluation
ext extract, external
F Fahrenheit
F female
F field (of vision)
F formula
FB foreign body
FBS fasting blood sugar
FD fatal dose
ff following
FH family history
fl fluid
FLD full lower denture
fld field
fl. dr. fluid dram
fl. oz. fluid ounce
FMS full mouth series
FMX full mouth x-ray examination

FR or **frac** fracture
frag fragment
frec or **freq** frequent, frequency
ft foot
ft let it be made (L., *fiat/fiant*)
FUD full upper denture
func function
Fx fracture
G gold
g gram
gal gallon
GF gold foil
GI gold inlay
ging gingiva, gingivectomy
glob globulin
gm gram
GP general practitioner
gr grain
gt drop (L., *gutta*)
gtt drops (L., *guttae*)
H, h, hr hour (L., *hora*)
H₂O water
Hb, hgb hemoglobin
HBP high blood pressure
Hdpc handpiece
h.d. at hour of lying down at bedtime (L., *hora decubitus*)
hosp hospital
hr hour
h.s. hour of sleep (L., *hora somni*)
ht height
Hx history
I & D incision and drainage
IA incurred accidentally
ibid. in the same place (L., *ibidem*)
id the same (L., *idem*)
i.e. that is (L., *id est*)
IH infectious hepatitis
IM intramuscular
imp impression
IMP impacted
in inch
inc incisal, incisive incise
in d. daily (L., *in dies*)
inf infected, inferior, infusion
inj injection, injury
inop inoperable, inoperative
int internal
IQ intelligence quotient
i.q. the same as (L., *idem quod*)
IS interspace
IV intravenous

kg, kgm kilogram
kilo kilogram
kV kilovolt
L Latin
L, l liter
lab laboratory
lac laceration
LASER (laser) light amplification by stimulated emission of radiation
lat lateral
lb pound (L., *libra*)
lig ligament
ling lingual
liq liquid, liquor
LLQ lower left quadrant
LN lymph node
LRQ lower right quadrant
lt left
m murmur
m meter
m. dict. as directed (L., *modo dictu*)
M male
M, mes mesial
ma milliampere
mand mandibular
MASER (maser) microwave amplification by stimulated emission of radiation
max maximum, maxillary
MDR minimum daily requirement
med medical, medicine
mg, mgm milligram
micro microscopic
min minute, minimum
ML midline
ml milliliter
MM mucous membrane
mm millimeter
MO mesiocclusal
MOD mesiocclusodistal
mo month
MS multiple sclerosis
msec millisecond
N negroid, negro
N₂O nitrous oxide
narc narcotic, narcotism
nc no change, no charge
NCP not clinically present
neg negative
non. rep. do not repeat
norm normal
NPC no previous complaint
NPH no previous history

n.p.o. nothing by mouth (L., *nil per os*)
NR normal record
n.r. not to be repeated (L., *non repetatur*)
N/S normal saline
O oxygen
O₂ oxygen gas
obl oblique
occ or **Occl** occlusal
ODC oral disease control
o.d. every day (L., *omni die*)
o.d. right eye
OH oral hygiene
OHI oral hygiene instructions
o.h. every hour (L., *omni hora*)
o.m. every morning (L., *omni mane*)
o.n. every night (L., *omni nocte*)
op operation
OPC outpatient clinic
OPD outpatient department
opp opposite, opposed
OR operating room
org organism, organic
oz ounce
P pulse
P after (L., *post*)
p- para-
PA posteroanterior
Pan panoral x-ray examination
PATH pituitary adrenotropic hormone
path pathology
p.c. after meal (L., *post cibum*)
PCN penicillin
PDR *Physicians' Desk Reference*
Ped Pediatrics
perf perforating
PLD partial lower denture
P.M. PM, p.m. after noon (L., *post meridiem*)
PM after death (L., *post mortem*)
PO, postop postoperative
p.o. by mouth (L., *per os*)
POH personal oral hygiene
pos positive
postop postoperative
prep preparation, prepare (for surgery)
preop preoperative
p.r.n. as required, as the occasion arises (L., *pro re nata*)
prog prognosis
pt patient
PUD partial upper denture
Px, Pro, Proph prophylaxis
q every (L., *quaque*)
q.d. every day (L., *quaque die*)

q.h. every hour (L., *quaque hora*)

q.2h every second hour (L., *quaque secunda hora*)

q.i.d. four times a day (L., *quater in die*)

q.l. as much as pleased (L., *quantum libet*)

q.n. every night (L., *quaque nocte*)

q.p. at will (L., *quantum placeat*)

q.q.h. every 4 hours (L., *quaque quarta hora*)

qt quart

q.v. as much as liked (L., *quantum vis*)

r roentgen

R respiration

R$_x$ take (thou) a recipe

rad radiograph

RC retruded contact position

RC root canal

R.D.A. Registered Dental Assistant

RDH Registered Dental Hygienist

reg regular

rem(s) roentgen-equivalent-man

req requires, required

rep(s) roentgen-equivalent-physical

resp respiration

Rh Rh factor in blood (L., *Rhesus*)

RHD rheumatic heart disease

RN Registered Nurse

ROA Received on Account

rt right

Rx treatment (L., *recipe*)

s without (L., *sine*)

SBE subacute bacterial endocarditis

SD sterile dressing

sec second, secondary

Sig. write on label

sol solution

spec specimen

s̄s̄ one half signs and symptoms (L., *semis*)

stat immediately (L., *statim*)

std standard

stim stimulator, stimulate

strep *Streptococcus*

sup superior

surg surgeon, surgery

Sx symptom

sym symmetric

symp symptom

sys system

T temperature

tab tablet

TAT Tetanus antitoxin

TB, TBC tuberculosis

TBI toothbrush instructions

tbsp tablespoon

temp temperature

t.i.d. three times a day (L., *ter in die*)

tinc tincture

TLC tender loving care

TM temporomandibular

TMJ temporomandibular joint

TPR temperature, pulse, respiration

TrP treatment plan

tsp teaspoon

U, u unit

ULQ upper left quadrant

ung ointment (L., *unguentum*)

unk unknown

URI upper respiratory infection

URQ upper right quadrant

USP *United States Pharmacopoeia*

ut. dict. as directed

V, v volt

VD venereal disease

vert vertebra, vertical

visc viscous

VIT vitamin

viz that is, namely (L., *videlicet*)

VO verbal order

vol volume

vs versus

WF white female

wh white

WM white male

w-n well-nourished

wnd wound

wt weight

x times: 4×, four times; ×4, times four yard; x-ray

xt extract, extracted

xyl, xylo Xylocaine

yd yard

YOB year of birth

yr year

SYMBOLS

& and

* birth

† death

↓ decrease

° degree

= equal

′ feet, minutes

♀ female

> greater than, or indicating increase

″ inches; seconds

↑ increase

< less than, or indicating decrease

♂ male

− minus, negative
\# number, pound
i, ii, iii one, two, or three (as in number of grams, etc.)
3 $\overline{\text{iss}}$ one and one-half drams
3 **T** one ounce
3 $\overline{\text{ss}}$ one-half ounce
/ per

% percent
+ plus, positive

Adapted from Zwemer TJ: *Boucher's clinical dental terminology,* ed 4, St Louis, 1993, Mosby.

Prefixes and Suffixes

PREFIXES

Prefixes, the most frequently used elements in the formation of medical-dental words, are one or more syllables placed before words or roots to show various kinds of relationships. They are never used independently, but when added before verbs, adjectives, or nouns, they modify the meaning. Most prefixes are a part of words in ordinary speech and do not refer specifically to medical-dental or scientific terminology, but there are many that occur frequently in medical terminology. Studying them is an important step in learning medical terms and building a medical-dental vocabulary.

Prefix	Translation	Examples
a- (an before vowel)	Without, lack of	Apathy (lack of feeling), anemia (lack of blood)
ab-	Away from	Abductor (leading away from), aboral (away from mouth)
ad-	To, toward, near to	Adductor (leading toward), adhesion (sticking to)
ambi-	Both	Ambidextrous (ability to use hands equally), ambilaterally (both sides)
amphi-	About, on both sides, both	Amphibious (living on both land and water)
ampho-	Both	Amphogenic (producing offspring of both sexes)
ana-	Up, back, again, excessive	Anatomy (a cutting up)
ante-	Before, forward	Antecubital (before elbow), anteflexion (forward bending)
anti-	Against, opposed to, reversed	Antisepsis (against infection)
apo-	From, away from	Aponeurosis (away from tendon), apochromatic (abnormal color)
bi-	Twice, double	Bilateral (two sides), bifurcation (two branches)
cata-	Down, according to, complete	Catabolism (breaking down), catalepsia (complete seizure)
circum-	Around, about	Circumference (surrounding), circumscribe (to draw around)
com-	With, together	Commissure (sending or coming together)
con-	With, together	Conductor (leading together), concentric (having a common center)
contra-	Against, opposite	Contraception (prevention of conception), contraindicated (not indicated)
de-	Away from	Dehydrate (remove water from), decompensation (failure of compensation)
di-	Twice, double	Diplopia (double vision), dichromatic (two colors)
dia-	Through, apart, across, completely	Diaphragm (wall across), diapedesis (ooze through), diagnosis (complete knowledge)
dis-	Reversal, apart from, separation	Disinfection (apart from infection), dissect (cut apart)
dys-	Bad, difficult, disordered	Dyspepsia (bad digestion), dyspnea (difficult breathing)
e-, ex-	Out, away from	Enucleate (remove from), exostosis (outgrowth of bone)
ec-	Out from	Ectopic (out of place), eccentric (away from center)
ecto-	On outside, situated on	Ectoderm (outer skin), ectoretina (outer layer of retina)
em-, en-	In	Empyema (pus in), encephalon (in the head)
endo-	Within	Endodont (within tooth)

Continued

Prefix	Translation	Examples
epi-	Upon, on	Epidural (upon dura), epidermis (on skin)
exo-	Outside, on outer side, outer layer	Exogenous (produced outside)
extra-	Outside	Extracellular (outside cell)
hemi-	Half	Hemiplegia (partial paralysis), hemianesthesia (loss of feeling on one side of body)
hyper-	Over, above, excessive	Hyperemia (excessive blood), hypertrophy (overgrowth), hyperplasia (excessive formation), hypertension (high blood pressure)
hypo-	Under, below, deficient	Hypotension (low blood pressure)
im-, in-	In, into	Immersion (act of dipping in), injection (act of forcing liquid into)
im-, in-	Not	Immature (not mature), involuntary (not voluntary), inability (not able)
infra-	Below	Infraorbital (below eye), infraclavicular (below clavicle or collarbone)
inter-	Between	Intercostal (between ribs), intervene (come between)
intra-	Within	Intracerebral (within cerebrum), intraocular (within eyes)
intro-	Into, within	Introversion (turning inward), introduce (lead into)
meta-	Beyond, after, change	Metamorphosis (change of form), metastasis (beyond original position)
opistho-	Behind, backward	Opisthotic (behind ears), opisthognathous (behind jaws)
para-	Beside, by side	Paraplegia (paralysis of both sides), paracentesis (puncture along side of)
per-	Through, excessive	Permeate (pass through), perforate (bore through)
peri-	Around	Periosteum (around bone), periatrial (around atrium)
post-	After, behind	Postoperative (after operation), postocular (behind eye)
pre-	Before, in front of	Premolar (in front of molars), preoral (in front of mouth)
pro-	Before, in front of	Prognosis (foreknowledge), prophase (appear before)
re-	Back, again, contrary	Reflex (bend back), revert (turn again to)
retro-	Backward, located behind	Retrograde (going backward), retrolingual (behind tongue)
semi-	Half	Semicartilaginous (half cartilage), semiconscious (half conscious)
sub-	Under	Subcutaneous (under skin), subungual (under nail)
super-	Above, upper, excessive	Supercilia (upper brows), supernumerary (excessive number)
supra-	Above, upon	Suprarenal (above kidney), suprascapular (on upper part of scapula)
sym-, syn-	Together, with	Symphysis (growing together), synapsis (joining together)
trans-	Across, through	Transection (cut across), transmit (send beyond)
ultra-	Beyond, in	Ultraviolet (beyond violet end of spectrum), ultrasonic (sound waves beyond the upper frequency of hearing by human ear)

SUFFIXES

Suffixes are the one or more syllables or elements added to the root, or stem, of a word (the part that indicates the essential meaning) to alter the meaning or indicate the intended part of speech.

To make it pronounceable the last letter or letters of the root to which the suffix is attached may be changed. The last vowel may be changed to an *o*, or *o* may be inserted if it is not already present before a suffix beginning with a consonant, as in *cardiology*. The final vowel in the root may be dropped before a suffix beginning with a vowel, as in *neuritis*.

Most suffixes are in common use in English, but there are some peculiar to medical science. The suffixes most commonly used to indicate disease are *-itis*, meaning "inflammation," *-oma*, meaning "tumor," and *osis*, meaning "a condition," usually morbid. The following suffixes occur often in medical-dental terminology, but they are also in use in ordinary language:

Suffix	Use	Examples
-ise, -ize, -ate	Add to nouns or adjectives to make verbs expressing to use and to act like; to subject to; make into	Visualize (able to see), hypnotize (put into state of hypnosis)

Continued

Suffix	Use	Examples
-ist, -or, -er	Add to verbs to make nouns expressing agent or person concerned or instrument	Anesthetist (one who practices the science of anesthesia), donor (giver)
-ent	Add to verbs to make adjectives or nouns of agency	Recipient (one who receives), concurrent (happening at the same time)
-sia, -y	Add to verbs to make nouns expressing action, process, or condition	Therapy (treatment), anesthesia (process or condition of feeling)
-ia, -ity	Add to adjectives or nouns to make nouns expressing quality or condition	Septicemia (poisoning of blood), disparity (inequality), acidity (condition of excess acid), neuralgia (pain in nerves)
-ma, -mata, -men, -mina, -ment, -ure	Add to verbs to make nouns expressing result of action or object of action	Trauma (injury), foramina (openings), ligament (tough, fibrous band holding bone or viscera together), fissure (groove)
-ium, -olus, -olum, -culus, -culum, -cule, -cle	Add to nouns to make diminutive nouns	Bacterium, alveolus (air sac), follicle (little bag), cerebellum (little brain), molecule (little mass), ossicle (little bone)
-ible, -ile	Add to verbs to make adjectives expressing ability or capacity	Contractile (ability to contract), edible (capable of being eaten), flexible (capable of being bent)
-al, -c, -ious, -tic	Add to nouns to make adjectives expressing relationship, concern, or pertaining to	Neural (referring to nerve), neoplastic (referring to neoplasm), cardiac (referring to heart), delirious (suffering from delirium)
-id	Add to verbs or nouns to make adjectives expressing state or condition	Flaccid (state of being weak or lax), fluid (state of being fluid or liquid)
-tic	Add to verbs to make adjectives showing relationships	Caustic (referring to burn), acoustic (referring to sound or hearing)
-oid, -form	Add to nouns to make adjectives expressing resemblance	Polypoid (resembling polyp), plexiform (resembling a plexus), fusiform (resembling a fusion), epidermoid (resembling epidermis)
-ous	Add to nouns to make adjectives expressing material	Ferrous (composed of iron), serous (composed of serum), mucinous (composed of mucin)

The following verbs or combining forms of verbs are derived from either Greek or Latin. They may be attached to other roots to form words, or suffixes and prefixes may be added to them to form words. In the following examples, the part or root of the word to which the verb is attached is underlined and the meaning, if not clear, is given in parentheses:

Root	Translation	Examples
-algia-	Pain	Cardialgia (heart), gastralgia (stomach), neuralgia (nerve)
-audi-, -audio-	Hear, hearing	Audiometer (measure), audiophone (voice instrument for deaf)
-bio-	Live	Biology (study of living), biogenesis (origin)

Continued

Root	Translation	Examples
cau-, -caus-	Burn	Caustic (suffix added to make adjective), cauterization, causalgia (burning pain), electrocautery
-centesis-	Puncture, perforate	Thoracentesis (chest), pneumocentesis (lung), arthrocentesis (joint), enterocentesis (intestine)
-clas-, -claz-	Smash, break	Osteoclasis (bone), odontoclasis (tooth)
-duct-	Lead	Ductal (suffix added to make adjective), oviduct (egg uterine tube or fallopian tube), periductal (peri means "around")
-dynia-	Pain	Mastodynia (breast), esophagodynia (esophagus)
-ecta-, -ectas-	Dilate	Venectasia (dilation of vein), cardiectasis (heart), ectatic (suffix added for adjective)
-edem-	Swell	Myoedema (muscle), lymphedema (lymph), (a is a suffix added to make a noun)
-esthes-	Feel	Esthesia (suffix added to make noun), anesthesia (an is a prefix)
-flex-, -flec-	Bend	Flexion (suffix added to make noun), flexor (suffix added), anteflect (prefix added meaning "before" bending forward)
-fiss-	Split	Fissure, fission (suffixes added to make nouns)
-flu-, -flux-	Flow	Fluctuate, fluxion, affluent (abundant flowing)
-geno-, -genesis-	Produce, origin	Genotype, homogenesis (same origin), pathogenesis (disease, origin of disease), heterogenesis (prefix added meaning "other," alteration of generation)
-iatro-, -iatr-	Treat, cure	Geriatrics (old age), pediatrics (children)
-kine-, -kino-, -kineto-, -kinesio-	Move	Kinetogenic (producing movement), kinetic (suffix added to make adjective), kinesiology (study)
-liga-	Bind	Ligament (suffix added to make noun) ligate, ligature
-logy-	Study	Parasitology (parasites), bacteriology (bacteria), histology (tissues)
-lysis-	Breaking up, dissolving	Hemolysis (blood), glycolysis (sugar), autolysis (self-destruction of cells)
-morph-, -morpho-	Form	Morphology, amorphous (not definite form), pleomorphic (more, occurring in various forms), polymorphic (many)
-olfact-	Smell	Olfactophobia (fear), olfactory (suffix added to make adjective)
-op-, -opto-	See	Amblyopia (dull, dimness of vision), presbyopia (old, impairment of vision in old age), optic, myopia (myo, to wink, half close the eyes)
-palpit-	Flutter	Palpitation
-pep-	Digest	Dyspepsia (bad, difficult), peptic (suffix added to make adjective)
-phag-, -phago-	Eat	Phagocytosis (eating of cells), phagomania (madness, mad craving for food or to eat), dysphagia (difficulty eating or swallowing)
-phan-	Appear, visible	Phanerosis (act of becoming visible), phantasia, phantasy
-pexy-	Fix	Mastopexy (fixation of breast), nephrosplenopexy (surgical fixation of kidney and spleen)
-phas-	Speak, utter	Aphasia (unable to speak), dysphasia (difficulty in speaking)
-phobia-	Fear	Hydrophobia (fear of water), claustrophobia (closeness, fear of closed places)
-phil-	Like, love	Hemophilia (blood, a hereditary disease characterized by delayed clotting of blood), acidophilia (acid stain, liking or straining with acid stains), philanthropy (love of mankind)
-phrax-, -phrag-	Fence off, wall off	Diaphragm (across, partition separating thorax from abdomen), phragmoplast (formed)
-plas-	Form, grow	Neoplasm (new growth), rhinoplasty (nose operation for formation of nose), otoplasty (ear)
-plegia-	Paralyze	Paraplegia (paralysis of lower limbs), ophthalmoplegia (eye), hemiplegia (partial paralysis)
-pne-, -pneo-	Breathe	Dyspnea (difficult breathing), apnea (lack of breathing), hyperpnea (overbreathing)
-poie-	Make	Hematopoiesis (blood), erythropoiesis (red blood cells), leukopoiesis (making white cells)
-rrhagia-	Burst forth, pour	Menorrhagia (abnormal bleeding during menstruation), hemorrhage (blood)
-rrhaphy-	Suture	Herniorrhaphy (suturing or repair of hernia), hepatorrhaphy (liver), nephrorrhaphy (kidney)
-rrhea-	Flow, discharge	Leukorrhea (white discharge from vagina), rhinorrhea (nasal discharge)
-rrhexis-	Rupture	Enterorrhexis (intestines), metrorrhexis (uterus)
-schiz-	Split, divide	Schizophrenia (mind, split personality), schizonychia (nails), schizotrichia (hair)
-scope-	Examine	Microscopic, cardioscope, endoscope (endo means "within," an instrument for examining the interior of a hollow internal organ)

Continued

Root	Translation	Examples
-stasis-	Stop, stand still	Hematostatic (pertaining to stagnation of blood), epistasis (checking or stopping of any discharge)
-stazien-	Drop	Epistaxis (nosebleed)
-teg-, -tect-	Cover	Tegmen, tectum (rooflike structure), integument (skin covering)
-therap-	Treat, cure	Therapy, neurotherapy (nerves), chemotherapy (chemicals), physiotherapy
-tomy-	Cut, incise	Phlebotomy (incision of vein), arthrotomy (joint), appendectomy (ectomy, meaning "cutout," excision of appendix)
-topo-	Place	Topography, toponarcosis (numbing, hence numbing of a part or localized anesthesia)
-tropho-	Nourish	Hypertrophy (enlargement or overnourishment), atrophy (undernourishment), dystrophy (difficult or bad)

The following roots and combining forms are derived from Greek or Latin adjectives. Adjectives will appear most often in compounds and will be joined to either nouns or verbs. Suffixes may be added to make them into nouns.

In the following examples, the part or root of the word the adjective modifies is underlined, and the meaning, if not clear, is given in parentheses:

Root	Translation	Examples
-auto-	Self	Autoinfection, autolysis, autopathy (disease), autopsy (view, postmortem examination)
-brachy-	Short	Brachycephalia (head), brachydactylia (fingers), brachychelia (lip), brachygnathous (jaw)
-brady-	Slow	Bradypnea (breath), bradypragia (action), bradyuria (urine), bradypepsia (digestion)
-brevis-	Short	Brevity, breviflexor (short flexor muscle)
-cavus-	Hollow	Cavity, cavernous, vena cava (vein)
-coel-	Hollow	Coelarium (lining membrane of body cavity), coelom (body cavity of embryo)
-cryo-	Cold	Cryotherapy, cryotolerant, cryometer
-crypto-	Hidden, concealed	Cryptorchid (testis), cryptogenic (origin obscure or doubtful), cryptophthalmos (eye)
-dextro-	Right	Ambidextrous (using both hands with equal ease), dextrophobia (fear of objects on right side), dextrocardia (heart)
-dys-	Difficult, bad, disordered, painful	Dysarthria (speech), dyshidrosis (sweat), dyskinesia (motion), dystocia (birth), dysphasia (speech), dyspepsia (digestion)
-eu-	Well, good	Euphoria (well-being), euphagia, eupnea (breath), euthyroid (normal thyroid), eutocia (normal birth)
-eury-	Broad, wide	Eurycephalic (head), euryopia (vision), eurysomatic (body, squat thickset body)
-glyco-	Sugar, sweet	Glycohemia (sugar in blood), glycopenia (poverty of sugar, low blood sugar level)
-gravis-	Heavy	Gravida (pregnant woman), gravidism (pregnancy)
-haplo-	Single, simple	Haploid (having a single set of chromosomes), haplodermatitis (simple inflammation of skin), haplopathy (simple uncomplicated disease)
-hetero-	Other, different	Heterogeneous (kind, dissimilar elements), heteroinoculation, heterology (abnormality of structure), heterointoxication
-homo-	Same	Homogeneous (same kind or quality throughout), homozygous (possessing identical pair of genes), homologous (corresponding in structure)
-hydro-	Wet, water	Hydronephrosis (kidney, collection of urine in kidney pelvis), hydrophobia (fear of water, water causes painful reaction in this disease)
-iso-	Equal	Isocellular (similar cells), isodontic (all teeth alike), isocytosis (equality of size of cells), isochromatic (having same color throughout)
-latus-	Broad	Latitude, latissimus dorsi (muscle adducting humerus)
-leio-	Smooth	Leiomyosarcoma (smooth muscle, fleshy malignant tumor), leiomyofibroma (tumor of muscle and fiber elements), leiomyoma (tumor of unstriped muscle)

Continued

Root	Translation	Examples
-lepto-	Slender	Leptosomatic (body), leptodactylous (fingers)
-levo-	Left	Levocardia (heart), levorotation (turning to left)
-longus-	Long	Adductor longus (muscle of thigh), longitude
-macro-	Large, abnormal size	Macrocephalic (head), macrochiria (hands), macromastia (breast), macronychia (nails)
-magna-	Large, great	Magnitude, adductor magnus (thigh muscle)
-malaco-	Soft	Malacia (softening), osteomalacia (bones)
-malus-	Bad	Malady, malaise, malignant, malformation
-medius-	Middle, median, medium	Gluteus medius (femur muscle)
-mega-	Great	Megacolon (large colon), megacephaly (head)
-megalo-	Huge	Megalomania (delusion of grandeur), hepatomegaly (enlarged liver), splenomegaly (enlarged spleen)
-meso-	Middle, mid	Mesocarpal (wrist), mesoderm (skin), mesothelium (a lining membrane of cavities)
-micro-	Small	Microglossia (tongue), microblepharia (eyelids), microorganism, microphonia (voice)
-minimus-	Smallest	Gluteus minimus (smallest muscle of hip), adductor minimus (muscle of thigh)
-mio-	Less	Mioplasmia (plasma, abnormal decrease in plasma in blood), miopragia (perform, decreased activity)
-mono-	One, single, limited to one part	Monochromatic (color), monobrachia (arm)
-multi-	Many, much	Multipara (bear, woman who has borne many children), multilobar (numerous lobes), multicentric (many centers)
-necro-	Dead	Necrosed, necrosis, necropsy (postmortem examination), necrophobia (fear of death)
-neo-	New	Neoformation, neomorphism (form), neonatal (first 4 weeks of life), neopathy (disease)
-oligo-	Few, scanty, little	Oligophrenia (mind), oligopnea (breath), oliguria (urine), oligodipsia (thirst)
-ortho-	Straight, normal, correct	Orthodont (teeth, normal), orthogenesis (progressive evolution in a given direction), orthograde (walk, carrying body upright), orthopnea (breath, unable to breathe unless in an upright position)
-oxy-	Sharp, quick	Oxyesthesia (feel), oxyopia (vision), oxyosmia (smell)
-pachy-	Thick	Pachyderm (skin), pachysulemia (blood), pachypleuritis (inflammation of pleura), pachycholia (bile), pachyotia (ears)
-paleo-	Old	Paleogenetic (origin in the past), paleopathology (study of diseases in mummies)
-platy-	Flat	Platybasia (skull base), platycoria (pupil), platycrania (skull)
-pleo-	More	Pleomorphism (forms), pleochromocytoma (tumor composed of different colored cells)
-poikilo-	Varied	Poikiloderma (skin mottling), poikilothermal (heat, variable body temperature)
-poly-	Many, much	Polyhedral (many bases or faces), polymastia (more than two breasts), polymelia (supernumerary limbs), polymyalgia (pain in many muscles)
-pronus-	Face down	Prone, pronation
-pseudo-	False, spurious	Pseudostratified (layered), pseudocirrhosis (apparent cirrhosis of liver), pseudohypertrophy
-sclero-	Hard	Sclerosis (hardening), arteriosclerosis (artery), scleronychia (nails), sclerodermatitis (skin)
-scolio-	Twisted, crooked	Scoliodontic (teeth), scoliosis, scoliokyphosis (curvature of spine)
-sinistro-	Left	Sinistrocardia, sinistromanual (left-handed), sinistraural (hearing better in left ear)
-supinus-	Face up	Supine, supination, supinator longus (muscle in arm)
-steno-	Narrow	Stenosis, stenostomia (mouth), mitral stenosis (mitral valve in heart)
-stereo-	Solid, three dimensions	Stereoscope, stereometer
-tachy-	Fast, swift	Tachycardia (heart), tachyphrasia (speech)
-tele-	End, far away	Telepathy, telecardiogram
-telo-	Complete	Telophase
-thermo-	Heat, warm	Thermal, thermometer, thermobiosis (ability to live in high temperature)
-trachy-	Rough	Trachyphonia (voice), trachychromatic (deeply staining)
-xero-	Dry	Xerophagia (eating of dry foods) xerostomia (mouth), xerodermia (skin)

PRONUNCIATION OF MEDICAL-DENTAL TERMS

Medical terms are hard to pronounce, especially if you have read them but have never heard them spoken. The following are some helpful shortcuts:

ch is sometimes pronounced like *k*. Examples: chromatin, chronic.

ps is pronounced like *s*. Examples: psychiatry, psychology.

pn is pronounced with only the *n* sound. Example: pneumonia.

c and *g* are given the soft sound of *s* and *j*, respectively, before *e, i,* and *y* in words of both Greek and Latin origin. Examples: cycle, cytoplasm, giant, generic.

c and *g* have a harsh sound before other letters. Examples: gastric, gonad, cast, cardiac.

ae and *oe* are pronounced *ee*. Examples: coelom, fasciae.

e and *es,* when forming the final letters or letter of a word, are often pronounced as separate syllables. Examples: rete (reetee), nares (nayreez).

i at the end of a word (to form a plural) is pronounced *eye*. Examples: alveoli, glomeruli, fasciculi.

Glossary of Dental Terminology

abrasion Mechanical wearing away of teeth by abnormal stresses. This could result from abnormal toothbrushing habits or other abnormal stresses on the teeth.

accessional Permanent teeth that do not replace deciduous teeth but rather become an accession (an addition) to the deciduous or succedaneous teeth, or both types.

accessory root canals Extra openings into the pulp; usually located on the sides of the roots or in the bifurcations.

acquired Pertaining to something obtained by oneself; not inherited.

ala Latin for ''wing,'' referring to the sides of the nostrils of the nose; plural *alae*.

alignment Arrangement of teeth in a row.

allergenic Being hypersensitive to something.

allergic reaction Body's reaction to an allergen; an example of such a reaction is hives.

alveolar bone Bone that forms the sockets for the teeth.

alveolar crest Highest part of the alveolar bone closest to the cervical line of the tooth.

alveolar eminences Bulges on the facial surface of alveolar bone that outline the position of the roots.

alveolar mucosa Mucosa between the mucobuccal fold and gingiva.

alveolar process Part of the bone in the maxillae and mandible that forms the sockets for the teeth.

alveolus (alveoli) Cavity, or socket, in the alveolar process in which the root of the tooth is held.

anatomical crown That part of the tooth covered by enamel.

angle of the mandible Point at the lower border of the body of the mandible where it turns up onto the ramus.

Angle's classification System of dental classifications based primarily on the relationship of the permanent first molars to each other and to a lesser degree on the relationship of the permanent canines to each other.

ankyloglossia See *tongue-tie*.

ankylosis Fusion of the cementum of a tooth with alveolar bone.

anodontia No teeth at all are present in the jaw.

anomaly Any noticeable difference or deviation from that which is ordinary or normal.

anterior Situated in front of; a term commonly used to denote the incisor and canine teeth or the area toward the front of the mouth.

anterior pillar Fold of tissue extending down in front of the tonsil.

antihistamine Drug that controls the body's histamine reaction, which causes congestion of tissues.

apex (apices) End point, or furthest tip, as of the tooth root.

apical foramen Aperture, or opening, at or near the apex of a tooth root through which the blood and nerve supply of the pulp enters the tooth.

arch, dental See *dental arch*.

atrophic Pertaining to the wasting away of a tissue, organ, or part from disease, defective nutrition, or lack of use.

atrophy Wasting away of a tissue, organ, or part from disease, defective nutrition, or lack of use.

attached gingiva Tightly adherent gingiva that extends from free gingiva to alveolar mucosa.

attrition Process of normal wear on the crown.

autonomic nervous system Automatic nervous system of the body that is not willfully controlled. It controls the functions of the glands and smooth and cardiac muscle.

bicuspid See *premolars*.

bifurcation Division into two parts or branches, as any two roots of a tooth.

body of the mandible Horizontal portion of the mandible, excluding the alveolar process.

bone Hard connective tissue that forms the framework of the body. The hardness is attributable to the hydroxyapatite crystal.

bruxism Abnormal grinding of the teeth.

bucca Latin word for cheek.

buccal Pertaining to the cheek; toward the cheek or next to the cheek. Also called facial.

buccal developmental groove Groove that separates the buccal cusps on a buccal surface.

buccal glands Small minor salivary glands in the cheek.

buccinator Muscle of facial expression that extends from the posterior buccal portion of the maxillae and mandible and pterygomandibular raphe, forward in the cheek to the corner of the mouth.

calcification Process by which organic tissue becomes hardened by a deposit of calcium salts within its substance. The term, in a liberal sense, denotes the deposition of any mineral salts that contribute to the hardening and maturation of hard tissue.

canal Long tubular opening through a bone.

canines Third teeth from the midline, at corner of mouth; used for grasping; also called cuspids.

capsule Fibrous band of tissue surrounding a joint.

cell Basic functioning component of the body; capable of reproducing itself in most instances. Tissues are made up of groups of cells.

cementoenamel junction (CEJ) Junction of enamel of the crown and cementum of the root. This junction forms the cervical line around the tooth.

cementoma Cementum tumor at root tip that destroys surrounding bone.

cementum Layer of bonelike tissue covering the root of the tooth.

central developmental groove Developmental groove that crosses the occlusal surface of a tooth from the mesial to the distal side; divides the tooth into buccal and lingual parts.

centric occlusion (central occlusion) Relationship of the occlusal surfaces of one arch to those of the other when the jaws are closed and the teeth are in maximum intercuspation.

centric relation Arch-to-arch relationship of the maxilla to the mandible when the condyles are in their most upward position and the mandible is in its most posterior position and the jaw is most braced by its musculature.

cervical The portion of a tooth near the junction of the crown and root. Pertaining to the neck region, for example, nerves of the neck.

cervical line Line formed by the junction of the enamel and cementum on a tooth.

cervical third That portion of the crown or root of a tooth at or near the cervical line.

cervicoenamel ridge Any prominent ridge of enamel immediately near the cervical line on the crown of a tooth.

cervix Constricted structure; the narrow region at the junction of the crown and root of the tooth.

circumvallate papillae Large V-shaped row of papillae lying on the posterior dorsum of the tongue.

class I occlusal relationship Normal relationship between maxillary and mandibular molars.

class II occlusal relationship When a mandibular molar is posterior to its normal position.

class III occlusal relationship When a mandibular molar is anterior to its normal position.

cleft lip Gap in the upper lip occurring during development.

cleft palate Lack of joining together of the hard or soft palates.

clinical crown That part of the tooth protruding out of the gingiva.

clinical root That part of the tooth embedded in the gingiva and socket.

concavity Depression in a surface.

congenital Occurring at or before birth; may or may not be hereditary.

contact area Area of contact of one tooth with another in the same arch.

contact point Specific point at which a tooth from one arch occludes with another tooth from the opposing arch.

cross-bite Condition in which the cusps of a tooth in one arch exceed the cusps of a tooth in the opposing arch, buccally or lingually.

cross section Cutting through a tooth perpendicular to the long axis.

crown That part of the tooth covered with enamel.

cusp Major pointed or rounded eminence on or near the occlusal surface of a tooth.

cusp of Carabelli Fifth lobe of a maxillary first molar.

cyst Sac of fluid lined by epithelium that may grow to varying sizes.

cytoplasm Fluid substance of cells.

debrided Having already accomplished the removal (debridement) of nerve tissue and other debris from the pulp cavity to leave a surgically cleaned area.

deciduous That which will be shed; specifically, the first dentition of human or animal.

deglutition Action of swallowing.

dental arch All the teeth in either the maxillary or mandibular jaw that form an arch.

dentin (formerly **dentine**) Hard calcified tissue forming the inside body of a tooth, underlying the cementum and enamel and surrounding the pulpal tissue.

dentinal tubule Space in the dentin occupied by ontoblastic process.

dentinocemental junction Location in root where the dentin joins the cementum.

dentinoenamel junction Line marking the junction of the dentin and the enamel.

dentinogenesis imperfecta Hereditary imperfect dentin formation.

dentition General character and arrangement of the teeth, taken as a whole, as in carnivorous, herbivorous, and omnivorous dentitions. Primary dentition refers to the deciduous teeth, secondary dentition to the permanent teeth. Mixed dentition refers to a combination of permanent and deciduous teeth in the same dentition.

depression Lowering of the mandible or opening of the mouth.

developmental depression Noticeable concavity on the formed crown or root of a tooth; occurs at the junction of two lobes, as on the mesial surface of maxillary first premolars, or at the furcation of roots.

developmental grooves Fine depressed lines in the enamel of a tooth that mark the union of the lobes of the crown.

diastema Any spacing between teeth in the same arch.

distal Distant; farthest from the median line of the face, or from the origin of a structure.

distal proximal surface Proximal surface on the posterior side of a tooth.

distal third Viewed from the facial or lingual surface, third of a surface farther from the midline.

distobuccal developmental groove Developmental groove that extends on the buccal surface of a lower first or third molar between the distobuccal and distal cusps.

distoclusion See *class II occlusal relationship.*

dorsum of the tongue Top or superior surface of the tongue.

edema Swelling of tissue.

edge, incisal See *incisal edge.*

embrasure Open space between the proximal surfaces of two

teeth where they diverge buccally, labially, or lingually and occlusally from the contact area.

enamel Hard calcified tissue that covers the dentin of the crown portion of a tooth.

enamel dysplasia Abnormalities of enamel growth.

enamel hypocalcification Enamel that is not as dense as regular enamel.

enamel hypoplasia Enamel that is thin or pitted.

endocrine Gland or type of secretion that is carried away from the producing cells by blood vessels; the secretion is used in other parts of the body to control certain functions; has no duct system.

enzyme Agent capable of producing chemical changes in processes such as the digestion of foods.

epiglottis Cartilage that helps cover laryngeal opening.

epinephrine Substance produced by the body or synthetically produced that causes many reactions; in dentistry, used to constrict blood flow in tissues.

epithelial Pertaining to epithelium.

epithelial attachment The substance produced by the reduced enamel epithelium that helps secure the attachment epithelium at the base of the gingival sulcus to the tooth.

epithelium Layer or layers of cells that cover the surface of the body or line the tubes or cavities inside the body; one of the four basic tissues.

equilibrium Sense of balance.

eruption Movement of the tooth as it emerges through surrounding tissue so that the clinical crown gradually appears longer.

eruptive stage Period of eruption from the completion of crown formation until the teeth come into occlusion.

exfoliation Shedding or loss of a primary tooth.

facial Term used to designate the outer surfaces of the teeth collectively (buccal or labial).

facial surface See *facial.*

facial third From a proximal view, the third of that surface closest to the facial side.

fauces Space between the left and right palatine tonsils.

FDI system The Federation Dentaire Internationale (International Dental Federation); system for tooth identification.

filiform papillae Small pointed projections that heavily cover most of the dorsum of the anterior two thirds of the tongue.

fissure Deep cleft; developmental line fault usually found in the occlusal or buccal surface of a tooth; commonly the result of the imperfect fusion of the enamel of the adjoining dental lobes.

flange Projecting edge; the edge of the denture.

fluorosis Discolored enamel resulting from excessive fluoride intake while crown is developing.

foliate papillae Poorly developed papillae that appear as small vertical folds in the posterior part of the sides of the tongue.

foramen Short circular opening through a bone.

fossa Round, wide, relatively shallow depression in the surface of a tooth as seen commonly in the lingual surfaces of the maxillary incisors or between the cusps of molars; also a shallow depression in bone.

free gingiva gingiva that forms the gingival sulcus.

frenulum Little frenum or fold of tissue.

frontal sinus Air sinus in frontal bone above the eye that opens into the hiatus semilunaris in the middle meatus.

fungiform papillae Small circular papillae scattered throughout the anterior two thirds of the dorsum of the tongue.

fusion Two teeth that fuse at the dentin while developing.

gingiva Part of the mucosal tissue that immediately surrounds the teeth and alveolar bone.

gingival crest Most occlusal or incisal extent of gingiva.

gingival crevice Subgingival space that, under normal conditions, lies between the gingival crest and the epithelial attachment.

gingival papillae That portion of the gingiva found between the teeth in the interproximal spaces gingival or inferior to the contact area; also called interdental papillae.

gingival sulcus Space between the free gingiva and the tooth surface.

gingivitis Inflammation involving the gingival tissues only.

hematoma Escape of blood from injured blood vessel into tissue spaces.

hemoglobin Component in red blood cells that carries oxygen.

hereditary Inherited through the genes of parents.

immunity Body's resistance to certain organisms or diseases.

impacted Teeth not completely erupted that are fully or partially covered by bone or soft tissue.

incisal edge Edge formed at the labioincisal line angle of an anterior tooth after an incisal ridge has worn down.

incisal ridge Rounded ridge form of the incisal portion of an anterior tooth.

incisal third From a proximal, lingual, or labial view of an anterior tooth, third of the surface closest to the incisal edge.

incisive papilla Small, rounded, oblong mound of tissue directly behind or lingual to the maxillary central incisors and lying over incisive foramen.

incisors Four center teeth in either arch; essential for cutting.

inflammatory reaction Body's mechanism to combat harmful organisms by bringing more plasma and blood cells to injured area.

inherited Passed on from parents or grandparents.

interdental Located between the teeth.

interdental papilla Projection of gingiva between the teeth.

interproximal Between the proximal surfaces of adjoining teeth in the same arch.

interproximal space Triangular space between adjoining teeth; the proximal surfaces of the teeth form sides of the triangle; the alveolar bone, the base, and the contact area of the teeth form the apex.

labia Latin word for lips; singular *labium.*

labial Of or pertaining to the lips; toward the lips.

labial frenum Fold of tissue that attaches the lip to the labial mucosa at the midline of the lips.

larynx Voice box; trachea begins just below it.

lingual Pertaining to or affecting the tongue; next to or toward the tongue.

lingual frenum Fold of tissue that attaches the undersurface of the tongue to the floor of the mouth.

lingual glands Minor salivary glands of the tongue.

lingual groove Developmental groove that occurs on the lingual side of the tooth.

lingual surface See *lingual.*

lingual third From a proximal view, third of a surface closest to the lingual side.

macrodontia Teeth are too large for the jaw.

malocclusion Abnormal occlusion of the teeth.

mamelon One of the three rounded protuberances of the incisal surface of a newly erupted incisor tooth.

mandible Lower jaw.

mandibular Pertaining to the lower jaw.

mandibular arch First pharyngeal arch that forms the area of the mandible and maxillae; the lower dental arch.

mandibular condyle Rounded top of the mandible that articulates with the mandibular fossa.

mandibular foramen Opening on the medial surface of the ramus of the mandible for entrance of nerves and blood vessels to the lower teeth.

mandibular process That portion of the mandibular pharyngeal arch that goes to form the mandible.

mandibular tori Bony growths on the lingual cortical plate of bone opposite the mandibular canines; also called torus mandibularis.

marginal ridge Ridge or elevation of enamel forming the margin of the surface of a tooth; specifically, at the mesial and distal margins of the occlusal surfaces of premolars and molars, and the mesial and distal margins of the lingual surfaces of incisors and canines.

mastication Act of chewing or grinding.

maxillae Paired main bone of the upper jaw.

maxillary Pertaining to the upper arch.

maxillary arch Upper dental arch.

maxillary sinus Largest of the paired paranasal sinuses, located in the maxillae.

maxillary tuberosity Bulging posterior surface of the maxillae behind the third molar region.

median line Vertical (central) line that divides the body into right and left; the median line of the face.

mesial Toward or situated in the middle, for example, toward the midline of the dental arch.

mesial drift Phenomenon of permanent molars continuing to move mesially after eruption.

mesial third From a facial or a lingual view, third of the surface closest to the midline.

microdontia Teeth are too small for the jaw.

mixed dentition State of having primary and permanent teeth in the dental arches at the same time.

molars Large posterior teeth used for grinding.

mucosa Moist epithelial linings of oral cavity and respiratory and digestive systems.

mucous Pertaining to mucus, the thick viscous secretion of a gland.

mulberry molars Molars with multiple cusps that are caused by congenital syphilis.

multiple root Root with more than one branch.

muscle One of the four basic tissues; has the property of contraction or shortening of the fibers, which accomplishes work. There are three types of muscle: skeletal, cardiac, and smooth.

nasal septum Wall between the left and right sides of the nasal cavity, made up of the ethmoid and vomer bones.

nervous tissue One of the four basic tissues. Groups of cells (neurons) carry messages to and from the brain and perform many other tasks.

neuron Nerve cell.

nonsuccedaneous Permanent teeth that do not succeed or replace deciduous teeth.

occluding Contacting opposing teeth.

occlusal Articulating or biting surface.

occlusal plane Side view of the occlusal surfaces.

occlusal relationship Way in which the maxillary and mandibular teeth touch each other.

occlusal third From a proximal, lingual, or buccal view of a posterior tooth, the third of a surface closest to the occlusal surface.

occlusal trauma Injury brought about by one tooth prematurely hitting another during closure of the jaws.

occlusion Relationship of the mandibular and maxillary teeth when closed or during excursive movements of the mandible; when the teeth of the mandibular arch come into contact with the teeth of the maxillary arch in any functional relationship.

odontoma A tumor made up of enamel, dentin, cementum, and pulp.

opaque Not easily able to transmit light.

open bite Space left between the teeth when the jaws close.

open contact Space between adjacent teeth in the same arch; an interproximal opening instead of a contact area where the teeth touch.

overbite Relationship of the teeth in which the incisal ridges of the maxillary anterior teeth extend below the incisal edges of the mandibular anterior teeth when the teeth are placed in a centric occlusal relationship.

overhanging restoration Excess of filling material extending past the confines of the tooth preparation; an overextension of filling material.

overjet Relationship of teeth in which the incisal ridges or buccal cusp ridges of the maxillary teeth extend facially to the incisal ridges or buccal cusp ridges of the mandibular teeth when the teeth are in a centric occlusal relationship.

palatal Pertaining to the palate or roof of the mouth.

Palmer notation system System of coding the teeth using brackets, numbers, and letters.

papillary gingiva Gingiva that forms the interdental papillae.

paramolar Small supernumerary tooth located buccally or lingually to a molar.

parasympathetic nervous system Part of the autonomic (automatic) nervous system that originates from some of the cranial nerves and some of the sacral nerves. It controls a number of functions, including stimulation of the salivary glands.

parathyroid gland Small gland embedded in the thyroid gland that helps control calcium metabolism in the body.

passive eruption Condition in which the tooth does not move but the gingival attachment moves farther apically.

peg-shaped lateral Poorly formed maxillary lateral incisor with a cone-shaped crown.

periapical Around the tip of a tooth root.

periodontal Surrounding a tooth.

periodontium Supporting tissues surrounding the teeth.

periosteum Fibrous and cellular layer that covers bones and contains cells that become osteoblasts.

periphery Circumferential boundary; outer border.

pharynx Throat area, from the nasal cavity to the larynx.

philtrum Small depression at the midline of the upper lip.

pillars Folds of tissue appearing in front of and behind the palatine tonsils.

pit Small pointed depression in dental enamel, usually at the junction of two or more developmental grooves; a small hole anywhere on the crown.

posterior Situated toward the back, as premolars and molars.

posterior pillars Folds of tissue behind the tonsil that contain the palatopharyngeus muscle.

posterior teeth Teeth of either jaw to the rear of the incisors and canines.

preeruptive stage Period of time when the crown of the tooth is developing.

premature contact area The area where an upper and a lower tooth touch and hit each other before the rest of the teeth occlude together.

premaxilla Bony area of the upper jaw that includes the alveolar ridge for the incisors and the area immediately behind it.

premolars Permanent teeth that replace the primary molars.

primary dentin Dentin formed from the beginning of calcification until tooth eruption.

primary dentition First set of teeth; baby teeth; milk teeth; deciduous teeth.

primary palate The early developing part of the hard palate that comes from the medial nasal process and forms a V-shaped wedge of tissue that runs from the incisive foramen forward and laterally between the lateral incisors and canines of the maxilla.

primary teeth See *deciduous.*

prosthetic appliance Any constructed appliance that replaces a missing part.

protrusion Condition of being thrust forward, as protrusion of the anterior teeth, referring to the teeth being too far labial; the forward movement of the mandible.

proximal Nearest, next, immediately adjacent to; distal or mesial.

proximal contact areas Proximal area on a tooth that touches an adjacent tooth on the mesial or distal side.

pulp canal Canal in the root of a tooth that leads from the apex to the pulp chamber. Under normal conditions it contains dental pulp tissue.

pulp cavity Entire cavity within the tooth, including the pulp canal and pulp chamber.

pulp chamber Cavity or chamber in the center of the crown of a tooth that normally contains the major portion of the dental pulp. The pulp canals lead into the pulp chambers.

pulp, dental Highly vascular and innervated connective tissue contained within the pulp cavity of the tooth. The dental pulp is composed of arteries, veins, nerves, connective tissues and cells, lymph tissue, and odontoblasts.

pulp horn (horn of pulp) Extension of pulp tissue into a thin point of the pulp chamber in the tooth crown.

pulp stones Small dentinlike calcifications in pulp.

quadrants One fourth of the dentition. The four quadrants are divided into right and left, maxillary and mandibular.

ramus of the mandible Vertical portion of mandible.

recession Migration of the gingival crest in an apical direction, away from the crown of the tooth.

referred pain Pain that seems to originate in one area but actually originates in another area.

reparative dentin Localized formation of dentin in response to local trauma such as occlusal trauma or caries.

resorption Physiological removal of tissues or body products, as of the roots of deciduous teeth, or of some alveolar process after the loss of the permanent teeth.

retromolar pad Pad of tissue behind the mandibular third molars.

retromolar triangle Triangular area of bone just behind the mandibular third molars.

retrusion Act or process of retraction or moving back, as when the mandible is placed in posterior relationship to the maxillae.

ridge Long narrow elevation or crest, as on the surface of a tooth or bone.

root That portion of a tooth embedded in the alveolar process and covered with cementum.

root canal See *pulp canal.*

root planing Process of smoothing the cementum of the root of a tooth.

rugae Small ridges of tissue extending laterally across the anterior of the hard palate.

sebaceous glands Small oil-producing glands that are usually connected to and lubricate hairs.

secondary dentin Dentin formed throughout the pulp chamber and pulp canal from the time of eruption.

secondary dentition Permanent dentition.

single root Root with one main branch.

slough Loss of dead cells from the surface of tissue; pronounced *sluff.*

soft tissue Noncalcified tissues, such as nerves, arteries, veins, and connective tissue.

spasm Constant contraction of muscle.

submucosa Supporting layer of loose connective tissue under a mucous membrane.

succedaneous Permanent teeth that succeed, or take the place of, the deciduous teeth after the latter have been shed, that is, the incisors, canines, and premolars.

sulcus Long V-shaped depression or valley in the surface of a tooth between the ridges and the cusps. A sulcus has a developmental groove at the apex of its V shape. Sulcus also refers to the trough around the teeth formed by the gingiva.

supplemental groove Shallow linear groove in the enamel of a tooth. It differs from a developmental groove in that it does not mark the junction of lobes; it is a secondary, or smaller, groove.

supplemental tooth Supernumerary tooth that resembles a regular tooth.

supraeruption Eruption of a tooth beyond the occlusal plane.

taste buds Small structures in vallate, fungiform, and foliate papillae that detect taste.

temporomandibular ligament Thickened part of the temporomandibular joint (TMJ) capsule on the lateral side.

tongue-tie, tongue-tied Condition when the lingual frenum is short and attached to the tip of the tongue, making normal speech difficult.

tonsillor pillars The vertical folds of tissue that lie in front of and behind the palatine tonsils in the lateral throat wall.

tooth germ Soft tissue that develops into a tooth.

tooth migration Movement of the tooth through the bone and gum tissue.

torus palatinus Large bony growth in hard palate.

transverse ridge Ridge formed by the union of two triangular ridges, transversing the surface of a posterior tooth from the buccal to the lingual side.

trauma Wound; bodily injury or damage.

trifurcation Division of three tooth roots at their point of junction with the root trunk.

Universal system, Universal Code System of coding teeth using the numbers 1 to 32 for permanent teeth and the letters A to T for the deciduous teeth.

uvula Small hanging fold of tissue in back of the soft palate.

vallate papillae See *circumvallate papillae*.

vascular Relating to blood supply.

vasoconstrictor Substance that constricts blood vessels.

vermillion zone Red part of the lip where the lip mucosa meets the skin.

vestibule Space between the lips or cheeks and the teeth.

From Brand RW, Isselhard DE: *Anatomy of orofacial structures,* ed 5, St Louis, 1994, Mosby.

Testbank

1 Which of the following duties is considered an advanced function for dental assistants in some states?
   a. Scaling teeth
   b. Oral evacuation
   c. Administration of local anesthetic
   d. Placing and carving amalgam restorations

2 Which of the following statements are *not* true regarding credentials for dental assistants?
   1. Dental assistants are licensed in all states.
   2. Credentials verify professional credibility.
   3. Certification from the Dental Assisting National Board is a prerequisite to be eligible for state licensure.
   4. General and specialty credentials are offered through the Dental Assisting National Board.
   a. 1 and 3
   b. 2 and 4
   c. 1, 2, 3
   d. 1, 2, 3, and 4

3 The _____ nerve innervates the muscles of facial expression.
   a. Maxillary
   b. Mandibular
   c. Occipital
   d. Zygomatic

4 The bones that make up the viscerocranium include which of the following?
   1. Maxilla
   2. Mandible
   3. Nasal
   4. Ethmoid
   5. Vomer
   6. Temporal
   7. Frontal
   8. Nasal conchae
   a. 1, 3, 6, and 7
   b. 1, 2, 4, and 6
   c. 1, 2, 3, 5, and 8
   d. 2, 3, 5, 7, and 8

In items 5-8, select the correct definition in column B for each term in column A.

Column A	Column B
_____ 5 Elevation	a. Raising or closing mandible
_____ 6 Retrusion	b. Moving forward
_____ 7 Lateral excursion	c. Moving back
_____ 8 Protrusion	d. Lowering or opening mouth
	e. Moving sideways

In items 9-11, select the correct term in column B for each definition in column A.

Column A	Column B
_____ 9 The suture between the frontal and parietal bones	a. Lambdoidal
	b. Sagittal
_____ 10 The suture between the parietal and temporal bones	c. Coronal
	d. Squamous
_____ 11 The suture between the parietal bones	e. Condyle

12 The central nervous system consists of which of the following?
   1. Brain
   2. Spine
   3. Spinal cord
   4. Parasympathetic system
   5. Sympathetic system
   a. 1 and 3
   b. 2 and 4
   c. 1, 3 and 5
   d. 1, 2, 3, and 4
   e. 1, 2, 3, 4, and 5

13 The chambers of the heart include the right and left
   1. Ventricle
   2. Aorta
   3. Atrium
   4. Jugular
   5. Carotid
   a. 1 and 2
   b. 1 and 3
   c. 2 and 4
   d. 3 only
   e. 4 only

In items 14-18, place an A for *True* or a B for *False* in the space provided for each statement.

_____ 14 A sagittal cut provides a cross section.

_____ 15 The mesial and distal surfaces of teeth are considered proximal surfaces.

_____ 16 The oral cavity can be divided into six segments and four quadrants.

_____ 17 The orbicularis oris functions to draw the lips together.

_____ 18 The minor salivary glands are basically found in clusters in the mouth.

19 Which of the following is *not* considered one of the three sets of tonsils?
   a. Palatine

b. Fauces
c. Pharyngeal adenoid
d. Lingual

20 Which of the following is *not* located in the vestibule?
  a. Maxillary frenum
  b. Sublingual caruncle
  c. Incisive foramen
  d. Vermilion border

21 The cells that produce bone are the
  a. Fibrocytes
  b. Osteoblasts
  c. Osteocytes
  d. Osteoclasts

22 A joint is a(n)
  a. Point of intersection of muscle and bone
  b. Junction of bones
  c. Overlapping of muscles
  d. Center of ossification

23 Joints that do not move are called
  a. Hinge joints
  b. Ball-and-socket joints
  c. Gliding joints
  d. Sutures

24 The types of muscle tissue are
  1. Smooth
  2. Elastic
  3. Striated
  4. Cardiac
  5. Extension
  a. 1, 3, and 4
  b. 2, 3, and 4
  c. 2, 4, and 5
  d. 3, 4, and 5

25 Tendons attach the
  a. Muscle to bone
  b. Muscle to nerve
  c. Nerve to bone
  d. Bone to bone

26 A reflex is
  a. An action that can always be controlled
  b. Always hormonal
  c. An involuntary response to a stimulus
  d. A response that bypasses the central nervous system

27 Where does gaseous exchange take place in the lungs?
  a. Larynx
  b. Bronchioles
  c. Alveoli
  d. Bronchi

28 Blood normally transports
  1. Fibrin
  2. Oxygen
  3. Cellulose
  4. Nutrients
  5. Hormones
  a. 1, 2, and 4
  b. 2, 3, and 5
  c. 2, 4, and 5
  d. 3, 4, and 5

29 The fluid portion of blood is known as
  a. Megakaryocytes
  b. Plasma
  c. Erythrocytes
  d. Lymph

30 Blood platelets are necessary for
  a. Carbon dioxide elimination
  b. Antigen-antibody reactions
  c. Allergic reactions
  d. Blood clotting

31 What types of tissue make up the heart?
  1. Muscle
  2. Epithelial
  3. Nervous
  4. Connective
  a. 1 and 3
  b. 2 and 4
  c. 1, 2, and 3
  d. 1, 2, 3, and 4
  e. 4 only

32 The major function of the large intestine is to
  a. Aid in protein metabolism
  b. Lubricate the food bolus
  c. Aid in water absorption
  d. Store nutrients

33 Chromosomes are made up of
  a. Fats
  b. Glycogen
  c. Carbohydrates
  d. Nucleic acids

34 Components of the urinary system are the
  1. Ureters
  2. Uterus
  3. Bladder
  4. Urethra
  5. Liver
  a. 1, 2, and 3
  b. 1, 3, and 4
  c. 2, 3, and 4
  d. 3, 4, and 5

35 The lungs are considered a part of which two systems?
  1. Circulatory
  2. Respiratory
  3. Urinary
  4. Excretory
  a. 1 and 2
  b. 1 and 3
  c. 1 and 4
  d. 2 and 3
  e. 2 and 4

36 The liver functions to
  a. Metabolize fat
  b. Detoxify harmful substances
  c. Manufacture bile
  d. All of the above

37 What do all microbes have in common?
  a. They have nucleic acid.

b. They have chloroplasts.

c. They are parasitic.

d. They cause disease.

In items 38-42, select the correct term in column B for each condition in column A.

	Column A	Column B
_____	**38** An existing space between the maxillary and mandibular teeth	a. Crossbite
_____	**39** Facially positioned mandibular teeth	b. Overjet
_____	**40** Lingually positioned mandibular teeth	c. Open bite
_____	**41** Deep or vertical overlap of the maxillary teeth on the mandibular teeth beyond what is considered normal edge	d. Overbite
_____	**42** Horizontal overlap creating protrusion between the labial surface of the mandibular incisors and the lingual surface of the maxillary incisors	e. Normal bite

43 Which of the following statements is/are true in relation to the development of the permanent incisors?

1. They develop apically from the primary incisors.

2. They develop inferiorly from the primary incisors.

3. Commonly erupt lingually to the primary incisors.

4. Commonly erupt labially to the primary incisors.

a. 1 and 3

b. 2 and 4

c. 1, 2, and 3

d. 4 only

44 The largest portion of the pulp found in the coronal portion of the tooth is the

a. Pulp chamber

b. Pulp canal

c. Pulp horn

d. Apical foramen

45 An embrasure is

a. Usually located toward the cervical aspect of the teeth

b. The small spot on the mesial or distal surface of teeth at the point of contact

c. The curvature toward or away from the contact area

46 Rounded elevations of enamel found on the incisal edges of anterior teeth at the time of eruption are known as

a. Lobes

b. Cusps

c. Enamel pearls

d. Mamelons

47 The retruded mandible profile is classified as

a. Distoocclusion

b. Mesioocclusion

c. Buccoocclusion

d. Neutroocclusion

48 Mastication is accomplished by means of impulses transmitted to the jaw muscles through the motor branch of the

a. Chorda tympani

b. Maxillary nerve

c. Trigeminal nerve

d. Glossopharyngeal nerve

49 The bone that lines the tooth socket in a radiographic examination is the

a. Lamina dura

b. Cancellous bone

c. Trabecular bone

d. Hypocalcified bone

50 The lateral pterygoid muscles function to

a. Retract the mandible

b. Elevate the mandible

c. Protract the mandible

d. Protract and elevate the mandible

51 The cells responsible for the formation of periodontal ligament are

a. Ameloblasts

b. Fibroblasts

c. Fibroclasts

d. Cementoblasts

In items 52-57, place an A for *Major* or a B for *Minor* (trace) for each mineral.

_____ **52** Calcium

_____ **53** Iron

_____ **54** Phosphorus

_____ **55** Iodine

_____ **56** Sodium

_____ **57** Copper

58 The primary function of protein is to

a. Contribute to energy metabolism

b. Play a significant role in the body's resistance to disease

c. Supply amino acids for building other essential protein substances

d. Aid the growth and maintenance of tissue

59 Vitamin K can cause

a. Blood clotting

b. Cheilosis

c. Beriberi

d. Anemia

60 Which of the following are considered simple sugars?

a. Fructose and glucose

b. Sucrose and cellulose

c. Lactose and galactose

d. Levulose and dextrose

61 Which of the following statements is true concerning diet?

a. Sugar is an essential ingredient in a diet for energy.

b. Brown sugar contains more essential nutrients than white sugar.

c. Refined sugar provides empty calories.

d. A banana is an example of a fibrous food.

62 What are the best sources of vitamin C?

a. Fresh fruits

b. Green, leafy vegetables

c. Milk and cheese

d. Egg yolk and yellow vegetables

63 Proteins are made up of

a. Adipose tissue

b. Amino acids

c. Glycogen

d. Lactose

64 Koplik's spots are associated with which of the following systemic diseases?

a. Leukemia

b. Diabetes

c. Measles

d. Pernicious anemia

65 The clinical symptoms of lichen planus resemble which of the following conditions?

a. Leukoplakia

b. Geographic tongue

c. Dental fluorosis

d. Squamous cell carcinoma

66 Oral conditions commonly seen in patients with AIDS include

1. Mucocele

2. Kaposi's sarcoma

3. Fordyce granules

4. Hairy leukoplakia

a. 1 and 3

b. 2 and 4

c. 1, 2, and 3

d. 4 only

67 Which of the following is an oral fungal infection?

a. Thrush

b. Herpes

c. Melanoma

d. Aphthous ulcer

68 The best protective measure against periodontal disease is to

a. Use hydrotherapy

b. Eat course, fibrous foods

c. Increase vitamin C intake

d. Brush teeth properly and regularly

e. Use supplementary stimulating aids

69 Which of the following statements is true of enamel hypoplasia?

a. It occurs during the formative stage of tooth development.

b. It may involve both deciduous and permanent dentitions.

c. It is basically a result of disturbed function of ameloblasts.

d. All of the above are correct.

70 Recurrent caries refers to

a. Decay that begins inside the tooth

b. Root caries only

c. Caries around the margins of restorations

d. Occlusal caries only

71 A cavity preparation that involves the buccal pit of a mandibular molar is classified as a _____ cavity preparation.

a. Class I

b. Class II

c. Class III

d. Class IV

72 Possible causes of irreversible pulpal damage include

1. Caries invasion

2. Trauma

3. X-rays

4. Use of irreversible hydrocolloid

5. Chemical irritation

a. 1, 2, and 4

b. 1, 2, and 5

c. 2, 4, and 5

d. 3, 4, and 5

73 Which of the following microorganisms is associated with the onset of dental caries in humans?

a. *Staphylococcus aureus*

b. *Streptococcus mutans*

c. *Candida albicnas*

d. *Lactobacilli*

e. None of the above

74 Plaque in the oral cavity is composed of

a. Saliva glycoproteins

b. Oral bacteria

c. Saliva glycoproteins and oral bacteria

d. None of the above

75 A cavity preparation found on the cervical one third of an anterior tooth is considered to be which class?

a. Class I

b. Class II

c. Class III

d. Class V

76 If teeth appear to have roots shorter than normal on a radiograph, the appearance is a result of

a. Attrition

b. Abrasion

c. Resorption

d. Normal growth for the individual

In items 77-84, place an A for *True* or a B for *False* in the space provided for each statement.

_____ **77** Calculus is usually removed during polishing.

_____ **78** A point angle is where three surfaces meet.

_____ **79** A line angle is where three surfaces meet.

_____ **80** A Class III cavity preparation is located only in anterior teeth.

_____ **81** A Class II cavity preparation is located only in posterior teeth.

_____ **82** Hairy leukoplakia is pathognomonic for periodontal disease.

_____ **83** Something that is erythematous is usually ulcerated.

_____ **84** Antibiotics are useful for treating oral infections.

In items 85-88, select the correct area of common occurrence in column B for each condition in column A.

Column A		*Column B*
_____ **85**	Erythroplakia	a. Floor of mouth
_____ **86**	Squamous cell carcinoma	b. Skin exposed to sun
		c. Any mucous membrane
_____ **87**	Basal cell carcinoma	d. Lateral border of tongue
_____ **88**	Leukoplakia	

In items 89-92, select the correct definition in column B for each term in column A.

Column A   *Column B*

_____ **89** Bilateral   a. Condition without clear path-
_____ **90** Unilateral   ogenesis
_____ **91** Idiopathic   b. Present at birth
_____ **92** Congenital   c. Decrease in size of an object
                d. Affecting one side
                e. Affecting two sides

In items 93-95, select the correct definition in column B for each term in column A.

Column A   *Column B*

_____ **93** Dysplastic   a. Malignant tumor in epithelial
_____ **94** Atrophy   tissue
_____ **95** Benign   b. Abnormally developed tissue
                c. Decrease size of an object
                d. Not recurrent or progressive

96 A condition in which the tongue is characterized by a nonuniform pattern of smooth areas resulting from a loss of the epithelium is
a. Black hairy tongue
b. Aphthous ulcers
c. Herpes simplex
d. Geographic tongue

97 A patient complains of bleeding and painful gingiva and a foul odor in the mouth. Evidence of poor oral hygiene indicates that this condition is probably
a. Periodontal disease
b. Leukoplakia
c. Geographic tongue
d. Acute necrotizing ulcerative gingivitis

98 Cleft lip is caused by a lack of fusion between the
a. Soft and hard palates
b. Maxillary process
c. Maxillary and median nasal processes
d. Frontonasal and median nasal processes

In items 99-103, place an A for *True* or a B for *False* in the space provided for each statement.

_____ **99** Eating in the sterilization area is permitted providing it is not in the area where instruments are processed.

_____ **100** The general-purpose solution used in an ultrasonic cleaner disinfects as well as cleans the instruments.

_____ **101** An omniclave provides steam under pressure, whereas an autoclave provides the same process in addition to dry-heat sterilization.

_____ **102** The use of autoclave heat-sensitive tape on a package is proof that the package is sterile.

_____ **103** If a disinfecting immersion-instrument solution has a 28-day reuse life, it is always used for 28 days.

104 Which of the following describes the surface after completion of a spray/wipe/spray/wipe procedure?
a. Clean
b. Sterile
c. Disinfected
d. Clean and disinfected

105 A protective, nongrowing form of a microorganism is referred to as a(n)

a. Spore
b. Crypt
c. Egg
d. Virus

106 Who can become infected from contaminated instruments?
a. The dentist
b. The dental assistant
c. The patient
d. All of the above

107 The instrument or device best cleaned with an iodophor wipe is a(n)
a. Amalgam plugger
b. Mobile cabinet
c. Rubber dam clamp
d. Suture needle

108 How can you tell whether a package of instruments has been processed in steam under pressure?
a. The processed spore strip indicates sterilization.
b. The temperature-sensitive tape changes color.
c. The instruments are a different color.
d. The bags are left open.

109 Sterilization by steam under pressure is accomplished at what temperature?
a. 175° F
b. 121° F
c. 250° F
d. 320° F

110 Metal instruments are best sterilized by
a. Dry heat
b. Steam under pressure
c. Disinfectants
d. Flaming

111 At what temperature are instruments dry-heat sterilized?
a. 200° to 212° F
b. 215° to 240° F
c. 250° to 260° F
d. 300° to 320° F

112 Conditions in steam sterilization that result in effective sterilization include which of the following?
1. A temperature of 250° F
2. 15 to 25 lb of pressure
3. A minimum of 10 to 20 minutes
4. Ultraviolet light
a. 1 and 3
b. 2 and 4
c. 1, 2, and 3
d. 1, 2, 3, and 4
e. 4 only

113 Which of the following diseases may result from the use and handling of contaminated instruments?
a. Hepatitis
b. Vincent's gingivitis
c. Anaphylaxis
d. Pneumonia cheilosis

114 The use of disposable materials is advantageous because they

a. Are cheaper
b. Save time in cleaning
c. Can be sterilized by dry heat
d. None of the above

115 Dry-heat sterilization requires a temperature of _____
a. 212° F for 30 minutes
b. 212° F for 1 hour
c. 250° F for 15 minutes
d. 320° F for 1 hour

116 Iodophores are effective against all of the following *except*
a. Bacterial spores
b. Gram-positive bacteria
c. Hepatitis virus
d. Bacterial spores and gram-positive bacteria
e. Gram-positive bacteria and hepatitis viruses

117 Which of the following are usually correct for operating a steam-under-pressure sterilization unit?
1. 250° F
2. 320° F
3. 1 hour
4. 20 minutes
5. 15-20 lb pressure
6. 0 lb pressure
a. 1, 3, and 5
b. 2, 3, and 5
c. 1, 3, and 6
d. 1, 4, and 5
e. 1, 4, and 6

118 Which of the following are usually correct for operating a dry-heat sterilizer?
1. 250° F
2. 320° F
3. 1 hour
4. 20 minutes
5. 15-20 lb pressure
6. 0 lb pressure
a. 1, 3, and 6
b. 1, 4, and 5
c. 2, 3, and 5
d. 2, 3, and 6
e. 1, 4, and 6

119 An example of medical waste is
a. Used gauze
b. Amalgam scrap
c. Fluid from the HVE trap

120 Poster 2203 is
a. Required only by the state agency
b. Mandated by federal standards
c. Found only in medical offices

121 In order of greatest exposure to the DHCW, which of the following applies to infection?
a. Most common
b. Less common
c. Rare

In items 122-124, select the correct description in column B for each term in column A. The descriptions relate to disease transmission in the dental office.

Column A	*Column B*
_____ **122** Direct transmission	a. Microorganisms in the air from a patient's blood or saliva while a hand piece is being used
_____ **123** Indirect transmission	b. Contact with contaminated items through a tear in a glove
_____ **124** Aerosolization	c. Contact with a lesion while wearing protective gloves
	d. Air that is contaminated by breathing
	e. Tissue contact with lesion during dental treatment

In items 125-134, select the best procedure in column B for handling each of the contaminated devices or materials in column A.

Column A	*Column B*
_____ **125** Explorer	a. Steam under pressure
_____ **126** Mouth mirror	b. Sharps container
_____ **127** Scissors	c. Spray/wipe/spray/ wipe with surface disinfection
_____ **128** Handpiece	d. Dry heat
_____ **129** HVE hose	e. Cold chemical immersion
_____ **130** Needle	
_____ **131** Orthodontic wire	
_____ **132** Blood-soaked gauze	
_____ **133** Medicament bottles	
_____ **134** Protective glasses	

135 The most common routes of transmission of disease is/are
1. Blood
2. Saliva
3. Aerosols
4. Splatter
5. Kissing
a. 1, 2, and 3
b. 1, 2, 3, and 4
c. 1, 2, 3, 4, and 5
d. 1 only

136 If done in accordance with OSHA guidelines, swabbing a dental unit, operating light, and cabinetry with gauze soaked in a surface disinfectant may be considered a
a. Cleaning procedure
b. Disinfectant procedure
c. Sterilization procedure
d. Cleaning and disinfectant procedure

137 Cephalometry is
a. Compression of the skull
b. The study of soft tissues of the head
c. A technique for maintaining orthodontic movement
d. Measurement of the skull's dimensions

138 In manual processing, an exposed radiographic film should remain in the fixer solution
a. For as long as it remained in the developer
b. Until the film first clears
c. For 5 minutes at 70° F
d. For at least 10 minutes

139 When fresh developing solution is used in a manual processor, the ideal developing time is

a. 3 minutes at 70° F
b. 4 minutes at 64° F
c. 4 1/2 minutes at 68° F
d. 4 minutes at 68.5° F
e. When an image becomes visible on the film

140 In most states, radiation protection laws require that the diameter of the dental x-ray beam directed at the patient's face be no more than
a. 2 3/4 inches
b. 3 1/4 inches
c. 3 1/2 inches
d. 4 inches

141 Which of the following structures appear radiopaque on a radiograph?
1. Nasal fossa
2. Mylohyoid ridge
3. External oblique line
4. Coronoid process of the mandible
a. 1 and 3
b. 1 and 4
c. 1, 2, and 3
d. 2 and 4
e. 2, 3, and 4

142 Distance from the x-ray tube to the film is increased from 8 to 16 inches. To what fraction of the original radiation intensity at 8 inches is the film now exposed at 16 inches?
a. One fifth
b. One fourth
c. One third
d. One half

143 The greatest total amount of radiation to which a worker of any age is permitted to be exposed is expressed by
a. REM
b. MAD
c. RBE
d. RAD
e. MPD

144 A film is properly exposed at 10 mA and 60 impulses. At how many impulses should 15mA film be exposed?
a. 30
b. 40
c. 45
d. 50
e. 90

145 When no radiation shield is available, the operator should stand out of the x-ray beam and at least _____ from the patient's head.
a. 2 feet
b. 4 feet
c. 6 feet
d. 8 feet
e. 10 feet

146 The ALARA concept endorses the use of the _____ possible exposure of the patient and operator to radiation to produce a diagnostically acceptable radiograph.
a. Highest
b. Lowest

147 The human cells and tissues most sensitive to radiation are the _____.
a. Cells of the embryo
b. Thyroid cells
c. Gonadal tissues
d. Epithelial tissues of the alimentary canal

148 A(n) _____ is an extension placed on the tube head.
a. Anode pole
b. Cathode pole
c. Tungsten target
d. Position indicator device

149 The best radiography image is from radiation that is
a. Leakage
b. Primary
c. Scatter
d. Secondary

150 A(n) _____ radiograph is used primarily for the detection of carious lesions.
a. Bitewing
b. Dual film
c. Occlusal
d. Periapical

In items 151-160, place an A for *True* and a B for *False* in the space provided for each statement.

_____ **151** Erythema is an early sign of overexposure to x-rays.

_____ **152** All x-rays in the beam from a dental x-ray machine have the same penetrating power.

_____ **153** Collimating the x-ray beam reduces the amount of tissue being irradiated.

_____ **154** The kVp controls the penetrating power of the x-ray beam.

_____ **155** Irradiation of patients beyond childbearing age has no deleterious effects.

_____ **156** The dental assistant should hold the film in the patient's mouth when the patient is unable to hold it steady.

_____ **157** The occlusal film is larger than the periapical film.

_____ **158** The rays that pass from the x-ray tube through the filter and enter the cone are called secondary x-rays.

_____ **159** All panoramic radiographs examine the same layer of tissue in the patient's head.

_____ **160** A bent film can show a white or black line artifact when the film is processed.

161 Inside the radiography tube the tungsten filament is heated to produce free electrons; this process is called
a. Electron generation
b. Thermionic emission
c. Conductivity
d. Threshold exposure

162 Small, positively charged particles are called
a. Atoms
b. Electrons
c. Protons
d. Neutrons

163 Dense material that absorbs x-rays, thereby appearing light on the radiographic film, is said to be

a. Radiolucent
b. Radiopaque
c. Irradiated
d. Phosphorescent

164 Thin material that allows x-rays to pass through, thereby appearing dark on the radiographic film, is said to be
a. Radiolucent
b. Radiopaque
c. Irradiated
d. Phosphorescent

165 Which of the following statements are true for the focusing cup? It:
1. Aims the electrons at the target.
2. Is made of tungsten.
3. Is made of molybdenum.
4. Is found in the anode.
5. Is found in the cathode.
a. 1, 2, and 5
b. 1, 3, and 4
c. 1, 3, and 5
d. 3 and 5

166 When positive angulation is used for examination of the maxillary teeth, the PID will be pointing
a. Up
b. Down
c. Perpendicular

167 Bitewing radiographs are taken at _____ angulation in both the bisecting and the paralleling techniques.
a. Zero
b. Plus 10
c. Plus 50
d. Negative 10

168 In the paralleling technique the film-to-tooth distance must be _____ to keep the film parallel to the tooth.
a. Increased
b. Decreased
c. Altered

In items 169-176, select from the accompanying radiographs the error in exposure or processing that is illustrated.

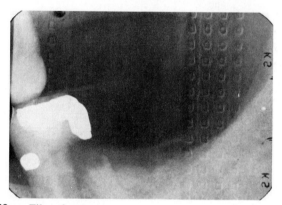

169 a. Film placement
b. Underprocessed
c. PID cutoff
d. Developer cutoff

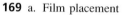

170 a. Film placement
b. Overexposure
c. Reversed film
d. Overdeveloped film

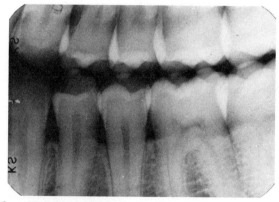

171 a. Horizontal angulation
b. Vertical angulation
c. Overlapped image
d. Both a and c

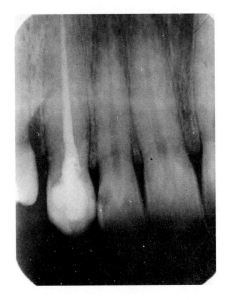

172 a. Vertical angulation
    b. Horizontal angulation
    c. Film placement
    d. Both a and c

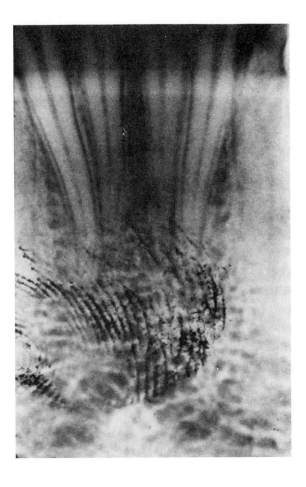

174 a. Bent film
    b. Film placement
    c. Human artifact
    d. Scratched film

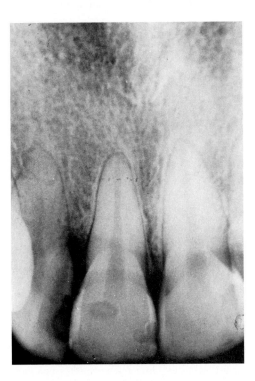

173 a. Film placement
    b. Foreshortened
    c. Elongated
    d. Both a and b

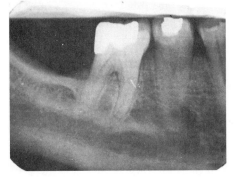

175 a. Developer cutoff
    b. PID cutoff
    c. Film placement
    d. Fixer cutoff

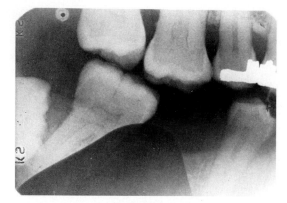

176 a. Light leak
   b. Fixer stain
   c. Films stuck together
   d. Radiation blocked by lead apron
177 Parenteral routes of drugs include
   1. Subcutaneous
   2. Intramuscular
   3. Intravenous
   4. Intradermal
   a. 1 and 3
   b. 1, 2, and 3
   c. 1, 2, 3, and 4
   d. 2 and 4
   e. 4 only
178 When determining the dosage of a drug to be prescribed, an important consideration is the
   a. Patient's weight
   b. Patient's height
   c. Patient's sex
   d. Frequency of the patient's meals
179 Which federal agency ensures public safety regarding drugs?
   a. Federal Safety Commission
   b. Food and Drug Administration
   c. National Health Commission
   d. American Medical Association
180 Antihistamines are used to
   a. Delay the effects of a narcotic
   b. Premedicate the patient and allay fears
   c. Enhance the effects of antibiotics
   d. Counteract allergic reactions
181 Caffeine is a(n)
   a. Depressant
   b. Tranquilizer
   c. Stimulant
   d. Irritant
182 Addictive analgesic drugs are known as
   a. Narcotics
   b. Antihistamines
   c. Tranquilizers
   d. Stimulants

183 Common barbiturates used in dentistry include
   1. Nitrous oxide
   2. Secobarbital
   3. Phenobarbital
   4. Pentobarbital
   5. Meperidine
   a. 1, 2, and 4
   b. 2, 3, and 4
   c. 2, 3, and 5
   d. 3, 4, and 5
184 The most commonly used analgesic is
   a. Codeine
   b. Aspirin
   c. Meperidine
   d. Morphine
185 Which antibiotic can cause staining of a child's primary teeth when taken by a pregnant woman during her last trimester of pregnancy?
   a. Tetracycline
   b. Penicillin
   c. Erythromycin
   d. Streptomycin
186 The use of drugs in cancer therapy is referred to as
   a. Radiotherapy
   b. Electrocautery
   c. Chemotherapy
   d. Psychotherapy
187 An agent that counteracts the action of a poison or drug is an
   a. Elixir
   b. Emetic
   c. Antidote
   d. Antibiotic
188 Which of the following would be the best treatment for a person showing the signs of an anaphylactic response after a penicillin injection?
   a. Intravenous cortisone
   b. Subcutaneous epinephrine
   c. Intramuscular epinephrine
   d. Intravenous diphenhydramine
   e. Intramuscular diphenhydramine
189 An antibody that neutralizes a toxin is a(n)
   a. Antibiotic
   b. Antitoxin
   c. Toxoid
   d. Vaccine
190 A patient may have _____ as a side effect of radiation therapy.
   a. Diabetes
   b. Heart disease
   c. Phlebitis
   d. Xerostomia
191 The following are drug reference texts commonly used during treatment of patients *except* for the
   a. DEA
   b. PDR
   c. USP
   d. NF

192 Which of the following is *not* one of the four main categories of drugs used in a dental practice?
  a. Analgesic
  b. Tranquilizer
  c. Antihistamine
  d. Antibiotic

In items 193-197, select the correct description in column B for each term in column A.

Column A	*Column B*
_____ **193** Antagonistic	a. Destroys microorganisms
_____ **194** Germicide	b. Federal regulatory agency
_____ **195** PDR	c. Pharmacopoeia reference
_____ **196** FDA	d. That which counteracts the
_____ **197** USP	action of something else
	e. Agent that soothes

In items 198-201, select the correct meaning in column B for each abbreviation in column A.

Column A	*Column B*
_____ **198** qh	a. Three times a day
_____ **199** stat	b. Immediately
_____ **200** qod	c. Capsule
_____ **201** cap	d. Every other day
	e. Every hour

202 Anaphylactic shock results from
  a. A reaction to mental depression
  b. A sudden, violent allergic reaction
  c. Aspiration of a foreign object
  d. A chronic allergic reaction

203 Parenteral refers to all routes of administration *except*
  a. Subcutaneous
  b. Intramuscular
  c. Intravenous
  d. Oral

204 A dentist wants a patient to take a prescribed drug three times a day. The signa of the prescription might include which of the following?
  a. Take one capsule tid.
  b. Take one capsule q8h.
  c. Take one capsule with breakfast, one with dinner, and one at bedtime.
  d. All of the above

205 Clinically objectionable dental fluorosis begins at what level of fluoride ion concentration in a domestic water supply?
  a. 2 ppm
  b. 3 ppm
  c. 4 ppm
  d. 1 ppm
  e. 0.8 ppm

206 Which of the following statements is always true of dental fluorosis?
  a. If it is going to occur, it will be present when the teeth erupt.
  b. It is as common in deciduous teeth as in permanent teeth.
  c. Affected teeth are always stained.
  d. It is an inevitable consequence of water fluoridation.

207 The full benefit of controlled fluoridation means a reduction in dental caries of
  a. 10% to 20% of all teeth
  b. 45% in deciduous teeth
  c. 60% of all teeth

208 _____ is the ability of a material to withstand permanent deformation under tensile stress without fracture.
  a. Ductility
  b. Malleability
  c. Ultimate strength

209 An investment material that expands when immersed in water is
  a. Malleable
  b. Hypothermic
  c. Plasticized
  d. Hygroscopic

210 When pouring an impression, stone should be added at only one corner of an impression to
  a. Prevent air or water from being trapped on the surface of the cast
  b. Prevent stone of poor quality from being present on the ridge area
  c. Prevent artifacts in the body of the cast

211 Inlay wax patterns should be invested as soon as possible after fabrication to minimize change in shape caused by
  a. Reduced flow
  b. Drying of the wax
  c. Relaxation of internal stress
  d. Continued expansion of the wax

212 To successfully solder two adjacent metal alloy structures, which of the following applies?
  a. At least one of the metal alloy structures should be heated to its fusion temperature.
  b. Both metal alloy structures to be joined should be heated to their fusion temperature.
  c. Neither adjoining metal alloy structure should be heated to its fusion temperature.

213 In polishing an acrylic resin denture, polishing should
  a. Be done at a slow speed to prevent overheating
  b. Leave a high gloss on all surfaces
  c. Be confined to peripheries only

214 Each impression tray should be deep enough to provide _____ mm of impression material beyond the occlusal surfaces and the tray.
  a. 1 to 2
  b. 2 to 3
  c. 3 to 4
  d. 4 to 5

215 To amalgamate means to
  a. Squeeze out excess mercury
  b. Mull material before condensation
  c. Measure each substance on a scale
  d. Unite a metal or an alloy with mercury

216 Which type of materials emit heat during a chemical reaction?
  a. Exothermic
  b. Hygroscopic

c. Endothermic

d. Thermoplastic

217 A benefit of using premeasured, prepackaged materials is

a. Lower cost

b. Assurance that proportions are correct

c. No need for temperature regulation

d. Ease of storage

218 Dentin bonding is based on _____ retention.

a. Chemical

b. Mechanical

219 The process by which mercury and alloy are mixed together to form amalgam for a dental restoration is referred to as

a. Casting

b. Investing

c. Mulling

d. Trituration

220 Ideally, dental materials should have a _____ rate of thermal conductivity.

a. High

b. Low

c. Moderate

221 To minimize the risk of retinal damage when using a visible light-cured unit, dental personnel should wear

a. OSHA-approved eyewear

b. Laboratory glasses

c. Safety eyewear

d. Special protective glasses

222 Most dental resins are hardened by a process called

a. Amalgamation

b. Crystallization

c. Polymerization

d. Trituration

223 A _____ rate of thermal conductivity is a disadvantage of amalgam restorations.

a. High

b. Low

224 Composite restorative materials may include elements to make them _____.

a. Radioactive

b. Radiolucent

c. Radiopaque

225 The _____ technique makes it possible to bond composite restorations to the enamel.

a. Acid etch

b. Monomer

c. Polymer

d. Autopolymerization

226 _____ is (are) not indicated for use under composite restorations.

a. Calcium hydroxide

b. Cavity liners

c. Copal cavity varnishes

d. Both a and c

227 _____ composites contain inorganic filler particle ranging in size from 1 to 5 μm. These composites produce a restoration with a semipolishable surface.

a. Hybrid

b. Macrofilled

c. Microfilled

228 When gypsum products are mixed, the _____ acts as a lubricant.

a. Agar

b. Calcium hemihydrate

c. Eugenol

d. Water

229 _____ impression materials are supplied as a heavy-bodied or putty form.

a. Polyether

b. Polysiloxane

c. Polysulfide

d. Both a and c

230 The phenomenon of relaxation and the resulting _____ is important in dentistry.

a. Adhesion

b. Distortion

c. Elasticity

231 The crystals of high-strength dental stone are _____.

a. Irregularly shaped

b. Large and spongy

c. Short and stubby

232 As a safety precaution, scrap amalgam should be stored under _____ in a closed non-breakable container.

a. Water

b. Acid etch solution

c. X-ray developer

d. X-ray fixer

233 In case of eye or skin contact with acid etch solution, rinse with a large amount of _____.

a. Boric acid solution

b. Saline solution

c. Water

Classify the following impression materials as rigid or elastic (place an A for *Rigid* or a B for *Elastic*).

_____ **234** Zinc oxide eugenol

_____ **235** Polyether

_____ **236** Addition silicone

_____ **237** Condensation silicone

_____ **238** Agar/alginate hydrocolloid

239 Which of the following impression materials is reversible?

a. Alginate hydrocolloid

b. Agar hydrocolloid

c. Addition silicone

240 _____ stress is not a mechanical property of dental materials.

a. Shear

b. Tensile

c. Compressive

d. Distortion

241 Dental amalgam alloy is mixed with _____ to form a dental restorative material.

a. Zinc

b. Aluminum

c. Mercury

242 Tearing of rubber impression materials when removing them from the mouth can be minimized by

a. Use of an alginate material instead of rubber

b. Allowing the impression to remain in the mouth an additional 2 minutes

c. Removal with a rapid, uniform motion

243 Cavity varnish is used to
1. Seal dentinal tubules
2. Provide an anodyne effect
3. Seal margins of cavity preparations
4. Provide insulation
   a. 1 and 3
   b. 2 and 4
   c. 1, 2, and 3
   d. 4 only

244 Syneresis refers to
   a. Intake of fluid
   b. Loss of fluid

245 An accelerator added to a dental material will _____ the working or setting time.
   a. Increase
   b. Decrease

246 Regarding an indirect technique for constructing a cast gold alloy restoration, which of the following statements are true?
1. A final impression is made of the prepared tooth.
2. A final impression is not made of the prepared tooth.
3. The wax pattern is made on the prepared tooth.
4. The wax pattern is made on the die.
   a. 1 and 3
   b. 1 and 4
   c. 1, 2, and 3
   d. 2 and 3

247 When the frozen slab technique is used in mixing zinc phosphate cement, setting time is _____.
   a. Increased
   b. Decreased

248 Which of the following statements about porcelain in dentistry is not true?
   a. It is used as an intracoronal restoration and is inserted directly into the tooth as is a composite restoration.
   b. It is more translucent than other materials.
   c. It is well tolerated by oral tissues.
   d. It is used for denture teeth, facings, laminates, and fusion to gold alloys.

249 Which of the following restorative materials has/have values of thermal conductivity similar to those of human enamel and dentin?
1. Dental amalgam
2. Composite plastics
3. Gold alloys
4. Zinc phosphate cement
   a. 1 and 3
   b. 2 and 4
   c. 1, 2, and 3
   d. 4 only

250 Which of the following conditions could lead to corrosion in restorative dentistry?
1. A chemical attack of a metal by components in food or saliva
2. Polished amalgams that have become dull and discolored with time

3. Adjacent restorations constructed of dissimilar metals
   a. 1 and 3
   b. 1, 2, and 3
   c. 2 only

251 Etching of the tooth surface is done primarily with
   a. Phosphoric acid
   b. Acetic acid
   c. Hydrochloric acid
   d. Nitric acid

252 Zinc phosphate is mixed over a large area of the glass slab to
   a. Dissipate the heat from the reaction
   b. Thin the mix
   c. Speed up the reaction
   d. Remove excess water

253 The major disadvantage of zinc phosphate cement is that it is too
   a. Thin
   b. Weak
   c. Acidic
   d. Difficult to place

254 An obtundent material is one that is
   a. Drying
   b. Soothing
   c. Cleansing
   d. Irritating

In items 255-259, place an A for *True* or a B for *False* in the space provided for each statement.

_____ **255** Moisture interferes with the retention of a sealant.

_____ **256** Percolation can cause irritation to the pulp and recurrent decay.

_____ **257** Dental compound in cake form could be used to take an impression of an edentulous arch.

_____ **258** A bite-registration impression is used to reproduce a single arch of a patient's occlusion.

_____ **259** Polymerization shrinkage of composite can be reduced by placing all of the polymer into the preparation at once.

In items 260-263, select the correct term from column B for each description in column A.

Column A	*Column B*
_____ **260** Movement of fluids and microorganisms into the space between the cavity preparation and the restoration	a. Microleakage
_____ **261** Force that causes unlike molecules to attach to one another	b. Ductility c. Adhesion d. Strain
_____ **262** Ability of a material to withstand permanent deformation under a compressive stress	e. Corrosion
_____ **263** Change in the length of a material as a result of force	

264 Which of the following sentences are correct?
1. Mary and I went to the seminar on infection control.
2. Me and Cindy didn't want to interrupt you.
3. Mary and me decided to visit the museum of modern dentistry.

4. Nancy and Ted are there children.
5. Ted Jenkins lost his bite splint.
   a. 2 and 3
   b. 1 and 5
   c. 2, 3, and 4
   d. 3 and 4

265 When supplies are received in the office, the form that accompanies the supplies but does not indicate charges is called a/an:
   a. Invoice
   b. Credit slip
   c. Packing slip
   d. Statement

266 Which of the following is *not* true of informed consent?
   a. Consent must be given freely.
   b. The patient has the right to ask questions.
   c. Risks, benefits, and alternative treatment must be presented.
   d. A minor has the right to give consent.

267 Checks *not* indicated on the monthly bank statement are known as _____ checks.
   a. Certified
   b. Canceled
   c. Outstanding
   d. Nonsufficient fund

268 Office policy should be determined by the
   a. Dentist
   b. State dental board
   c. Local dental society
   d. Auxiliary personnel

269 During malpractice litigation, the person who provides firsthand knowledge during testimony is referred to as the
   a. Fact witness
   b. Expert witness

270 Which of the following is *not* one of the most common bookkeeping systems used in dentistry?
   a. Accounts receivable/accounts payable
   b. Computerized system
   c. Peg-Board system

271 All of the following are true of a patient ledger card *except*
   a. It contains all financial information for each patient but not the family.
   b. It contains only treatment information for the patient and family.
   c. It contains all financial information for each patient or family.
   d. It is completed at the end of each procedure to indicate charges, credit, and balance.

272 You receive the following phone call: "Hello, this is Mrs. Perez. I'm having some pain in a tooth and need an appointment." Which of the following questions should you ask?
   1. May I have the correct spelling of your first and last name?
   2. How long has it been bothering you?
   3. Is it a sharp pain? Dull ache? Continuous or periodic?
   4. What is your social security number?
   5. What is your age?
   a. 1 and 3
   b. 2 and 4
   c. 1, 2, and 3
   d. 1, 2, 3, and 4

273 Which of the following statements applies to professional use of an answering machine or a professional answering service?
   1. Your message on an answering machine should be as caring as possible.
   2. Your message on an answering machine should indicate specific instructions as to what the patient should do in case of emergency.
   3. If an answering service is used, follow-up of messages should be as prompt as possible.
   4. Dental offices should use an answering service instead of a machine to provide immediate response to a problem.
   5. Dental offices that rely on answering machines violate basic ethics principles.
   a. 1 and 3
   b. 2 and 4
   c. 1, 2, and 3
   d. 1, 2, 3, and 4
   e. 5 only

274 Transmission of information from one site to another by electronic means is referred to as a
   a. Fax
   b. UPS
   c. Fed Ex
   d. Xerox

275 An appointment book entry includes the
   1. Patient's complete name
   2. Treatment to be provided
   3. Business and home phone numbers
   4. Amount of time needed
   5. Cross-reference when needed
   a. 1 and 3
   b. 2 and 4
   c. 1, 2, 3, and 4
   d. 1, 2, 3, 4, and 5

276 Which of the following items is nonexpendable?
   a. Anesthetic needle
   b. Dental cement
   c. Computer
   d. Surgical forceps

In items 277-282, place an A for *True* and a B for *False* in the space provided for each statement.

_____ **277** A financial record is generally kept for each patient.

_____ **278** A code system used in bookkeeping is a form of shorthand that denotes specific treatment or payments in an abbreviated form.

_____ **279** An appointment matrix is an outline of routine events in the office, such as meetings, buffer periods, and holidays.

_____ **280** Appointment book entries should always be made in ink.

_____ **281** A ledger card is kept separate from the clinical record.

_____ **282** A recall system is a preventive program that recalls patients to the office for various reasons.

In items 283-287, select the term in column B that best fits each description in column A.

Column A

_____ **283** A dentist fails to schedule a patient for completion of treatment prior to moving out of town.

_____ **284** A patient is held in the dental chair without his or her permission.

_____ **285** Treatment is performed on a patient that a reasonable, careful person under similar circumstances would not do.

_____ **286** A patient is seen routinely for several years in an office. Periodontal disease continues to bother the patient, but the dentist never discusses the problem.

_____ **287** Publicly, you denounce the morals of a patient.

Column B
a. Abandonment
b. Assault
c. False imprisonment
d. Negligence
e. Defamation

288 Which of the following is *not* considered a positive characteristic in a manager?
a. Good listener
b. Exercises self-control
c. Makes all decisions
d. Delegates authority
e. Avoids delays in decision making

289 Which is the most desirable management style in health occupations?
a. Authoritarian
b. Participatory
c. Free rein

290 The lowest level on Maslow's hierarchy is
a. Physiologic
b. Security
c. Social
d. Self-actualization

291 The seated assistant's eye level should be
a. Even with that of the operator
b. 4 to 6 inches below that of the dentist
c. 4 to 6 inches above the patient's shoulder
d. 4 to 6 inches above that of the dentist

292 To say that the members of the operating team have balanced posture means that
a. They are practicing sit-down dentistry.

b. They are using proper equipment.
c. They are practicing ergonomic techniques.
d. Both b and c are correct.

In items 293-296, place an A for *True* or a B for *False* in the space provided for each statement.

_____ **293** A dental auxiliary is used to transfer instruments, provide oral evacuation, prepare dental materials, and diagnose in four-handed dentistry.

_____ **294** Disorganized treatment areas, poor appointment scheduling, and lack of standardized procedures are examples of poor time management resulting in inefficiency.

_____ **295** Efficient instrument transfer greatly reduces the amount of movement for the dentist.

_____ **296** Unnecessary instrument exchange can be eliminated if the dentist uses an instrument to its maximum before returning it to the assistant.

In items 297-300, select the correct description in column B for each term in column A.

Column A

_____ **297** HVE system
_____ **298** Fixed cabinetry
_____ **299** Operating light
_____ **300** Mobile cabinetry

Column B
a. Mounted
b. Adjustable for operator or assistant
c. Movable
d. Removes fluids only by immersion
e. Removes fluids without immersion

In items 301-304, select the correct description in column B for each term in column A.

Column A

_____ **301** Omniclave
_____ **302** Vacuum pump
_____ **303** Amalgamator
_____ **304** Ultrasonic scaler

Column B
a. Required in an HVE system
b. Mixes restorative material
c. Uses water to operate
d. Cures by light
e. Sterilizes

305 Which of the following is *not* used to perform treatment with indirect vision?
a. Mirror
b. Change in operator position
c. Change in assistant position
d. Change in patient position

In items 306-311, place an A for *True* or a B for *False* in the space provided for each statement.

_____ **306** In a supine position a patient's legs and head should be at the same level.

_____ **307** The operator's zone for a right-handed dentist is from 8 to 12 o'clock.

_____ **308** The static zone for a left-handed operator is from 12 to 2 o'clock.

_____ **309** The assistant's zone changes depending on which arch is being treated.

_____ **310** A distance of 4 to 6 inches between the operator's nose and the patient's oral cavity should be maintained to avoid encroaching on the patient's breathing space.

_____ **311** Once the patient is supine and the operating team is seated, the chair base is lowered to place the head of the patient in the lap of the dentist.

312 Which instrument is used in the pen grasp?
a. High-speed handpiece
b. Scissors
c. Wedelstaedt chisel
d. Anesthetic syringe

313 When working with a right-handed dentist, which hand does the assistant use to transfer instruments?
a. Right
b. Left
c. Either

314 All of the following are shanks in which hand-cutting instruments may be supplied _except_ the _____ shank.
a. Curved
b. Binangle
c. Monangle
d. Triple angle

In items 315-318, select the correct function in column B for each instrument in column A.

Column A	Column B
_____ **315** Large condenser	a. Condense last incre-ment of amalgam
_____ **316** Ball burnisher	b. Check pocket depth
_____ **317** Small condenser	c. Place cement
_____ **318** Plastic instrument	d. Compress first incre-ment of amalgam
	e. Anatomic smoothing

In items 319-322, select the correct function in column B for each instrument in column A.

Column A	Column B
_____ **319** Periodontal	a. Remove calculus
_____ **320** Curet scaler	b. Check for caries
_____ **321** Explorer	c. Check pocket depth
_____ **322** Cotton forceps	d. Transfer small items
	e. Retrieve instruments

323 Which of the following instruments has/have a four-numbered instrument formula?
1. Angle former
2. Enamel hatchet
3. Gingival marginal trimmer
4. Chisel
a. 1 and 3
b. 2 and 4
c. 3 only
d. 4 only

324 A gingival marginal trimmer is used to place bevels on the
1. Proximal cervical floor
2. Axial wall
3. Point angle
4. Pulpal floor
a. 1 and 3
b. 1 and 4
c. 2 only
d. 4 only

325 Which of the following instruments is used to remove soft debris from a cavity preparation?
a. Angle former
b. Gingival marginal trimmer
c. Spoon excavator
d. Wedelstaedt chisel

In items 326-329, select the correct series number from column B for each bur in column A.

Column A	Column B
_____ **326** End cutting	a. 1/4 to 10
_____ **327** Inverted cone	b. 55 to 64
_____ **328** Round	c. 900 to 902
_____ **329** Straight fissure, plain cut	d. 33 1/2 to 39
	e. 555 to 564

In items 330-332, select the correct series number from column B for each bur in column A.

Column A	Column B
_____ **330** Straight fissure, cross cut	a. 555 to 564
_____ **331** Tapered fissure, plain cut	b. 33 1/2 to 39
	c. 699 to 708
_____ **332** Tapered fissure, cross cut	d. 169 to 172
	e. 69 to 72

In items 333-336, select the correct term in column B for each description in column A.

Column A	Column B
_____ **333** May aid in elimi-nation of pulp ex-posures	a. Pediatric handpiece
	b. Diamond disk
	c. Prophylaxis brush
_____ **334** Attached to an an-gle for polishing coronal surfaces with pumice	d. Screw-type mandrel
	e. Straight handpiece
_____ **335** Accepts pinhole-type disks	
_____ **336** Makes a slice on a tooth with maxi-mum efficiency	

337 Which of the following can be attached to a low-speed handpiece?
1. High-speed attachment
2. Latch-type contra-angle
3. Friction-grip bur
4. Prophylaxis angle
5. Latch-type bur
a. 1 and 3
b. 1, 2, 3, and 5
c. 2, 3, 4, and 5
d. 1, 2, 3, 4, and 5

338 Which of the following can be attached to a high-speed handpiece?
1. High-speed attachment
2. Latch-type contra-angle
3. Friction-grip bur
4. Prophylaxis angle
5. Latch-type bur
a. 1 and 3
b. 2 and 4
c. 3 only

d. 1, 2, 3, and 5

e. 1, 2, 3, 4, and 5

In items 339-349, place an A for *True* or a B for *False* in the space provided for each statement (all are about rotary instruments).

_____ **339** A screw-type mandrel may have an RA, FG, or HP shank.

_____ **340** Water-spray devices on a handpiece are used to reduce frictional heat and help remove debris from the cavity preparation.

_____ **341** When a high-speed handpiece is used with a water coolant, it becomes the responsibility of the dental assistant to remove the accumulated water in the patient's mouth and the water drops on the operator's mirror.

_____ **342** A carborundum disk is the same device as a lightning disk.

_____ **343** Fiberoptic capabilities on a handpiece provide not only additional illumination but also increased speed.

_____ **344** When the operator uses the A/W syringe, the assistant passes it by holding the syringe beneath the control buttons near the hose.

_____ **345** The operator must adjust his or her hand position when receiving some instruments, such as rubber dam forceps or scissors.

_____ **346** When it is determined that an instrument will not be needed again by the operator, it is returned to the far right side of the tray to prevent it from being used again.

_____ **347** When a maxillary right second premolar is being worked on, the working end of the instrument is placed in a downward position.

_____ **348** Instruments should never be passed over the patient's face.

_____ **349** Simultaneous delivery of the mirror and cotton pliers should occur at the beginning of most procedures.

350 All of the following are common instrument grasps *except* the

a. Pen grasp

b. Palm grasp

c. Modified pen grasp

d. Modified palm grasp

In items 351-355, select from column B the term that denotes the proper surface on which the suction tip is placed when the right handed operator is using the handpiece for each location in column A.

Column A		*Column B*
_____ **351**	#14³	a. Labial
_____ **352**	Lingual surface of #8	b. Occlusal
_____ **353**	#19°	c. Lingual
_____ **354**	Lingual surface of #19	d. Buccal
_____ **355**	Occlusal surface of #31	

356 If treatment is to be performed on tooth #19, which teeth would be isolated with a rubber dam?

a. #19 through #27

b. #18 through #27

c. #19 through #26

d. #18 through #30

357 The diastolic blood pressure is the pressure exerted by blood on the walls of the

a. Arteries when the heart is at rest

b. Veins when the heart pumps

c. Arteries when the heart pumps

d. Veins when the heart is at rest

358 To determine the pulse in the patient's wrist, palpate the _____ artery.

a. Brachial

b. Facial

c. Radial

d. Ulnar

359 The blood pressure of a patient who is considered hypotensive might be

a. 80/120

b. 110/52

c. 210/104

d. 132/80

360 The temporomandibular joint is palpated by gently placing the fingers just anterior to the _____ of the ear.

a. Ala

b. Pinna

c. Tragus

d. Zygoma

361 Which of the following factors would not affect temperature?

a. Excitement

b. Lack of exercise

c. Time of the day

d. Process of digestion

362 Diastole is the

a. Device with a bladder used to register blood pressure

b. Highest pressure that is registered

c. Lowest pressure that is registered

d. Device placed in the ears to hear the blood pressure

363 Which of the following would *not* be used to determine tooth vitality

1. Electronic pulp tester

2. Ice pencil

3. Percussion

4. Mobility

5. Heat

6. Transillumination

a. 1, 2, and 3

b. 1, 2, 3, and 5

c. 1, 2, 3, 4, and 5

d. 4 only

e. 6 only

364 When a patient's health history is being reviewed, illnesses or conditions that might require alteration in medication or premedication for a routine prophylaxis might include which of the following?

1. Rheumatic fever

2. Prolapsed valve

3. Joint replacement

4. Diabetes

5. A prescription for coumadin

a. 1, 2, and 5
b. 1, 2, 3, and 5
c. 1, 2, 3, 4, and 5
d. 4 only

365 Which of the following are components of a thorough clinical examination?
1. Photographs
2. Laboratory studies
3. Radiographic findings
4. Diagnostic findings
5. Complete intraoral and extraoral examinations
6. Complete personal, dental and health histories
   a. 1, 2, and 3
   b. 1, 2, 3, 4, and 5
   c. 2, 3, 4, 5, and 6
   d. 1, 2, 3, 4, 5, and 6

In items 366-370, place an A for *True* or a B for *False* in the space provided for each statement.

_____ 366 Intraoral imaging illustrates for a patient precise oral conditions in high detail with magnification.

_____ 367 Cosmetic imaging provides the patient with a before-and-after visual image of existing conditions, generating an image of what the tooth will look like when restored with various types of restorations.

_____ 368 When taking diagnostic impressions, the maxillary impression should be obtained first.

_____ 369 Temperature, pulse rate, respiration, and blood pressure should be obtained at every appointment.

_____ 370 Prognosis is the foretelling of the probable course of a disease.

371 If a patient has dry mouth with breath that smells of acetone, complains of thirst, and has a weak pulse, the most likely cause is
a. Kidney stone attack
b. Diabetic coma
c. Hypertension
d. Petit mal seizure

372 A mother calls about her young child, who just fell off his skateboard and lost a front tooth. What would you direct the mother to do at this point?
a. Immediately make an appointment for the child the next day.
b. Wrap the tooth in a clean, moist cloth and place it in the refrigerator until the appointment.
c. Wrap the tooth in a clean, moist cloth and immediately bring the child in for an appointment.
d. Place gauze or a piece of cloth over the socket and have the child bite down on it.
e. Both c and d are correct.

373 Opposition to the fluoridation of a community water supply is usually based on the premise that it will
1. Cause mottled enamel
2. Be hazardous
3. Produce skeletal damage
4. Violate personal rights
5. Cause mental disorders
   a. 1 and 3
   b. 1, 2, and 3
   c. 2 and 4
   d. 1, 2, and 4
   e. 3, 4, and 5

374 Which of the following techniques for using dental floss is correct?
a. The floss is snapped through the contact.
b. The floss is held parallel to the occlusal surfaces of the teeth.
c. The floss is removed by pulling it through the embrasure against the papilla.
d. All of the above are correct.

375 Which fluoride is administered in a series of four applications approximately 1 week apart?
a. Sodium fluoride
b. Stannous fluoride
c. Acidulated phosphate fluoride
d. Monofluorophosphate

376 The most effective way to provide fluoride to a tooth is
a. Systemic, by way of community drinking water
b. Systemic, by way of school drinking water
c. Topical, in a dental office
d. Topical, in a dentifrice

377 Which of the following is the literal definition of dental prophylaxis?
a. Teeth cleaning
b. Prevention of dental disease
c. Polishing the teeth

378 What condition would be visible in the mouth of a patient who has excess fluoride in his or her system?
a. Gray stains
b. Mottled enamel
c. Decalcification
d. Mottled dentin

379 Disclosing a patient's mouth should
1. Be done before brushing
2. Be done before and after brushing
3. Indicate areas of calculus
4. Indicate areas of plaque
5. Indicate areas of plaque and calculus
   a. 1 and 3
   b. 2 and 4
   c. 2 and 3
   d. 2 and 5
   e. 1 and 5

380 Coronal polishing involves treating only the
a. Clinical crown
b. Anatomic crown
c. Crown and subgingival areas

381 Contraindications for coronal polishing include
a. Tuberculosis
b. Abraded tooth surfaces
c. History of prolapsed valve
d. History of joint replacement
e. All of the above

382 A rotary bristle brush is used because it
a. Can easily remove stain from the gingival areas

b. Is only used on deep pits and fissures

c. Is kinder to the tooth surfaces

383 Which of the following devices could be used for caries removal?

1. #2 bur on slow speed
2. #1/4 bur on high speed
3. Spoon excavator
4. Enamel hatchet
5. Explorer

a. 1 and 2

b. 1 and 3

c. 2 and 4

d. 1, 3, and 4

e. 1, 3, and 5

384 Which of the following statements is/are true regarding the acid etching process during placement of a composite restoration?

1. In a class III preparation a celluloid matrix is placed before etching to protect adjacent tooth enamel.
2. After the bonding material is placed, the surface is rinsed for 30 seconds.
3. After etching, the celluloid matrix is removed and a new matrix is inserted before composite insertion.
4. In a class III preparation a celluloid matrix is not needed.

a. 1 and 3

b. 2 and 4

c. 1, 2, and 3

d. 4 only

385 Which instrument is used after the first increment of amalgam is placed in the preparation?

a. Ball burnisher

b. Small condensor

c. Larger condensor

d. Anatomic burnisher

In items 386-389, select the appropriate description in column B for each term in column A.

Column A	Column B
_____ **386** Wedge	a. Cervical caries
_____ **387** Hatchet	b. Is used to place bevels
_____ **388** Class I	c. Separates teeth
_____ **389** Class V	d. Occlusal caries
	e. Removes unsupported enamel

In items 390-392, select the appropriate description in column B for each term in column A.

Column A	Column B
_____ **390** Mesial gingival marginal trimmer	a. Is circumferential
_____ **391** Tofflemire retainer	b. Is used to place bevels
_____ **392** Ivory retainer	c. Assists in restoring single proximal wall
	d. Removes unsupported enamel

In items 393-403, place an A for *True* or a B for *False* in the space provided for each statement.

_____ **393** A mesial and distal marginal trimmer is used during the procedure for a preparation on #30mo.

_____ **394** A spirec drill is an instrument common to all pin procedures.

_____ **395** A #34 or #35 bur is preferred to make the initial pinhole opening.

_____ **396** The autoclutch chuck contra-angle is used in placing threaded pins.

_____ **397** Threaded pins must be precut with a wire cutter.

_____ **398** A twist drill and a spirec drill are the same.

_____ **399** Capillary-like fibers can be embedded in a denture base to recreate a lifelike appearance of oral mucosa.

_____ **400** Zinc phosphate mixed to secondary consistency may be used for final cementation of a cast restoration.

_____ **401** A specialized carbonized paper is used to check occlusal clearance during a crown preparation.

_____ **402** A die made from metal or stone is a positive reproduction of a tooth.

_____ **403** The pontic is the artificial tooth that replaces the missing natural tooth.

404 Baseplates should be on their respective casts when wax occlusal rims are attached, so as to

a. Minimize warping

b. Adjust the wax rim more easily

c. Establish vertical dimension

405 A function of a fixed bridge is to

a. Help move teeth

b. Prevent movement of teeth

c. Make cleaning easier

d. All of the above

406 The restoration used to reinforce an endodontically treated tooth before a crown is fabricated is a(n)

a. Acrylic core

b. Copper band

c. Aluminum shell

d. Metal post

407 How is the maxillary denture retained in place?

a. By cohesion

b. By adhesion

c. By close adaptation to the tissue surface

d. All of the above

408 The part of the partial denture that lies over the ridge is called the

a. Saddle

b. Rigid connector

c. Surveyor

d. Clasp

409 A surveyor is used in the construction of partial dentures to

a. Attach wax rims

b. Determine the placement of clasps

c. Determine the mould of artificial teeth

410 The function of the preliminary impression in full-denture construction is to

a. Construct wax rims

b. Help mount final casts

c. Construct a custom-made tray

d. Help make adjustments after insertion

411 After dentures are inserted, sore spots are

a. Common

b. Infrequent
c. Nonexistent
d. Ignored

In items 412-415, select the appropriate description in column B for each term in column A.

Column A	Column B
___ **412** Border molding	a. One side of the mouth
___ **413** Unilateral partial	b. Add warm compound to peripheries of tray, and adapt the compound to the patient's mucobuccal and muccolabial folds.
___ **414** Posterior palatal seal	c. Replaces the gingival tissue
___ **415** Bilateral partial	d. Both sides of the mouth
	e. Provides retention

In items 416-418, select the appropriate description in column B for each term in column A.

Column A	Column B
___ **416** Tenon	a. Female joint of precision attachment
___ **417** Mortise	b. Device for processing a denture
___ **418** Flask	c. Precision attachment
	d. Replaces the gingival tissue
	e. Male joint of precision attachment

419 The purpose of relining a denture is to
a. Alter the occlusion
b. Construct a custom-made tray
c. Take bite registration
d. Readapt the denture base to the existing tissue conditions

In items 420-423, select the appropriate definition in column B for each term in column A.

Column A	Column B
___ **420** Bite registration	a. Space between the adjacent teeth
___ **421** Draw	b. Uniform taper of preparation
___ **422** Final impression	c. Replica of the opposing arches as they occlude
___ **423** Occlusal clearance	d. Space between the prepared and opposing teeth
	e. Accurate impression of the prepared tooth and surroundling tissues

In items 424-427, select the appropriate description in column B for each term in column A.

Column A	Column B
___ **424** Occlusal clearance	a. Displaced gingiva
___ **425** Margin finish	b. Space between the prepared and opposing teeth
___ **426** Lost-wax technique	c. Chamfer with gradual transitions to all surfaces
___ **427** Gingival retraction	d. Burnout and centrifugal force
	e. Wax pattern

In items 428-430, select the appropriate description in column B for each term in column A.

Column A	Column B
___ **428** Laminate	a. Support usually on one abutment only
___ **429** Cantilever	b. Only two surfaces of the tooth are involved.
___ **430** Porcelain fused	c. Requires minimal reduction of tooth structure on the facial surface
	d. Small dovetail retainers on abutment teeth
	e. Neck of metal usually seen at cervical line

431 Which of the following would *not* be used to remove a temporary restoration during a cementation procedure?
a. Explorer
b. Modified sickle scaler
c. Spoon excavator
d. Broken instrument with blunted end

432 Which of the following is a problem that can be created by the loss of a single tooth?
a. Loss of esthetics
b. Hypereruption
c. Difficulty with mastication
d. Appearance of premature aging
e. All of the above

433 Which of the following is *not* correct for the procedures commonly used for the insertion of an immediate denture?
a. Removal of posterior teeth followed by tissue healing
b. Setup try-in is completed with anterior teeth intact
c. All teeth are extracted followed by tissue healing
d. Denture restricts edema after extractions

434 A pulpectomy is the
a. Removal of the coronal portion of the pulp
b. Removal of the entire pulp
c. Entrance into the pulp chamber
d. Slow degeneration of the pulp

435 Regarding instruments during treatment of a root canal, which of the following is important?
a. Extending the instrument 2 mm beyond the apex of the tooth
b. Forcing the instrument to the apex of the root
c. Sequential use of instruments
d. Rotary motion of the instrument

436 Various medicaments are used in endodontic therapy to
1. Irrigate canals
2. Strengthen the coronal portion of the tooth
3. Increase asepsis
4. Fit the master point
5. Aid instrumentation
a. 1, 2, and 3
b. 1, 3, and 5
c. 3, 4, and 5
d. 2, 4, and 5

437 When a solution such as sodium hypochlorite is used in a canal during endodontic treatment, which of the following are its functions?
1. Cleanse canal

2. Act as biomechanical agent
3. Soften dentin
4. Provide sterile work environment
5. Medicate canal
   a. 1 and 2
   b. 1, 2, and 3
   c. 2 and 3
   d. 3 and 4
   e. 3, 4, and 5

438 Which of the following is *not* a diagnostic tool commonly used in endodontics?
   a. Endo Ice
   b. Radiograph
   c. Mirror handle
   d. Hot dental compound
   e. Study model

439 A vitalometer reading of 9 to 10 indicates that the tooth is
   a. Within normal range
   b. Nonvital
   c. Pyrexic
   d. Near death

From the accompanying diagram, identify each instrument in items 440-443.

_____ **440** K-style file
_____ **441** Gates Glidden drill
_____ **442** Reamer
_____ **443** Hedstrom file

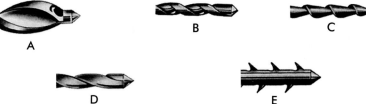

444 If the instruments listed are part of an endodontic tray setup, the procedure will likely be which of the following?

   Burs #34, #57, #4, or #6
   Rubber dam setup
   Sterile cotton pellets
   Formocresol
   Temporary crown setup

   a. Pulpotomy
   b. Apicoectomy
   c. Opening for pulpectomy
   d. Obturation for pulpectomy

445 Which of the following is *not* a type of bleaching technique?
   a. Internal
   b. External
   c. Iatrogenic
   d. Home bleaching

446 Which of the following statements regarding mouth guards is *not* true?
   a. They are important when a child participates in a team sport.
   b. They act as a cushion.
   c. They cannot be purchased over the counter.
   d. They reinforce the concept of maintaining teeth for a lifetime.

447 Which of the following statements is *not* true as it applies to luxated teeth?
   a. They may be intruded.
   b. They may be extruded.
   c. They are usually extracted to protect permanent teeth.
   d. They are usually allowed to remain in place to maintain space for permanent teeth.

448 A pediatric handpiece is used for a child because
   a. A larger handpiece may frighten a child.
   b. It allows for access from the occlusal because it has a smaller head.
   c. It provides greater access to the buccal and occlusal areas.

449 Placing a temporary crown on a primary tooth is important because it
   a. Protects the tooth from additional trauma
   b. Maintains space for the permanent tooth
   c. Protects during endodontic treatment
   d. All of the above

450 Interceptive treatment provides all *except* which of the following?
   a. Stops deleterious habits
   b. Avoids drifting into space after loss of primary tooth
   c. Improves existing problems
   d. Avoids impaction of permanent teeth

451 Which of the following is an environmental factor in orthodontic care?
   a. Size of teeth
   b. Size of jaw
   c. Supernumerary teeth
   d. Thumb sucking

452 A periodontal splint
   a. Prevents hypereruption of teeth
   b. Distributes force over a broader area
   c. Is only bonded on teeth when it is used

453 Which of the following are considered basic in periodontal surgery?
   1. Patient rapport
   2. Medical and dental histories
   3. Hygienist's role
   4. Restorative treatment
   5. Case presentation
   6. Treatment
   7. Evaluation
   8. Postoperative care
   9. Continuing care
   a. 1, 2, 3, 5, 6, and 8
   b. 1, 2, 5, 6, 7, and 9
   c. 1, 2, 4, 5, 7, 8, and 9

d. 2, 3, 4, 5, 6, 7, and 8
e. 1, 2, 3, 4, 5, 6, 7, 8, and 9

454 Which of the following instruments is/are *not* used for periodontal examination?
a. Mirror, explorer, periodontal probe, air syringe, floss
b. Pain sensitivity range

c. Sulcus electrical gauge
d. Automated bite recorder

455 An oxygenating agent
a. Increases respirated oxygen
b. Kills microorganisms
c. Systemically creates healthy tissue

Name _____

Date _____

(T)	(F)		KEY
[%]	[2]	[3]	[5]

1 [A] [B] [C] [D] [E]
2 [A] [B] [C] [D] [E]
3 [A] [B] [C] [D] [E]
4 [A] [B] [C] [D] [E]
5 [A] [B] [C] [D] [E]
6 [A] [B] [C] [D] [E]
7 [A] [B] [C] [D] [E]
8 [A] [B] [C] [D] [E]
9 [A] [B] [C] [D] [E]
10 [A] [B] [C] [D] [E]
11 [A] [B] [C] [D] [E]
12 [A] [B] [C] [D] [E]
13 [A] [B] [C] [D] [E]
14 [A] [B] [C] [D] [E]
15 [A] [B] [C] [D] [E]
16 [A] [B] [C] [D] [E]
17 [A] [B] [C] [D] [E]
18 [A] [B] [C] [D] [E]
19 [A] [B] [C] [D] [E]
20 [A] [B] [C] [D] [E]
21 [A] [B] [C] [D] [E]
22 [A] [B] [C] [D] [E]
23 [A] [B] [C] [D] [E]
24 [A] [B] [C] [D] [E]
25 [A] [B] [C] [D] [E]
26 [A] [B] [C] [D] [E]
27 [A] [B] [C] [D] [E]
28 [A] [B] [C] [D] [E]
29 [A] [B] [C] [D] [E]
30 [A] [B] [C] [D] [E]
31 [A] [B] [C] [D] [E]
32 [A] [B] [C] [D] [E]
33 [A] [B] [C] [D] [E]
34 [A] [B] [C] [D] [E]
35 [A] [B] [C] [D] [E]
36 [A] [B] [C] [D] [E]
37 [A] [B] [C] [D] [E]
38 [A] [B] [C] [D] [E]
39 [A] [B] [C] [D] [E]
40 [A] [B] [C] [D] [E]
41 [A] [B] [C] [D] [E]
42 [A] [B] [C] [D] [E]
43 [A] [B] [C] [D] [E]
44 [A] [B] [C] [D] [E]
45 [A] [B] [C] [D] [E]
46 [A] [B] [C] [D] [E]
47 [A] [B] [C] [D] [E]
48 [A] [B] [C] [D] [E]
49 [A] [B] [C] [D] [E]
50 [A] [B] [C] [D] [E]

(T)	(F)		KEY
[%]	[2]	[3]	[5]

51 [A] [B] [C] [D] [E]
52 [A] [B] [C] [D] [E]
53 [A] [B] [C] [D] [E]
54 [A] [B] [C] [D] [E]
55 [A] [B] [C] [D] [E]
56 [A] [B] [C] [D] [E]
57 [A] [B] [C] [D] [E]
58 [A] [B] [C] [D] [E]
59 [A] [B] [C] [D] [E]
60 [A] [B] [C] [D] [E]
61 [A] [B] [C] [D] [E]
62 [A] [B] [C] [D] [E]
63 [A] [B] [C] [D] [E]
64 [A] [B] [C] [D] [E]
65 [A] [B] [C] [D] [E]
66 [A] [B] [C] [D] [E]
67 [A] [B] [C] [D] [E]
68 [A] [B] [C] [D] [E]
69 [A] [B] [C] [D] [E]
70 [A] [B] [C] [D] [E]
71 [A] [B] [C] [D] [E]
72 [A] [B] [C] [D] [E]
73 [A] [B] [C] [D] [E]
74 [A] [B] [C] [D] [E]
75 [A] [B] [C] [D] [E]
76 [A] [B] [C] [D] [E]
77 [A] [B] [C] [D] [E]
78 [A] [B] [C] [D] [E]
79 [A] [B] [C] [D] [E]
80 [A] [B] [C] [D] [E]
81 [A] [B] [C] [D] [E]
82 [A] [B] [C] [D] [E]
83 [A] [B] [C] [D] [E]
84 [A] [B] [C] [D] [E]
85 [A] [B] [C] [D] [E]
86 [A] [B] [C] [D] [E]
87 [A] [B] [C] [D] [E]
88 [A] [B] [C] [D] [E]
89 [A] [B] [C] [D] [E]
90 [A] [B] [C] [D] [E]
91 [A] [B] [C] [D] [E]
92 [A] [B] [C] [D] [E]
93 [A] [B] [C] [D] [E]
94 [A] [B] [C] [D] [E]
95 [A] [B] [C] [D] [E]
96 [A] [B] [C] [D] [E]
97 [A] [B] [C] [D] [E]
98 [A] [B] [C] [D] [E]
99 [A] [B] [C] [D] [E]
100 [A] [B] [C] [D] [E]

(T)	(F)		KEY
[%]	[2]	[3]	[5]

101 [A] [B] [C] [D] [E]
102 [A] [B] [C] [D] [E]
103 [A] [B] [C] [D] [E]
104 [A] [B] [C] [D] [E]
105 [A] [B] [C] [D] [E]
106 [A] [B] [C] [D] [E]
107 [A] [B] [C] [D] [E]
108 [A] [B] [C] [D] [E]
109 [A] [B] [C] [D] [E]
110 [A] [B] [C] [D] [E]
111 [A] [B] [C] [D] [E]
112 [A] [B] [C] [D] [E]
113 [A] [B] [C] [D] [E]
114 [A] [B] [C] [D] [E]
115 [A] [B] [C] [D] [E]
116 [A] [B] [C] [D] [E]
117 [A] [B] [C] [D] [E]
118 [A] [B] [C] [D] [E]
119 [A] [B] [C] [D] [E]
120 [A] [B] [C] [D] [E]
121 [A] [B] [C] [D] [E]
122 [A] [B] [C] [D] [E]
123 [A] [B] [C] [D] [E]
124 [A] [B] [C] [D] [E]
125 [A] [B] [C] [D] [E]
126 [A] [B] [C] [D] [E]
127 [A] [B] [C] [D] [E]
128 [A] [B] [C] [D] [E]
129 [A] [B] [C] [D] [E]
130 [A] [B] [C] [D] [E]
131 [A] [B] [C] [D] [E]
132 [A] [B] [C] [D] [E]
133 [A] [B] [C] [D] [E]
134 [A] [B] [C] [D] [E]
135 [A] [B] [C] [D] [E]
136 [A] [B] [C] [D] [E]
137 [A] [B] [C] [D] [E]
138 [A] [B] [C] [D] [E]
139 [A] [B] [C] [D] [E]
140 [A] [B] [C] [D] [E]
141 [A] [B] [C] [D] [E]
142 [A] [B] [C] [D] [E]
143 [A] [B] [C] [D] [E]
144 [A] [B] [C] [D] [E]
145 [A] [B] [C] [D] [E]
146 [A] [B] [C] [D] [E]
147 [A] [B] [C] [D] [E]
148 [A] [B] [C] [D] [E]
149 [A] [B] [C] [D] [E]
150 [A] [B] [C] [D] [E]

Name _____
Date _____

	(T)	(F)			KEY
	[%]	[2]	[3]		[5]

	(T)	(F)			KEY			(T)	(F)			KEY			(T)	(F)			KEY
151	[A]	[B]	[C]	[D]	[E]		201	[A]	[B]	[C]	[D]	[E]		251	[A]	[B]	[C]	[D]	[E]
152	[A]	[B]	[C]	[D]	[E]		202	[A]	[B]	[C]	[D]	[E]		252	[A]	[B]	[C]	[D]	[E]
153	[A]	[B]	[C]	[D]	[E]		203	[A]	[B]	[C]	[D]	[E]		253	[A]	[B]	[C]	[D]	[E]
154	[A]	[B]	[C]	[D]	[E]		204	[A]	[B]	[C]	[D]	[E]		254	[A]	[B]	[C]	[D]	[E]
155	[A]	[B]	[C]	[D]	[E]		205	[A]	[B]	[C]	[D]	[E]		255	[A]	[B]	[C]	[D]	[E]
156	[A]	[B]	[C]	[D]	[E]		206	[A]	[B]	[C]	[D]	[E]		256	[A]	[B]	[C]	[D]	[E]
157	[A]	[B]	[C]	[D]	[E]		207	[A]	[B]	[C]	[D]	[E]		257	[A]	[B]	[C]	[D]	[E]
158	[A]	[B]	[C]	[D]	[E]		208	[A]	[B]	[C]	[D]	[E]		258	[A]	[B]	[C]	[D]	[E]
159	[A]	[B]	[C]	[D]	[E]		209	[A]	[B]	[C]	[D]	[E]		259	[A]	[B]	[C]	[D]	[E]
160	[A]	[B]	[C]	[D]	[E]		210	[A]	[B]	[C]	[D]	[E]		260	[A]	[B]	[C]	[D]	[E]
161	[A]	[B]	[C]	[D]	[E]		211	[A]	[B]	[C]	[D]	[E]		261	[A]	[B]	[C]	[D]	[E]
162	[A]	[B]	[C]	[D]	[E]		212	[A]	[B]	[C]	[D]	[E]		262	[A]	[B]	[C]	[D]	[E]
163	[A]	[B]	[C]	[D]	[E]		213	[A]	[B]	[C]	[D]	[E]		263	[A]	[B]	[C]	[D]	[E]
164	[A]	[B]	[C]	[D]	[E]		214	[A]	[B]	[C]	[D]	[E]		264	[A]	[B]	[C]	[D]	[E]
165	[A]	[B]	[C]	[D]	[E]		215	[A]	[B]	[C]	[D]	[E]		265	[A]	[B]	[C]	[D]	[E]
166	[A]	[B]	[C]	[D]	[E]		216	[A]	[B]	[C]	[D]	[E]		266	[A]	[B]	[C]	[D]	[E]
167	[A]	[B]	[C]	[D]	[E]		217	[A]	[B]	[C]	[D]	[E]		267	[A]	[B]	[C]	[D]	[E]
168	[A]	[B]	[C]	[D]	[E]		218	[A]	[B]	[C]	[D]	[E]		268	[A]	[B]	[C]	[D]	[E]
169	[A]	[B]	[C]	[D]	[E]		219	[A]	[B]	[C]	[D]	[E]		269	[A]	[B]	[C]	[D]	[E]
170	[A]	[B]	[C]	[D]	[E]		220	[A]	[B]	[C]	[D]	[E]		270	[A]	[B]	[C]	[D]	[E]
171	[A]	[B]	[C]	[D]	[E]		221	[A]	[B]	[C]	[D]	[E]		271	[A]	[B]	[C]	[D]	[E]
172	[A]	[B]	[C]	[D]	[E]		222	[A]	[B]	[C]	[D]	[E]		272	[A]	[B]	[C]	[D]	[E]
173	[A]	[B]	[C]	[D]	[E]		223	[A]	[B]	[C]	[D]	[E]		273	[A]	[B]	[C]	[D]	[E]
174	[A]	[B]	[C]	[D]	[E]		224	[A]	[B]	[C]	[D]	[E]		274	[A]	[B]	[C]	[D]	[E]
175	[A]	[B]	[C]	[D]	[E]		225	[A]	[B]	[C]	[D]	[E]		275	[A]	[B]	[C]	[D]	[E]
176	[A]	[B]	[C]	[D]	[E]		226	[A]	[B]	[C]	[D]	[E]		276	[A]	[B]	[C]	[D]	[E]
177	[A]	[B]	[C]	[D]	[E]		227	[A]	[B]	[C]	[D]	[E]		277	[A]	[B]	[C]	[D]	[E]
178	[A]	[B]	[C]	[D]	[E]		228	[A]	[B]	[C]	[D]	[E]		278	[A]	[B]	[C]	[D]	[E]
179	[A]	[B]	[C]	[D]	[E]		229	[A]	[B]	[C]	[D]	[E]		279	[A]	[B]	[C]	[D]	[E]
180	[A]	[B]	[C]	[D]	[E]		230	[A]	[B]	[C]	[D]	[E]		280	[A]	[B]	[C]	[D]	[E]
181	[A]	[B]	[C]	[D]	[E]		231	[A]	[B]	[C]	[D]	[E]		281	[A]	[B]	[C]	[D]	[E]
182	[A]	[B]	[C]	[D]	[E]		232	[A]	[B]	[C]	[D]	[E]		282	[A]	[B]	[C]	[D]	[E]
183	[A]	[B]	[C]	[D]	[E]		233	[A]	[B]	[C]	[D]	[E]		283	[A]	[B]	[C]	[D]	[E]
184	[A]	[B]	[C]	[D]	[E]		234	[A]	[B]	[C]	[D]	[E]		284	[A]	[B]	[C]	[D]	[E]
185	[A]	[B]	[C]	[D]	[E]		235	[A]	[B]	[C]	[D]	[E]		285	[A]	[B]	[C]	[D]	[E]
186	[A]	[B]	[C]	[D]	[E]		236	[A]	[B]	[C]	[D]	[E]		286	[A]	[B]	[C]	[D]	[E]
187	[A]	[B]	[C]	[D]	[E]		237	[A]	[B]	[C]	[D]	[E]		287	[A]	[B]	[C]	[D]	[E]
188	[A]	[B]	[C]	[D]	[E]		238	[A]	[B]	[C]	[D]	[E]		288	[A]	[B]	[C]	[D]	[E]
189	[A]	[B]	[C]	[D]	[E]		239	[A]	[B]	[C]	[D]	[E]		289	[A]	[B]	[C]	[D]	[E]
190	[A]	[B]	[C]	[D]	[E]		240	[A]	[B]	[C]	[D]	[E]		290	[A]	[B]	[C]	[D]	[E]
191	[A]	[B]	[C]	[D]	[E]		241	[A]	[B]	[C]	[D]	[E]		291	[A]	[B]	[C]	[D]	[E]
192	[A]	[B]	[C]	[D]	[E]		242	[A]	[B]	[C]	[D]	[E]		292	[A]	[B]	[C]	[D]	[E]
193	[A]	[B]	[C]	[D]	[E]		243	[A]	[B]	[C]	[D]	[E]		293	[A]	[B]	[C]	[D]	[E]
194	[A]	[B]	[C]	[D]	[E]		244	[A]	[B]	[C]	[D]	[E]		294	[A]	[B]	[C]	[D]	[E]
195	[A]	[B]	[C]	[D]	[E]		245	[A]	[B]	[C]	[D]	[E]		295	[A]	[B]	[C]	[D]	[E]
196	[A]	[B]	[C]	[D]	[E]		246	[A]	[B]	[C]	[D]	[E]		296	[A]	[B]	[C]	[D]	[E]
197	[A]	[B]	[C]	[D]	[E]		247	[A]	[B]	[C]	[D]	[E]		297	[A]	[B]	[C]	[D]	[E]
198	[A]	[B]	[C]	[D]	[E]		248	[A]	[B]	[C]	[D]	[E]		298	[A]	[B]	[C]	[D]	[E]
199	[A]	[B]	[C]	[D]	[E]		249	[A]	[B]	[C]	[D]	[E]		299	[A]	[B]	[C]	[D]	[E]
200	[A]	[B]	[C]	[D]	[E]		250	[A]	[B]	[C]	[D]	[E]		300	[A]	[B]	[C]	[D]	[E]

Name _____
Date _____

(T)	(F)		KEY		(T)	(F)		KEY		(T)	(F)		KEY
[%]	[2]	[3]	[5]		[%]	[2]	[3]	[5]		[%]	[2]	[3]	[5]
301 [A] [B] [C] [D] [E]					353 [A] [B] [C] [D] [E]					405 [A] [B] [C] [D] [E]			
302 [A] [B] [C] [D] [E]					354 [A] [B] [C] [D] [E]					406 [A] [B] [C] [D] [E]			
303 [A] [B] [C] [D] [E]					355 [A] [B] [C] [D] [E]					407 [A] [B] [C] [D] [E]			
304 [A] [B] [C] [D] [E]					356 [A] [B] [C] [D] [E]					408 [A] [B] [C] [D] [E]			
305 [A] [B] [C] [D] [E]					357 [A] [B] [C] [D] [E]					409 [A] [B] [C] [D] [E]			
306 [A] [B] [C] [D] [E]					358 [A] [B] [C] [D] [E]					410 [A] [B] [C] [D] [E]			
307 [A] [B] [C] [D] [E]					359 [A] [B] [C] [D] [E]					411 [A] [B] [C] [D] [E]			
308 [A] [B] [C] [D] [E]					360 [A] [B] [C] [D] [E]					412 [A] [B] [C] [D] [E]			
309 [A] [B] [C] [D] [E]					361 [A] [B] [C] [D] [E]					413 [A] [B] [C] [D] [E]			
310 [A] [B] [C] [D] [E]					362 [A] [B] [C] [D] [E]					414 [A] [B] [C] [D] [E]			
311 [A] [B] [C] [D] [E]					363 [A] [B] [C] [D] [E]					415 [A] [B] [C] [D] [E]			
312 [A] [B] [C] [D] [E]					364 [A] [B] [C] [D] [E]					416 [A] [B] [C] [D] [E]			
313 [A] [B] [C] [D] [E]					364 [A] [B] [C] [D] [E]					417 [A] [B] [C] [D] [E]			
314 [A] [B] [C] [D] [E]					366 [A] [B] [C] [D] [E]					418 [A] [B] [C] [D] [E]			
315 [A] [B] [C] [D] [E]					367 [A] [B] [C] [D] [E]					419 [A] [B] [C] [D] [E]			
316 [A] [B] [C] [D] [E]					368 [A] [B] [C] [D] [E]					420 [A] [B] [C] [D] [E]			
317 [A] [B] [C] [D] [E]					369 [A] [B] [C] [D] [E]					421 [A] [B] [C] [D] [E]			
318 [A] [B] [C] [D] [E]					370 [A] [B] [C] [D] [E]					422 [A] [B] [C] [D] [E]			
319 [A] [B] [C] [D] [E]					371 [A] [B] [C] [D] [E]					423 [A] [B] [C] [D] [E]			
320 [A] [B] [C] [D] [E]					372 [A] [B] [C] [D] [E]					424 [A] [B] [C] [D] [E]			
321 [A] [B] [C] [D] [E]					373 [A] [B] [C] [D] [E]					425 [A] [B] [C] [D] [E]			
322 [A] [B] [C] [D] [E]					374 [A] [B] [C] [D] [E]					426 [A] [B] [C] [D] [E]			
323 [A] [B] [C] [D] [E]					375 [A] [B] [C] [D] [E]					427 [A] [B] [C] [D] [E]			
324 [A] [B] [C] [D] [E]					376 [A] [B] [C] [D] [E]					428 [A] [B] [C] [D] [E]			
325 [A] [B] [C] [D] [E]					377 [A] [B] [C] [D] [E]					429 [A] [B] [C] [D] [E]			
326 [A] [B] [C] [D] [E]					378 [A] [B] [C] [D] [E]					430 [A] [B] [C] [D] [E]			
327 [A] [B] [C] [D] [E]					379 [A] [B] [C] [D] [E]					431 [A] [B] [C] [D] [E]			
328 [A] [B] [C] [D] [E]					380 [A] [B] [C] [D] [E]					432 [A] [B] [C] [D] [E]			
329 [A] [B] [C] [D] [E]					381 [A] [B] [C] [D] [E]					433 [A] [B] [C] [D] [E]			
330 [A] [B] [C] [D] [E]					382 [A] [B] [C] [D] [E]					434 [A] [B] [C] [D] [E]			
331 [A] [B] [C] [D] [E]					383 [A] [B] [C] [D] [E]					435 [A] [B] [C] [D] [E]			
332 [A] [B] [C] [D] [E]					384 [A] [B] [C] [D] [E]					436 [A] [B] [C] [D] [E]			
333 [A] [B] [C] [D] [E]					385 [A] [B] [C] [D] [E]					437 [A] [B] [C] [D] [E]			
334 [A] [B] [C] [D] [E]					386 [A] [B] [C] [D] [E]					438 [A] [B] [C] [D] [E]			
335 [A] [B] [C] [D] [E]					387 [A] [B] [C] [D] [E]					439 [A] [B] [C] [D] [E]			
336 [A] [B] [C] [D] [E]					388 [A] [B] [C] [D] [E]					440 [A] [B] [C] [D] [E]			
337 [A] [B] [C] [D] [E]					389 [A] [B] [C] [D] [E]					441 [A] [B] [C] [D] [E]			
338 [A] [B] [C] [D] [E]					390 [A] [B] [C] [D] [E]					442 [A] [B] [C] [D] [E]			
339 [A] [B] [C] [D] [E]					391 [A] [B] [C] [D] [E]					443 [A] [B] [C] [D] [E]			
340 [A] [B] [C] [D] [E]					392 [A] [B] [C] [D] [E]					444 [A] [B] [C] [D] [E]			
341 [A] [B] [C] [D] [E]					393 [A] [B] [C] [D] [E]					445 [A] [B] [C] [D] [E]			
342 [A] [B] [C] [D] [E]					394 [A] [B] [C] [D] [E]					446 [A] [B] [C] [D] [E]			
343 [A] [B] [C] [D] [E]					395 [A] [B] [C] [D] [E]					447 [A] [B] [C] [D] [E]			
344 [A] [B] [C] [D] [E]					396 [A] [B] [C] [D] [E]					448 [A] [B] [C] [D] [E]			
345 [A] [B] [C] [D] [E]					397 [A] [B] [C] [D] [E]					449 [A] [B] [C] [D] [E]			
346 [A] [B] [C] [D] [E]					398 [A] [B] [C] [D] [E]					450 [A] [B] [C] [D] [E]			
347 [A] [B] [C] [D] [E]					399 [A] [B] [C] [D] [E]					451 [A] [B] [C] [D] [E]			
348 [A] [B] [C] [D] [E]					400 [A] [B] [C] [D] [E]					452 [A] [B] [C] [D] [E]			
349 [A] [B] [C] [D] [E]					401 [A] [B] [C] [D] [E]					453 [A] [B] [C] [D] [E]			
350 [A] [B] [C] [D] [E]					402 [A] [B] [C] [D] [E]					454 [A] [B] [C] [D] [E]			
351 [A] [B] [C] [D] [E]					403 [A] [B] [C] [D] [E]					455 [A] [B] [C] [D] [E]			
352 [A] [B] [C] [D] [E]					404 [A] [B] [C] [D] [E]								

Answers to Testbank

#	Ans	#	Ans	#	Ans	#	Ans	#	Ans	#	Ans	#	Ans	#	Ans	#	Ans	#	Ans
1	D	51	B	101	B	151	A	201	C	251	A	301	E	351	D	401	B	451	D
2	A	52	A	102	B	152	B	202	B	252	A	302	A	352	A	402	A	452	B
3	B	53	B	103	B	153	A	203	D	253	C	303	B	353	D	403	A	453	B
4	C	54	A	104	D	154	A	204	D	254	B	304	C	354	D	404	A	454	C
5	A	55	B	105	A	155	B	205	A	255	A	305	C	355	C	405	B	455	B
6	C	56	A	106	D	156	B	206	A	256	A	306	A	356	B	406	D		
7	E	57	B	107	B	157	A	207	C	257	A	307	A	357	A	407	A		
8	B	58	D	108	B	158	B	208	A	258	B	308	A	358	C	408	A		
9	C	59	A	109	C	159	B	209	D	259	B	309	B	359	B	409	B		
10	D	60	A	110	B	160	A	210	A	260	A	310	B	360	C	410	C		
11	B	61	C	111	D	161	A	211	C	261	C	311	A	361	B	411	A		
12	A	62	B	112	C	162	C	212	B	262	B	312	A	362	C	412	B		
13	B	63	B	113	A	163	B	213	A	263	D	313	B	363	D	413	A		
14	B	64	C	114	B	164	A	214	B	264	B	314	A	364	B	414	E		
15	A	65	A	115	D	165	A	215	D	265	C	315	A	365	D	415	D		
16	A	66	B	116	C	166	B	216	A	266	D	316	E	366	A	416	E		
17	A	67	A	117	D	167	B	217	B	267	C	317	D	367	A	417	A		
18	A	68	D	118	D	168	A	218	A	268	A	318	C	368	B	418	B		
19	B	69	D	119	B	169	C	219	D	269	A	319	C	369	B	419	D		
20	D	70	C	120	B	170	C	220	B	270	A	320	A	370	A	420	C		
21	B	71	A	121	C	171	D	221	D	271	B	321	B	371	B	421	B		
22	B	72	B	122	E	172	A	222	C	272	C	322	D	372	E	422	E		
23	D	73	B	123	B	173	D	223	A	273	C	323	A	373	D	423	D		
24	A	74	C	124	A	174	C	224	C	274	A	324	B	374	B	424	B		
25	A	75	A	125	A	175	A	225	A	275	D	325	C	375	A	425	C		
26	C	76	C	126	A	176	C	226	C	276	D	326	C	376	A	426	D		
27	C	77	B	127	A	177	C	227	B	277	B	327	D	377	B	427	A		
28	C	78	A	128	A	178	A	228	D	278	A	328	A	378	B	428	C		
29	B	79	B	129	C	179	B	229	B	279	A	329	B	379	B	429	A		
30	D	80	A	130	B	180	D	230	B	280	B	330	A	380	A	430	E		
31	D	81	A	131	B	181	C	231	C	281	A	331	D	381	E	431	A		
32	C	82	B	132	B	182	A	232	A	282	A	332	C	382	B	432	E		
33	D	83	A	133	C	183	B	233	C	283	A	333	A	383	B	433	C		
34	B	84	A	134	E	184	B	234	A	284	C	334	C	384	A	434	B		
35	E	85	A	135	B	185	A	235	B	285	D	335	D	385	B	435	C		
36	D	86	D	136	D	186	C	236	B	286	D	336	B	386	C	436	B		
37	A	87	B	137	D	187	C	237	B	287	E	337	C	387	E	437	B		
38	C	88	C	138	D	188	C	238	B	288	C	338	C	388	D	438	E		
39	A	89	E	139	C	189	B	239	B	289	B	339	A	389	A	439	D		
40	E	90	D	140	A	190	D	240	D	290	A	340	A	390	B	440	B		
41	D	91	A	141	D	191	A	241	C	291	D	341	A	391	A	441	A		
42	B	92	B	142	B	192	C	242	C	292	D	342	B	392	C	442	D		
43	B	93	B	143	E	193	D	243	A	293	B	343	B	393	B	443	C		
44	A	94	C	144	B	194	A	244	B	294	A	344	B	394	A	444	A		
45	C	95	D	145	C	195	C	245	B	295	A	345	A	395	B	445	C		
46	D	96	D	146	B	196	B	246	B	296	A	346	B	396	A	446	C		
47	A	97	D	147	A	197	C	247	A	297	E	347	B	397	A	447	C		
48	C	98	D	148	D	198	E	248	A	298	A	348	A	398	A	448	C		
49	A	99	B	149	B	199	B	249	B	299	B	349	B	399	A	449	D		
50	C	100	B	150	A	200	D	250	B	300	C	350	D	400	B	450	C		

Index

Vasodilator, in emergency, 285
Vasopressors, in emergency, 284
Vein, 33, 34
Ventral, 24
Vermilion, 36
Vermilion border, 35, 36
Vertical dimension, 343
Vesicle, 77
Vestibule, 35, 37
Vibrator, 468
Vincent's gingivitis, 89
Vincent's gingivostomatitis, 89
Vincent's inflammation, 89
Vinyl plastics, 176
Viscosity, 164
Vision, 209
Vital bleaching technique, 384
Vitality, symbol for, 266
Vital signs, in oral and maxillofacial surgery, 391
Vitamins, 69
    sources, functions and effects of, 67

Voice-activated recording system, 442
Voice control in behavior management, 432
Voluntary standards, 18
Vomer bone, 31

W

Walking bleach technique, 384
Water, 69
    sources, functions and effects of, 66
Water irrigation device, 296
Water-soluble vitamins, 69
Wax, 180-181
    microcrystalline wax, 374
Waxing unit, 468
Wettability, 164
Wharton's duct, 33
Wheezing, 262
White lesions, 77
Winged or wingless clamp, 238
Wood stimulator on toothbrush, 296
Written communication, 193-195

X

Xerostomia, radiation and, 122
X-ray film, 116-117, 120, 124-125
    ALARA concept and, 123
    quality control factors, 127

Y

Yield point, 163

Z

Zinc, 66, 181
Zinc oxide-eugenol cement, 351
Zinc oxide-eugenol impression material, 177
Zinc phosphate cement, 351
Zones of activity, 209-210, 212
Zygomatic bones, 31
Zygomaticus minor and major muscles, 32